ELECTRONICS FOR NEUROBIOLOGISTS

Paul B. Brown
Bruce W. Maxfield
Howard Moraff

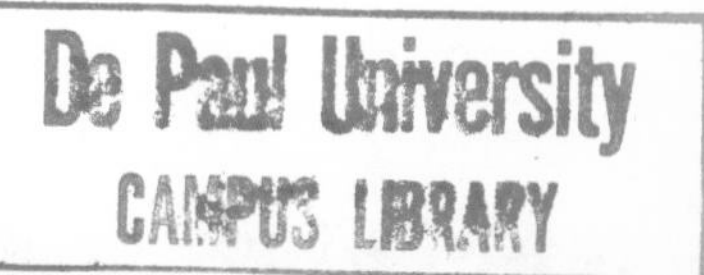

This book was set in Monophoto Baskerville,
printed on Finch Publishers Offset
and bound in Columbia Millbank Vellum MBV-4585
by Halliday Lithograph Corporation
in the United States of America.

Library of Congress Cataloging in Publication Data

Brown, Paul Burton 1942–
Electronics for neurobiologists.

Includes bibliographies.
1. Electronics. 2. Electronics in biology.
3. Neurobiology. I. Maxfield, Bruce W. II. Moraff,
Howard. III. Title.
[DNLM: 1. Biomedical engineering. 2. Electronics,
Medical. 3. Neurophysiology. QT 34 B883e 1973]
TK7816.B76 621.381 73-3193
ISBN 0-262-02094-7

ELECTRONICS FOR NEUROBIOLOGISTS

The MIT Press
Cambridge, Massachusetts, and London, England

CONTENTS

PREFACE

During the late 1960s, the cost of integrated circuits (ICs) had dropped sufficiently, and their variety and quality had increased sufficiently, to make it possible for the first time to begin compiling material for a book in which the designs for the more common neurobiological electronics devices could be based on this new technology. The advent of small, reliable "black boxes" that were inexpensive and easy to use, and that performed a large variety of analog and digital functions, made it possible to present in a single volume all the theory and practical circuits needed to construct, service, and design much of the equipment used by neurobiologists, excluding some display and electromechanical recording devices.

This volume is intended for use both as a textbook and a handbook of useful circuits. It is assumed that the reader has a standard college mathematics and physical sciences background, and of course, training in neurophysiology.

There is no discussion of electron tubes in this text, except for a brief discussion of cathode ray tubes, and there is only a superficial treatment of discrete transistor design principles. Both of these subjects would require a more extensive treatment than we could possibly give here, and several excellent texts are already available. It is our conviction that the utility of discrete components, especially tubes, will continue to diminish relative to that of integrated circuits and modules.

For purposes of mutual compatibility and compatibility with the majority of devices commercially produced, all analog circuits have been designed with

± 15 V supply requirements, except in those applications where no devices were available which operated on these voltages at the time of design testing. All digital functions are performed by TTL (Transistor-Transistor Logic) devices, which operate on $+5$ V. It seems safe to assume that these will remain the industry standards.

Developments in electronics are proceeding at a rapid pace. The reader is encouraged to keep informed of new developments, in order to optimize designs in terms of cost, performance, and design simplicity. We hope to revise this text at regular intervals, in order to keep abreast of technology. All other texts and manuals with which the authors are familiar are obsolete with respect to electronics for neurobiologists. Some do not even use transistors but rely on outmoded tube designs; others make use of transistors but present no IC designs.

We hope that this book will stimulate the use of more quantitative methods in neurobiological research. Most researchers impose limits on the sophistication of their methods that are based either on their conception of the state of the art or their own lack of technical expertise; frequently these limitations are unnecessarily modest. We hope that this book will also help the neurophysiologist gain an added perspective on the quality and cost of commercial instrumentation and that indirectly the industry will be stimulated to give the researcher a better buy in electronics devices.

We have tried as much as possible to develop theory and practical applications in parallel, on the grounds that the theory is best retained by immediate applications, and in the hope that the conventional biologist's fear of electronic circuit design will be overcome by providing opportunities to build equipment as quickly as possible. The experimenter who can implement simple circuit modifications in commercial equipment, or that of his own design, as his needs change, has an immeasurable advantage in terms of flexibility.

Although this book is geared toward the needs of neurobiologists, other biologists will undoubtedly find the material useful. The neurobiologist is perhaps the most dependent on electronics because of the very nature of his research.

In order to ensure that subsequent editions are suited to the needs of the readers, we invite suggestions for future improvements. These should be addressed to Dr. P. B. Brown, Neurological Unit, Boston State Hospital, 591 Morton Street, Boston, Massachusetts 02124.

Much of the present edition was made possible through the assistance of various individuals. Special thanks go to Leonard Smithline, Bruce Halpern, Maxwell Mozell, Daniel Tapper, Frederick Hiltz, Robert Capranica, Jay Goldberg, and Dario Domizi. The following organizations graciously permitted us to reprint material from their publications: Allen-Bradley Company; Analog Devices, Inc.; AP, Inc.; Cambridge Thermionic Corporation; Corning Glass Works; Fairchild Camera and Instrument Corporation; Gardner-Denver Company; Hayden Publishing Company; Hewlett-Packard Company; Holden-Day, Inc.; John Wiley & Sons, Inc.; Lansing Research Corporation; McGraw-Hill Book Company; Mentor Corporation; Microtran Co., Inc.; MIT Press; Monsanto Company; National Semiconductor Corporation; Oak Manufacturing Company; Ohmite Manufacturing Company; ORTEC, Inc.; Simpson Electric Company; Sprague Electric Company; Tektronix, Inc.; Teledyne Philbrick; Testronic Development Laboratory; and Texas Instruments, Inc.

Texas Instruments requested that the following notice be included in reference to material from their publication: "These device descriptions are reported, courtesy of Texas Instruments, Incorporated, Dallas, Texas. Material herein is excerpted from complete data sheets in Texas Instruments Catalog CC-401 which provides more detailed information. Texas Instruments reserves the right to make changes at any time in order to improve design and to supply the best possible product. TI cannot assume any responsibility for any circuit shown or represent that they are free from patent infringement."

Although none of the other manufacturers whose data sheets are reproduced here requested a statement of this nature, the reader should assume that similar reservations apply.

Dr. Brown was a U.S. Public Health Service Postdoctoral Trainee Fellow (Grant No. 2-FO2-NS-40,636-02), and Dr. Moraff received support from U.S. Public Health Service Grant No. RR 326 during the preparation of this book.

Paul B. Brown
Bruce W. Maxfield
Howard Moraff
Cornell University

January 1973

1 PASSIVE CIRCUIT ELEMENTS AND NETWORKS

B. W. Maxfield

1.1 Current, Voltage, and Resistance

Many materials, such as metals and semiconductors, contain charges that are free to move under the influence of an applied force. If an electric field E or voltage V is produced between two points, the electric force (electromotive force, EMF) on the free charges produces a current I, defined as the rate of charge flow through a cross section of the material, that is,

$$I = \frac{\Delta q}{\Delta t} \tag{1.1}$$

where Δq is the amount of charge that moves through a cross section in a time increment Δt. The current is given in amperes A if Δq is expressed in coulombs and t in seconds.

For a variety of reasons, the free charges cannot accelerate indefinitely under the application of a constant electric force. At constant temperature, all metals and semiconductors pass a steady current when a constant voltage or electric field is applied to them. The ratio of voltage to current is called the resistance R.

In some materials, R is independent of the magnitude of the applied voltage. Such materials are said to obey Ohm's law, which can be written as

$$V = IR. \tag{1.2}$$

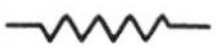

Figure 1.1
Symbol for a resistor.

A circuit element that obeys Ohm's law as given by Equation 1.2 is called a resistor and is represented by the symbol in Figure 1.1.

A constant voltage applied to a resistor produces a current flowing in one direction. By convention, the current flows in an external circuit (in this case the resistor) from positive (high potential) to negative (low potential). Inside a voltage source, the current flow is from negative to positive. The unit of potential difference (voltage) is the volt V. A resistance of one volt per ampere is called an ohm, represented by the symbol Ω. Decade and fractional decade multiples of these units (as well as others) are often used. Table 1.1 shows the accepted abbreviations of various powers of ten.

A quantity called resistivity should not be confused with resistance. *Resistivity* is a means of specifying the electrical conduction property of a material. Hence we speak of the resistivity of copper or carbon. *Resistance* is a property of a particular piece of material. For example, equal lengths of copper wire of different diameter will have different resistances, but the copper in each wire will have the same resistivity.

Materials having a very large resistivity are called *insulators;* they cannot pass any appreciable amount of current. Some structures that are made of insulating materials are also called insulators. These structures usually serve as tie points for electrical connections and thus insulate the components from some other portion of the circuit.

The applied voltage does work on the charge carriers, and therefore the source of this voltage must be able to deliver power to the resistor. The power P dissipated in the resistor (and therefore the power supplied by the voltage source) is

Table 1.1
Accepted abbreviations of powers of ten.

G	giga	10^9
M	mega	10^6
k	kilo	10^3
m	milli	10^{-3}
μ	micro	10^{-6}
n	nano	10^{-9}
p	pico	10^{-12}

given by

$$P = IV. \tag{1.3}$$

When Ohm's law is obeyed, Equation 1.3 becomes

$$P = I^2R = V^2/R. \tag{1.4}$$

If the current is expressed in amperes and potential difference in volts, then the power is given in watts W.

The power dissipated in the resistor appears as heat. The steady power input due to a constant current flowing through a resistor causes the element to reach a temperature such that the power radiated or conducted to its surroundings is equal to the power input to the resistor. Obviously, resistors that must dissipate considerable power (say 5 to 100 W) must get very warm (even hot!) to touch. It is often necessary to provide a specific means for cooling resistors (as well as any other elements that dissipate power). For an element to be useful as a power resistor, its resistance must not change appreciably when powers up to its rated value are dissipated.

1.2 Alternating or Time-Dependent Current

So far, only unidirectional or direct current (dc) flow has been considered. Even when the applied voltage changes with time, the current at any instant through a resistor is given by Ohm's law, namely $i = \xi/R$, where now i and ξ are instantaneous values of current and voltage, respectively. In one very important and very common situation, ξ is a sinusoidal function of time. This implies that i must also be a sinusoidal function of time although ξ and i need not be in phase. Thus the current alternately flows in one direction and then the other, according to the time dependence shown in Figure 1.2; it always changes at the same uniform rate defined by the frequency f or the period $T = 1/f$. Note that ξ and i as shown in Figure 1.2 are in phase; that is, at every instant, the voltage is directly proportional to the current.

This simple time variation is normally referred to as an alternating voltage or current (ac). For discussion purposes in this chapter, we will use the term ac voltage or current to imply a voltage or current state whose time variation can be specified by a single frequency (such as given by Equations 1.5 through 1.8). It should, of course, be remembered that the term ac voltage or ac current need not be so restrictive. Here, it is very important that R be independent of V, because the voltage is changing constantly in magnitude. The instantaneous power dissipated in the resistor is $P_i = i\xi$. If the current and voltage are both in phase (as

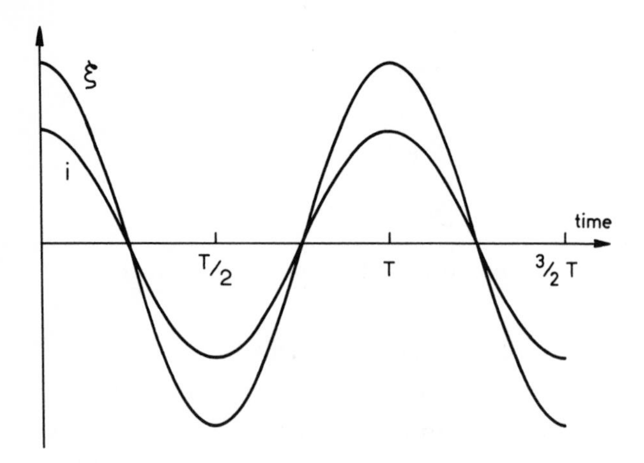

Figure 1.2
A sinusoidal or ac current and voltage of frequency $f = 1/T$.

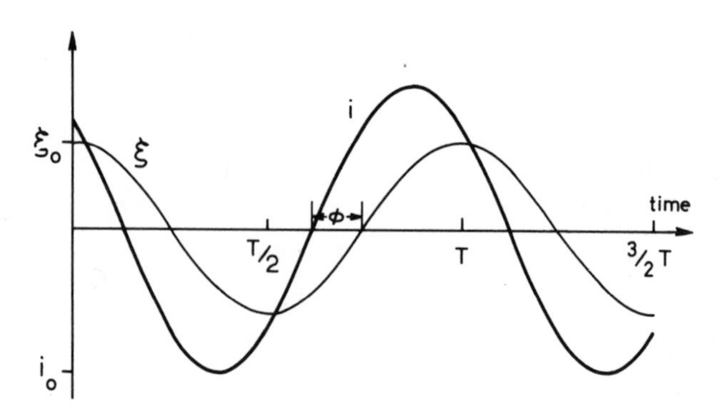

Figure 1.3
A current and voltage of the same frequency $f = 1/T$ but the voltage lags the current by ϕ.

shown in Figure 1.2) and are sinusoidal functions of time, we can write

$$i = i_0 \cos \omega t \tag{1.5}$$

$$\xi = \xi_0 \cos \omega t \tag{1.6}$$

where $\omega = 2\pi f$ and i_0 and ξ_0 are referred to as peak values. Often, however, i and ξ are not in phase but instead ξ is shifted backward (or forward) in time by a constant, time-independent amount that can be represented by a phase angle ϕ. This is illustrated in Figure 1.3, where the heavy line represents current and the light line represents voltage. It may seem peculiar that the current does not increase at the same instant as the voltage increases, but, in fact, we will see that this is a very common situation in ac circuits. In Figure 1.3, the voltage lags the current by the phase angle ϕ; these curves are represented by

$$\xi = \xi_0 \cos \omega t \tag{1.7}$$
$$i = i_0 \cos (\omega t + \phi). \tag{1.8}$$

The instantaneous power dissipation P_i is then given by

$$P_i = i_0 \xi_0 \cos \omega t \cos (\omega t + \phi), \tag{1.9}$$

which when averaged over 1 period gives an average power dissipation of

$$P = \tfrac{1}{2} i_0 \xi_0 \cos \phi, \tag{1.10}$$

where $\cos \phi$ is referred to as the power factor. For a resistor, the current and voltage are in phase, that is, $\phi = 0$ ($\cos \phi = 1$). Since $\xi_0 = i_0 R$, the power dissipation is given by

$$P = \tfrac{1}{2} i_0^2 R. \tag{1.11}$$

Further discussion of the origin and significance of ϕ will be delayed until more properties of alternating currents have been discussed.

Since the current or voltage is changing constantly, what should be used as a number to describe "alternating current" or "alternating voltage" (referred to as ac current and ac voltage)? The instantaneous values are of little use because the time must also be specified. Clearly, one number that characterizes the strength of an ac voltage or current is the maximum value, more commonly referred to as the *peak value*. From Figure 1.3 or Equations 1.5 and 1.6, the peak current and voltage values are i_0 and ξ_0, respectively. The *peak-to-peak* (ptp) value of any sinusoidal current or voltage is twice the peak value. Another meaningful and useful number is the value of either the current or voltage averaged over a half cycle (the average over a full cycle is, of course, zero). From Equations 1.5, 1.6, or 1.7, 1.8, the *average current* and *voltage* over one half cycle are, respectively:

$$i_{av} = \bar{i} = \frac{2}{\pi} i_0, \tag{1.12}$$

and

$$\xi_{av} = \bar{\xi} = \frac{2}{\pi} \xi_0. \tag{1.13}$$

Yet another means of specifying an ac voltage or current is through the *root mean square* (rms) value that is defined in terms of the equivalent dc power delivered to a resistor by an ac source. The rms current is therefore defined in terms of the average ac power delivered to a resistor by

$$P = i_{\mathrm{rms}}^2 R \tag{1.14}$$

or from Equation 1.11, the rms and peak values are related by

$$i_{\mathrm{rms}} = i_0/\sqrt{2}, \tag{1.15}$$

$$\xi_{\mathrm{rms}} = \xi_0/\sqrt{2}. \tag{1.16}$$

The ac rms current delivers the same power to a resistor as a dc current of the same magnitude. At this point, it is worth emphasizing that these relationships between peak, peak-to-peak, average, and rms quantities are only true for sinusoidal currents and voltages.

1.3 Alternating Current Circuit Elements; Impedance

1.3.1 Capacitance and Inductance

So far we have dealt only with a single circuit element, the resistor. It can be used with both ac and dc voltage sources. For a resistor, the voltage developed across the terminals is proportional to the rate of charge flow (current) through it. There are other circuit elements that prove to be very useful in ac circuits. Two such elements are the capacitor and the inductor.

A capacitor, which is represented by the symbol in Figure 1.4, develops a terminal voltage V_C proportional to the charge q that is stored in the capacitor, that is,

$$V_C = \frac{q}{C} \tag{1.17}$$

where C is the capacitance in farads F (or some appropriate smaller unit such as μF, nF) if q is the charge in coulombs and V_C is the potential difference in volts.

An inductor, represented by the symbol in Figure 1.5, has a terminal voltage V_L proportional to the rate of change of the current di/dt through it; that is,

$$V_L = -L\frac{di}{dt}. \tag{1.18}$$

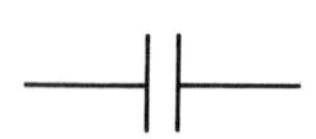

Figure 1.4
Symbol for a capacitor.

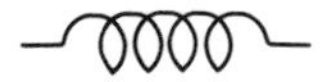

Figure 1.5
Symbol for an inductor.

Equation 1.18 is written with a minus sign to describe the fact that a current changing in one direction gives rise to a voltage that changes in the opposite direction. The inductance L is measured in Henrys H (or some convenient smaller unit such as mH) if V_L is in volts and di/dt is in amperes per second.

In the capacitor, energy is stored in the form of an electric field (static charge) and in the inductor, energy is stored in the form of a magnetic field (moving charge, that is, current). Further discussion of capacitance and inductance can be found in the Halliday and Resnick reference at the end of this chapter.

Seldom in real life do circuit elements closely approximate ideal behavior under all conditions. For instance, a resistor may have some inductance associated with it or an inductor may also have some capacitance. Initial discussions will be concerned with ideal elements so that we learn something about their basic properties. However, in practice, we must always be on the alert for nonideal behavior; it is everywhere, so always remember it cannot be assumed *a priori* that any circuit element will exhibit its ideal behavior in a particular circuit.

1.3.2 Impedance

Suppose a sinusoidal voltage source $\xi = \xi_0 \cos \omega t$ is connected to the terminals of a capacitor. The current through the capacitor is then given by (differentiate Equation 1.17)

$$i = C\frac{d\xi}{dt} = C\xi_0\omega \sin \omega t. \tag{1.19}$$

Notice that the current through a capacitor is zero unless the voltage across it is changing. By analogy with our discussion of the resistor, the ratio of voltage to current is then

$$\frac{\xi}{i} = \frac{1}{\omega C}\frac{\cos \omega t}{\sin \omega t}. \tag{1.20}$$

On the surface this appears to have little meaning because Equation 1.20 includes a time-dependent term. Are we to infer that a generalized form of Ohm's law is not valid for a capacitor? Let us look at this more closely by referring to the time-dependence of ξ and i shown in Figure 1.6. Certainly if we take the ratio of maximum values of ξ and i we get a number that is time-independent and appears to

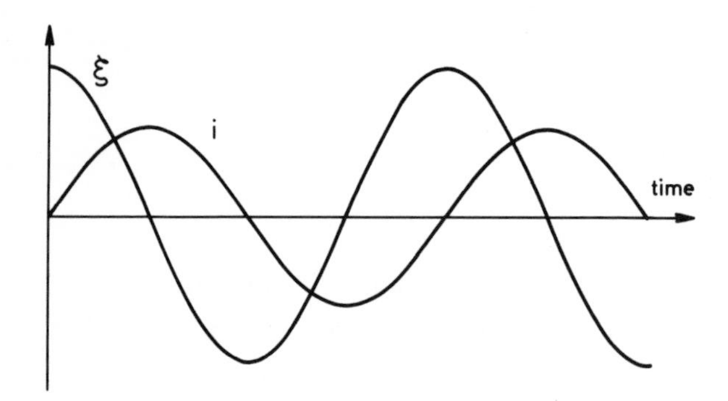

Figure 1.6
The current through a capacitor when driven by a voltage source, $\xi = \xi_0 \cos \omega t$.

be a meaningful way of describing the current and voltage in a capacitor, namely,

$$\frac{\xi_0}{i_0} = \frac{1}{\omega C}. \tag{1.21}$$

It is clear, however, that this number does not describe completely the current and voltage wave forms in Figure 1.6. The ratio of maximum values given by Equation 1.21 is the ratio of ξ to the value of the current at a time a quarter period $T/4$ later. Thus the current-voltage characteristics of a capacitor are only completely specified by two pieces of information, a magnitude (such as given by Equation 1.21) and a phase angle (the amount that either the current or voltage must be shifted in time to make the two maxima coincide).

Why does such a simple concept appear to be mathematically so complex? The main difficulty lies with the particular number system that we have been using; it does not permit easy representation of a two-component number (such as magnitude and phase). Complex numbers, however, provide a very convenient representation of two-component numbers. The appendix to this chapter gives all the basic rules for manipulating complex numbers. In particular, the relationship between complex numbers and two-dimensional vectors may help many readers recall quickly the properties of complex numbers. Because of the enormous simplification that they introduce, complex numbers will be used whenever needed in the discussions that follow. However, only the real part of a voltage or current can be determined in any individual measurement.

The ratio of voltage to current in an ac circuit is called *impedance;* in general, it is a complex number with both the real and imaginary parts having significance. The imaginary part of the impedance determines the phase angle *between the voltage across a circuit and the current through it.*

Thus the sinusoidal voltage connected to the capacitor terminals may be written as

$$\xi = \xi_0 e^{j\omega t}. \tag{1.22}$$

(Note: Re $\xi = \xi_0 \cos \omega t$ as before. Re stands for "the real part of," see the appendix at the end of this chapter.) The current through the capacitor is (from Equation 1.19)

$$i = j\omega C\xi. \tag{1.23}$$

Thus the impedance of a capacitor Z_C, defined as the voltage across the capacitor divided by the current through it, is given by

$$Z_C = \frac{1}{j\omega C}. \tag{1.24}$$

It is easy to see that Equation 1.24 represents what was argued less clearly earlier. Since $-j = \exp(-j\pi/2)$ and $j^{-1} = -j$ (the magnitude of j is unity), the ratio of the maximum values of ξ and i is $1/\omega C$, and the phase angle between the current and voltage is $\pi/2$; that is, one wave form is shifted with respect to the other by a quarter period or a time $T/4$.

Work must be done by the voltage source in order to build up a charge on a capacitor. However, during discharge, the capacitor does work on the voltage source. Averaged over a complete cycle, no work is done by the voltage source; therefore, no net power is dissipated by the capacitor. Whenever the current and the voltage in a circuit are 90° out of phase, the circuit does not draw any net power from the voltage source. Thus, the instantaneous power delivered to a capacitor is

$$P_i = \text{Re}\,\xi \times \text{Re}\,i. \tag{1.25}$$

From Equations 1.22 and 1.23, Equation 1.25 becomes

$$P_i = (\xi_0 \cos \omega t) \times (-\omega C\xi_0 \sin \omega t) \tag{1.26}$$

or, averaged over one cycle, the power delivered to a capacitor is

$$P = \frac{\omega C i_0 \xi_0}{T} \int_0^T \cos \omega t \sin \omega t \, dt = 0. \tag{1.27}$$

The previous arguments can be extended very easily to the analysis of the current-voltage characteristic of an inductor. Equation 1.18 is written so that a positive di/dt gives the correct sign for the voltage drop across the inductor. If the inductance is driven by a voltage given by Equation 1.22 (that is, the terminal volt-

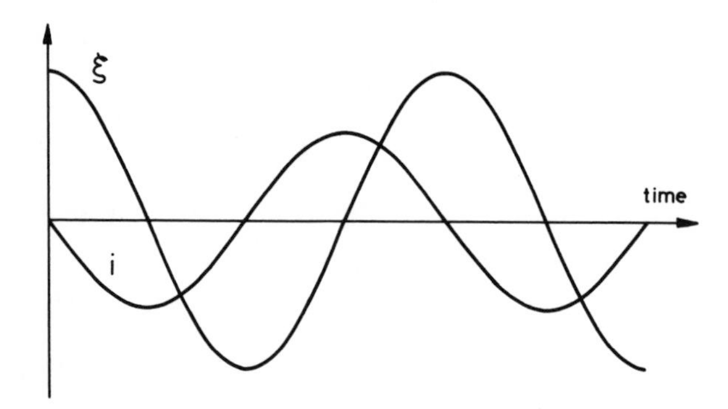

Figure 1.7
The current through an inductor when driven by a voltage source, $\xi = \xi_0 \cos \omega t$.

age is forced to follow Equation 1.22), then it follows from Equation 1.18 that the current through it is as shown in Figure 1.7.

Since the maximum value of di/dt is ω times the maximum value of i, the ratio of the maximum voltage drop across the inductance to the maximum rate of change of current through it is given by

$$\frac{\xi_0}{\omega i_0} = L. \tag{1.28}$$

The current wave form must be shifted forward in time by 90° in order to be in phase with the voltage wave form; this shift is expressed by

$$\xi = i\omega L e^{j\pi/2}, \tag{1.28}$$

which is equivalent to

$$\xi = ij\omega L. \tag{1.29}$$

Therefore, the impedance of an inductor is defined as

$$Z_L = j\omega L. \tag{1.30}$$

An ideal inductance does not dissipate any power, because the voltage and current are 90° out of phase. It takes energy to build up current in either direction in an inductor, but the same energy is pumped back into the circuit when the current is decreasing. Averaged over a complete period, no power is dissipated in an ideal inductor.

Figure 1.8 is a photograph of the many types of resistors, capacitors, and inductors that are commonly used for circuit construction.

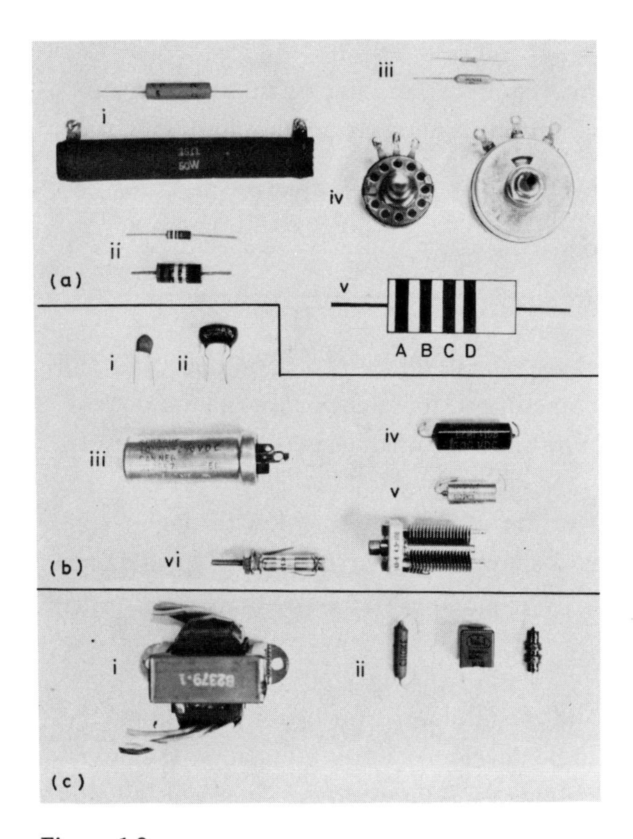

Figure 1.8
Some of the numerous types of resistors, capacitors, and inductors that are commonly used for circuit construction.

(a) Resistors: (i) wire-wound resistors (can dissipate large amounts of power), (ii) medium power ($\frac{1}{8}$ to 2 W) carbon composition resistors (these are low-cost, moderate-tolerance components), (iii) metal film resistors (low-power components having a small temperature coefficient), (iv) carbon composition and wire-wound potentiometers or variable resistors (normally 1 or 2 W rating), (v) the composition and metal film resistance code: Band A, first significant digit; Band B, second significant digit; Band C, power of ten multiplier; and Band D, the resistor tolerance rating (gold = 5%, silver = 10%, none = 20%). On metal film resistors, the first three numbers are the significant figures, and the fourth number is the power of ten multiplier. For example, brown, red, green is $12 \times 10^5 = 1.2$ MΩ and 1002 is $100 \times 10^2 = 10$ kΩ. Resistor color code: black, 0; brown, 1; red, 2; orange, 3; yellow, 4; green, 5; blue, 6; violet, 7; gray, 8; and white, 9.

(b) Capacitors: (i) ceramic, and (ii) dipped mica (reasonably low cost, moderate voltage (< 1 kV) low capacitance ($\leqq 0.1\ \mu$F)), (iii) molded tubular of paper or polyester dielectric (low-cost, medium capacitance, and moderate voltage ratings), (iv) metal can electrolytic (large capacitance (< 10 mF) and moderate voltage), and (v) solid tantalum capacitors (large capacitance, low voltage), (vi) variable capacitors.

(c) Inductors: (i) low-frequency transformer (many henries inductance), (ii) a variety of radio frequency inductors ranging from 1 μH to 100 mH with moderate (< 1 amp) current rating.

1.4 Some Useful Circuit Theorems

Resistors, capacitors, and inductors are frequently used in combination. To facilitate the analysis of multicomponent circuits, it is necessary to develop some basic rules.

1.4.1 Kirchhoff's Rules

The conservation of charge or junction rule is

The algebraic sum of all currents into a junction at any instant must be zero.

A junction is defined as a connection between circuit elements and does not itself act in any way as a circuit element. Sometimes a junction is also called a node. Leads connecting circuit elements are assumed to introduce no additional resistance, capacitance, or inductance into the circuit.

This rule is illustrated in Figure 1.9. Currents i_1, i_2, and i_3 flow through R_1, R_2, and R_3, respectively, in directions as shown by the arrows. Point *a* is the junction between the resistors (R_1, R_2, R_3). The junction rule states that

$$i_1 + i_2 + i_3 = 0.$$

If this were not true, then charge would accumulate at (or be removed from) the junction. By definition, no voltage can be developed across a junction. If charge accumulated at the junction, then a voltage would have to exist across it (recall the discussion of a capacitor). This is contrary to the definition of a junction. If it is found, through measurement, that a voltage exists across a "junction," then the appropriate circuit element (R, L, or C) must be inserted at an appropriate point and a new set of junctions defined.

For the general case of N currents flowing into or out of a junction, we have

$$\sum_{n=1}^{N} i_n = 0. \tag{1.31}$$

Current flowing into a junction is the same as the negative of that current flowing out of the junction and vice versa.

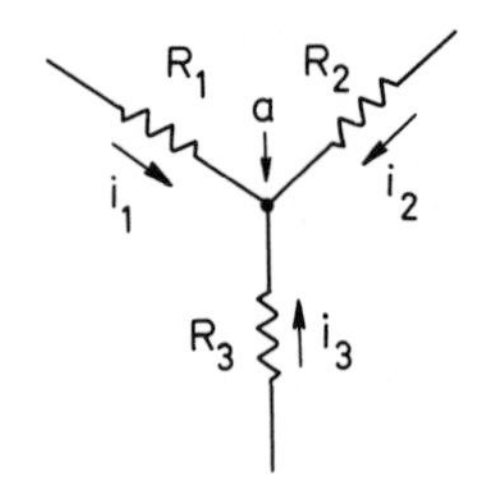

Figure 1.9
Currents i_1, i_2, and i_3 flowing into junction *a*.

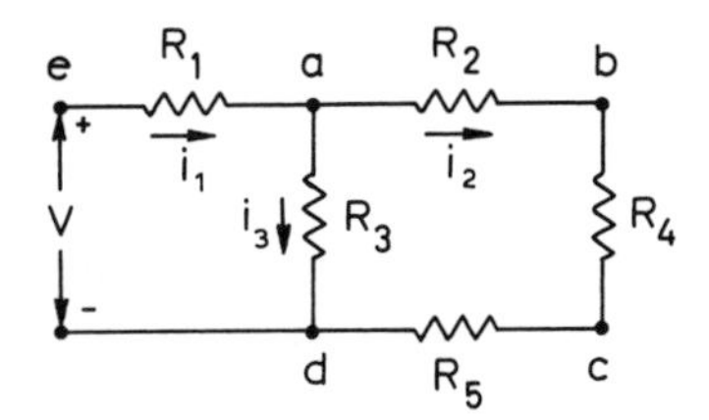

Figure 1.10
A circuit with two independent loops and five junctions.

The single-valuedness or loop rule is

The algebraic sum of all voltage sources in any closed loop must equal the algebraic sum of the voltage drops across all the circuit elements in the same closed loop.

Stated more explicitly, for a loop having N sources and M circuit elements, we have

$$\sum_{n=1}^{N} \xi_n - \sum_{m=1}^{M} i_m Z_m = 0 \tag{1.32}$$

where i_m is the current through the mth impedance Z_m, and a loop is any closed path through which currents flow. The direction that is chosen for current flow through the circuit elements is arbitrary. Currents that turn out to be negative are simply flowing in a direction opposite to that assumed. To illustrate this, consider the multielement circuit in Figure 1.10. This circuit contains five junctions (a, b, c, d, and e) and two independent loops, *adea* and *abcda*. An independent loop is one that cannot be constructed from a combination of other loops. The loop *abcdea* is not independent because it can be constructed from the above two independent loops. The number of independent loops determines the number of independent equations that must be solved in order to determine the current through each resistance (impedance). This, of course, assumes that the voltages are known.

The loop rule may also be stated as "the potential drop around any closed loop is zero." If this were not true, the potential of any junction could be multivalued. Because measurement must always yield a unique potential for each junction, the potential drop around any closed loop must be zero.

Applying the junction rule to junction a in Figure 1.10, we have

$$i_1 - i_2 - i_3 = 0.$$

The loop rule for loops *adea* and *abcda* yields, respectively,

$$-i_3 R_3 + V - i_1 R_1 = 0$$

and

$$-i_2R_2 - i_2R_4 - i_2R_5 + i_3R_3 = 0.$$

These rules are valid for ac as well as for dc currents, that is, for impedances as well as resistances. However, at high frequencies (say $f > 10^7$ Hz $= 10$ MHz) a real circuit junction may be significantly different from the ideal junction used in our examples. For example, the inductance of a 12 inch length of wire may be significant at such a high frequency; in this instance a 12 inch length of resistanceless wire forming a common point between three circuit elements (e.g. resistors) could not be considered as a simple junction whereas for a direct current it would be an ideal junction.

1.4.2 Impedance Combinations

Unless there is some reason to label the performance of a particular circuit element as either a resistor, capacitor, or inductor, it will be represented by the symbol in Figure 1.11. This is the same symbol as used previously for the resistor; from now on this symbol will be used to represent either a resistor or a general impedance Z.

Suppose that we have two impedances connected in *series*, that is, connected so that *the same current flows through each element* as indicated in Figure 1.12a. Such a combination of impedances is equivalent to the single series equivalent impedance Z_{seq}, shown in Figure 1.12b. We wish to obtain a relationship between Z_1, Z_2, and Z_{seq}. Any two combinations of impedances are equivalent if they produce exactly the same effect in a circuit. In this example then, a voltage ξ applied to the series

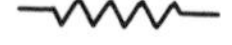

Figure 1.11
Symbol for a general impedance.

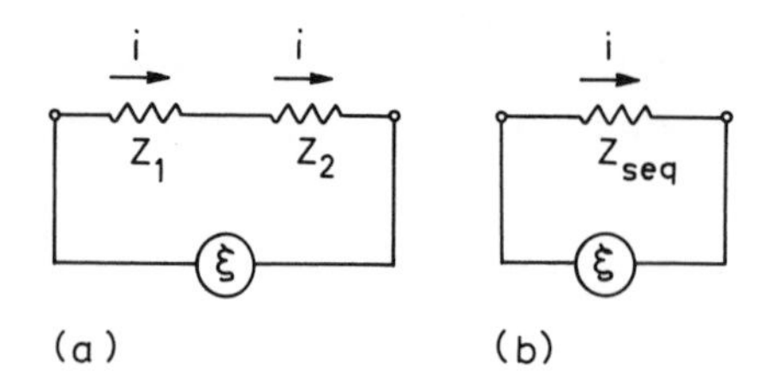

Figure 1.12
(a) Two general impedances connected in series, and
(b) their series equivalent impedance.

combination of Z_1 and Z_2 should produce the same current as the voltage ξ applied to Z_{seq}. Since a generalized form of Ohm's law is obeyed by all passive circuit elements (resistors, capacitors, and inductors), the circuit in Figure 1.12a yields

$$\xi = iZ_1 + iZ_2 \tag{1.33}$$

for any impedance, and the circuit in Figure 1.12b yields

$$\xi = iZ_{seq}. \tag{1.34}$$

Thus, for the two circuits and therefore Equations 1.33 and 1.34 to be equivalent, we must have

$$Z_{seq} = Z_1 + Z_2. \tag{1.35}$$

This gives the series impedance addition rule:

The equivalent impedance of any number of circuit elements all of which are connected in series is the algebraic sum of the individual impedances.

Therefore, the equivalent series resistance of two resistors is

$$R_{seq} = R_1 + R_2; \tag{1.35a}$$

the equivalent series inductance of two inductors is

$$L_{seq} = L_1 + L_2; \tag{1.35b}$$

and the equivalent series capacitance of two capacitors is

$$\frac{1}{C_{seq}} = \frac{1}{C_1} + \frac{1}{C_2}. \tag{1.35c}$$

Circuit elements may also be connected in *parallel*, that is, with *the same voltage applied across all the elements.* Consider two impedances Z_1 and Z_2 connected in parallel and the parallel equivalent impedance Z_{peq}, both shown in Figure 1.13.

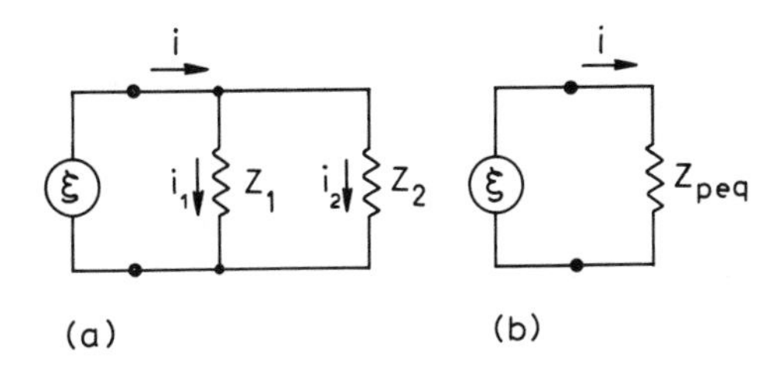

Figure 1.13
(a) Two impedances connected in parallel, and
(b) their parallel equivalent impedance.

From Kirchhoff's rules, we require that

$$i = i_1 + i_2 \tag{1.36}$$

and

$$\xi = i_1 Z_1 = i_2 Z_2 \tag{1.37}$$

for the circuit in Figure 1.13a and

$$\xi = iZ_{\text{peq}} \tag{1.38}$$

for the circuit in Figure 1.13b. For these two circuits and, therefore, for Equations 1.37 and 1.38 to be equivalent, we must have

$$\frac{1}{Z_{\text{peq}}} = \frac{1}{Z_1} + \frac{1}{Z_2}. \tag{1.39}$$

Equation 1.39 gives the parallel impedance addition rule:

The reciprocal of the equivalent impedance of any number of circuit elements all of which are connected in parallel is the algebraic sum of the reciprocals of the individual impedances.

Therefore, the equivalent parallel resistance of two resistors is

$$\frac{1}{R_{\text{peq}}} = \frac{1}{R_1} + \frac{1}{R_2}; \tag{1.39a}$$

the equivalent parallel inductance of two inductors is

$$\frac{1}{L_{\text{peq}}} = \frac{1}{L_1} + \frac{1}{L_2}; \tag{1.39b}$$

and the equivalent parallel capacitance of two capacitors is

$$C_{\text{peq}} = C_1 + C_2. \tag{1.39c}$$

Often, calculations are easier to carry out in terms of reciprocal impedance, which is called *admittance*. The admittance addition rules follow directly from the impedance addition rules. Clearly, the admittance of a circuit must be complex if the impedance is complex. The impedance Z of any circuit can be written as the sum of real and imaginary parts (the resistance and *reactance*, respectively); namely

$$Z = R + jX, \tag{1.40}$$

where X is the reactance.

Similarly, the admittance Y can be represented by

$$Y = G + jB \tag{1.41}$$

where G is the *conductance* and B the *susceptance*. The unit of admittance (and therefore of conductance and susceptance) is the mho; one mho is one ampere per volt; it is often abbreviated Ω^{-1}. For example, an admittance of 20 μmho is exactly the same as an impedance of 50 kΩ and a conductance of 10 mmho is exactly the same as a resistance of 100 Ω.

Thus,

$$G = \frac{R}{R^2 + X^2} = \frac{R}{|Z|^2}; \qquad B = \frac{-X}{R^2 + X^2} = \frac{-X}{|Z|^2}; \tag{1.42}$$

$$R = \frac{G}{G^2 + B^2} = \frac{G}{|Y|^2}; \qquad X = \frac{-B}{G^2 + B^2} = \frac{-B}{|Y|^2}. \tag{1.43}$$

1.5 Voltage and Current Sources

We have referred extensively to voltage sources without ever really saying what they are. Voltages are normally generated by either chemical or electromagnetic means. The lead-acid wet cell, carbon-zinc dry cell, and mercury cell are examples of chemical generators of electrical energy and are conventionally denoted by the symbol in Figure 1.14a. Lead-acid batteries are used when large dc currents are required, carbon-zinc batteries are the most economical means of obtaining moderate battery currents (<1000 mA) or large battery voltages, say up to 300 V. Mercury batteries are stable voltage sources, but they can only deliver relatively small currents. Batteries are sometimes represented as stacked cells; this is how large-voltage batteries are constructed: by placing voltage sources in series.

Time-varying or alternating voltages are generated either electronically or electromagnetically (by rotating loops of wire in a magnetic field). However, for our purposes, we can regard the 60 Hz electrical outlet as an ac voltage source. The symbol in Figure 1.14b is normally used to denote an ac voltage source.

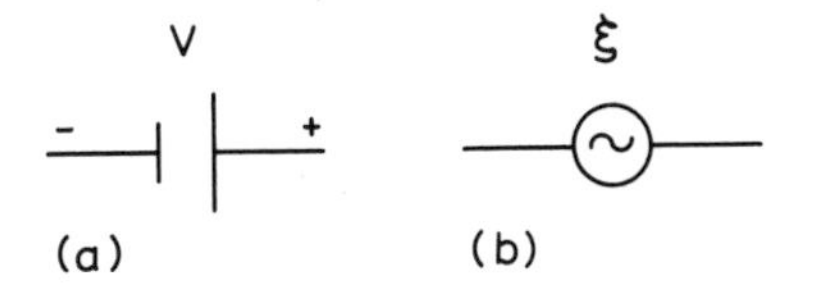

Figure 1.14
(a) Symbol for a battery, and
(b) symbol for an ac voltage source.

Somewhat later, we will discuss a means of converting an ac voltage to a dc voltage. This process, called *rectification*, is actually the most common means of obtaining a dc voltage. Units performing this function are called power supplies. Although batteries must be used in truly portable equipment, they are a much more expensive source of dc power than is rectified ac power.

The reader may have noted that it has been assumed the voltage source can deliver any necessary current to the load. In general this is not true; something other than the output voltage of a voltage source must be specified so that the current delivering capacity of the power source can be determined. All real voltage sources (dc or ac) contain a finite internal resistance that limits the output current. Thus a battery may be represented by the equivalent circuit shown in Figure 1.15a. The internal resistance r_o limits the current that the battery can deliver to any external load. The output voltage V_o across the battery output terminals when a current I is delivered to a load R_L is given by (see Figure 1.15b)

$$V_o = IR_L. \tag{1.44}$$

It follows from Ohm's law, Equation 1.2, and from Kirchhoff's rules that

$$I = \frac{V}{R_L + r_o}. \tag{1.45}$$

Combining Equations 1.44 and 1.45, we obtain

$$V_o = V\left[\frac{R_L}{R_L + r_o}\right] = V\left[\frac{1}{1 + r_o/R_L}\right] \tag{1.46}$$

where V is the open circuit (zero output current) voltage of the battery. An *ideal* voltage source, that is, one with zero internal resistance, has a terminal or output voltage that does not depend upon the load resistance; the current delivered to the load resistance is determined only by V and R_L. The current limiting internal resistance in a nonideal voltage source is referred to as the output resistance.

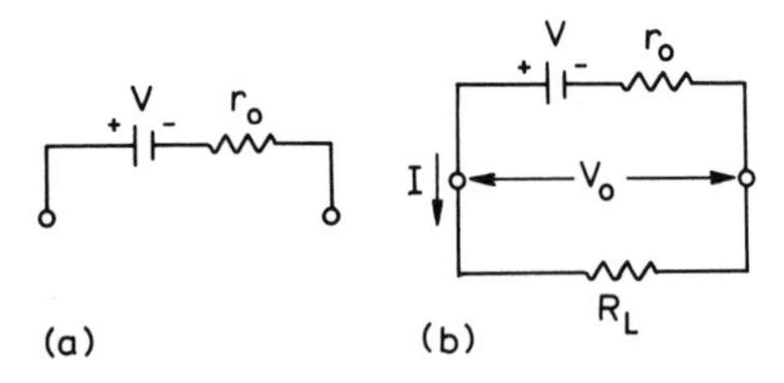

Figure 1.15
(a) The equivalent circuit of a battery with internal resistance r_o, and
(b) a load resistance R_L connected to such a voltage source.

For ac sources, the output characteristics are determined by the output impedance rather than just the output resistance. By identical arguments, an ac voltage source of open circuit voltage ξ and output impedance z_o connected to a load Z_L will have a terminal voltage given by

$$\xi_o = \frac{\xi}{1 + z_o/Z_L}. \tag{1.47a}$$

Frequently, it is necessary to optimize the amount of either current, voltage, or power that is transferred from the source to the load. From the circuit in Figure 1.15b, it should be clear that maximum current is transferred to the load when $R_L \ll r_o$ (the maximum load current is $I_{L_{max}} = V/r_o$) and that maximum voltage transfer occurs when $R_L \gg r_o$ (the maximum voltage across the load is V). Maximum power transfer from source to load is obtained when $r_o = R_L$, that is, when the output resistance is equal to the load resistance. Similar results are obtained for ac power sources; V, r_o, and R_L are replaced by ξ, z_o, and Z_L, respectively.

A battery cannot deliver a specified current indefinitely, regardless of its internal resistance, because only a limited amount of energy is stored in the battery. Thus an energy storage rating is needed if one is to determine the battery lifetime for any particular application; lifetime is commonly expressed in ampere-hours A h. Power supplies are specified for operation at some maximum power output (usually with separate upper limits on both current and voltage), because the internal components have a limited ability to dissipate power. More will be said about specifications of power supplies when they are discussed in detail in Chapter 11.

Many electronic circuits to be discussed in the following chapters behave more like current sources than voltage sources. A *voltage source* is a power source where the output voltage remains reasonably constant under changing load conditions (that is, the output current changes with load but the output voltage does not). A *current source* is a power source where the output current remains reasonably constant under changing load conditions (the output voltage changes but the output current does not). Any voltage source can be converted into a current source and vice versa. The voltage source shown in Figure 1.16a is equivalent to (indistinguishable from) the current source in Figure 1.16b if the current generator has an output current $i = \xi/z_o$. This can be verified easily, because when $i = \xi/z_o$, the open circuit ($Z_L = \infty$) output voltage and the short circuit ($Z_L = 0$) output current are identical for both circuits. Maximum current transfer from source to load for both networks in Figure 1.16 occurs for $Z_L \ll z_o$, and maximum voltage transfer occurs for $Z_L \gg z_o$. Equation 1.47a describes the output voltage for the

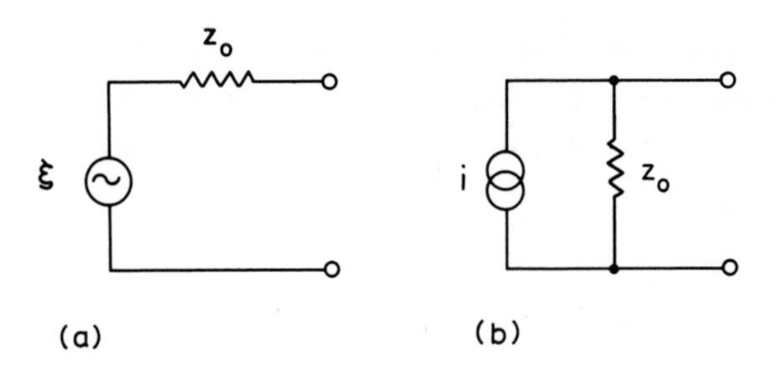

Figure 1.16
(a) A voltage source of internal impedance r_o, and
(b) a current source of internal impedance r_o. These two networks are equivalent if the ideal current generator output is $i = \xi/z_o$.

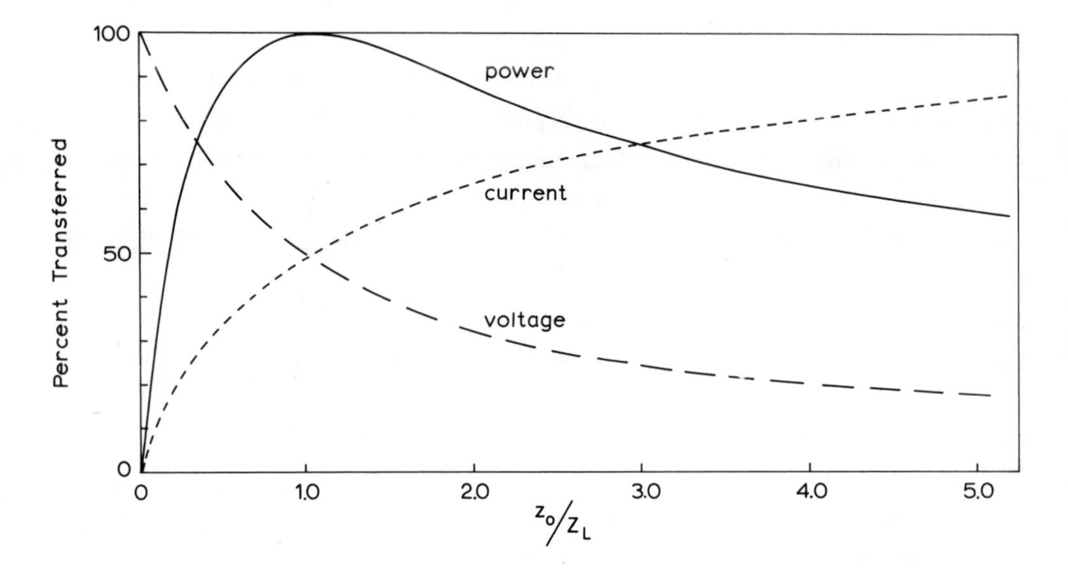

Figure 1.17
Percentage transfer of current, voltage, and power from source to load as a function of the output and load resistance. For these curves, both the output and load impedances are assumed to be real; (a) for the voltage source in Figure 1.16a, and (b) for the current source in Figure 1.16b.

circuit in Figure 1.16a; maximum power transfer takes place when $Z_L = z_o$. The output current for the circuit in Figure 1.16b is given by

$$i_o = \frac{i}{1 + Z_L/z_o}. \tag{1.47b}$$

From this expression, it is easy to show that maximum power transfer also occurs when $Z_L = z_o$. Curves for determining the current, voltage, or power that is transferred from source to load (for real output and load impedances) are given in Figure 1.17.

1.6 Alternating Current Circuits

An ideal capacitor blocks direct current flow in a circuit (in fact, this is one very important use of a capacitor), and no voltage drop exists across an ideal inductor carrying a direct current. Therefore, it is not surprising that capacitors and inductors find their greatest use in circuits involving time-dependent currents.

All useful voltages do not have a sinusoidal time-dependence. For example, wave forms such as the square, triangular, and sawtooth time-dependence illustrated in Figure 1.18 are encountered frequently. However, a general principle of

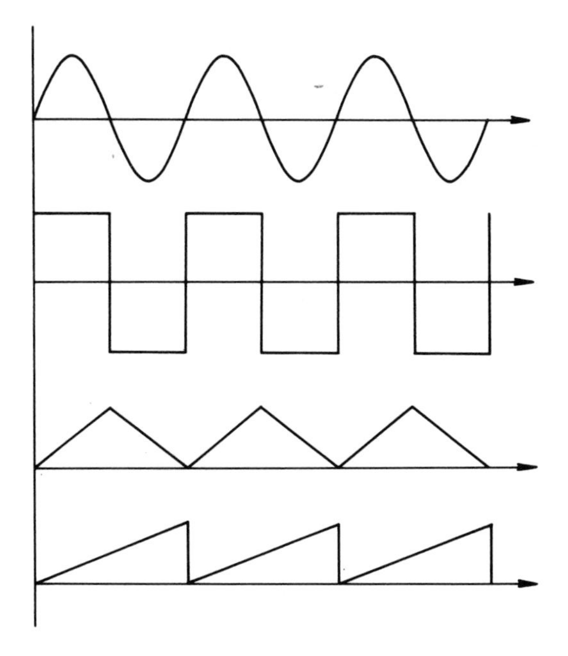

Figure 1.18
Sinusoidal and other voltage wave forms that are commonly encountered. All wave forms have the same period or repetition time.

superposition that applies particularly to periodic signals permits one to divide any time-dependent voltage into an appropriate sum of sinusoidal voltages, each component having a different frequency and specifiable amplitude. The existence of this superposition principle means that a discussion of the response of circuits to a sinusoidal voltage becomes a very general discussion of circuit response. Although the square wave response (often referred to as the transient response) can be obtained from an appropriate sum of sinusoidal responses, it is more convenient to treat this particular example directly; this is done in Section 1.7.

The discussion of impedance in Section 1.3 provides all the necessary background to solve for current-voltage relationships at various points in any circuit consisting of passive elements driven by a sinusoidal voltage source. When used in a generalized form of Ohm's law, the concept of impedance can be expressed as

$$\xi = iZ. \tag{1.48}$$

The rules governing series and parallel combinations of impedances are developed in Section 1.4.

1.6.1 Relative Gain: The Decibel

In general, the output of any network will have a magnitude that is different from the input, and the output voltage will be shifted in phase with respect to the input voltage. However, if Equation 1.48 is valid for the network, then the actual signal magnitude is not important; only the network impedance will determine the change in magnitude and phase of the signal between input and output. The change in magnitude (gain or attenuation) of a signal is often most conveniently expressed in decibels dB. The voltage gain A in decibels is defined as

$$A = 20 \log_{10} (\xi_o/\xi_i) \tag{1.49a}$$

where ξ_i and ξ_o refer to the peak input and output voltages, respectively. If $\xi_o < \xi_i$, the gain in dB is negative; negative gain is often referred to as *attenuation*. The power gain in dB is defined as

$$A_p = 10 \log_{10} (p_o/p_i). \tag{1.49b}$$

Gain or attenuation of ξ_o is expressed as A dB *re* ξ_i; similar notation is used for A_p.

1.6.2 The High-Pass Filter

To illustrate the general procedure for determining the frequency response of a network of passive elements, let us analyze the high-pass filter shown in Figure 1.19. We will assume that the output is connected to some very high impedance so that the load cannot affect the circuit operation. The input-output relationship

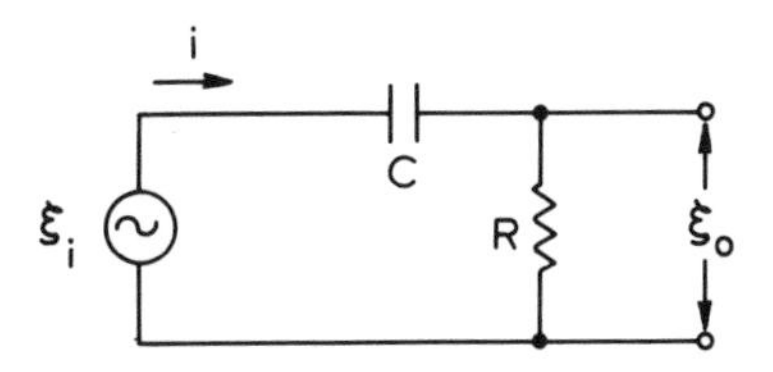

Figure 1.19
A high-pass *RC* network driven by a sine wave generator of frequency ω.

is determined from $\xi_o = iR$ and the loop rule (Equation 1.32), which gives

$$\xi_i - iZ = 0, \tag{1.50}$$

where Z is the impedance of the resistor R in series with the capacitor C. The rule for series addition of impedances, Equation 1.35, gives

$$Z = R + \frac{1}{j\omega C}, \tag{1.51}$$

a complex number representing both a magnitude and a phase. Combining Equations 1.50 and 1.51, we obtain

$$\frac{\xi_o}{\xi_i} = \frac{j\omega RC}{1 + j\omega RC}. \tag{1.52}$$

Equation 1.52 is clearer if the complex number ξ_o/ξ_i is shown explicitly in terms of a magnitude and a phase; that is,

$$\frac{\xi_o}{\xi_i} = \frac{R}{|Z|} \exp\,(-j\phi) \tag{1.53}$$

where

$$|Z| = [R^2 + 1/\omega^2 C^2]^{\frac{1}{2}} \tag{1.54}$$

and

$$\phi = \tan^{-1}\,(-1/\omega RC). \tag{1.55}$$

This means that the output voltage is phase-shifted with respect to the input voltage by an amount ϕ (the phase angle between ξ_o and ξ_i is ϕ), and the magnitude of the output voltage divided by the magnitude of the input voltage (the network gain) is given by $R/|Z|$.

Both the current i and the voltages ξ_i and ξ_o have the same frequency. As is evident from Equation 1.53, both the gain and the phase angle between the current and the voltage are frequency dependent. It is important to realize that only

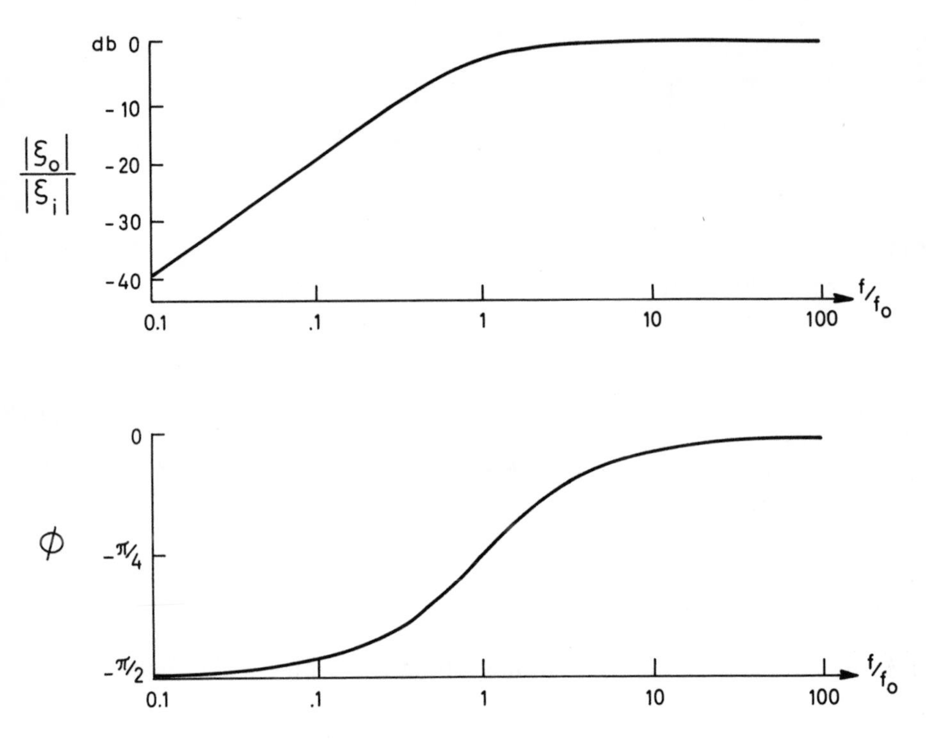

Figure 1.20
Frequency dependence of both the magnitude and phase angle of the output of a high-pass filter.

phase angles between two quantities (relative phase angles), such as between ξ_i and i or between ξ_o and ξ_i, can be measured.

Figure 1.20 shows the frequency dependence of both the gain and phase angle. Logarithmic scales have been used for the gain and frequency axes. For convenience, the frequency is plotted in units of f_0, that is, the frequency axis is normalized to f_0, where $f_0 = 1/2\pi RC$.

At a frequency determined by $\omega RC = 1$ (where $f = f_0$), we have

$|\xi_o| = 1/\sqrt{2}\,|\xi_i|$.

Therefore, at $f = f_0$, we have

$$A(f_0) = -20 \log \sqrt{2} \cong -3 \text{ dB}$$

and

$$\phi(f_0) = \tan^{-1}(-1) = -45°.$$

It is common to refer to f_0 as the characteristic, corner, or -3 dB frequency. For frequencies up to about f_0, the output is proportional to frequency (assuming the input remains constant), and above f_0 the output is independent of frequency.

1.6.3 Vector Representation

The real and imaginary parts of a complex number are independent quantities and therefore (as described in the appendix to this chapter) a complex number may be represented as the vector position of a point on a plane. Hence ac circuits may also be analyzed using standard vector notation. Although the actual circuit analysis is more easily accomplished using complex numbers, it is often useful to use ideas inherent in the vector representation when doing measurements. Figure 1.21 shows the vector addition of voltages for the circuit shown in Figure 1.20. Standard sign conventions have been used in determining the directions of voltages; a positive reactance gives a positive imaginary voltage, and a negative reactance gives a negative imaginary voltage for a positive current, and so on (see end of Section 1.4 for definition of reactance). Because the reactance of a capacitor is negative, ξ_C is negative. From Figure 1.21 it follows that

$$\tan \phi = -|\xi_C|/|\xi_R| \tag{1.56}$$

and

$$|\xi_i| = (|\xi_R|^2 + |\xi_C|^2)^{\frac{1}{2}}. \tag{1.57}$$

Since $\xi_C = iZ_C$, $\xi_R = iR$, $\xi_i = iZ$, and $Z_C = -jX_C$, we have $|\xi_i| = |i|\,|Z|$ with

$$|Z| = (R^2 + 1/\omega^2C^2)^{\frac{1}{2}} \tag{1.58}$$

and

$$\tan \phi = -1/\omega RC. \tag{1.59}$$

Equations 1.58 and 1.59 are, of course, identical to Equations 1.54 and 1.55 that were obtained by using complex numbers. Often it is convenient to use the

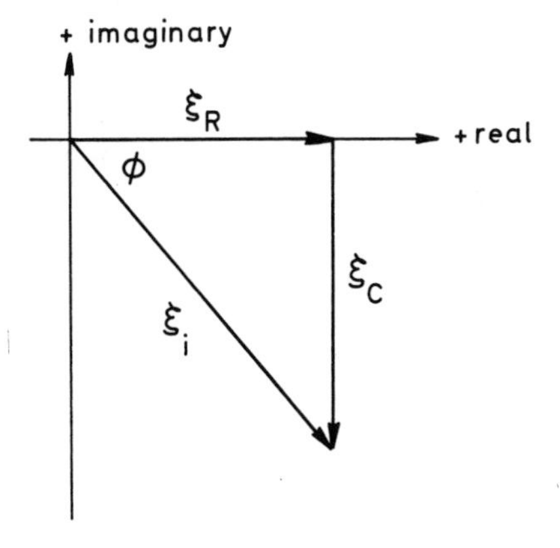

Figure 1.21
Vector addition of voltages for the high-pass filter shown in Figure 1.19.

relationship

$$\cos \phi = |\xi_R|/|\xi_i| \qquad (1.60)$$

to determine the phase angle. Both the phase and amplitude of ac voltages can be easily measured using an oscilloscope. The operation and use of the oscilloscope is discussed in some detail in Chapter 6.

1.6.4 Other Simple Impedance Combinations

As another example of circuit analysis, consider the series combination of a resistance and inductance as shown in Figure 1.22. Such a network will pass low frequencies very effectively, because the inductive reactance is small at low frequencies. Analysis follows along lines identical to those used for the high-pass filter. The series LR combination is represented by an impedance, $Z = R + j\omega L$ and, therefore,

$$\xi_o = \xi_i \frac{R}{|Z|} \exp(-j\phi) \qquad (1.61)$$

where

$$\phi = \tan^{-1}(\omega L/R) \qquad (1.62)$$

and

$$|Z| = [R^2 + \omega^2 L^2]^{\frac{1}{2}}. \qquad (1.63)$$

Figure 1.23 shows the frequency response of this low-pass network; in this case, the frequency is scaled by the characteristic frequency or -3 dB frequency, $f_0 = R/2\pi L$. (Note again the use of log scales.)

Two other common circuits, a low-pass and high-pass, respectively, are shown in Figure 1.24. From the properties of capacitors and inductors, it is easy to deduce that the low-pass RC network in Figure 1.24a has the same frequency characteristics as those of the low-pass LR network shown in Figure 1.22; in this RC case, the characteristic frequency is $f_0 = 1/2\pi RC$. Likewise, the high-pass LR network shown in Figure 1.24b has the frequency characteristics shown in Figure 1.20

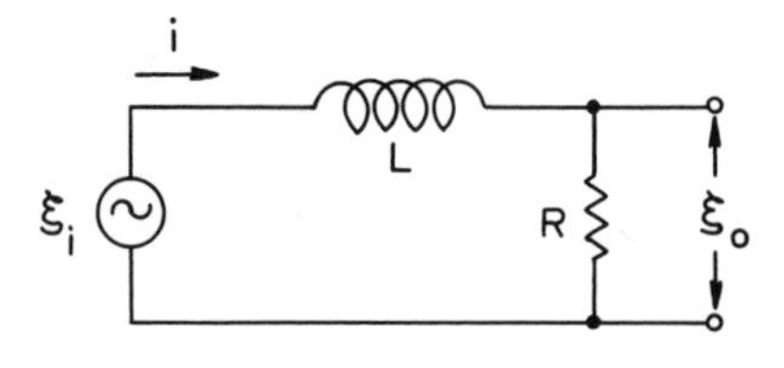

Figure 1.22
A low-pass LR network.

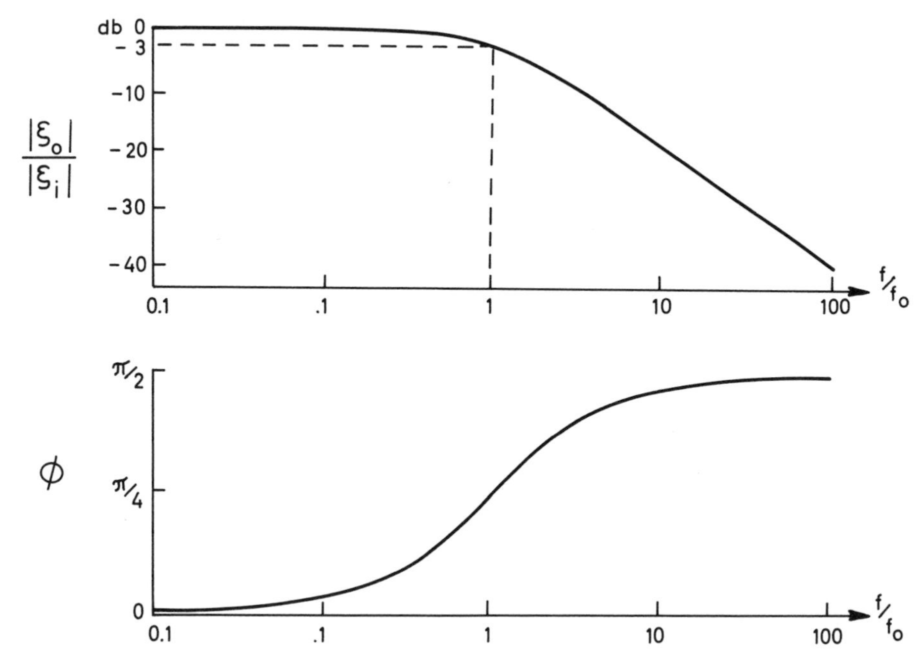

Figure 1.23
The frequency response of the low-pass LR network in Figure 1.11; $f_0 = R/2\pi L$.

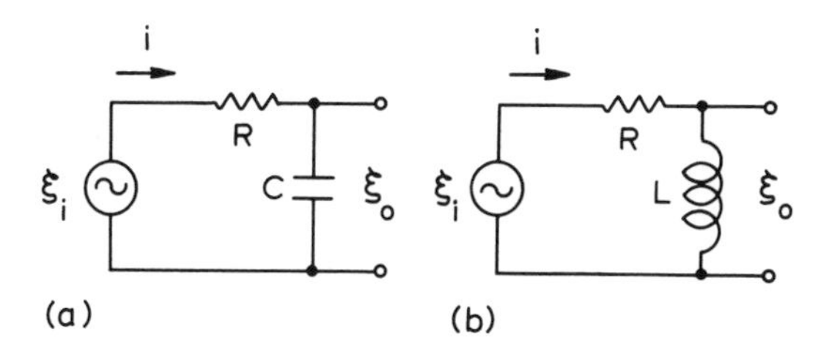

Figure 1.24
(a) A low-pass RC network, and
(b) a high-pass LR network.

with $f_0 = R/2\pi L$. Note, however, that the LR networks have dc continuity between the voltage source and ground whereas the RC networks do not. Except where the dc pass characteristic of an LR circuit must be exploited, it is best to use RC networks. At low frequencies (below 100 kHz) capacitors are usually more economical than inductors. In addition, the performance of real resistors and capacitors can be made to approximate ideal behavior very closely. This is seldom true of inductors.

1.6.5 Resonance Circuits

Much more striking input-output (transfer) relationships are obtained by using combinations of all three circuit elements. The series combination of R, L, and C

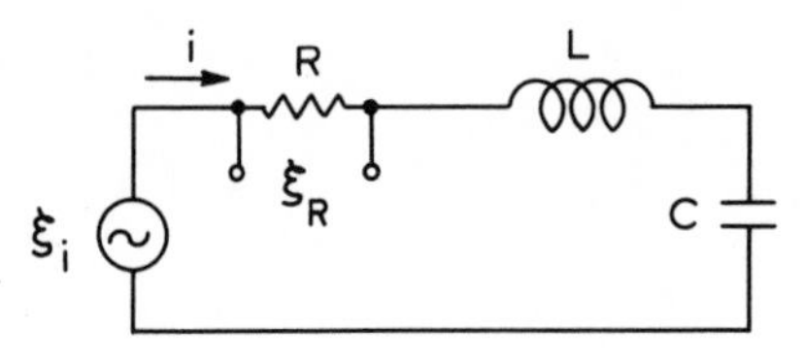

Figure 1.25
A series resonant circuit.

is shown in Figure 1.25. Because series impedances add, we have

$$Z = Z_R + Z_L + Z_C$$
$$= R + j\omega L + \frac{1}{j\omega C}. \tag{1.64}$$

The magnitude of this impedance is given by

$$|Z| = R^2 + [(\omega L - 1/\omega C)^2]^{\frac{1}{2}} \tag{1.65}$$

and of the phase angle by

$$\phi = \tan^{-1}\left[\frac{\omega L - 1/\omega C}{R}\right]. \tag{1.66}$$

Examination of Equations 1.65 and 1.66 shows that at a frequency $\omega = \omega_0$, where $\omega_0 = 1/\sqrt{LC}$, the phase angle is zero and the magnitude of the impedance is a minimum. Most of the frequency dependence actually occurs in the vicinity of ω_0. When written in terms of ω_0, Equations 1.65 and 1.66 become

$$|Z| = R\left[1 + \left(\frac{\omega_0 L}{R}\right)^2\left(\frac{\omega}{\omega_0} - \frac{\omega_0}{\omega}\right)^2\right]^{\frac{1}{2}} \tag{1.67}$$

and

$$\phi = \tan^{-1}\left[\frac{\omega_0 L}{R}\left(\frac{\omega}{\omega_0} - \frac{\omega_0}{\omega}\right)\right]. \tag{1.68}$$

This type of frequency response is referred to as *resonance; $f_0 = \omega_0/2\pi$* is called the *resonant frequency*. In general, the resonant frequency is defined by the condition

$$\text{Im } Z = 0 \tag{1.69}$$

where Im Z refers to the imaginary part of Z. Equation 1.69 must be used to determine the resonant frequency of more complex networks. At resonance, the current through this series circuit is in phase with the voltage across it (that is, ξ_i is in phase with ξ_R); in fact, this is the fundamental definition of the resonant frequency as expressed by Equation 1.69. In the vicinity of ω_0, the frequency dependence is determined by the scaling factor $\omega_0 L/R$. For instance, if $\omega_0 L/R$ is large, only a small change in ω/ω_0 is required to produce a large change in either $|Z|$ or ϕ. From the frequency dependence of Equation 1.67 given in Figure 1.26, it is clear that inherent in a series resonant circuit is a degree of frequency selectivity.

The factor $\omega_0 L/R$ is a measure of the frequency selectivity or sharpness of frequency separation that is obtained; it is known as the quality factor Q_s of the series resonant circuit. That is,

$$Q_s = \frac{\omega_0 L}{R}. \tag{1.70}$$

In real circuits, the Q is limited by the self-resistance of the inductor (coil). Values of Q up to 1000 are possible if well-designed components are used, but values less than 100 are much more typical. An inherently high-Q inductor can, of course, be used in a low-Q circuit since a series resistance can be added.

The frequency dependence of Equations 1.67 and 1.68 is shown in Figure 1.26. This same functional form for the frequency response is encountered frequently; for future convenience these equations have been plotted on both linear and logarithmic frequency scales.

It follows from the definition of Z that ϕ is the phase angle between ξ_i and i (see Figure 1.25). However, because the voltage across a resistor is in phase with the current through it, ϕ is also the phase angle between ξ_i and ξ_R. The ξ_R and ξ_i can be measured directly.

These circuits and others having a similar frequency response are very useful in many areas of signal processing. For convenience in future work, we define two additional quantities, one a reduced or normalized frequency,

$$x = \frac{\omega}{\omega_0}, \tag{1.71}$$

and the other quantity,

$$y = \frac{\omega}{\omega_0} - \frac{\omega_0}{\omega}, \tag{1.72}$$

which is related to the fractional difference between ω and ω_0. Using Equations 1.70, 1.71, and 1.72, we reduce Equations 1.64, 1.67, and 1.68 to

$$Z = R(1 + jQ_s y); \tag{1.73}$$

$$|Z| = R(1 + Q_s^2 y^2)^{\frac{1}{2}}; \tag{1.74}$$

$$\phi = \tan^{-1}(Q_s y). \tag{1.75}$$

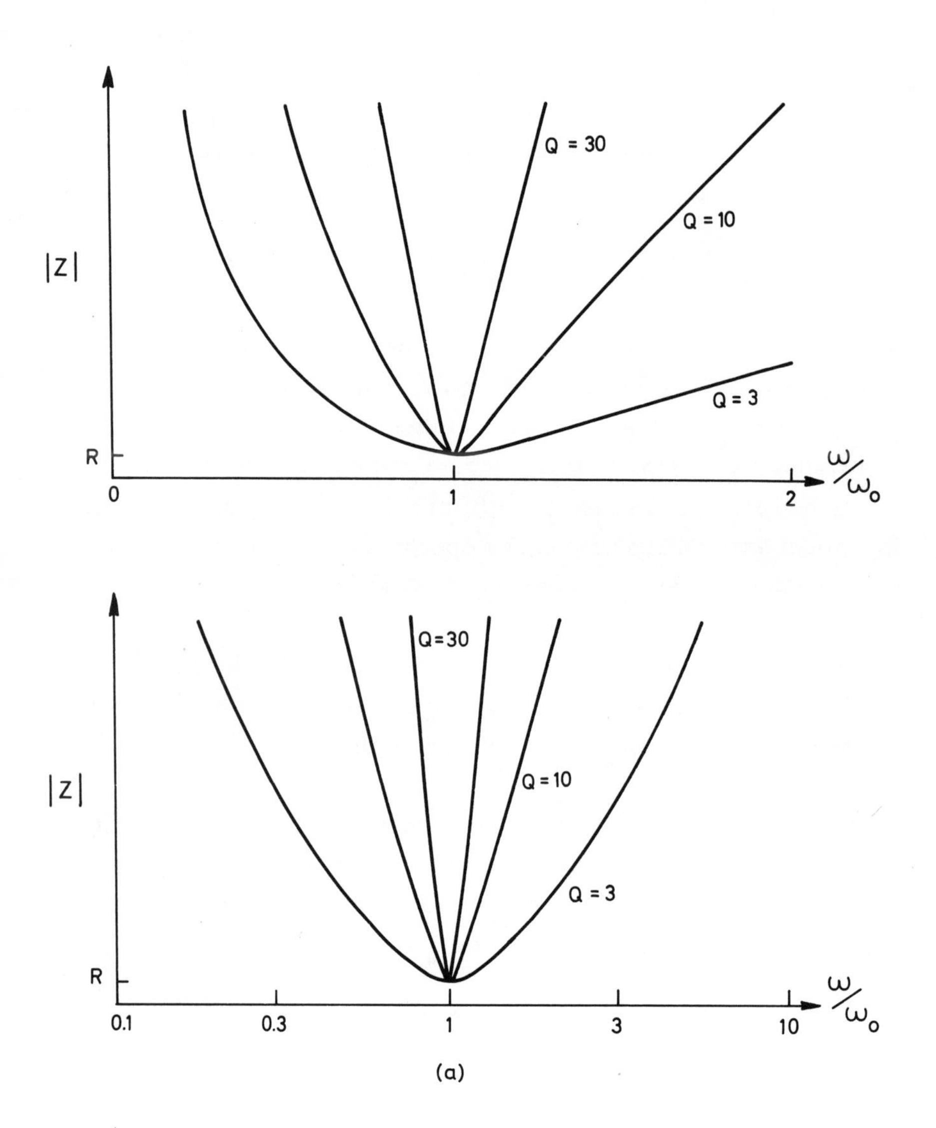

Figure 1.26

The frequency dependence of (a) the magnitude and (b) the phase angle of the impedance of a series resonant circuit shown in terms of reduced frequency units $\omega/\omega_0 = 1/\sqrt{LC}$. Both quantities are shown for linear and logarithmic frequency scales.

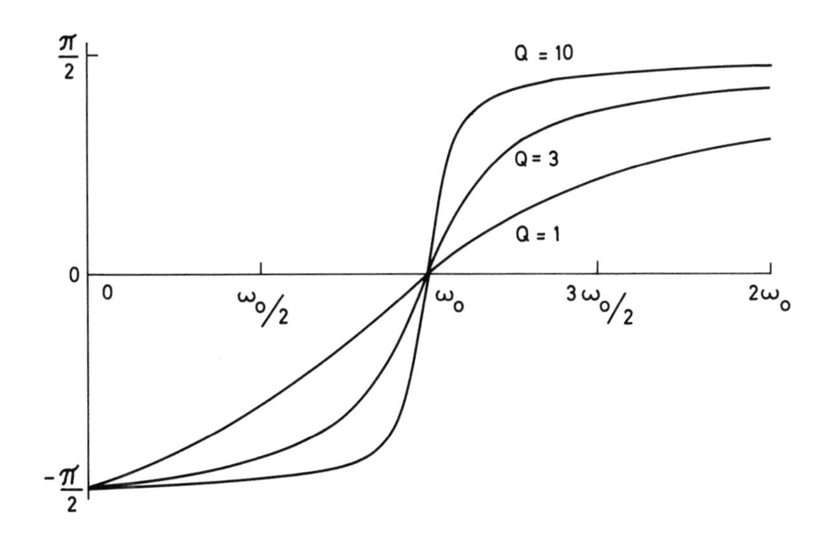

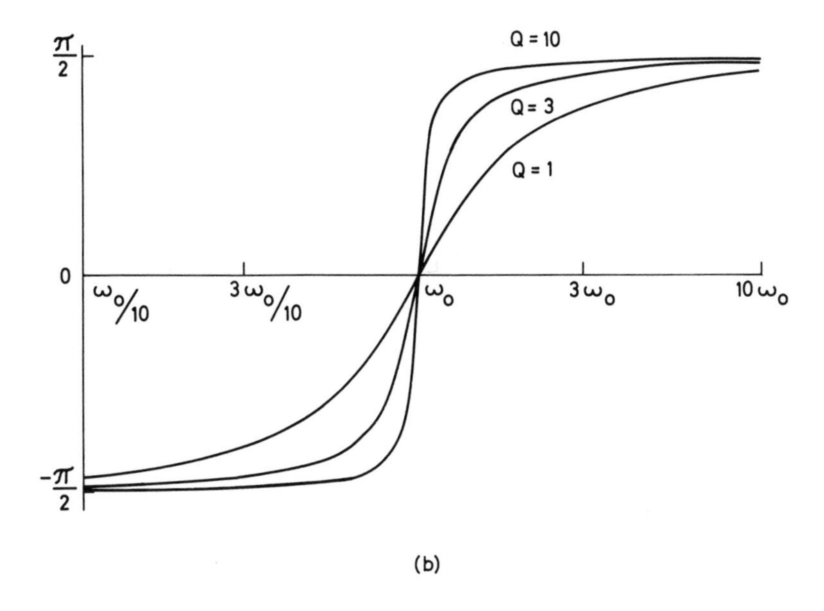

(b)

Figure 1.26 (continued)

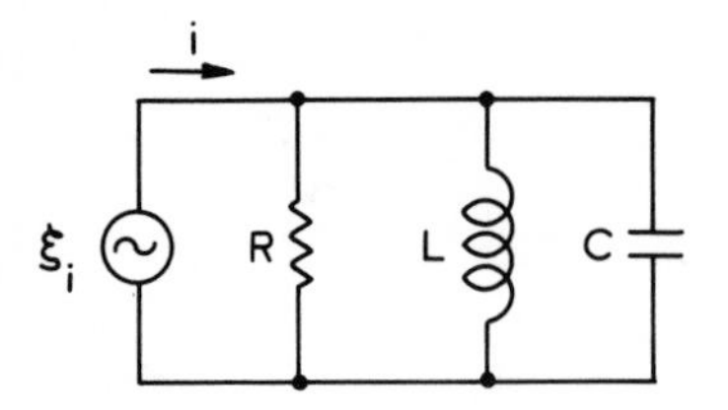

Figure 1.27
One form of a parallel resonant circuit.

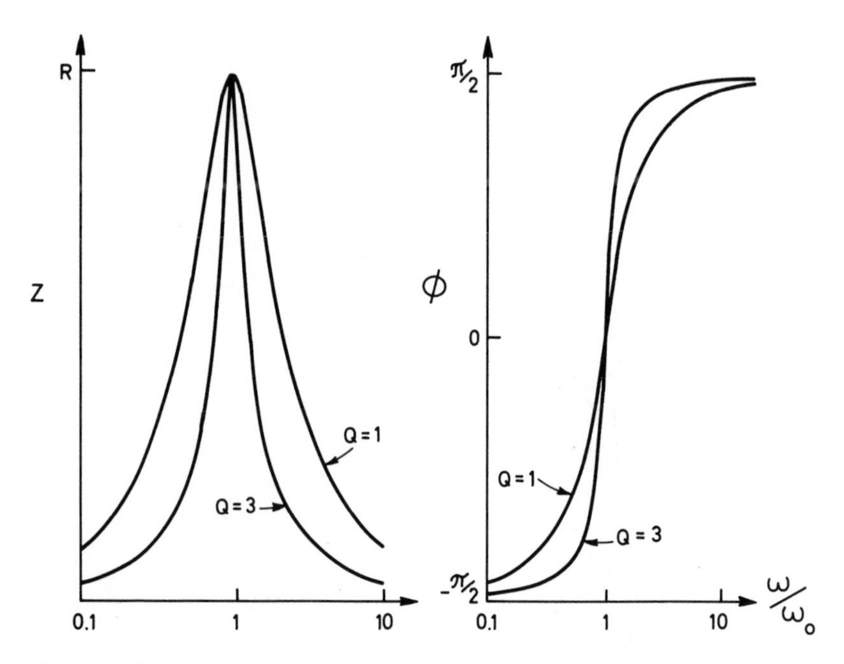

Figure 1.28
Frequency response of the parallel resonant circuit shown in Figure 1.27.

A parallel combination of L, R, and C such as that shown in Figure 1.27 has a different kind of resonant behavior. From Equation 1.39, it follows that the impedance of this circuit is given by

$$\frac{1}{Z} = \frac{1}{Z_R} + \frac{1}{Z_C} + \frac{1}{Z_L}$$

$$= \frac{1}{R} + j\omega C + \frac{1}{j\omega L}. \quad (1.76)$$

Using Equation 1.72 and introducing the parallel resonance quality factor, we obtain

$$Q'_p = \frac{R}{\omega_0 L} \quad (1.77)$$

where the resonant frequency, $\omega_0 = 1/\sqrt{LC}$, is determined from Equation 1.69,

$$Z = \frac{R}{1 + jQ'_p y}. \quad (1.78)$$

For a parallel resonant circuit, Z is a maximum and the current and voltage are in phase at $\omega = \omega_0$.

Figure 1.28 shows the frequency response of a parallel resonant circuit as given by Equation 1.78. In this case, a large parallel (shunt) resistance produces a high-Q circuit. The impedance at resonance is the main difference between series and parallel resonant circuits; at resonance the series combination is a low impedance circuit while the parallel circuit is a high impedance at resonance. Note also that a parallel resonant circuit is a short circuit for dc currents whereas the series resonant circuit has an infinite dc resistance (blocks the flow of dc current).

1.7 Transient Response

The response of various impedance combinations to an abrupt, steplike change in the applied voltage is called the *transient response of a circuit.* A knowledge of such behavior is necessary to understand the response of a circuit to a square wave voltage. A square wave can be represented as a sum of sinusoidal voltages each of a different frequency and amplitude. It follows, therefore, that the transient response of a circuit can be determined from the sinusoidal voltage responses by summing the contribution from each of the sinusoidal voltages that make up the square wave. However, an alternative procedure exists: The circuit equations as determined from Kirchhoff's rules can be solved directly for response to an abrupt change in the applied voltage. In practice, transient response is encountered quite frequently.

1.7.1 Series *RC* Circuit

An easy circuit to analyze is the series *RC* combination shown in Figure 1.29. Closing the switch *S* produces an abrupt voltage change across the *RC* network; we wish to determine the current that flows in this circuit after *S* is closed. Using Kirchhoff's rules, Ohm's law, and Equation 1.17, we find that the voltage-current relationship at any instant after the switch is closed is given by

$$V - iR - q/C = 0$$

or

$$V = \frac{q}{C} + R\frac{dq}{dt}. \tag{1.79}$$

The general solution to such a first-order, linear, differential equation can be found elsewhere (see references at the end of this chapter). The solution of Equation 1.79 is

$$q(t) = VC(1 - e^{-t/RC}), \tag{1.80}$$

from which it follows that

$$i(t) = \frac{V}{R}e^{-t/RC}. \tag{1.81}$$

Direct substitution of $q(t)$ (in Equation 1.80) and $i(t)$ (in Equation 1.81) into Equation 1.79 will verify that the correct solution has been obtained.

However, even without all this mathematics it is possible to see intuitively that Equations 1.80 and 1.81 are correct. Immediately after closing the switch, charge flows from the battery through the resistor and onto the capacitor. Initially, there is no voltage drop across C (no charge on it); so the current must be given by $i(t = 0) = V/R$. The voltage drop across R decreases as the charge (potential) on the capacitor increases (see Equation 1.17); hence as C charges less current can flow. Eventually (after a long time compared to RC), C is charged to a potential very close to the potential V, and therefore no current can flow through R. All of these conclusions follow directly from Equations 1.80 and 1.81. This description

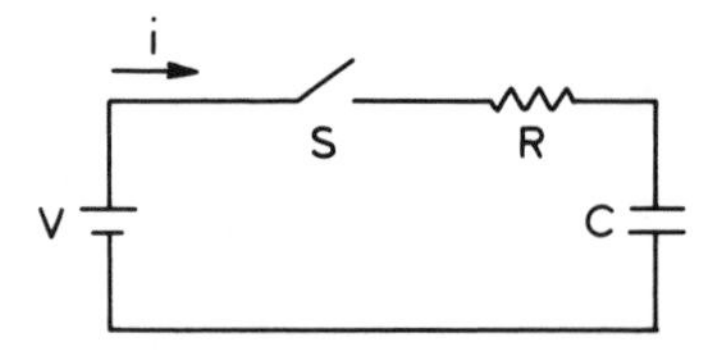

Figure 1.29
A circuit that can be used to determine the transient response of a series *RC* network.

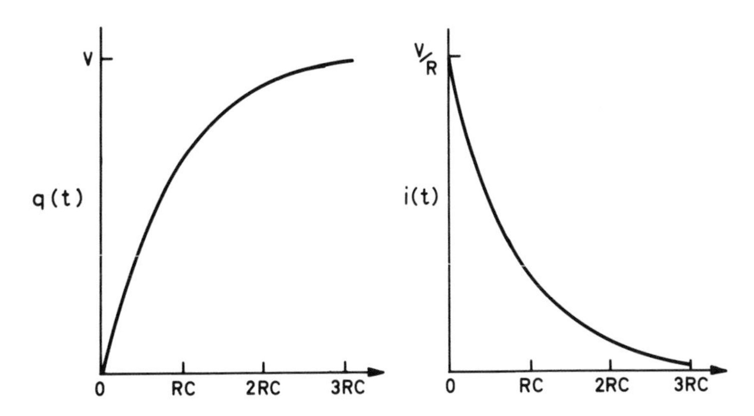

Figure 1.30
Charge build-up on the capacitor and current decrease through the resistor when a steady voltage is applied to the *RC* network in Figure 1.27.

is also consistent with our previous discussion of a capacitor; a current can flow in a series circuit containing a capacitor only if the voltage across the capacitor is time-dependent. Once the capacitor is charged to the potential V, the voltage across it does not change; hence no current flows.

Figure 1.30 shows the relationship between charge build-up on a capacitor and the current flow through the resistor. The saturating exponential characteristic is governed by the time constant

$$\tau_{RC} = RC. \tag{1.82}$$

If R is in ohms and C in farads, then τ_{RC} is in seconds.

It is reasonable that the charging time should be determined by RC because R determines the rate at which charge can flow onto C, and C determines the total amount of charge that must flow. Of course, a battery and switch are not the only means of producing an abrupt voltage change. The same effect is produced by a square wave voltage generator. The sharp increase in applied voltage that occurs every period corresponds to closing a switch, and thus allows C to charge. The rapid decrease in applied voltage, which also occurs once per period in a square wave generator, corresponds to discharging a charged capacitor through the resistance. With a real generator, both charging and discharging take place through the generator output impedance. Figure 1.30 shows the time dependence of the current through R and the charge on C for a series RC network driven from a voltage source of output resistance r_o that is much smaller than R. If the output resistance is not small, it should be clear that the time constant becomes $\tau_{RC} = C(R + r_o)$ and $i(t = 0) = V/(R + r_o)$.

1.7.2 Series *LRC* Circuit

Following an analytical procedure similar to that in the previous example, we find that charge flow for the series *LRC* circuit in Figure 1.31 is described by the equation

$$\frac{d^2q}{dt^2} + \frac{R}{L}\frac{dq}{dt} + \frac{q}{LC} - \frac{V}{L} = 0. \tag{1.83}$$

Equation 1.83 has the solution

$$q(t) = VC[1 - e^{-\gamma t} \cos \omega t] \tag{1.84}$$

where

$$\gamma = R/2L \tag{1.85}$$

and

$$\omega^2 = \left(\frac{1}{LC} - \frac{R^2}{4L^2}\right). \tag{1.86}$$

Substitution will verify that this is the correct solution. Therefore, the current in this series *LRC* network is given by

$$i(t) = VCe^{-\gamma t}(\omega \sin \omega t + \gamma \cos \omega t), \tag{1.87}$$

which as shown in Figure 1.32 is an oscillating function with an exponentially decreasing amplitude.

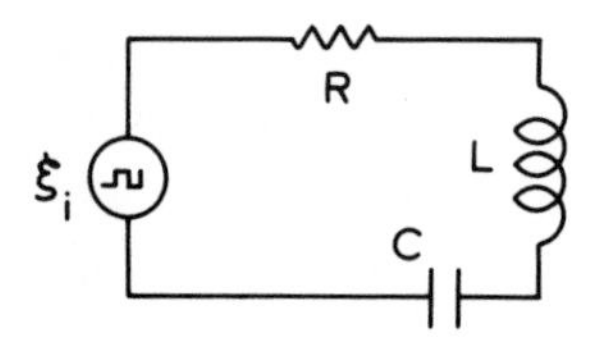

Figure 1.31
A series *LRC* network driven by an ideal square wave generator.

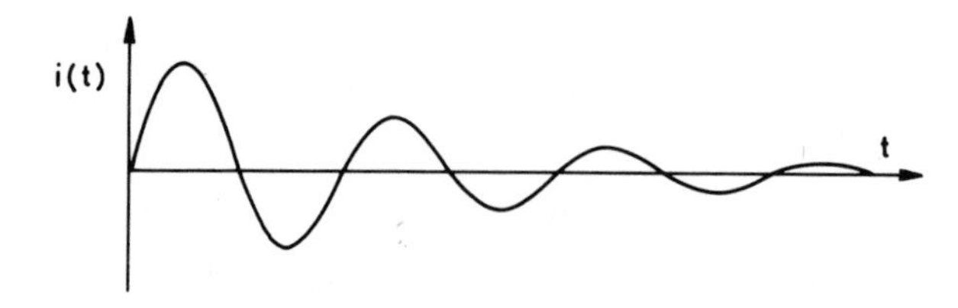

Figure 1.32
Exponentially damped oscillations that result when a constant voltage is applied abruptly to a series *LRC* network.

Appendix: The Use of Complex Numbers

As used in this book, complex numbers are simply a means whereby calculations involving quantities described by both a magnitude and a phase (for example, impedance) can be greatly simplified. No proofs of any statements will be given; these can be found in numerous introductory mathematical textbooks.

A *complex quantity* is defined as a quantity that can be expressed as the sum of a purely *real* term and a purely *imaginary* term. A purely imaginary number is a purely real number multiplied by $j = \sqrt{-1}$. The square root of a negative number is a very useful quantity.

Let us see how j and complex quantities are used in practice. First, we define two complex quantities α and β by

$$\alpha = a + jb$$

$$\beta = c + jd$$

where a, b, c, and d are defined to be purely real quantities (and therefore jb and jd are purely imaginary quantities). In order to handle complex quantities properly, we must know how to add one to another and how to multiply or divide one by another.

The operation of *addition* is defined by

$$\alpha + \beta = (a + c) + j(b + d);$$

that is, the real and imaginary terms are added separately. It follows that

$$\alpha - \beta = (a - c) + j(b - d).$$

Multiplication is defined by the operation

$$\alpha\beta = (a + jb)(c + jd).$$

Purely real and purely imaginary quantities multiply just like ordinary numbers; therefore, we have

$$\alpha\beta = ac + jad + jbc + j^2bd.$$

Because $j = \sqrt{-1}$, we must have $j^2 = -1$. Thus

$$\alpha\beta = (ac - bd) + j(ad + bc)$$

where $(ac - bd)$ and $(ad + bc)$ are purely real quantities.

The operation of *division*, defined by

$$\frac{\alpha}{\beta} = \frac{(a + jb)}{(c + jd)},$$

is a little more complicated, because both numerator and denominator are complex quantities. Because a fraction is unchanged if both numerator and denominator are multiplied by the same factor, we can write

$$\frac{\alpha}{\beta} = \frac{(a + jb)(c - jd)}{(c + jd)(c - jd)}.$$

Carrying out the respective multiplications, we obtain

$$(a + jb)(c - jd) = (ac + bd) + j(bc - ad);$$
$$(c + jd)(c - jd) = c^2 - jcd + jdc - j^2d.$$

Because $cd = dc$ and $-j^2 = 1$, we have

$$(c + jd)(c - jd) = c^2 + d^2$$

and

$$\frac{\alpha}{\beta} = \left[\frac{ac + bd}{c^2 + d^2}\right] + j\left[\frac{bc - ad}{c^2 + d^2}\right].$$

The preceding are the basic definitions that are needed in order to manipulate complex quantities. However, there are a number of additional useful terms that make discussions about complex numbers much more succinct.

The *complex conjugate* of a complex number is obtained by a transformation from j to $-j$. Thus the complex conjugate of α, denoted by α^*, is

$$\alpha^* = a - jb.$$

Note that the quantity $\alpha\alpha^*$ is real, namely,

$$\alpha\alpha^* = a^2 + b^2.$$

The *magnitude* of a complex number, denoted by $|\alpha|$ is defined by

$$|\alpha| = (\alpha\alpha^*)^{\frac{1}{2}}.$$

Hence if $\alpha = a + jb$,

$$|\alpha| = (a^2 + b^2)^{\frac{1}{2}}.$$

It also follows that $(\alpha\beta)^* = \alpha^*\beta^*$.

The *real* part of a complex quantity is usually represented by Re and the *imaginary* part by Im; thus if $\alpha = a + jb$ (with a and b real),

$$\text{Re}\,\alpha = a \quad \text{and} \quad \text{Im}\,\alpha = b.$$

It follows from $j = \sqrt{-1}$ that $j^2 = -1; j^3 = j^2j = -j; j^4 = j^2j^2 = 1; j^5 = j;$

etc. What about the quantity $\sqrt{j}$ or other nonintegral powers of j? Let the complex quantity $z = 1 + j$; then $z^2 = 1 + 2j - 1 = 2j$. Therefore, $z = (2j)^{\frac{1}{2}}$ and

$$\sqrt{j} = \frac{1 + j}{\sqrt{2}}.$$

Other powers are most easily determined from the identity

$$e^{jxp} = \cos px + j \sin px$$

where x is a real number and p is either an integer ($p = 1, 2, 3, \ldots$) or the inverse of an integer ($p = 1, 1/2, 1/3, \ldots$). For $p = 1$, we have

$$e^{jx} = \cos x + j \sin x.$$

Using our previous definitions, we have (where x and y are real quantities)

$$(e^{jx})^* = e^{-jx} = \cos x - j \sin x$$

$$e^{jx}e^{jy} = e^{j(x+y)} = \cos (x + y) + j \sin (x + y)$$

$$\frac{e^{jx}}{e^{jy}} = e^{j(x-y)} = \cos (x - y) + j \sin (x - y)$$

$$e^{jx} + e^{jy} = \cos x + \cos y + j \sin x + j \sin y$$

$$|e^{jx}| = |e^{jx}e^{-jx}|^{\frac{1}{2}} = 1.$$

Thus, the representation of a complex quantity as an *exponential function* is very useful when complex numbers must be multiplied or divided.

Using polar coordinates, we can also write the complex quantity α as

$$\alpha = re^{j\theta}$$

where r and θ are real quantities. How are r and θ related to our previous representation $\alpha = a + jb$ with a and b both real?

$$\alpha = a + jb = re^{j\theta} = r(\cos \theta + j \sin \theta);$$

$$\alpha^* = a - jb = re^{-j\theta} = r(\cos \theta - j \sin \theta).$$

Therefore, $|\alpha| = (a^2 + b^2)^{\frac{1}{2}} = r$;

$$a = r \cos \theta,$$

$$b = r \sin \theta.$$

Combining the last two expressions, we obtain

$$\tan \theta = \frac{b}{a} \quad \text{or} \quad \theta = \tan^{-1} (b/a).$$

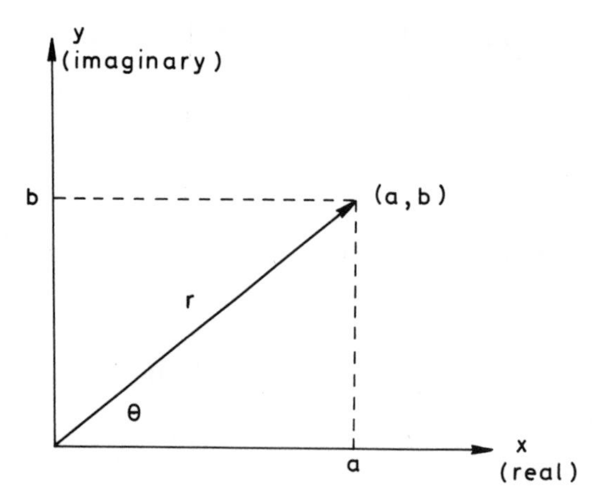

Figure 1.A1
The relationship between a complex quantity and a two-dimensional vector.

Hence r is the *magnitude* of the complex quantity, and θ is called the *phase* of the complex quantity.

Complex quantities are two-component numbers just like a vector that represents the position of a point in a plane. Consider the location of the point (a, b) in Figure 1.A1; it is a distance r from the origin and makes an angle θ with the x-axis. Suppose we called the x-axis the real axis and the y-axis the imaginary axis. Then the location z of the point (a, b) could be written as

$$z = a + jb,$$

meaning that to reach z we must go a distance a in the x-direction and then a distance b in the y-direction. The location of point z can also be described by

$$z = re^{j\theta},$$

meaning to go a distance r at an angle θ to the x-axis (real axis) to reach the point z. From our previous discussions, it follows that these two descriptions are equivalent and that a two-dimensional vector has the same properties as a complex number.

Selected References

For a more complete description of the mechanisms giving rise to resistance, see:

Halliday, D., and R. Resnick. 1962. *Physics for Students of Science and Engineering*. New York: John Wiley & Sons, Chapter 30: Capacitance; Chapter 31: Resistance; and Chapter 36: Inductance.

For methods of solving differential equations see:

Spiegel, Murray R. 1967. *Applied Differential Equations*, second edition. Englewood Cliffs, N.J.: Prentice-Hall.

2 ACTIVE CIRCUIT ELEMENTS

B. W. Maxfield

In Chapter 1, a number of circuit elements with voltage and current independent characteristics were discussed. This chapter describes a set of circuit elements in which even the ideal characteristics depend upon the applied voltages and/or currents. These are called *active elements*, and circuits incorporating them are referred to as *active circuits* or *active networks*.

2.1 Semiconductors

With the important exception of one element (a type of field-effect transistor), all the active elements that are used in this book depend upon specific properties of one or more *pn* junctions. Properties of these junctions are described in Section 2.2, and later sections describe the use of these junctions. Vacuum tubes, another type of active element, have been omitted from discussions in this book, because, for all applications of interest here, vacuum tubes have been superceded completely by various semiconductor circuit elements. A description of the *pn* junction helps in understanding the operation of most active elements. The particular limitations and nonideal characteristics inherent in each active element follow directly from the properties of the *pn* junction. Prior to a discussion of *pn* junctions and related active elements, however, it is necessary to describe some of the properties of semiconductors, the materials that are used to fabricate these junctions.

In isolated atoms, it is well known that the electrons around the nucleus exist in discrete energy levels. In a solid, the atoms are very close together; the outer

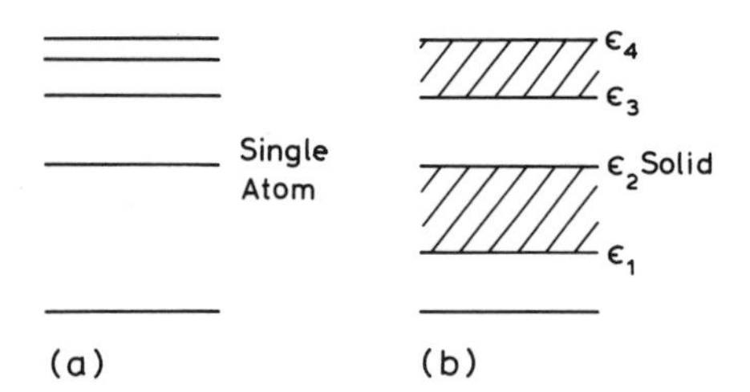

Figure 2.1
(a) Possible energy levels of single atoms; many narrow levels.
(b) Possible energy levels in a solid; continuous bands separated by forbidden regions.

electrons of one atom are influenced strongly by the presence of the outer electrons of neighboring atoms (that is, they interact strongly with them). This strong interaction alters dramatically the energy level structure; the many discrete atomic energy levels in the gas become a few bands in the solid. The different energy level diagrams of an isolated atom (such as in a gas) and a solid are illustrated in Figure 2.1.

In a solid there may exist electrons having a continuous range of energies between ϵ_1 and ϵ_2 and between ϵ_3 and ϵ_4, but no electrons may have energies between ϵ_2 and ϵ_3. These bands are *available* for electrons, but they need not be filled or even partially filled. In a perfect solid at low temperatures, the number of electrons in each band depends only upon the number of valence electrons. As will be shown later, both a finite temperature and the presence of impurity atoms can modify these energy bands in a very important way.

Since empty bands have no electrons, they cannot give rise to an electrical current. Full bands also cannot produce an electrical current, because there is no available energy state into which the more energetic electron in a full band may move. (Recall that an electron will gain energy when accelerated by an applied electric field.)

For our purposes, electrical conduction in a crystalline solid can be described in terms of two bands, a lower energy or *valence band* and a higher energy or *conduction band* as shown in Figure 2.2a. These bands are separated by an energy gap E_g. A semiconductor is a material that, in the pure single-crystal form at absolute zero, has a full valence band and empty conduction band such as shown in Figure 2.2b. At finite temperatures, an electron can be thermally excited from the valence band into the conduction band. If T is the absolute temperature, the probability of any electron being thermally excited into the conduction band depends exponentially on E_g/kT; namely,

$$P_{ex} = P_0 \exp(-E_g/kT). \tag{2.1}$$

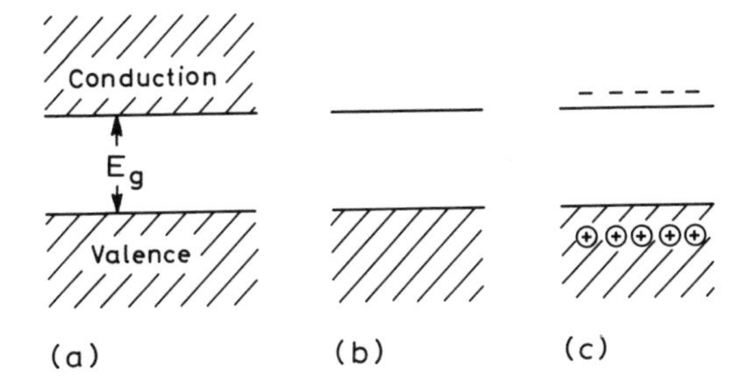

Figure 2.2
(a) General two-band representation of a crystalline solid.
(b) Energy band diagram for a pure semiconductor at absolute zero, and
(c) for a pure semiconductor at a finite temperature, say, room temperature.

At room temperature, the thermal energy kT is about 0.025 eV. For a semiconductor, E_g is typically about 1 eV; therefore, $P \sim e^{-40} \sim 10^{-17}$. In practice, this thermal excitation results in a resistivity the order of one ohm-meter (1 Ω-m). This should be compared with 10^{-8} Ω-m for metals and greater than 10^{+10} Ω-m for insulators; hence the name semiconductor.

Figure 2.2c illustrates the small number of electrons that are thermally excited into the conduction band at a finite temperature. These electrons are free to move when an electric field is applied. The empty states, or holes, left behind when the electrons leave the valence band are also free to move in an applied electric field; hence they also contribute to electrical conduction. Thermal excitation produces an equal number of holes and electrons. Such a pure semiconductor is termed intrinsic. Pure germanium and silicon are examples of intrinsic semiconductors.

The conduction properties of a semiconductor are changed markedly if a few impurity atoms are substituted for some of the material (host) atoms. This is not normally true for a metal. Consider for instance a small amount of a valence-five impurity (for example, phosphorus) uniformly distributed throughout a single crystal of silicon (the silicon atom has four valence electrons). Because of the impurities, the energy bands are a little more complex. Four of the valence electrons on each impurity atom essentially replace the four "lost" silicon valence electrons. This forms a full valence band (neglecting a small amount of thermal excitation across E_g). The extra electron on the impurity goes into a narrow band that forms just below the conduction band. This impurity band is easily depleted by thermal activation; therefore these impurity band electrons end up in the conduction band. For this reason the impurity band is called a *donor level*. Therefore, the addition of higher valence impurity atoms to a host places electrons in the conduction band without the simultaneous addition of holes to the valence band. The addition of

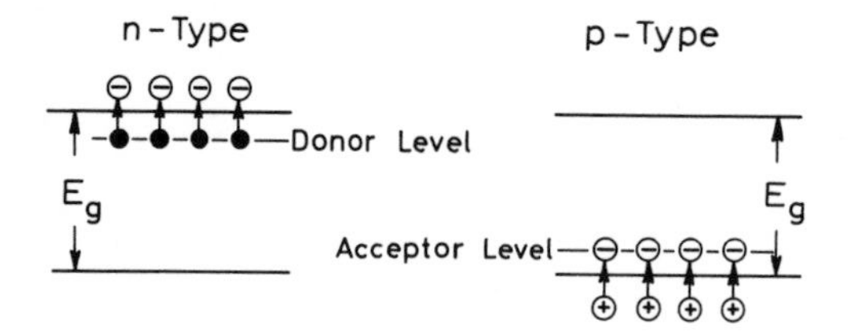

Figure 2.3
Donor and acceptor levels that result from doping with *n*-type and *p*-type impurities, respectively. Thermal excitation at room temperature readily depopulates the donor level and populates the acceptor level to create electrons in the conduction band or holes in the valence band. The arrows show the result of thermal excitation.

impurities, known as *doping*, produces an extrinsic semiconductor. Doping with higher valence or donor impurities gives an *n*-type semiconductor, so called because the charge carriers added by doping are negative.

If a valence-three impurity (for example, indium) is added to silicon, there are not enough electrons to fill the valence band. The holes that result can contribute to an electrical current. In fact, the behavior is not quite this simple. The impurities create an additional narrow energy band called an *acceptor level* that lies just above the valence band. At room temperature, thermal excitation from the valence band completely fills the acceptor level. This leaves holes in the valence band without producing electrons in the conduction band. Doping with lower valence or acceptor impurities produces a *p*-type semiconductor, so called because the charges induced by doping are positive. The thermal population of the acceptor level and depopulation of the donor level is illustrated in Figure 2.3.

2.2 The *pn* Junction

The transition from a *p*-type region to a *n*-type region (each created by doping) in the same semiconductor single crystal (that is, both *p* and *n* regions are in the same host) is called a *pn* junction. At this junction, some electrons from the *n* region are attracted into the *p* region, and some holes in the *p* region are attracted into the *n* region. The electron and hole currents that result are very similar; it is only necessary to describe one of these currents in detail. The electron currents are described below.

Both the *n* and *p* regions are extrinsic; the electron density in the *n* region is much greater (because it is due to doping) than the electron density in the *p* region (which is due to thermal effects). Attraction of electrons into the *p* region and holes into the *n* region results in two regions of opposite charge separated by a small distance; this means that a potential difference is set up across the junction.

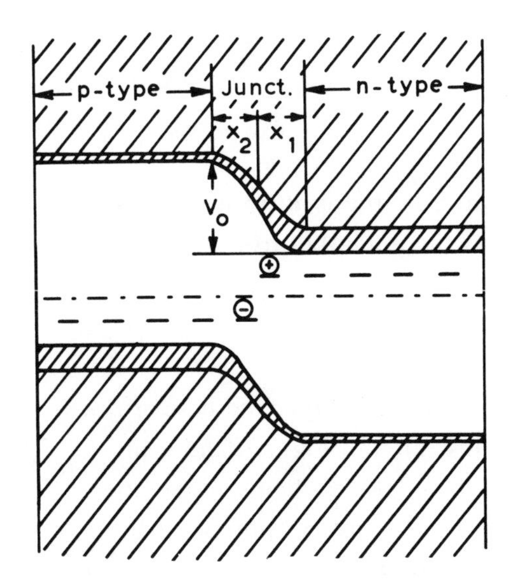

Figure 2.4
Energy band model for a *pn* junction (from *Basic Electronics for Scientists*, by James J. Brophy. Copyright 1966 by McGraw-Hill, Inc. Used with permission of McGraw-Hill Book Co.).

These characteristics of a *pn* junction are all described by the energy band model of a *pn* junction shown in Figure 2.4. The magnitudes of the quantities V_0, I_1, and I_2 are determined primarily by the host material, doping level and the temperature. In equilibrium (steady state), this potential difference is such that no net current flows across the junction. The small flow of electrons into the *p* region is just balanced by the small flow of holes from the *p* region into the *n* region.

As shown in Figure 2.4, the junction is divided into two parts, one of width x_1 that lies in what was originally the *n* region and other of width x_2 that is in the original *p* region. Here, N_a and N_d are respectively, the acceptor and donor doping levels. Since the semiconductor must remain uncharged, it is necessary to have the total negative charge in the *p* region equal to the total positive charge in the *n* region; this gives $x_1 N_d = x_2 N_a$. By solving Poisson's equation in the junction, it is possible to determine the potential distribution in each region as well as the junction width $d = x_1 + x_2$. In terms of fundamental and controllable parameters, we obtain

$$d = \left[\frac{2K_e\epsilon_0 V_0}{e(N_a + N_d)}\right]^{\frac{1}{2}}\left[\left(\frac{N_a}{N_d}\right)^{\frac{1}{2}} + \left(\frac{N_d}{N_a}\right)^{\frac{1}{2}}\right] \tag{2.2}$$

where $K_e\epsilon_0$ is the dielectric constant of the host material and other quantities are as defined previously. Normally, one impurity concentration is chosen to be much greater than the other. Therefore, if $N_a \ll N_d$, then

$$d = \left[\frac{2K_e\epsilon_0 V_0}{eN_a}\right]^{\frac{1}{2}}; \tag{2.3}$$

that is, the junction width is determined primarily by the *smaller* impurity concentration, in this case N_a. It can be shown that the potential drop V_0 is confined almost completely to the region of width d.

2.3 Biasing a *pn* Junction

A potential difference may be applied to a *pn* junction to either increase or decrease the intrinsic junction potential V_0. As illustrated in Figure 2.5a, if the *p* region is made slightly positive with respect to the *n* region, then the potential drop across the junction decreases. Under such conditions, the junction conducts more easily. A voltage that increases the conduction of current is called a *forward bias*. With increasing forward bias, the junction resistance defined by $R = V/I$ actually decreases, so the *pn* junction does not obey Ohm's law. When the *p* region is made slightly negative with respect to the *n* region, the potential drop across the junction increases. A junction that conducts less easily is said to be *reverse biased*. The resistance of a reverse biased junction increases as the voltage drop across the junction increases. Possible uses of such a strongly voltage-dependent resistance will be investigated in Sections 2.4, 2.5, and 2.6. First, let us obtain a slightly more quantitative description of current flow in a *pn* junction.

Because of the smaller potential barrier in the forward biased junction shown in Figure 2.5b, there is an increased flow of electrons from the *n* region into the

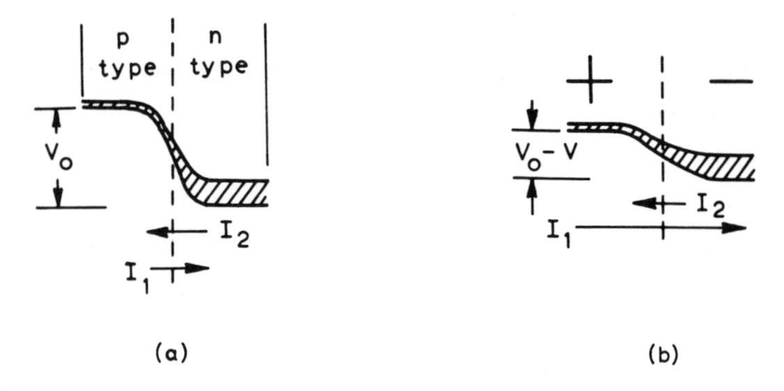

Figure 2.5
Simple energy band diagram of a *pn* junction:
(a) an unbiased junction where $I_1 = -I_2$, and
(b) a junction forward biased by potential V (from *Basic Electronics for Scientists*, by James J. Brophy. Copyright 1966 by McGraw-Hill, Inc. Used with permission of McGraw-Hill Book Co.).

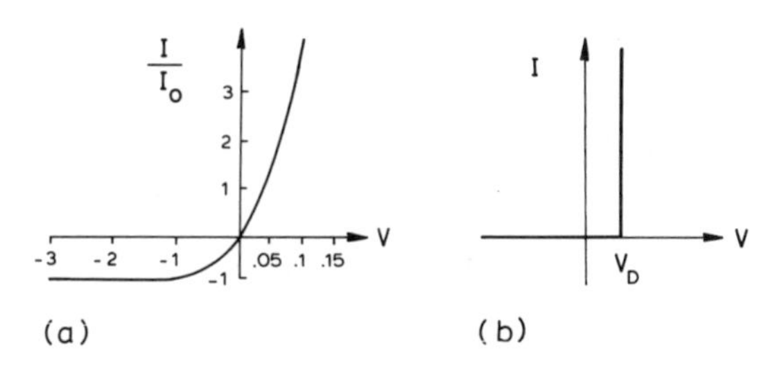

Figure 2.6
(a) Graphical representation of the diode equation (note the expanded voltage scale for reverse bias).
(b) One approximation to the real diode characteristics; the diode is a voltage-dependent switch that is on for voltages greater than V_D. ($V_D \simeq 0.3$ V for germanium diodes and $V_D \simeq 0.6$ V for silicon diodes.)

p region. The current I_1 in Figure 2.5b represents the increased electron flow from *n* to *p*, because, by convention, current flow is opposite in direction to electron flow. The electron flow from the *p* region into the *n* region is not affected appreciably by the forward bias; therefore, the total current will be determined by thermal activation across the potential barrier $V_0 - V$, where V is the forward bias voltage. This same forward bias will also increase the flow of holes from the *p* region valence band to the *n* region valence band.

The total current flow through the junction, of course, consists of both electron and hole contributions. The magnitude of each contribution depends upon the doping densities (number of impurities per cm^3) in the *n* and *p* regions, respectively. A complete analysis shows that the total current through the junction is given by

$$I = I_0[\exp(eV/kT) - 1], \tag{2.4}$$

where

$$I_0 = C(n, p) \exp(eV_0/kT), \tag{2.5}$$

and $C(n, p)$ is a constant that depends upon the host material, the type, and density of the *n* and *p* impurities, and the junction area. The constant V_0 is a property of the host material; for germanium $V_0 = 26$ mV and for silicon $V_0 = 50$ mV. Equation 2.4 is called the diode equation or rectifier equation; notice that the current depends strongly upon the sign of the bias potential V. Figure 2.6a shows the behavior of Equation 2.4 for $V_0 = 50$ mV. A reasonable approximation to this behavior is given in Figure 2.6b, that is, a *pn* junction can sometimes be approximated by a strongly voltage-dependent resistor having zero resistance for forward bias and infinite resistance for reverse bias.

There is an upper limit to the amount of reverse bias that can be applied to any *pn* junction. When the electric field exceeds some critical value, the host material will arc or break down. Under breakdown conditions, the *pn* junction conducts very well. Often the large current that accompanies reverse bias breakdown causes severe heating and permanently damages the junction. Junction active elements have specified voltages above which breakdown is likely to occur. If these breakdown voltages are exceeded, the active element will usually fail or burn out. Most junction active elements also have a maximum current rating for operation in the forward bias mode. Excessive forward bias current also damages an element through excessive heating.

2.4 Diodes

The simplest active element designed to make use of the strong polarity dependence of a *pn* junction is the diode. A general-purpose diode is represented by the symbol in Figure 2.7. The *I-V* characteristics of this element are shown in Figure 2.6a and are given by the diode equation, Equation 2.4. With large reverse bias, the diode current $-I_0$ is essentially voltage independent. Therefore, I_0 is called the saturation current or reverse bias leakage current. For germanium, V_0 is smaller than for silicon ($V_0 = 26$ mV for Ge and $V_0 = 50$ mV for Si), and therefore leakage currents are larger in germanium diodes. The reverse bias current often represents nonideal behavior (not a perfect switch) in a diode (and, in fact, in many *pn* junction devices). It is frequently necessary to use diodes that have very small leakage currents. Silicon diodes can have I_0 as small as 10^{-10} A $= 0.1$ nA and germanium diodes as small as 10^{-6} A $= 1$ μA at room temperature. Silicon diodes can sometimes be operated with junction temperatures as high as 200°C, while germanium diodes are limited to about 100°C. Diodes are rated according to a maximum permissible reverse bias (peak inverse voltage PIV), maximum power dissipation within the diode P_{max}, and a maximum current through the diode I_{max}. Most diodes are destroyed rapidly if the PIV rating is exceeded; this is especially true if the diode is working near the maximum rated power or current (and is therefore hot). Exceptions to this are the Zener diode and thyristor; both of these devices are designed to operate stably under reverse bias breakdown conditions.

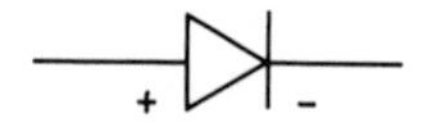

Figure 2.7
The symbol used to represent a conventional diode. Current flow in the conventional sense is from the anode (+) to the cathode (−). A diode is often referred to as a rectifier. These are discussed in more detail in Chapter 11.

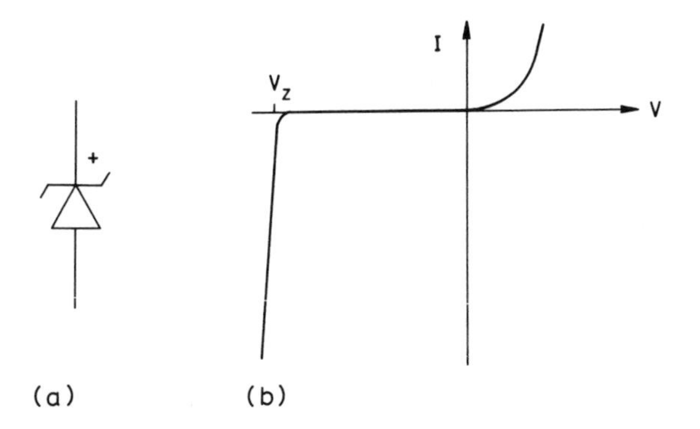

Figure 2.8
(a) The standard symbol for a Zener diode, and
(b) the *I-V* characteristics of a typical Zener diode.

From Equations 2.4 and 2.5 it follows that the current through a diode depends upon the carrier concentration in both the n and p regions. There are means other than doping that can be used to change the carrier concentration. One very useful method is through optical excitation; light incident upon the junction can increase the carrier concentration in one or both regions. A *photodiode* is a *pn* junction device that is designed to exploit this feature. Normally a photodiode is operated under reverse bias conditions where the current is essentially independent of the applied voltage. Photodiodes are used in some circuits in succeeding chapters.

A *Zener diode* is a *pn* junction that is designed to operate stably under reverse bias breakdown conditions. The diode is constructed so that breakdown always occurs at the same voltage V_Z. This voltage is almost independent of the current through the diode. Since the diode resistance is very small under breakdown conditions, a series current limiting resistance must always be used. The standard symbol and a typical *I-V* characteristic for a Zener diode are shown in Figure 2.8.

Zener diodes are specified according to breakdown voltage and maximum power dissipation P_M. General purpose Zener diodes are available with breakdown voltages ranging from 1.8 to 200 V and power ratings of 50 W or lower (the maximum current is $I_M = P_M/V_Z$). Normally, V_Z will change by less than 1% for operation at a nearly constant temperature within the recommended power range and less than 10% for operation within the specified temperature range.

2.5 Transistors

Transistors of various types comprise another very large class of active elements. All of these elements permit some small input signal (current or voltage) to control a larger output signal that is in some way related to the input. Transistors fall into two distinct groups: the *field-effect* or unipolar transistor (FET) in which a *voltage* controls the current that flows through the transistor, and the *junction* or bipolar transistor where an input *current* controls the current through the transistor. Often these latter units are just called transistors. Each of these two main types of transistors can be subdivided further into smaller groups. All of these devices have their particular merits. The remaining sections of this chapter discuss some of the more general transistor characteristics as well as some of the specific applications and limitations of some common types of transistors.

2.5.1 The Field-Effect Transistor (FET)

Figure 2.9 is a pictorial representation of one variety of field-effect transistor. The gate G and channel C are insulated electrically to form essentially a parallel-plate capacitor. A voltage applied to the gate induces charge of the opposite sign in the lightly doped channel region. Depending upon the type of doping (n or p) and the sign of the gate voltage, the net charge density in the channel region is either increased (enhanced) or decreased (depleted). Under some gate voltage bias conditions, it is possible for a current to flow in the transistor when a voltage is applied between the source S and drain D terminals. When a current flows, its magnitude is determined by the charge density in the channel region and therefore by the gate potential. Hence it is possible for the charge on the gate to control the current that flows through the transistor, that is, the drain current.

A more quantitative description of a field-effect transistor can be obtained by considering the circuit given in Figure 2.10. An FET having highly n-doped source and drain regions and a lightly p-doped channel is connected to external drain and gate voltage sources having polarities as indicated in Figure 2.10. For zero gate-to-source potential ($V_{GS} = 0$), the drain-channel pn junction is reverse biased. As the drain-to-source potential V_{DS} is increased, the drain current I_D decreases rapidly to zero (actually to the reverse bias leakage current). First, let us take the potential V_{DS} to be at a constant on the order of 10 V and investigate the behavior of I_D when V_{GS} is increased from zero. The positive gate voltage induces negative charge in the p-type channel; this decreases the net charge density

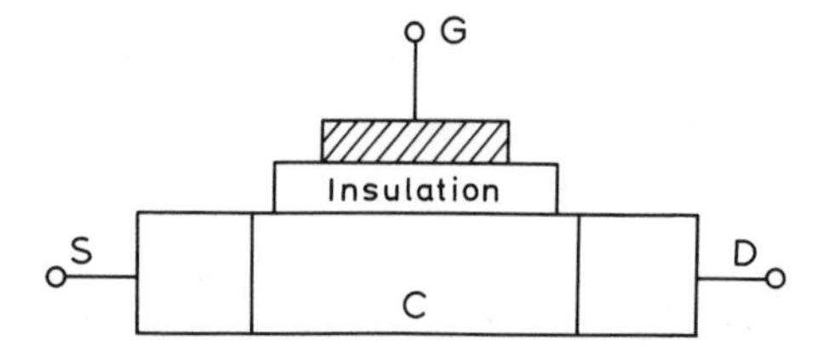

Figure 2.9
Pictorial representation of an FET.

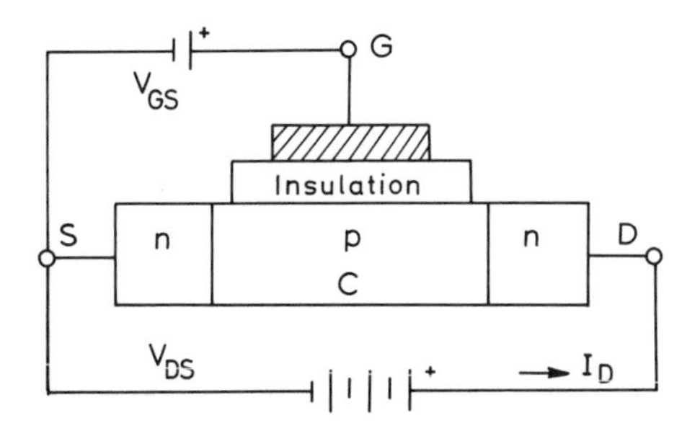

Figure 2.10
Gate and drain potentials connected to an FET having *n*-doped source and drain regions and a *p*-doped channel region.

in the channel. Eventually, the induced charge density will exceed the doping (hole) density and the channel will behave like an *n*-type region. When this happens, a *pn* junction no longer exists and drain current can flow. The transition from zero current to a large drain current is rapid but not discontinuous. A small gate voltage can be used to control the drain current. Moreover, a small change in gate voltage can produce a large change in drain current.

Next we take the gate potential to be constant and consider what happens when V_{DS} is increased from zero. Provided the gate is sufficiently positive, the induced charge turns the *p*-doped channel region into an *n* region. When this is the case, there is no drain-channel *pn* junction; for small V_{DS}, the drain current is proportional to V_{DS}. This means that for small V_{DS} an FET behaves like a resistor ($V_{DS} \propto I_D$) where the resistance (proportionality constant) is determined by the gate potential. As the current increases, however, the voltage drop within the channel becomes comparable to V_{GS}. Under these conditions, the charge on the channel side of the gate is not distributed uniformly. More charge accumulates at the low potential (source) end of the channel than at the drain end. The total charge in the channel remains constant, because it is determined by the fixed value of V_{GS}. Therefore, the drain end becomes depleted of charge. This decrease in the induced carrier density increases the channel resistance near the channel-drain junction. This resistance increases with the drain current, because the charge depletion increases with drain current. In a well designed and constructed FET, there is some point above which increasing V_{DS} causes only a very small increase in drain current. This effect is known as ***pinch-off***. The value of V_{DS} at which I_D becomes almost independent of V_{DS} is called the ***pinch-off voltage*** V_P. This results in the current-voltage characteristic shown in Figure 2.11. Above the pinch-off voltage, the drain current is nearly independent of V_{DS}. The rapid increase in I_D above V_{BR} is due to a type of breakdown effect within the channel region.

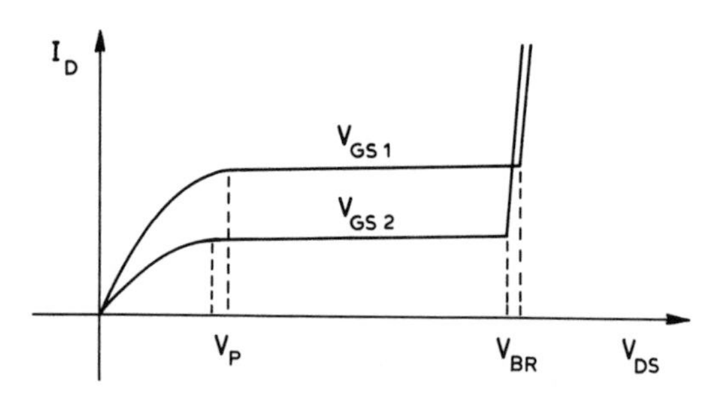

Figure 2.11
The general behavior of the current-voltage (I-V) characteristics of an FET for two gate potentials. Both the pinch-off and breakdown potentials are indicated.

The device just described is called an *n*-channel, enhancement mode field-effect transistor, because conduction in the channel is enhanced by inducing *n*-type charges (carriers). It is also possible to start with a lightly doped *n*-channel and achieve control of the drain current by *decreasing* conduction in the channel. This is done by inducing positive charge through a gate that is negative with respect to the source. Such a device is referred to as an *n*-channel depletion mode FET, because conduction is controlled by depleting *n*-type charges from the channel. From a knowledge of the basic properties of a *pn* junction, the enhancement mode FET is easier to understand than the depletion mode. For this reason, the operation of an enhancement mode FET was described. However, the operating principles of both enhancement and depletion types are very similar. In most important respects, a depletion mode FET behaves in exactly the same manner as an enhancement mode FET. The main circuit difference is that a negative gate potential is used to decrease conduction in a depletion mode FET instead of a positive potential being used to enhance conduction. For zero gate voltage, the drain current is essentially zero (the reverse bias leakage current) in an enhancement mode FET for all values of V_{DS}, whereas for $V_{GS} = 0$, the I_D is relatively large in a depletion mode FET. Characteristics such as those in Figure 2.11 are obtained for $V_{GS} = 0$ to a few volts negative for an *n*-channel depletion type and for V_{GS} between about $+2$ and $+6$ V for an *n*-channel enhancement type.

It is also possible to have *p*-channel enhancement and depletion mode types. They operate in exactly the same manner as the *n*-channel devices except that the polarity of both V_{GS} and V_{DS} are opposite to those used for the *n*-channel devices.

An electrically insulated gate electrode is not the only means of depleting the channel region. Under reverse bias conditions, charge is depleted from the junction region of a *pn* junction; the depletion region is of thickness *d*, where *d* is given

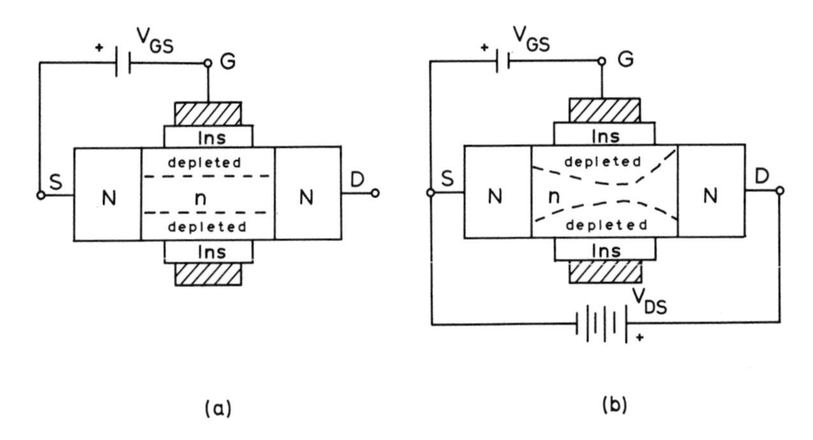

Figure 2.12
(a) An *n*-channel, depletion mode MOSFET biased with a gate potential, and
(b) the charge distribution when V_{GS} and V_{DS} give operation in the pinch-off region.

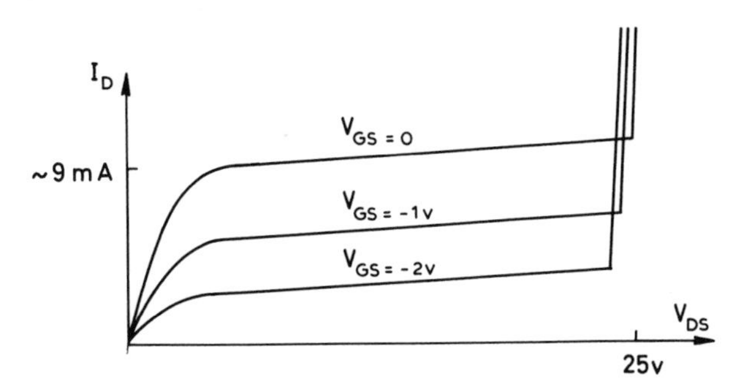

Figure 2.13
The *I-V* characteristics of an *n*-channel depletion mode MOSFET, the MPF 122.

by Equation 2.2. A junction restricts current flow in the channel in much the same manner as described above. A more extensive discussion of these junction field-effect transistors (JFETs) is included at the end of this section.

Field-effect transistors that have an insulating layer between the gate and the channel are called insulated gate FETs (IGFETs). Since the layered structure is a metal-oxide-semiconductor sandwich, these are also referred to as MOSFETs. Figure 2.12a is a pictorial representation of the structure of an *n*-channel, depletion mode MOSFET with moderate gate voltage (say $V_{GS} = -2$ V) and $V_{DS} = 0$, while Figure 2.12b shows the charge distribution within the channel region for a value of V_{GS} and V_{DS} such that operation is above the pinch-off voltage. A typical set of *I-V* characteristics for such a device is shown in Figure 2.13.

The drain characteristics shown in Figure 2.13 are also known as the *output characteristics*, because they represent relationships between the output current and

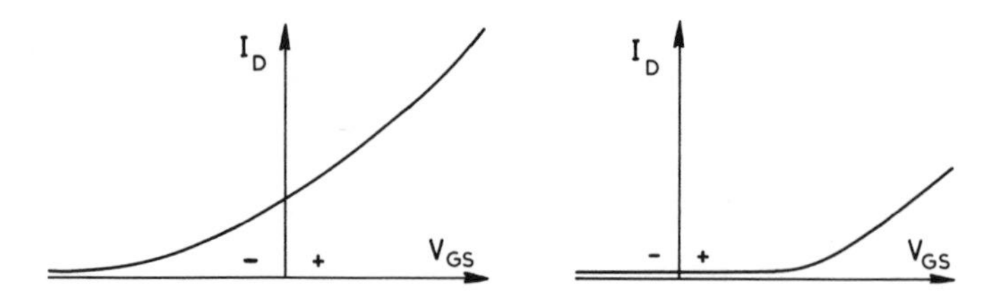

Figure 2.14
The transfer characteristics for an MPF 122 depletion mode MOSFET (left) and a 3N 172 enhancement mode MOSFET (right).

Figure 2.15
Pictorial representation of a JFET.

output voltage. Another set of parameters, the transfer characteristics, relate the input signal (gate voltage) to the output signal (drain current). Figure 2.14 shows the transfer characteristics of the MPF 122 depletion mode MOSFET and the 3N172 enhancement mode MOSFET over the useful range of gate voltages and drain currents. Each transistor has a set of maximum voltage differences that are permitted between various parts of the transistor. Exceeding these rated values will normally destroy the device.

The insulated gate FET uses an electric field in the capacitorlike region between the gate and channel to control the number of available charge carriers in the channel. The depletion layer in the vicinity of a reverse biased *pn* junction can also be used to control conduction in the channel. A pictorial representation of a junction field-effect transistor (JFET) is shown in Figure 2.15. The nomenclature is the same as that used in discussing MOSFETs. In this *n*-channel device, the channel is a rather lightly doped *n* region (of doping density N_d). A heavily doped *p* region (of doping density N_a) forms the gate terminal. Since the *p* region is highly doped, most of the depletion around the *pn* junction occurs in the channel region. As the gate *pn* junction reverse bias voltage is increased, the depletion region extends deeper and deeper into the channel. A sufficiently large depletion region (that is, a sufficiently large reverse bias) can cut off current flow completely. From Equation 2.3 it follows that the depletion layer has a thickness given by

$$d = \left[\frac{2\epsilon_0 K_e}{eN_d}(V + V_0)\right]^{\frac{1}{2}} \tag{2.6}$$

where V is the inverse bias and $N_d \ll N_a$. Thus, at a constant V_{DS}, the transfer characteristic (drain current as a function of gate-to-source voltage difference) is shown in Figure 2.16. Increasing the gate reverse bias decreases the drain current until the channel is pinched off completely. Because a reverse biased *pn* junction is used, the junction FET can be used for only one polarity of gate potential. The input current (gate current) is very small because of the reverse biased *pn* junction. Hence the input impedance (gate voltage divided by gate current) is very high.

The amount of reverse bias on the gate junction (at constant V_{GS}) increases with increasing drain current. Because of the channel resistance, the reverse bias is not uniform within the channel region. As shown in Figure 2.17, the reverse bias is greatest at the drain end of the channel. This pinches off current flow through the channel in much the same manner as occurred in MOSFETs. Well designed and constructed JFETs have output characteristics similar to those of the depletion mode MOSFET shown in Figure 2.13. The only major difference is the different dependence of V_P on V_{GS}. For small drain current, V_{DS} is proportional to I_D, that is, the channel behaves as a simple resistor. The magnitude of the resistance depends upon V_{GS}.

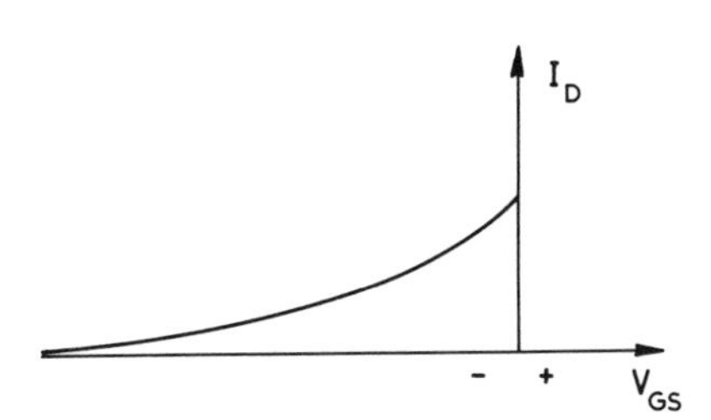

Figure 2.16
Transfer characteristics of an *n*-channel JFET; note that a JFET cannot be operated with a forward bias.

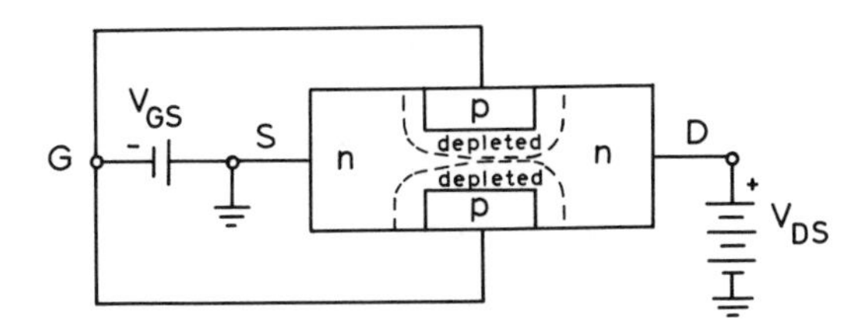

Figure 2.17
Pictorial illustration of drain current pinch-off in an *n*-channel JFET.

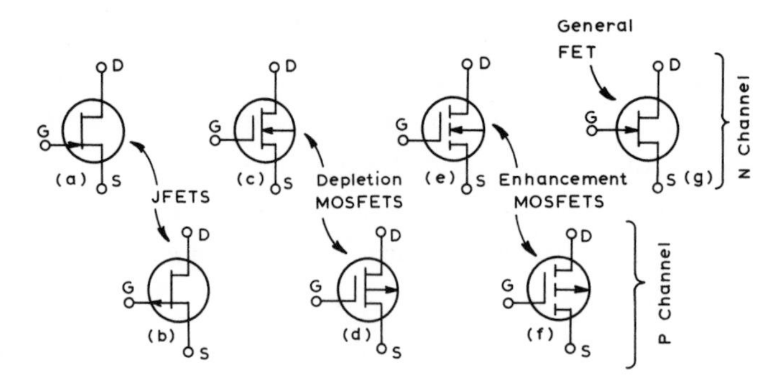

Figure 2.18
FET symbols.

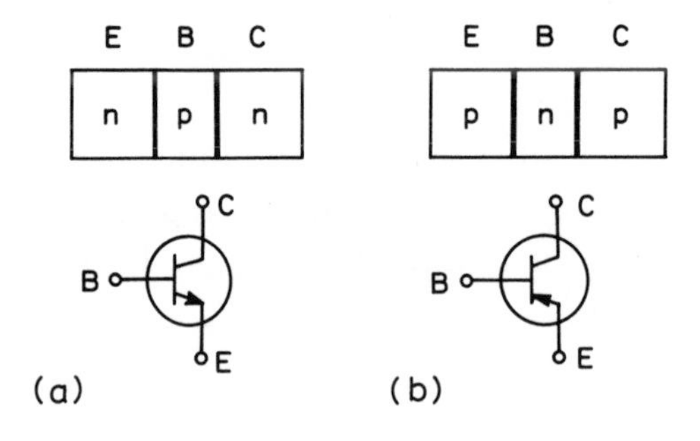

Figure 2.19
Pictorial and symbolic representation of (a) *npn*, and (b) *pnp* transistors. The heavy lines represent *pn* junctions.

Symbols that are commonly used to indicate the various types of FETs are given in Figure 2.18.

2.5.2 The Junction Transistor

The junction transistor is an active element consisting of two *pn* junctions that are separated by a narrow region called the base B. The two possible combinations, *pnp* and *npn*, are shown in Figure 2.19 along with the standard symbolic representation of each type. One can obtain *npn* and *pnp* transistors using either silicon or germanium as a host material.

For discussion purposes, we will consider a *pnp* transistor. Referring to Figure 2.19b, we see that holes from the left or emitter region E are forced to enter (injected into) the narrow base region. This is accomplished by forward biasing the emitter-base junction. The current through the junction is a strong function of the emitter-base voltage difference V_{BE}. This forward bias gives a sensitive means of

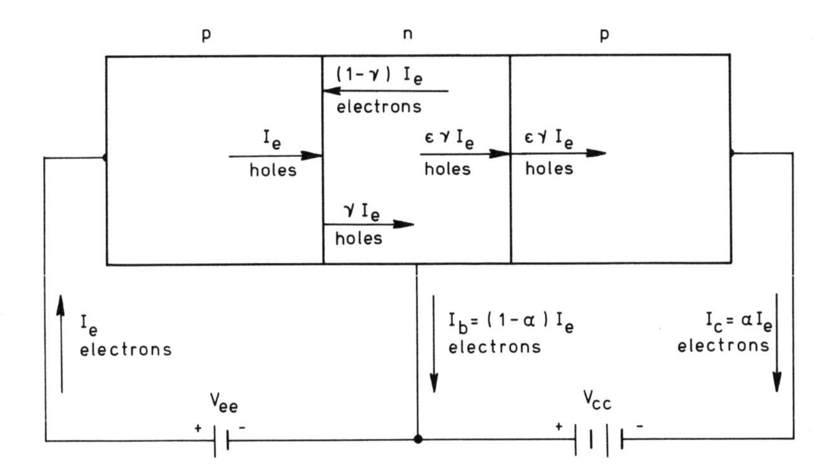

Figure 2.20
The bias voltage and resulting current flow in a *pnp* transistor (from *Basic Electronics for Scientists*, by James J. Brophy. Copyright 1966 by McGraw-Hill, Inc. Used with permission of McGraw-Hill Book Co.).

controlling the current flow across the first junction. How, in a practical circuit, can this control feature be utilized? If the second junction is reverse biased, then holes cannot flow from the right-hand region (collector C) into the base. However, it is very easy for holes to flow in the opposite direction, that is, from the base into the collector. A very narrow base region will permit nearly all the holes that leave the emitter to cross the base and thus to enter the collector. Therefore, the forward bias voltage V_{BE} makes it possible to control the current through this two-junction active element. Holes injected from the emitter into a sufficiently narrow base region are picked up by the collector.

Doping levels in the emitter, base, and collector regions are chosen to minimize numerous undesirable effects. The emitter is quite highly doped to provide the necessary hole current, while the base is both thin and lightly doped so that it is unlikely for a hole to encounter an electron and therefore combine with it (recombination effects). The collector region is doped simply to keep the resistance down and therefore prevent needless power loss. Also, if the emitter region has a high resistance, the ohmic resistance in this region and not the exponential thermal activation effect will determine the hole current at large currents.

Figure 2.20 illustrates one possible biasing arrangement for a *pnp* transistor. The emitter region is positive with respect to the base, and the collector is negative with respect to the base. This ensures the proper combination of a forward biased BE junction and a reverse biased BC junction. Energy band diagrams corresponding to zero bias and forward bias conditions are shown in Figure 2.21.

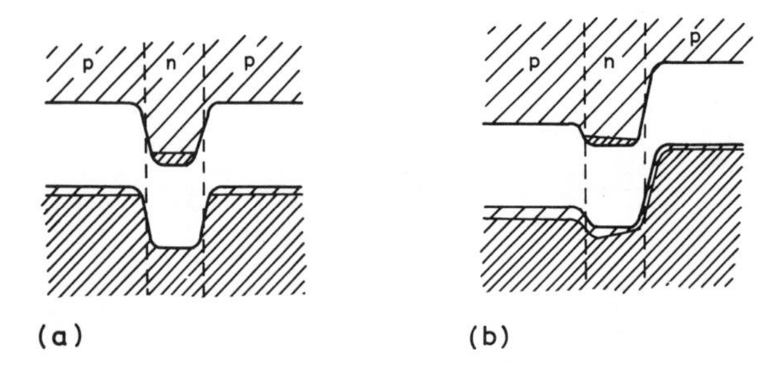

Figure 2.21
A simplified energy band diagram for a silicon *pnp* transistor (a) for zero bias, and (b) for a base-emitter forward bias (from *Basic Electronics for Scientists*, by James J. Brophy. Copyright 1966 by McGraw-Hill, Inc. Used with permission of McGraw-Hill Book Co.).

The emitter current I_e is supplied by the voltage source V_{BE}. The current flowing across the emitter-base junction consists of both holes going into the base and electrons flowing from the base into the emitter region. Only that fraction γ, which is a hole current, has any chance of getting into the collector region. The electron current flowing from the base region into the emitter region $(1 - \gamma)I_e$ is waste for our purposes. Light doping of the base region minimizes this electron current. Some doping, however, is necessary in order to keep the resistance sufficiently low. A fraction $(1 - \epsilon)$ of the holes entering into the base region are lost through recombination processes. Therefore, only a fraction $\alpha = \epsilon\gamma$ of the original emitter current is eventually collected by the collector. In practice α ranges from 0.9 in power transistors to greater than 0.997 in small-signal, low-power transistors.

The injected current of holes is given by the diode equation (Equation 2.4). The holes injected into the base region diffuse across the base to the base-collector junction. In the base region, holes can combine with electrons and hence be removed from the hole current. Therefore, the base region must be very narrow if recombination effects are to be kept at a minimum. Fewer holes reach the right (*BC*) junction than enter at the left (*BE* junction). However, once a hole reaches the base-collector junction, it is accelerated into the collector by the electric field in the *BC* junction. This two-junction element permits controlled injection of carriers (minority) across the base region where most of them are collected by a suitably large potential.

A current must flow in the base-emitter circuit if the forward bias voltage on the base-emitter junction is to be maintained. (Charge build-up in the base region would decrease the amount of forward bias.) For this reason a junction transistor is basically a current-operated active element. Referring to Figure 2.20, we can see that

$$I_b + I_c = I_e. \tag{2.7}$$

From previous arguments, we have $I_c = \alpha I_e$ so that Equation 2.7 becomes

$$I_b = \left(\frac{1}{\alpha} - 1\right) I_c = I_c/\beta. \tag{2.8}$$

This is the control current necessary to operate the junction transistor; a base current I_b produces a collector current β times as large. Typical values of β range from 10 in power transistors to as much as 500 in high-gain, low-power transistors. The emitter-base circuit has a small resistance because of the forward biased emitter-base junction. Hence the power loss in this circuit is small. Holes from the emitter region are shot across to the collector region that they can enter easily. The base-collector circuit has a high resistance because of the reverse biased base-collector junction. The collector current, therefore, comes from a source of high internal resistance. The combination of low input resistance and high output resistance means that a large power gain can be achieved rather easily. The collector circuit behaves very much like a constant current source (that is, I_c is nearly independent of V_{BC}). The collector characteristics (collector current as a function of collector-emitter voltage) for a 2N3904 transistor are shown in Figures 2.22 and 2.23. The constant-current behavior that is characteristic of transistors is very clear at small base currents.

The transfer characteristic for a junction transistor is the collector current (output) as a function of the base current (input). At very small base currents, the collector current is determined by the reverse leakage current through the collector-base junction. For base currents well above the collector leakage current, I_{CO},

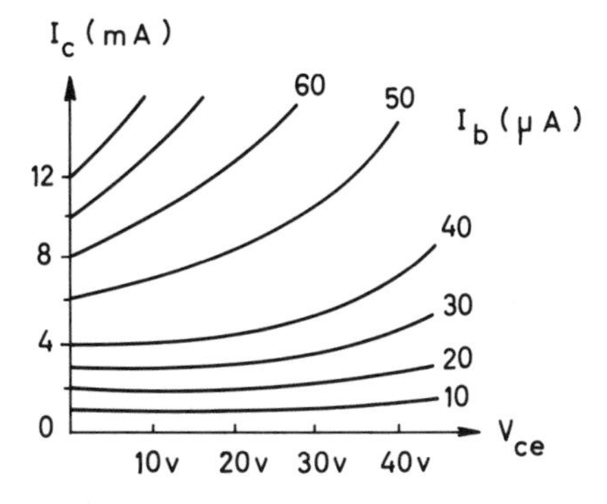

Figure 2.22

A complete set of collector characteristics for the 2N3904 *pnp* silicon transistor. Only for base currents below about 30 μA is β a constant independent of I_C.

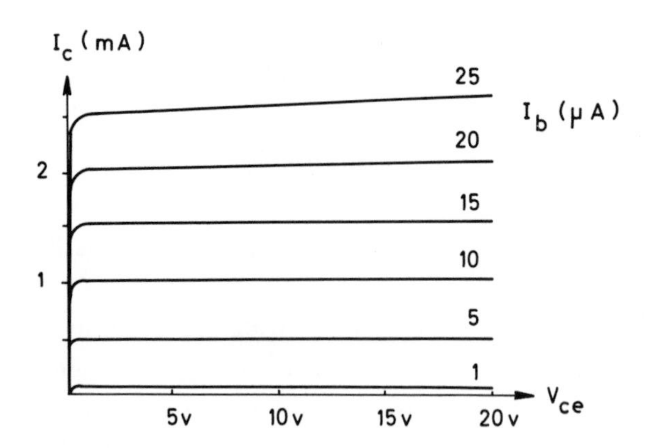

Figure 2.23
Collector characteristics for the 2N3904 transistor at small base current where it is normally used.

there is a large linear region where the collector current is proportional to the base current. Above this linear region, β depends upon I_C. At very large collector currents, there is severe heating. The collector current may also be limited by the static resistance in the emitter region. These features are evident in the collector characteristics given in Figures 2.22 and 2.23. With the exception that an electron current is injected across the base region, the previous discussion follows through for the *npn* transistor if the polarities of V_{BE} and V_{BC} are simply reversed. There are only minor differences between *pnp* and *npn* transistors.

Optical excitation can be used to generate a base current; that is, light energy incident upon the base region can create carriers of the appropriate sign that in turn give rise to a base current. In most transistors, the base region is protected from exposure to light by encapsulation. However, in phototransistors, the base can be exposed to light. In some such devices, there is a base lead that can be used for added control purposes, and in others, external connection is provided to only the emitter and collector. Some uses of phototransistors are described in later chapters.

2.5.3 Some Transistor Circuits

We will now direct our attention to some circuits in which transistors are used. No attempt is made to describe how the following circuit designs are derived. Readers interested in these aspects of electronics should consult the references at the end of this chapter.

There are three basic transistor amplifier configurations. Each has its own set of advantages and disadvantages. In the remainder of this section the distinguishing characteristics of each are described.

The Common-Source and Common-Emitter Amplifiers

A common-source (CS) or common-emitter (CE) amplifier is one where the source (in an FET circuit) or the emitter (in a junction transistor circuit) is common to both the input and output signals. Many different circuit configurations for CS and CE amplifiers are possible; one widely used version of each is shown in Figure 2.24. For the CE circuit in Figure 2.24a, resistors R_1 and R_2 supply the necessary forward bias on the base-emitter junction. The small emitter resistance R_E is not always necessary but its presence does provide improved dc stability. Without R_E, the emitter is grounded and hence is common to both the input and output signals. The collector current is controlled by the input signal; the output voltage is developed by the collector current passing through the load resistance R_L. For the CS amplifier in Figure 2.24b, the gate resistor R_G simply prevents charge from accumulating on the gate terminal and thereby maintains the gate very close to ground potential; typically, R_G is many megohms. The output voltage is developed by the drain current through the load resistance. The dc voltage level about which the output voltage changes is often referred to as the *operating point* (that is, the operating point is the collector or drain potential with zero input signal).

Both these circuits are capable of large current and voltage gains. The actual gain is a complicated function of the circuit and transistor parameters. The output impedance of both the CE and CS amplifiers is about R_L; for large voltage gains, this is a rather large output impedance (from 1 to 50 kΩ). A CE amplifier has a relatively low input impedance. It is never greater than R_1 and often much smaller, say around 10 to 50 kΩ. On the other hand, a CS amplifier has an input impedance nearly equal to R_G; this can easily be in excess of 10 MΩ.

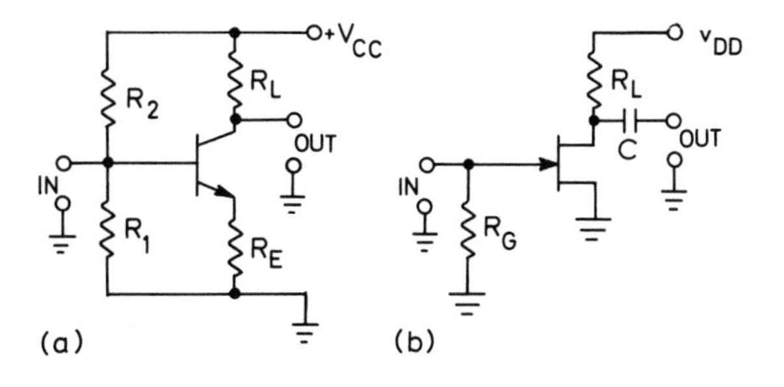

Figure 2.24
(a) A common-emitter, and
(b) a common-source amplifier.

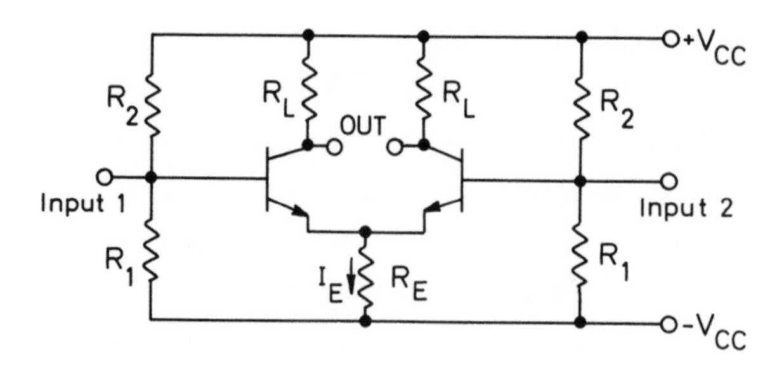

Figure 2.25
An emitter-coupled, differential amplifier.

Amplifier gains in excess of 50 are normally achieved by using more than one stage of gain. When the collector of the first stage is connected to the base of the second stage, the proper dc bias levels must be maintained. This can be a difficult task. However, if only ac signals must be amplified, then input, output, and interstage coupling can be done using capacitive coupling. This is illustrated in Figure 2.24b where the output voltage is capacitively coupled to whatever instrument is connected to the output terminal. One consequence of capacitive coupling is that each stage can be biased independently of the other stages and of the input and output connections. The low frequency response of an ac coupled amplifier is determined by the load and bias resistors as well as the coupling capacitor. For fixed resistance values, the larger the coupling capacitor, the better the low frequency response.

One particular version of a CE amplifier shown in Figure 2.25 is very widely used and deserves further discussion. It is usually referred to as an emitter-coupled pair. Resistors R_1 and R_2 establish the proper bias voltages. The emitter resistance R_E is normally many times larger than the load resistance R_L. This means that V_{CC} and R_E almost completely determine the current I_E that flows through R_E. If the very small base current is neglected, I_E is the sum of the two collector currents. Therefore, if the collector current in one transistor is to increase, the collector current in the other must decrease. This can be an extremely useful feature. If the same ac or dc voltage is supplied to each input, then both collector currents will tend to change in the same direction. The large emitter resistance does not permit this to occur; the collector currents do not change, and therefore there is no change in the output voltage. The output is determined by the difference in voltage between the two input terminals.

Because, ideally, an output is produced only if there is a difference in voltage between the two input terminals, the emitter-coupled amplifier is also known as a *differential amplifier*. A differential amplifier can always be used as a single-input or single-ended amplifier by applying the input signal between either input and ground.

The same signal applied to both inputs of a differential amplifier is known as a common-mode signal. The rejection of a common mode voltage is, in practice, never perfect; for a real amplifier the common mode rejection ratio (CMRR) determines the fraction of a common mode signal that appears on the output. For instance, a CMRR of 80 dB means that a 1 V common mode signal will result in the same output voltage as a 100 μV signal applied between the two input terminals (100 μV is 80 dB down from 1 V).

The Common-Drain and Common-Collector Amplifiers

The common-drain (CD) and common-collector (CC) amplifiers shown in Figure 2.26 have large current gain but, at best, the voltage gain is unity. These circuits are used primarily as impedance-matching devices (impedance transformers), because each is capable of a relatively high input impedance and low output impedance. The CC amplifier in Figure 2.26a is also known as an emitter-follower. Here R_b supplies the necessary base current. The collector current develops the output voltage across R_E. If R_b is very large, the input impedance is about $Z_{in} = \beta R_E$ and the output impedance about $Z_{out} = R_E/\beta$. The input impedance of the source follower in Figure 2.26b is about $Z_{in} = R_G$ while the output impedance is a very small fraction ($\sim 10^{-2}$) of R_S.

The Common-Gate and Common-Base Amplifiers

Both the common-gate (CG) and common-base (CB) amplifier have a current gain near unity. These circuits are not encountered very often in low-frequency (below a few hundred kHz) applications. However, at high frequencies where many of the nonideal characteristics of transistors create serious design problems, the CG and CB amplifiers have many advantages. These are covered in the references at the end of this chapter.

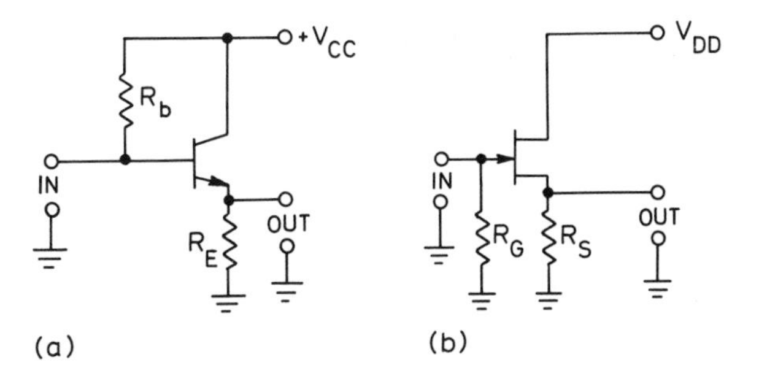

Figure 2.26
(a) A common-collector or emitter-follower amplifier, and
(b) a common-drain or source-follower amplifier.

2.6 Thyristors (Silicon-Controlled Rectifiers) and Triacs

A controller rectifier is used when it is desired to turn diode action on or off by means of an external voltage or current. There are many ways of doing this; the simplest is the silicon controlled rectifier (SCR) shown in Figure 2.27. It is a four-layer, three *pn* junction element. When the anode is made positive with respect to the cathode, junction 2 is reverse biased so very little current will flow. However, a sufficiently large positive voltage applied between the gate and cathode will cause junction 2 to break down and therefore allow a current to flow through the SCR. Once breakdown occurs, a current will flow until the cathode is made positive with respect to the anode. Since the only way to stop current flow is to reverse bias the whole device, SCRs are used primarily for the control of ac voltages. The ac automatically shuts the SCR off every cycle. Control is then achieved by turning the SCR on at some appropriate point on each cycle. An SCR can also be used to trigger the discharge of a capacitor or to short out a load if the voltage across it reaches a preset level. The standard symbol for an SCR is given in Figure 2.28 and the *I-V* characteristics in Figure 2.29. Note from these characteristics that above some voltage the center junction breaks down even at zero gate voltage. Hence if a complete range of control is desired, an SCR must be chosen with V_{crit} greater than the *peak* voltage applied across the SCR. As the gate current increases, breakdown occurs at lower applied (anode-cathode) voltages. Once the SCR has switched to the "on" state, there is a small forward resistance and conduction continues until the anode potential becomes negative. This is true even

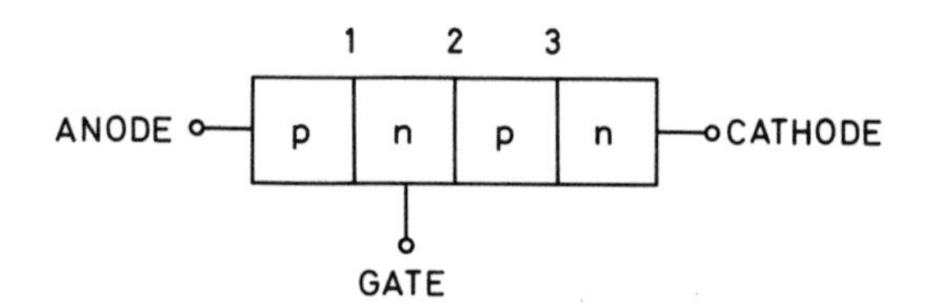

Figure 2.27
Pictorial representation of a silicon controlled rectifier.

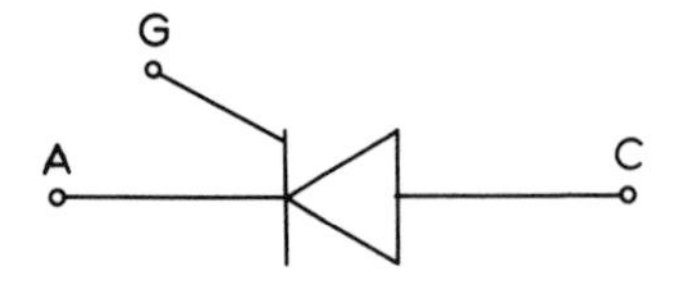

Figure 2.28
Symbol for an SCR.

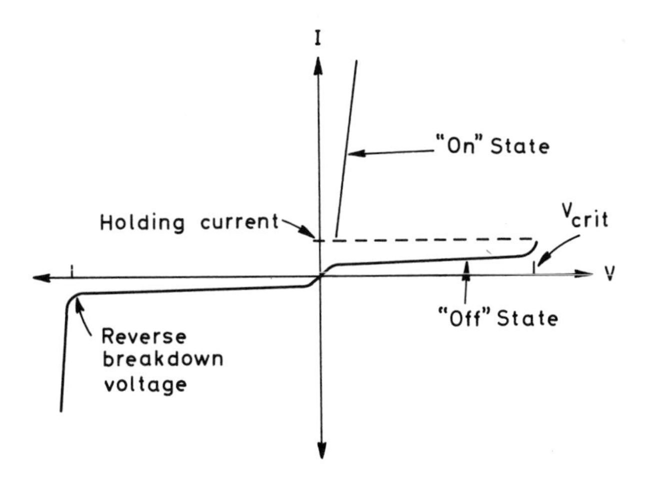

Figure 2.29
I-V characteristics of an SCR.

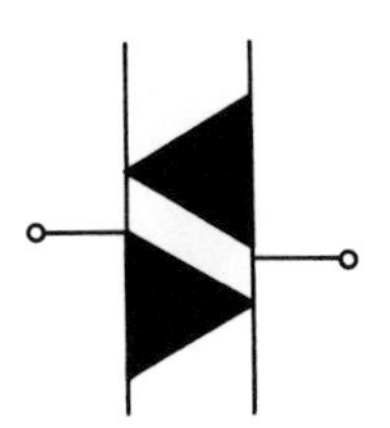

Figure 2.30
Symbol for a triac.

when the gate voltage is removed. In the "on" state, current flow is limited primarily by the load resistance. It is usually necessary to limit the current in the gate circuit with a series resistor in order to prevent damage to the gate. Clearly, a minimum current must be supplied if the junction is to break down. SCRs are rated for a peak anode-cathode voltage (the maximum blocking voltage), which ranges from 10 V to nearly 1 kV, and a maximum current.

The triac is similar to an SCR except that it can pass either positive or negative current and can be triggered by a voltage of either polarity. Figure 2.30 shows the symbol for a triac. Since the transfer characteristics are not polarity dependent, the input terminals cannot be designated by "anode" and "cathode."

Although any combination of input polarity and gate voltage can be used to initiate conduction, some combinations are much more sensitive than others. Manufacturer's specification sheets must be consulted to determine the best mode of operation for any particular device. Triacs are useful only at relatively low frequencies such as the 60 Hz line frequency, whereas SCRs are useful to about 100 kHz.

Selected References

There are a number of good but considerably more advanced textbooks dealing with electronic circuit analysis and design. Some of these are (order not significant) the following:

American Radio Relay League. 1970. *The Radio Amateur's Handbook*. Newington, Connecticut 06111.

Brophy, James J. 1966. *Basic Electronics for Scientists*. New York: McGraw-Hill Book Co.

Gray, Paul E., and Campbell L. Searle. 1969. *Electronic Principles, Physics, Models, and Circuits*. New York: John Wiley & Sons.

Romanowitz, H. Alex, and Russel E. Puckett. 1970. *Introduction to Electronics*. New York: John Wiley & Sons.

Smith, Ralph J. 1971. *Circuits, Devices and Systems*. New York: John Wiley & Sons.

Much useful information is contained in manuals produced by the various electronic component manufacturers, for example, the *Transistor Manual*, General Electric Company, Semiconductor Products Department, Syracuse, New York.

3 OPERATIONAL AMPLIFIERS

Paul B. Brown

3.1 Introduction to Operational Amplifiers; Negative Resistive Feedback

Neurobiologists encounter two situations in which they must process continuously variable (analog) signals, namely, when recording bioelectric phenomena and when synthesizing signal wave forms in the course of generating various types of stimuli. Separate chapters are devoted to these tasks. To facilitate these discussions, a general approach to signal processing will be developed, based on the use of negative feedback in high-gain amplifiers. High-gain amplifiers designed to be used with strong negative feedback for the purpose of modifying ("operating on") an input signal are called *operational amplifiers* (op amps) and are usually designated by the symbol shown in Figure 3.1. The amplifier itself can be very complex and must be specified by many parameters. However, to illustrate the general utility of op amps, let us consider an idealized version of the real entity, in which we define an ideal op amp as an amplifier whose only effect is to multiply the difference between voltages applied across the positive and negative inputs by the

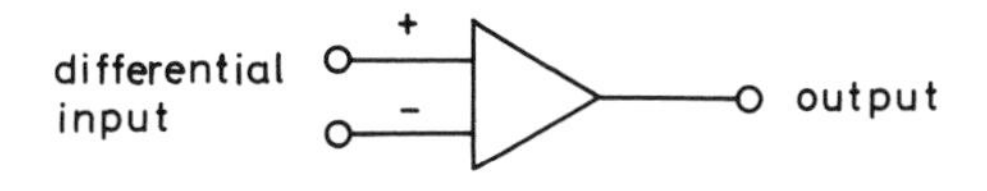

Figure 3.1
Operational amplifier symbol.

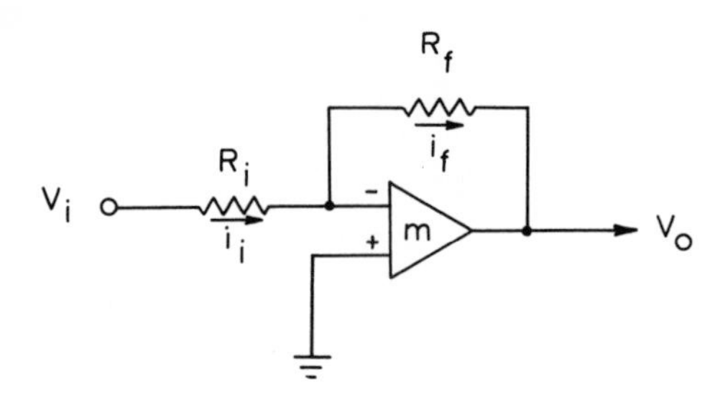

Figure 3.2
An op amp with negative resistive feedback.

amplifier gain m. Referring to the circuit in Figure 3.2 and applying Kirchhoff's rules, we can develop a relationship between V_i and V_o. Let the potential of the negative input be V^-, and let the potential of the positive input be V^+. For convenience and simplicity, the positive input will initially be considered grounded, that is, $V^+ = 0$. Therefore by definition:

$$-mV^- = V_o. \tag{3.1}$$

Also, by assumption, the amplifier input does not draw any current, in which case the Kirchhoff junction rule specifies

$$i_i = i_f. \tag{3.2}$$

Ohm's law yields

$$V_i - V^- = i_i R_i \tag{3.3}$$

and

$$V^- - V_o = i_f R_f. \tag{3.4}$$

Combining Equations 3.1 through 3.4, we obtain

$$\frac{R_f}{R_i}\left(V_i + \frac{V_o}{m}\right) = \frac{V_o}{m} - V_o, \tag{3.5}$$

or

$$V_o\left(\frac{1}{m} - \frac{R_f}{R_i}\frac{1}{m} - 1\right) = \frac{R_f}{R_i} V_i. \tag{3.6}$$

At first sight, this hardly looks like a simple relationship between V_i and V_o. However, let us consider a real example. In practice, it is very easy to obtain $m = 10^4$ in a commercial op amp, and gains of 10^5 and 10^6 are common. Thus terms of order $1/m$ may be neglected and Equation 3.6 reduces, with negligible error, to

$$\frac{V_o}{V_i} = \frac{-(R_f/R_i)}{1 + \dfrac{R_f}{mR_i}}. \tag{3.7}$$

Further simplification is possible if

$$m \gg \frac{R_f}{R_i}. \tag{3.8}$$

This is also an easy condition to meet. Furthermore, it will be pointed out later that much is gained if the inequality given by Equation 3.8 is satisfied. Suppose we choose $R_f = 100\ R_i$, that is, $R_f/mR_i \leqq 0.01$. Thus, to a good approximation,

$$\frac{V_o}{V_i} = -\frac{R_f}{R_i} = m' \tag{3.9}$$

when $m \geqq 100\ R_f/R_i$. Therefore, under the assumptions that have been stated, Equation 3.9 gives the signal gain m' or, as it is commonly called, the *closed-loop gain*. By contrast, m is usually referred to as the *open-loop gain*, that is, the gain without the feedback loop R_f connected. Feedback refers to any connection between output and input. Inspection of Equations 3.7 and 3.9 will reveal some of the many useful features of negative feedback, the type of feedback that has been incorporated in Figure 3.2. The signal gain is determined primarily by passive components, resistors, which are inherently very stable elements. This is not true of amplifiers, where the gain always changes with temperature and usually drifts with time (component aging). Thus, using negative feedback and satisfying the inequality given by Equation 3.8, we can obtain an amplifier with a signal gain that is controlled, for all practical purposes, by stable passive elements. This only requires that the open-loop gain be at least 100 times the closed-loop gain. More precisely, the theoretical closed-loop gain obtained by the calculation of Equation 3.9 will always be in error by a small amount, called the *closed-loop gain error*. This error is closely approximated by the reciprocal of the *gain margin*, which is simply the ratio of open-loop gain to closed-loop gain. Thus, for 1% error or less, assuming R_i and R_f to be exactly their nominal values (see Chapter 6 for computation of performance tolerances from component tolerances), the gain margin must be at least 100, or 40 dB.

Notice another point: from Equations 3.1 and 3.9,

$$V^- = V_i R_f/mR_i,$$

or under the assumptions of Equation 3.8,

$$|V^-| \ll |V_i|.$$

Hence for practical purposes, V^- is very small indeed. As the open-loop gain increases, V^- decreases; in the limit of m becoming infinite, V^- approaches zero. Because V^- is typically very small in practical situations, it is common to refer to the negative input as a virtual ground, in applications where V^+ is grounded. This does not mean that any current flows to ground at this point. In the idealized example discussed so far, this virtual ground is isolated from the real circuit ground by an infinite resistance (impedance). However, for practical purposes the negative input is at ground potential. This greatly simplifies circuit analysis. For example, the circuit in Figure 3.2 readily yields

$$V_i = i_i R_i;$$
$$V_o = -i_f R_f.$$

Since $i_i = i_f$, Equation 3.9 follows immediately. Of course, it has been assumed that m is large (see Equation 3.8).

But now what about a real amplifier which, most probably, will not behave like the idealized version discussed above? All ops amps have a finite input impedance, that is, they all draw some current from the virtual ground. How important is this factor?

First, note that the input current i_i is no longer equal to the feedback current i_f. The amplifier input impedance Z_i and the feedback resistance R_f act as a current divider, therefore it is reasonable to expect that a finite input impedance affects circuit operation when Z_i becomes comparable to R_f. Exact analysis confirms this expectation. In many applications it is easy to avoid the complication of considering a finite input impedance by choosing a unit that has

$$100\ R_i < Z_i > 100\ R_f.$$

We will, however, encounter situations where this rule may be ignored.

Op amps are normally designed to act as voltage sources, although units with current source outputs are available. In practice, the output impedance that characterizes the voltage source (or current source) is seldom the limiting feature of an op amp. However, the output impedance together with the maximum output voltage and current ratings are part of the usual op amp specifications. The influence of a finite output impedance has been discussed (see Chapter 1).

Usually the most troublesome nonideal characteristic is the finite frequency response of an op amp. Typical response of a common, useful integrated circuit

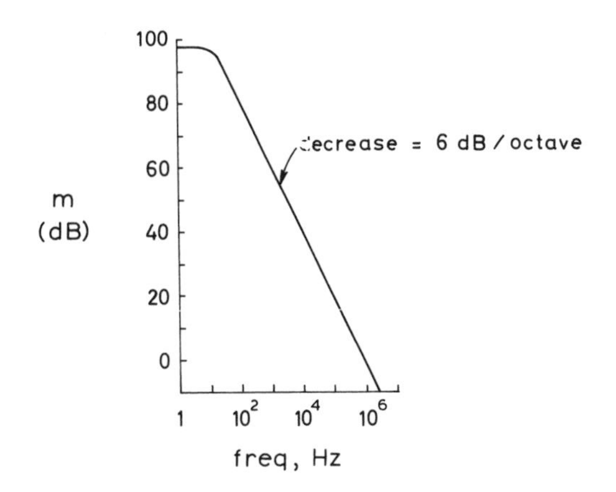

Figure 3.3
Frequency response of a 741 IC op amp (from *Semiconductor Integrated Circuits Data Catalog, 1970*, by Fairchild Semiconductor. Used with permission of Fairchild Camera and Instrument Corporation.)

op amp is shown in Figure 3.3. Note that log scales are used. Most new op amps are designed to have unconditionally stable frequency characteristics. This means that the amplifier will not break spontaneously into oscillation with purely resistive feedback. To accomplish this, it is necessary to decrease the gain with increasing frequency; a typical decrease, or *roll-off* as it is commonly called, is 6 dB/octave or 10 dB/decade. The roll-off is obtained by internal compensation in some op amps; others require external frequency compensation networks. In the case of external frequency compensation requirements, the manufacturer recommends that compensation components be attached to certain pins for different closed-loop gains; unfortunately, other factors sometimes influence the choice of compensation components, such as source or feedback impedance, presence of capacitances in the feedback or input circuits, and so forth. We will indicate the compensation required in practical circuits designed for actual laboratory use, and op amps that are internally compensated will be used wherever possible.

The open-loop gain m that is quoted in op amp specifications always refers to the dc (low-frequency) value. Open-loop gains at all other frequencies may be calculated from the unity gain frequency f and an assumed 6 dB/octave roll-off unless stated otherwise. The maximum unity gain frequency is usually referred to as the *gain-bandwidth product.*

Any op amp will exhibit a short time delay between input and output. This is composed of a constant component and a frequency-dependent component. For application of op amps in processing analog signals varying at rates under 100 kHz, the time delay does not influence circuit operation. However, in high-frequency applications this time delay can be very important. Further comments on the finite frequency response and other nonideal characteristics of op amps will be deferred until the particular limitations are discussed as part of the operation of some real circuit; also, nonidealities are discussed in the last section of this chapter.

From the basic concepts already presented, it is possible to analyze the behavior of numerous feedback component combinations. The remainder of this chapter consists of a discussion of important and useful feedback configurations. Some useful general discussions are included in the description of the next four circuits; an adder-subtracter, an integrator, a differentiator, and an absolute-value circuit.

3.2 Addition, Subtraction, Differentiation, and Integration of Signals

3.2.1 Adder-Subtracter

A circuit that provides the sum or difference of various input voltages is shown in Figure 3.4a. Assuming the operation of an ideal op amp, and using the concept

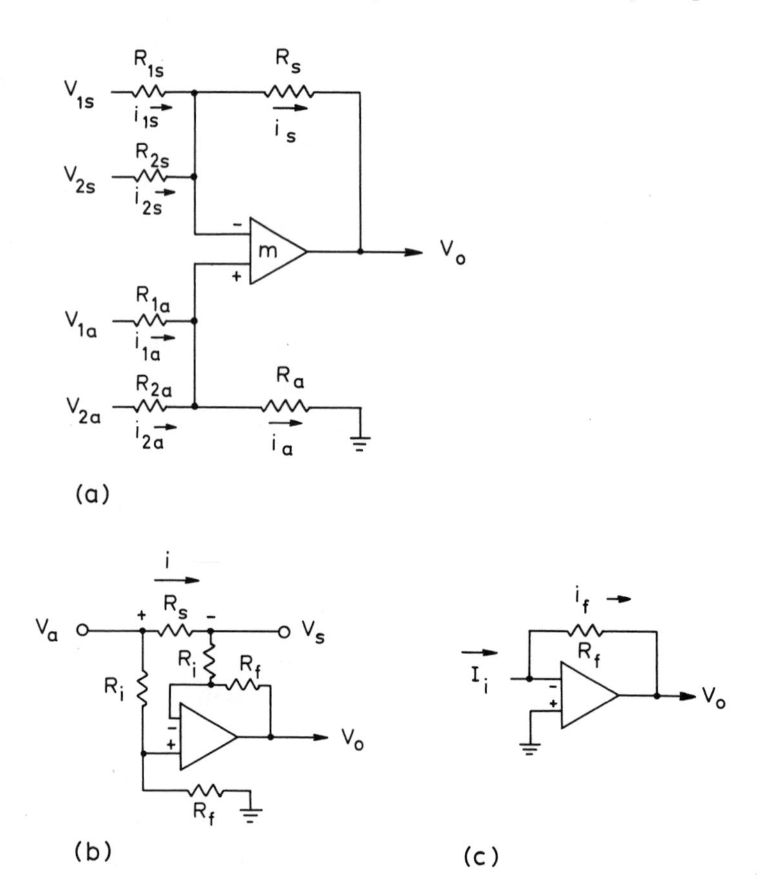

Figure 3.4
Resistive negative feedback applications: (a) 4-input adder-subtracter network; (b) current monitor; (c) current-voltage conversion.

of a virtual null, wherein the voltage difference between V^+ and V^- is rendered essentially zero by the negative feedback, we can apply Kirchhoff's rules to the various resistor networks to yield the following equations:

(a) $V^- = V^+ = i_a R_a$

(b) $i_{1s} + i_{2s} = i_s$

(c) $i_{1a} + i_{2a} = i_a$

(d) $V_{1s} - V^- = i_{1s} R_{1s}$

(e) $V_{2s} - V^- = i_{2s} R_{2s}$

(f) $V_o = V^- - i_s R_s$

(g) $V_{1a} - V^+ = i_{1a} R_{1a}$

(h) $V_{2a} - V^+ = i_{2a} R_{2a}$.

Using (d) and (e) to substitute for i_{1s} and i_{2s} in (b), we have

(i) $$\frac{1}{R_{1s}}(V_{1s} - V^-) + \frac{1}{R_{2s}}(V_{2s} - V^-) = i_s.$$

Similarly, using (g) and (h) to substitute for i_{1a} and i_{2a} in (c), we have

(j) $$\frac{1}{R_{1a}}(V_{1a} - V^+) + \frac{1}{R_{2a}}(V_{2a} - V^+) = i_a.$$

The relationship (a) can be used to substitute for V^- in (f):

(k) $V_o = i_a R_a - i_s R_s$.

It is possible to replace i_a and i_s in (k), using (i) and (j):

(l) $$V_o = \frac{R_a}{R_{1a}}(V_{1a} - V^+) + \frac{R_a}{R_{2a}}(V_{2a} - V^+) - \frac{R_s}{R_{1s}}(V_{1s} - V^-) - \frac{R_s}{R_{2s}}(V_{2s} - V^-).$$

Regrouping the terms, and using (a) to substitute $i_a R_a$ for V^+ and V^-, we have

(m) $$V_o = R_a\left(\frac{V_{1a}}{R_{1a}} + \frac{V_{2a}}{R_{2a}}\right) - R_s\left(\frac{V_{1s}}{R_{1s}} + \frac{V_{2s}}{R_{2s}}\right) - i_a R_a\left(\frac{R_a}{R_{1a}} + \frac{R_a}{R_{2a}} - \frac{R_s}{R_{1s}} - \frac{R_s}{R_{2s}}\right).$$

If we stipulate that

$$R_a\left(\frac{1}{R_{1a}} + \frac{1}{R_{2a}}\right) = R_s\left(\frac{1}{R_{1s}} + \frac{1}{R_{2s}}\right), \tag{3.10}$$

the last term of (m) drops out and we are left with a simple solution for V_o,

$$V_o = R_a\left(\frac{V_{1a}}{R_{1a}} + \frac{V_{2a}}{R_{2a}}\right) - R_s\left(\frac{V_{1s}}{R_{1s}} + \frac{V_{2s}}{R_{2s}}\right). \tag{3.11}$$

We will find, below, that restriction 3.10 actually simplifies construction of an adder-subtracter network.

Thus the output voltage is the appropriately scaled sum of the voltages applied to the positive input section (adder inputs $1a$ and $2a$) minus the appropriately scaled sum of voltages applied to the negative input section (subtracter inputs $1s$ and $2s$). A generalization of Equations 3.11 and 3.10 to an adder of n inputs and a subtracter with m inputs gives

$$V_o = R_a \sum_{i=1}^{n} \frac{V_{ia}}{R_{ia}} - R_s \sum_{j=1}^{m} \frac{V_{js}}{R_{js}}, \tag{3.12}$$

subject to the condition

$$R_a \sum_{i=1}^{n} \frac{1}{R_{ia}} = R_s \sum_{j=1}^{m} \frac{1}{R_{js}}. \tag{3.13}$$

This requirement is easily met. Simply choose

$$R_a = R_s \tag{3.14}$$

and apply adder and subtracter voltages through series input resistors adjusted such that

$$R_{ia} = \frac{R_a}{a_i}, \tag{3.15}$$

and

$$R_{js} = \frac{R_s}{s_j}, \tag{3.16}$$

where a_i and s_j are coefficients described in Equation 3.18, below. Add one more resistor R_x such that

$$\frac{1}{R_x} = \left| \sum_{i=1}^{n} \frac{1}{R_{ia}} - \sum_{j=1}^{m} \frac{1}{R_{js}} \right|. \tag{3.17}$$

If the quantity within the absolute-value bars is negative, R_x goes from the adder junction to ground. If it is positive, tie R_x between the subtracter junction and ground. If R_x is zero, no additional resistor is required.

Thus, the constraint of Equation 3.13 is met, and

$$V_o = \sum_{i=1}^{n} a_i V_i - \sum_{j=1}^{m} s_j V_j. \tag{3.18}$$

Thus, an algebraic sum of weighted terms, Equation 3.18, can be obtained, using Formulas 3.14 to 3.17 to determine values of resistors in an adder-subtracter network. A simple rule of thumb is to select $R_a = R_s = Z_i/100$, and proceed from there. Keep in mind the fact that each R_{ia} and R_{js} is composed of both the series input resistor *and* the output impedance of the voltage source V_{ia} or V_{js}. If the calculated R is smaller than $Z_o \times 100$, either lower Z_o with a current amplifier (described below) or select an op amp for the adder-subtracter that has a higher Z_i, in order to allow larger R_a and R_s and hence larger R_{ia} and R_{js}. Note that where it is necessary to sum currents, it is possible to use an op amp to convert accurately currents to voltages and then add the resulting voltages.

Two methods of current-to-voltage conversion are illustrated in Figure 3.4b, c. In 3.4b, the voltage across a resistor connected in series with the current path is amplified differentially. If $R_i \gg R_s$ and R_s is small in order to minimize alteration of the current path resistance, the current drawn by the measuring device is insignificant. This circuit is the basis of the current monitoring techniques used in ammeters and output compensated constant-current sources.

If true current sources are available, and current-to-voltage conversion is necessary, the circuit of Figure 3.4c can be used to convert a current to a voltage

A special case of the adder-subtracter circuit is the unity-gain voltage follower. We will consider this configuration in the last section of this chapter, as well as some other resistive negative feedback techniques.

The gain of a resistive feedback circuit is only as accurate as the resistance values used in the circuit. Error values can be calculated by expressing resistances as $R \pm \Delta R$, where ΔR is the maximum error expected for the type of resistor used: all resistors are coded for degree of precision. Thus, substituting $R \pm \Delta R$ for all R in a circuit's gain expression, we have a solution for $V \pm \Delta V$. Metal film and wire-wound resistors generally have better temperature stability than carbon resistors. The metal film resistors have the least capacitance and inductance.

3.2.2 Differentiation and Integration

From Equation 1.19, the current-voltage relationship for a capacitor is

$$i = C\frac{d\xi}{dt}.$$

Suppose that a capacitor and resistor are used in a feedback loop as shown in

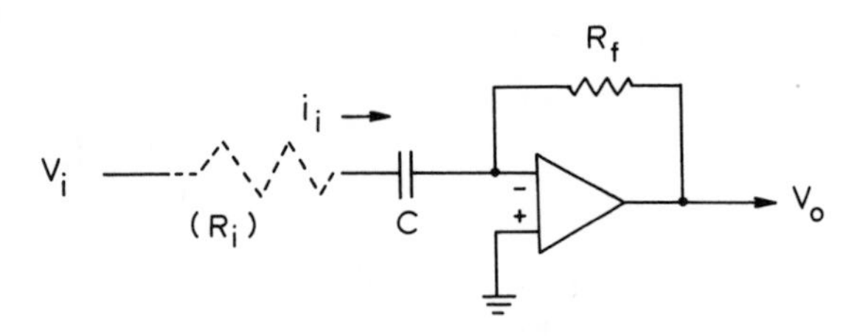

Figure 3.5
Differentiator.

Figure 3.5. Ignore, for the moment, the resistance in broken lines R_i. Assuming an ideal amplifier ($V^- = 0$), this circuit is described by

$$i_i = C\frac{dV_i}{dt}, \tag{3.19}$$

and

$$-V_o = i_f R. \tag{3.20}$$

Since $i_i = i_f$, Equations 3.19 and 3.20 give

$$V_o = -RC\frac{dV_i}{dt}. \tag{3.21}$$

That is, the output voltage is the time derivative of the input voltage.

Previous discussions of the limitations imposed by finite input and output impedances also apply to this example. It is obvious that the frequency response of an op amp can greatly influence its operation as a differentiator, because high frequencies are enhanced by a differentiator, but only within the bandpass limits of the device. Frequency response is most easily analyzed in terms of harmonic voltages. This approach is valid, because any time-varying voltage may be expressed as an appropriate sum of voltages varying at many different frequencies, that is, as the sum of harmonic voltages.

An extension of the analysis used in Figure 3.1 to the case of general impedances Z_i and Z_f in the feedback loop yields

$$\frac{V_o}{V_i} = -\frac{Z_f}{Z_i}. \tag{3.22}$$

For the differentiator shown in Figure 3.5, this gives

$$\frac{V_o}{V_i} = -j\omega RC, \tag{3.23}$$

which also follows directly from Equation 3.21 for an input voltage of frequency $f = \omega/2$. The j in Equation 3.23 represents a phase shift between input and output voltages. Figure 3.6 shows the frequency response of a differentiator (curve *b*) with $R = 100\ \mathrm{k}\Omega$ and $C = 0.1\ \mu\mathrm{F}$ along with the open-loop response of a 741 op amp (curve *a*).

Notice that the gain is eventually limited by the open-loop characteristics. At high frequencies the gain margin, that is, the difference between open-loop and closed-loop gain, decreases. Most of the useful features of op amps stem from a large gain margin. Therefore, as the closed-loop characteristics approach the open-loop characteristics, any discussions based upon the concept of a virtual ground become increasingly less valid. If the gain margin is greater than 40 dB, errors in differentiator operation due to finite gain will be less than 1%.

It is important to use "good" values for *R* and *C*. An *RC* product that is too small can give the signal a gain of less than unity, while a large *RC* might not have sufficient gain margin. Since any high-frequency noise (unwanted voltages) will be amplified more than low-frequency components, it is useful to limit the gain of a differentiator above the frequency range of interest. One way of accomplishing this is by a resistor (R_i, in broken lines) in series with the input capacitor as shown in Figure 3.5. The dashed line in Figure 3.6 (curve *c*) represents the resulting closed-loop characteristics for $R_i = 1\ \mathrm{k}\Omega$.

Reversing the feedback roles of the resistor and capacitor, one produces the operation that is the inverse of differentiation, namely integration. Figure 3.7

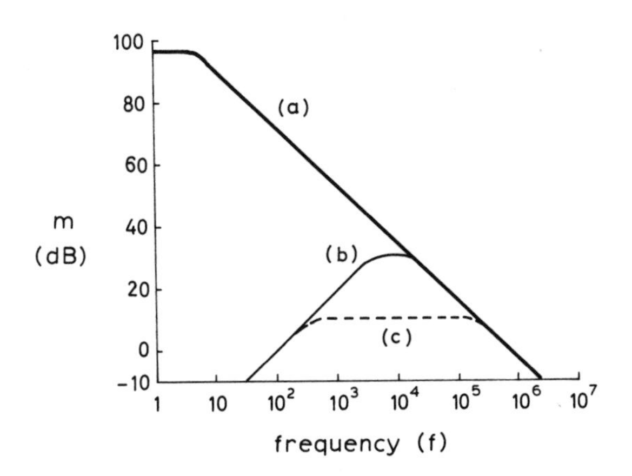

Figure 3.6
Frequency response for differentiators in Figure 3.5. Heavy solid line (a) is response of open-loop op amp configuration; thin solid line (b) is the differentiator response in the absence of R_i; dashed line is response of the differentiator with R_i included. $R = 100\ \mathrm{k}\Omega$, $C = 0.1\ \mu\mathrm{F}$ ($RC = 10^{-2}$ sec), and $R_i = 1\ \mathrm{k}\Omega$.

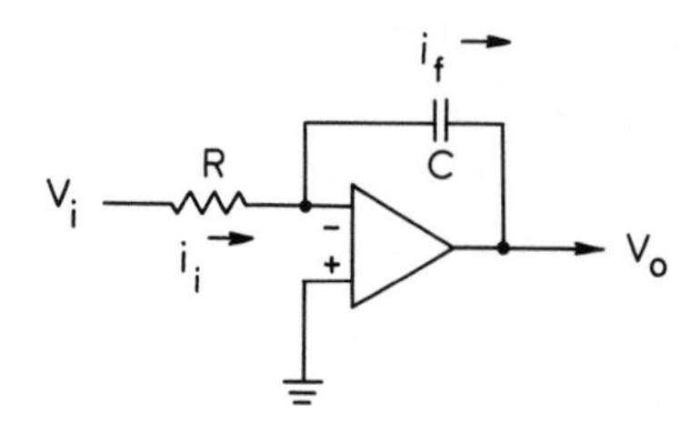

Figure 3.7
Integrator.

shows an ideal integrator; this circuit is described (assuming $V^- = 0$) by

$$V_i = i_i R \tag{3.24}$$

and

$$i_f = C\frac{dV_o}{dt}, \tag{3.25}$$

from which it follows that

$$\frac{V_i}{RC} = \frac{dV_o}{dt}$$

or

$$V_o = \frac{1}{RC}\int V_i \, dt. \tag{3.26}$$

Thus the output voltage is the integral over time of the input voltage.

Previous discussions of the limitations imposed by finite input and output impedances apply to the integrator. The frequency response of the op amp imposes limitations on its use as an integrator. Again, frequency response can be considered in terms of harmonic voltages. Equation 3.22 is also valid for the integrator; in this case $Z_f = 1/j\omega C$ and $Z_i = R$. This gives

$$\frac{V_o}{V_i} = \frac{1}{j\omega RC}, \tag{3.27}$$

a result which also follows from Equation 3.26 for harmonic voltages. As pointed out before, the j represents a phase difference of $\pi/2$ between input and output (with the output lagging the input). In fact, integrating a sine wave is a very useful means of producing a voltage that is accurately 90° out of phase with the input sine wave.

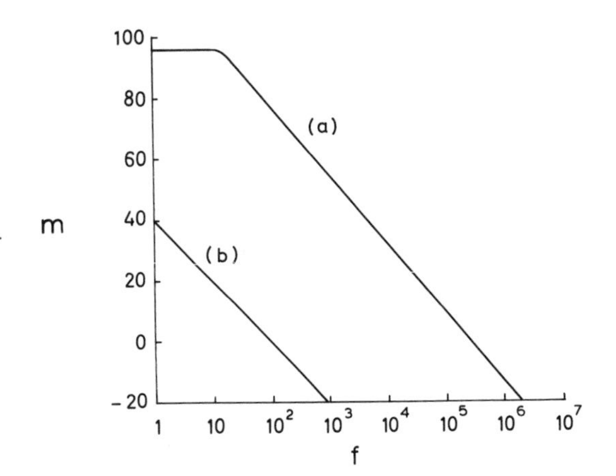

Figure 3.8
Response characteristics for integrator of Figure 3.7: (a) open loop; (b) closed loop, with $R = 100$ kΩ, $C = 0.1\ \mu$F ($RC = 10^{-2}$ sec).

The frequency response of an integrator with $R = 100$ kΩ and $C = 1.0\ \mu$F is shown in Figure 3.8 (curve *b*). For comparison, the open-loop characteristics of a 741 op amp are also shown (curve *a*).

Care should be taken to choose an *RC* value that is compatible with the open-loop characteristics and the frequency range of interest. Since the gain is very large at low frequencies, small-amplitude low-frequency voltage components may produce a dominant contribution to the output voltage. In particular, a small dc voltage at the input will eventually saturate the output, that is, drive it as far as possible in either the positive or negative direction. This is highly undesirable. A large capacitor may be inserted in series with R to block dc and attenuate low-frequency voltages or a resistor may be used in parallel with C to limit the low-frequency gain to a constant value. Combining these two features produces a combined differentiator-integrator; input voltages are differentiated at low frequencies and integrated at high frequencies. This is illustrated in Figure 3.9 where

$$Z_i = R_1 + 1/j\omega C_2$$
$$Z_f = R_2/(1 + j\omega R_2 C_1),$$

from which it follows that

$$\frac{V_o}{V_i} = \frac{-j\omega R_2 C_2}{(1 + j\omega R_2 C_1)(1 + j\omega R_1 C_2)}. \tag{3.28}$$

For large ω, this reduces to the expression for an integrator, Equation 3.27, and for small ω, to the expression for a differentiator, Equation 3.23. The frequency

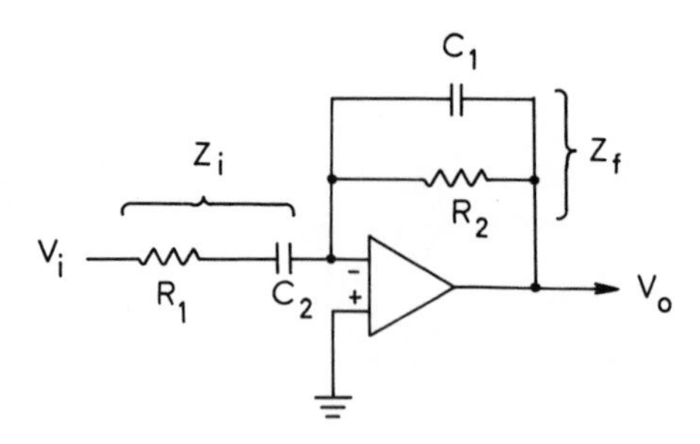

Figure 3.9
Differentiator-integrator.

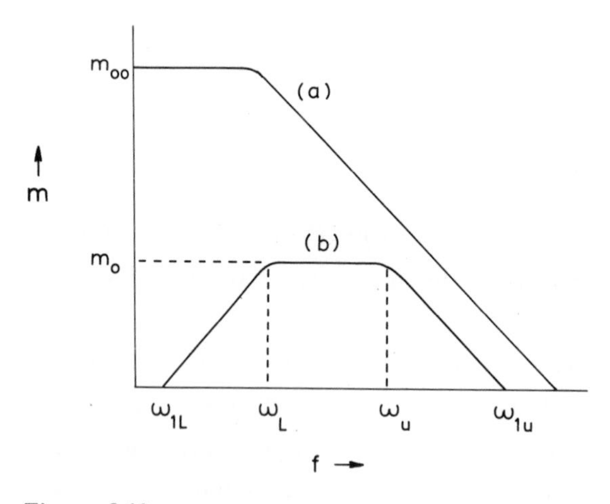

Figure 3.10
Frequency response of differentiator-integrator: (a) open-loop characteristic; (b) closed-loop characteristic.

response for this circuit is shown in Figure 3.10 (curve *b*). The frequency and gain scales are set by the relationships

$$\omega_{1L} R_2 C_2 = 1 \tag{3.29a}$$

$$\omega_L R_1 C_2 = 1 \tag{3.29b}$$

$$\omega_U R_2 C_1 = 1 \tag{3.29c}$$

$$\omega_{1U} R_1 C_1 = 1 \tag{3.29d}$$

$$m' = R_2/R_1, \qquad \text{if } \omega_L < \omega_U. \tag{3.29e}$$

In a real op amp, a small dc voltage is present at the input terminals due to "battery" action in the device itself. This input offset voltage is an unavoidable feature of all op amps. For linear amplifiers, this is no problem as it only causes a constant shift of the input. The differentiator generally has low dc gain and hence the input offset voltage is of no concern. However, in the integrator, Figure

3.7, the open-loop dc gain will rapidly cause the output voltage to saturate. For example, the 741 has a typical input offset voltage of 1.0 mV. The amplifier will therefore take about 100 sec to reach the saturation output voltage, around 10 V, with zero input, if $R = 100\ \text{k}\Omega$ and $C = 0.1\ \mu\text{F}$.

Derivatives of input voltages can be added and subtracted, as can integrated input voltages, by using multiple inputs connected to the negative input (subtraction) or positive input (addition). This is a direct extension of Equations 3.12 and 3.13 developed for the voltage adder-subtracter. The multiple differentiator shown in Figure 3.11 is described by

$$V_o = R_a \sum_{i=1}^{n} \frac{V_{ia}}{Z_{ia}} - R_s \sum_{j=1}^{m} \frac{V_{js}}{Z_{js}}. \quad (3.30)$$

Since $Z_{1a} = 1/j\omega C_{1a}$, $Z_{1s} = 1/j\omega C_{1s}$, and so forth,

$$V_o = j\omega R_a \sum_{i=1}^{n} C_{ia} V_{ia} - j\omega R_s \sum_{j=1}^{m} C_{js} V_{js} \quad (3.31)$$

for harmonic input voltages, or

$$V_o = R_a \sum_{i=1}^{n} C_{ia} \frac{dV_{ia}}{dt} - R_s \sum_{j=1}^{m} C_{js} \frac{dV_{js}}{dt} \quad (3.32)$$

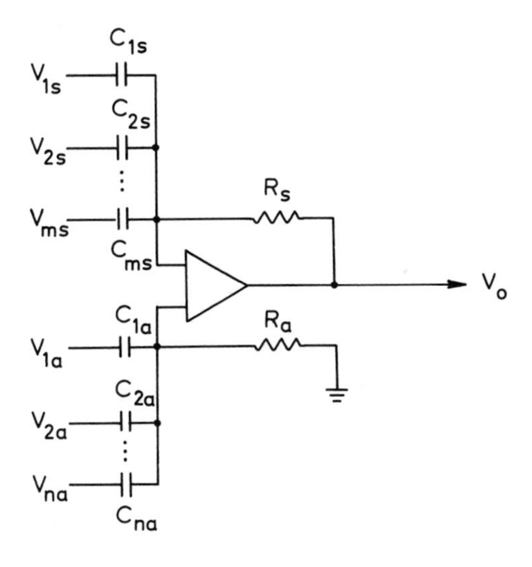

Figure 3.11
Multiple-input differentiator.

for a general time-varying input voltage. Equations 3.30, 3.31, and 3.32 are all subject to the condition

$$R_a \sum_{i=1}^{n} C_{ia} = R_s \sum_{j=1}^{m} C_{js}. \tag{3.33}$$

Again, by analogy with the equations for the adder-subtracter, we can realize the sum

$$V_o = \sum_{i=1}^{n} a_i V_i' - \sum_{j=1}^{m} s_j V_j', \tag{3.34}$$

if

$$R_a = R_s, \tag{3.35}$$

selecting C_{ia} and C_{js} such that

$$C_{ia} = \frac{a_i}{R_a} \tag{3.36}$$

and

$$C_{js} = \frac{s_j}{R_s}. \tag{3.37}$$

Then add one more capacitor C_x such that

$$C_x = \left| \sum_{i=1}^{n} C_{ia} - \sum_{j=1}^{m} C_{js} \right|, \tag{3.38}$$

tying it from the negative input to ground if the quantity

$$\left(\sum_{i=1}^{n} C_{ia} - \sum_{j=1}^{m} C_{js} \right)$$

is positive, and from the positive input to ground if the quantity is negative.

Figure 3.12 shows an integrator with n adder inputs and m subtractor inputs. Again, a generalization of linear voltage adder-subtracter equations (Equations 3.12 and 3.13) gives

$$V_o = \frac{1}{j\omega C_a} \sum_{i=1}^{n} \frac{V_{ia}}{R_{ia}} - \frac{1}{j\omega C_s} \sum_{j=1}^{m} \frac{V_{ja}}{R_{ja}} \tag{3.39}$$

for harmonic input voltages and

$$V_o = \int \frac{1}{C_a} \sum_{i=1}^{n} \frac{V_{ia}}{R_{ia}} - \frac{1}{C_s} \sum_{j=1}^{m} \frac{V_{js}}{R_{js}}\, dt \tag{3.40}$$

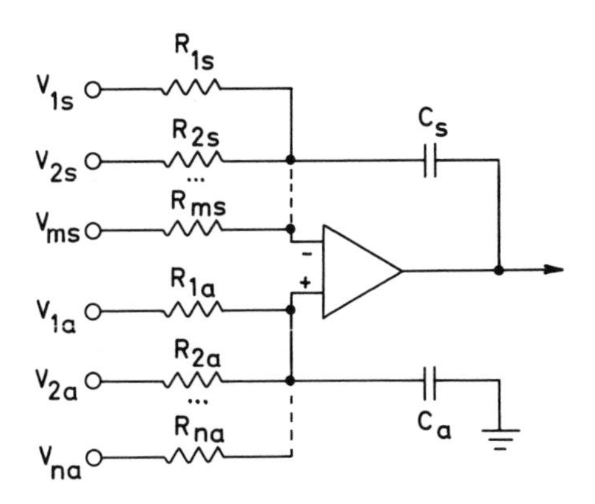

Figure 3.12
Multiple-input integrator.

for a general time-varying input voltage. Both Equations 3.39 and 3.40 are subject to the condition

$$C_a \sum_{i=1}^{n} \frac{1}{R_{ia}} = C_s \sum_{j=1}^{m} \frac{1}{R_{js}}. \tag{3.41}$$

We can realize the integral

$$\int \left(\sum_{i=1}^{n} a_i V_i - \sum_{j=1}^{m} s_j V_j \right) dt \tag{3.42}$$

if

$$C_a = C_s, \tag{3.43}$$

$$R_{ia} = \frac{C_a}{a_i}, \tag{3.44}$$

$$R_{js} = \frac{C_s}{s_j}. \tag{3.45}$$

Add one more resistor R_x such that

$$\frac{1}{R_x} = \left| \sum_{i=1}^{n} \frac{1}{R_{ia}} - \sum_{j=1}^{m} \frac{1}{R_{js}} \right|,$$

tying it from the negative input to ground if the quantity within the bars is positive, and from the positive input to ground if the quantity is negative.

3.3 Other Useful Functions

Nonlinear functions can be obtained by using nonlinear feedback elements. For example, we can easily obtain absolute values by the addition of diodes that

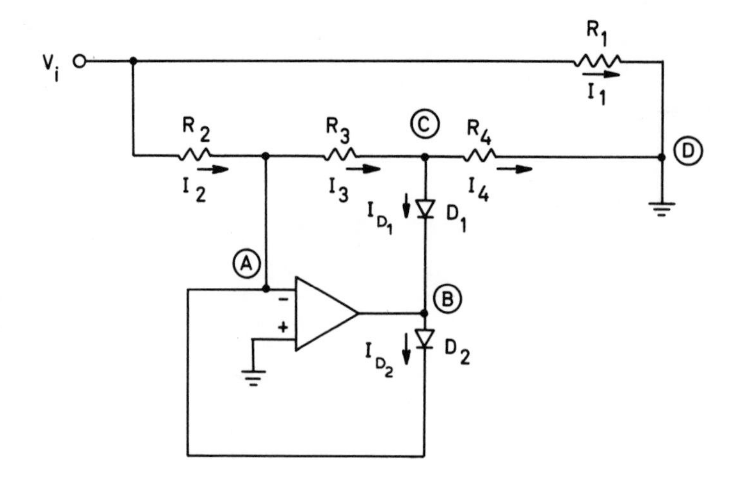

Figure 3.13
Absolute-value circuit (after Figure 2.42d, in *Application Manual for Operational Amplifiers*, 1968, by Philbrick/Nexus Research. Used with permission of Teledyne Philbrick.). Arrows indicate current flow with V_i positive. $R = R_1 = R_2 = R_3 = 2R_4$.

"steer" the output of the amplifier through different parts of the network, depending on the polarity of the amplifier output (Figure 3.13).

Let us examine the behavior of the circuit with opposite polarity inputs.

Positive voltage at the input: Currents into node A must sum to zero, because the positive input of the amplifier is grounded. The diode D_2 is nonconducting (output of the amplifier is negative), and D_1 conducts. Therefore, $I_1 = I_2 = V_i/R$ because nodes A and D are at ground. Since the voltage at node C drops to ground through R_4 and to virtual ground through R_3, $I_4 = 2I_3 = 2I_2 = 2V_i/R$. Therefore, current into node D must be $I_D = I_1 + I_4 = I_1 - 2I_2 = -V_i/R$.

Negative voltage at the input: D_2 is conducting, keeping node A at ground; D_1 is not conducting (amplifier output is positive), therefore nodes A and C are both at ground. Therefore, $I_4 = I_3 = 0$. So current into D must be only from I_1: $I_D = I_1 = V_i/R$.

Therefore, the general I/O equation for the circuit is: $I_D = -|V_i/R|$, which can be converted to an output voltage by the current-to-voltage output circuit of Figure 3.14.

In the modification of Figure 3.14, we have attached node D to a virtual ground, thus the current relations just derived still hold. But now the current I_D determines the output of the second amplifier:

$$V_o = \frac{R_f}{R}|V_i|. \tag{3.46}$$

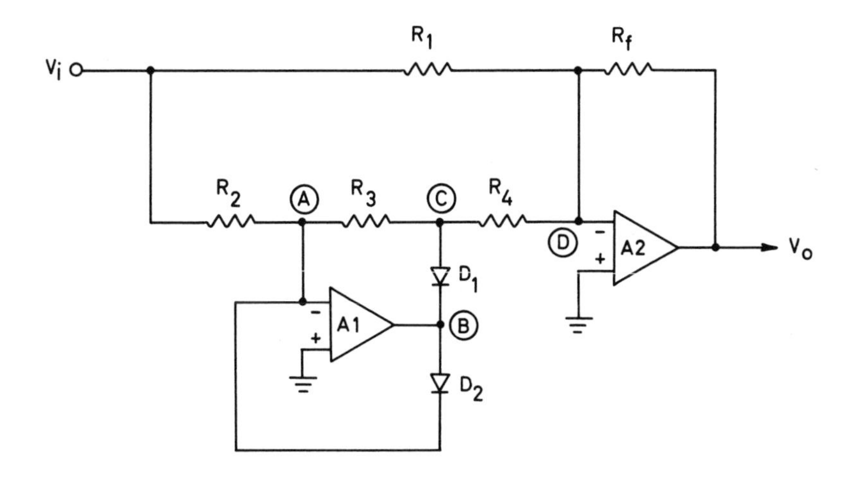

Figure 3.14
Output stage added to absolute-value circuit (after Figure 2.42d, in *Application Manual for Operational Amplifiers*, 1968, by Philbrick/Nexus Research. Used with permission of Teledyne Philbrick.). $R = R_1 = R_2 = R_3 = 2R_4$.

For our purposes, a practical value of R is 10 kΩ; for a gain of 0 to 10, R_f is a 0.1 MΩ pot. For unity gain, $R_f = R$.

Having established a method for addition and subtraction of voltages and for taking absolute values with op amps, let us now consider multiplication and division. The gain of a negative feedback circuit is a multiplier factor; by putting a pot in the feedback circuit, we obtain a variable multiplier. But how do we vary the gain of a circuit as a function of another input voltage? In other words, how do we realize the function $V_o = V_A \cdot V_B$?

It has been experimentally established that the emitter-to-base voltage of a forward-biased silicon transistor closely approximates the log of its collector current over a range of as many as nine decades. Therefore, we should be able to multiply and divide by using transistors in feedback circuits to obtain logarithmic voltage outputs. These voltages can then be added or subtracted, and the antilog obtained with a circuit in which the transistor is the input resistance element.

Figure 3.15 shows a working log circuit, which is included here only for purposes of illustration. For most applications, it is cheaper to buy commercially available log IC op amps or logarithmic modules. The first amplifier develops an emitter-to-base voltage on the feedback transistor which is proportional to the log of the input voltage, since the collector current must vary with $-V_i/10$ kΩ. This voltage difference is fed differentially to the second amplifier, which is a unity-gain inverter, isolating the transistor from output loading, correcting the algebraic sign, and providing a ground-referenced output. Only positive input voltages will

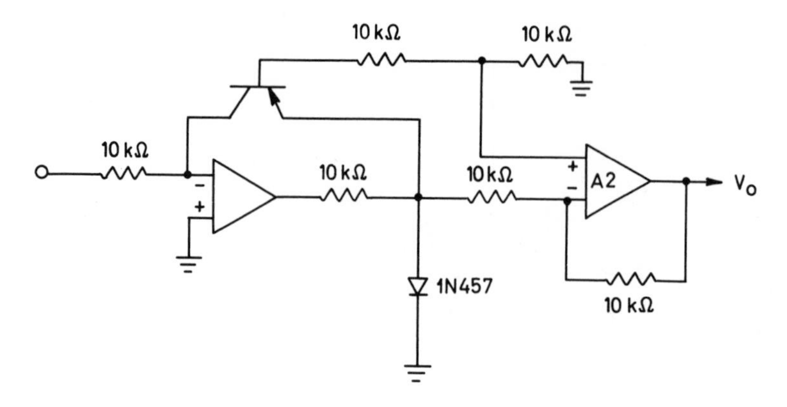

Figure 3.15
Log circuit.

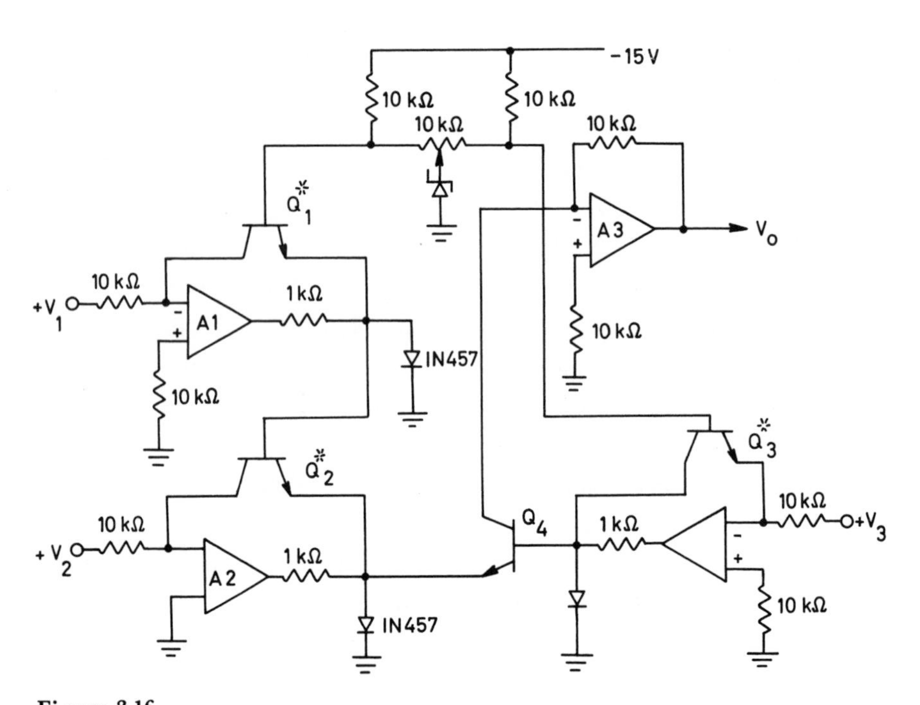

Figure 3.16
Multiplier-divider (after Figure 2.10, in *Designing with Linear Integrated Circuits*, 1969, by Jerry Eimbinder (ed.). Used with permission of John Wiley & Sons, Inc.).
$Q_1 - Q_4$ = dual transistors: 2N3728 matched pairs, mounted on a common heat-sink (*).

work in this design, because a negative input would drive the output positive and reverse bias the feedback transistor, which would not conduct. This would mean we would have no negative feedback, and the amplifier would operate at full open-loop gain, possibly damaging the feedback transistor. For this reason, the diode is added to the output of the first stage to shunt any positive output to ground.

We can now proceed to the somewhat more complicated circuit of Figure 3.16, a multiplier-divider. The input-output relation of this circuit is $V_o = \frac{V_1 \cdot V_2}{V_3}$. It has the advantage that it is designed to be temperature compensated: changes in I/O characteristics for one part of the circuit will compensate for corresponding changes in other parts of the circuit. To guarantee this, the transistors should be mounted on a common heat-sink with good thermal coupling among them.

$A1$ and $A2$ take the negative log of their respective inputs. Since the base-emitter junctions of the two transistors are in series, the voltage drops developed across them are summed. The potentiometer is used to adjust the offset voltages on all four transistors simultaneously. The next series transistor is inserted in the chain with the base-emitter junction pointed the opposite way; its voltage drop is subtracted, and therefore the log of V_3 is subtracted from the summed logs of V_1 and V_2. The transistor $Q4$ is the antilog generator: Because the base-emitter voltage equals the log of the collector current, it follows that collector current equals $e^{V_{be}}$, where V_{be} is the base-emitter voltage drop.

Therefore, the input to the final inverting amplifier $A4$ is proportional to $-e^{(\log V_1 + \log V_2 - \log V_3)}$, or $\frac{V_1 \cdot V_2}{V_3}$, and the output must be $V_o = \frac{V_1 \cdot V_2}{V_3}$.

Unfortunately, these designs do not handle negative voltages. They are "one-quadrant" devices. A "four-quadrant" multiplier (one that handles all four possible sign combinations of two input voltages) is block diagrammed in Figure 3.17a. Figure 3.17b illustrates one method for construction of a squaring network. A configuration for analog division is shown in Figure 3.18.

The entire device, like many of the circuits described here, can be replaced by a single quarter-squares multiplier module or IC, such as the Texas Instruments SN76502, which has an 80 dB input range and DC-40 MHz bandwidth. We recommend this approach wherever possible.

Since we have developed a technique for squaring and multiplication, it is not unreasonable to seek a technique for extracting algebraic roots. This can be accomplished by dividing the log of a voltage by a factor equal to the desired root and then taking the antilog (Figure 3.19).

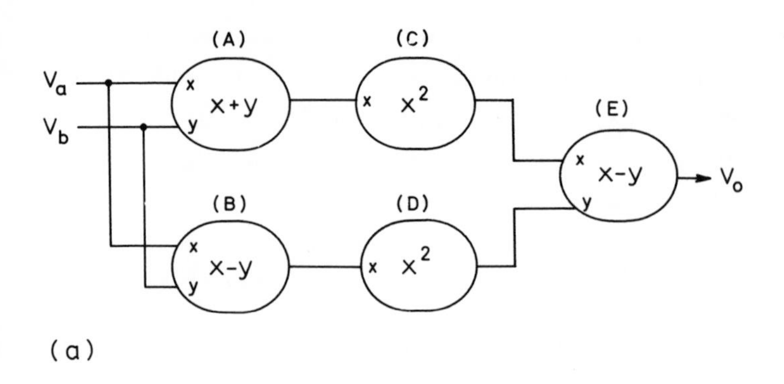

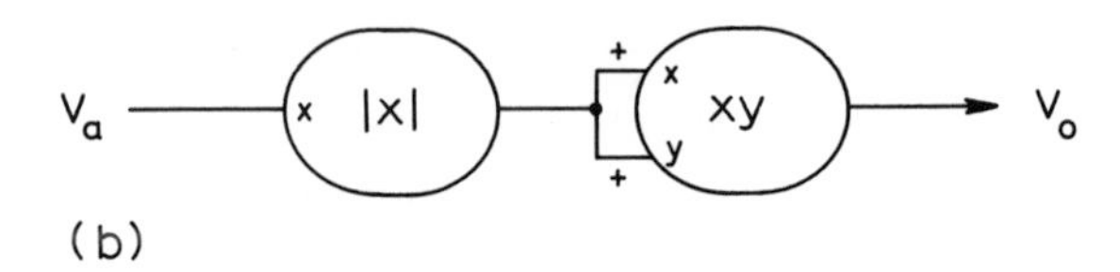

Figure 3.17
(a) Quarter-squares multiplier.
Output of adder (A): $V_a + V_b$
Output of subtracter (B): $V_a - V_b$
Output of squaring circuit (C): $(V_a + V_b)^2 = V_a^2 + 2V_aV_b + V_b^2$
Output of squaring circuit (D): $(V_a - V_b)^2 = V_a^2 - 2V_aV_b + V_b^2$
Output of subtracter (E): $V_o = (V_a + V_b)^2 - (V_a - V_b)^2 = 4V_aV_b$.
(b) Squaring circuit. For another method of squaring, use root extractor of Figure 3.19. $V_o = |V_a|^2 = V_a^2$.

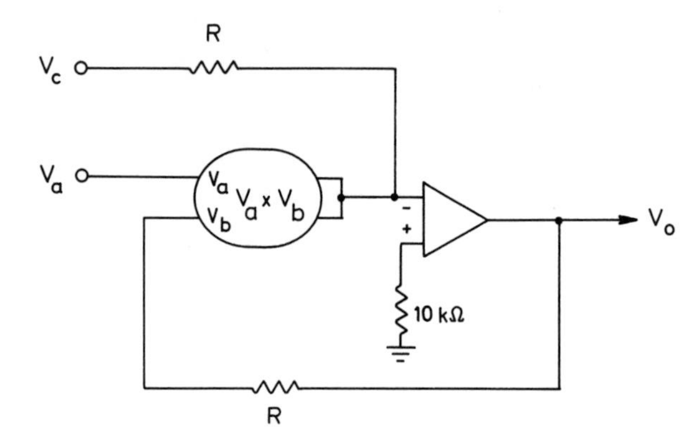

Figure 3.18
Multiplier operated as divider. $V_o = V_c/V_a$.

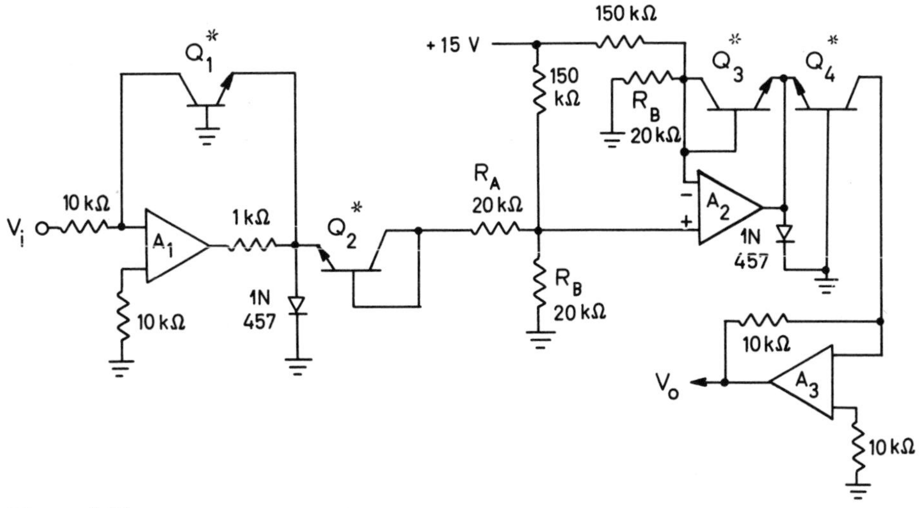

Figure 3.19
Root extractor. R_A and R_B are co-varied to determine the inverse power (root) (after Figure 2.11, in *Designing with Linear Integrated Circuits*, 1969, by Jerry Eimbinder (ed.). Used with permission of John Wiley & Sons, Inc.). With all resistors equal,

$$V_o = V_i^{(+)} \exp\left(\frac{R_A}{R_A + R_B}\right)$$

A_1–A_3 are LM101 operational amplifiers.
Q_1–Q_4 are 2N3728 matched pairs on common heat sink (*).

Here the log element is in the $A1$-$Q1$ pair; $Q2$ is just a level shifter (because we now go into the positive input of $A2$). The root is determined by the one R_A and the two R_B. A second level shifter $Q3$ allows proper voltage range into $Q4$, the antilog element. The input voltage range is 0.5–50 V (1% accuracy); for other voltage ranges, shift levels and gains accordingly. A simpler technique, which we recommend, is to use log and divider modules.

Log-of-ratio circuits are often useful for modeling membrane phenomena. Such a circuit is illustrated in Figure 3.20. We recommend the use of log-of-ratio modules, or the combined use of multiplier-divider and log modules.

All circuits using transistor transconductors (that is, using transistors in the feedback or other portions of the analog circuit) require some means of assuring that temperature variations will not affect circuit performance. In some circuits, it is only necessary to ensure that all the transistors are at the same temperature, because they mutually compensate each other. For this purpose, there are dual transistors available in the same metal case, assuring good thermal coupling. For circuits where transistors must be maintained at a constant temperature, the classical solution to the problem has been actually to put them in miniature ovens whose temperatures are thermostatically controlled. Fairchild has recently come

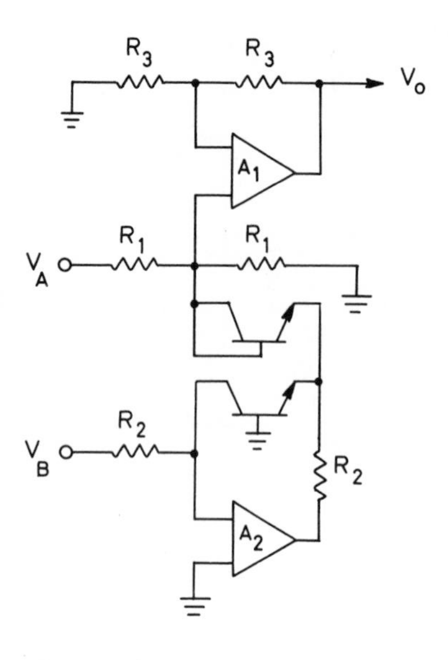

Figure 3.20
Log-of-ratio circuit (after Figure 2.28c, in *Application Manual for Operational Amplifiers*, 1968, by Philbrick/Nexus Research. Used with permission of Teledyne Philbrick).

$$V_o = \log V_1 - \log V_2 = \log \frac{V_1}{V_2}.$$

Vary resistors for changes in gain, baseline, and weighting of input values.

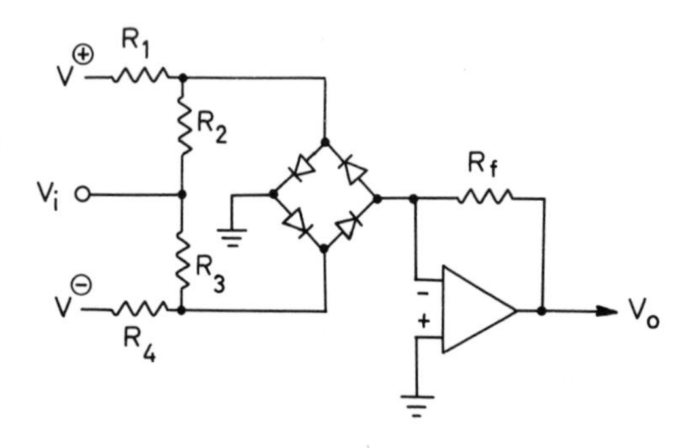

Figure 3.21
"Dead-zone" amplifier (after Figure 2.44a, in *Application Manual for Operational Amplifiers*, 1968, by Philbrick/Nexus Research. Used with permission of Teledyne Philbrick.).

When $V^- \dfrac{R_2}{R_1} < V_i < V^+ \dfrac{R_4}{R_3}$, $\quad V_o \cong 0.$

When $V_i < V^- \dfrac{R_2}{R_1}$, $\quad V_o = -\left(\dfrac{V_i}{R_2} + \dfrac{V^-}{R_1}\right) R_f.$

When $V_i > V^+ \dfrac{R_4}{R_3}$, $\quad V_o = -\left(\dfrac{V_i}{R_4} + \dfrac{V^+}{R_3}\right) R_f.$

up with an ingenious solution to the problem: the temperature-controlled transistor pair, the 726, an integrated circuit that consists of two NPN transistors on the same integrated circuit chip with a temperature-regulating circuit. The temperature regulator consists of a circuit that passes a large amount of current at lower temperatures and lesser amounts of current at higher temperatures. The current flow produces heat, which warms the integrated circuit chip. An external resistor is used to set the operating temperature of the device, and the geometry of the integrated circuit is such that the two NPN transistors are held at the same temperature. Fairchild has also developed an operational amplifier on a chip with integral temperature control. This allows extremely low-drift dc operation in environments with fluctuating ambient temperatures.

Two more nonlinear circuits which are of use to neurophysiologists are the "dead-zone" amplifier and the "clipper" circuit shown in Figures 3.21 and 3.22, respectively. The dead-zone amplifier prevents voltages below a certain value from being amplified; voltages above this level are amplified with constant gain; thus, voltages near zero are not "seen" at the output, and voltages farther from zero are amplified as the positive or negative input voltage minus the threshold, times the gain of the circuit.

The clipping circuit does the converse: Voltages near zero are amplified at a constant gain, and voltages beyond the lower and upper limits V^+ and V^- are

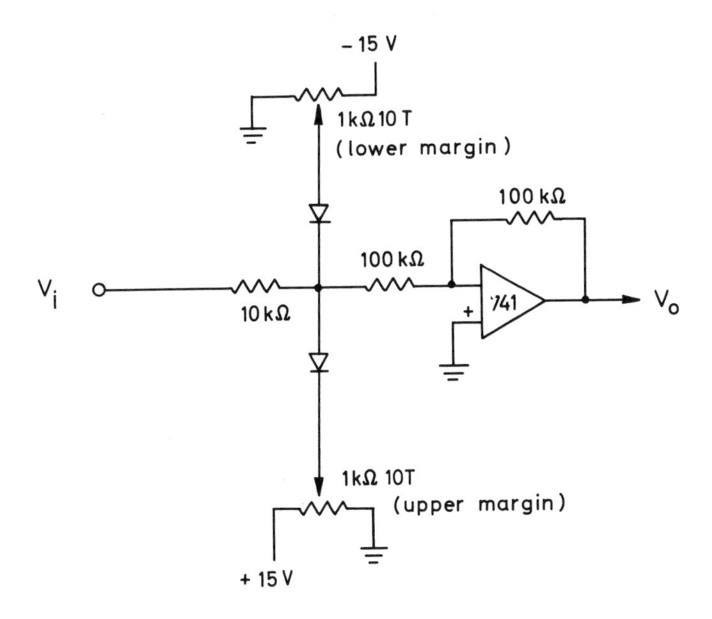

Figure 3.22
Clipping circuit.

"clipped" at the limiting levels minus the diode voltage drops. The positive and negative limits are independently controlled in this circuit.

Since op amps are not really the ideal elements we have described, it is necessary to take into account their nonideal characteristics. We have already discussed some of these. Some useful guides to the use of op amps are also included.

3.4 Simple Modifications of Input, Output, and Feedback Circuits

There are various means of modifying the input and output properties of op amp circuits and means that can be used to protect them against accidental faults, such as short circuits or deteriorating components. Such techniques are essentially specialized compensations for nonideal circuit parameters, especially input and output impedances.

The two most common requirements for the input stage of an analog circuit are (a) input protection from common-mode and single-ended overvoltages (*note:* the limits on positive or negative voltages at each input usually do not define the com-

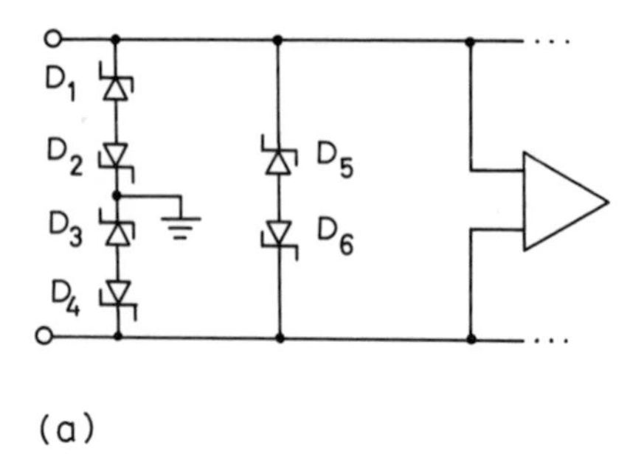

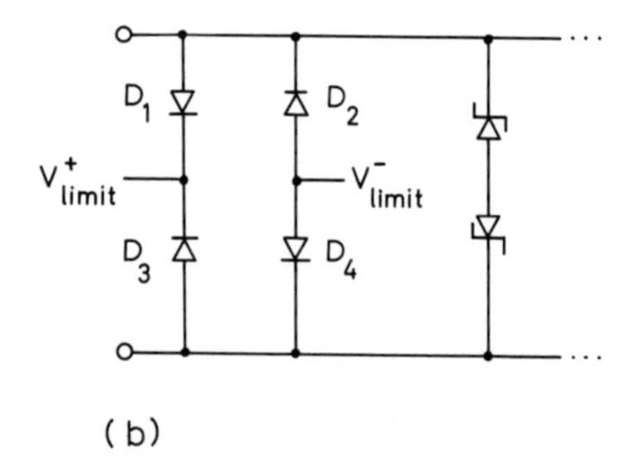

Figure 3.23
Input overvoltage protection: (a) using zener diodes; (b) using diodes and limiting voltages.

mon-mode voltage limit), and (b) sufficiently high input impedance to prevent overloading the signal source.

Figure 3.23a illustrates the use of diodes to protect an amplifier from excess voltages on either input (D_1–D_2 and D_3–D_4) and common-mode excess voltage (D_5–D_6). Each zener is prevented from conducting in its forward direction by the other zener in series with it. When the reverse bias on either zener of a pair is in excess of the zener breakdown voltage, the diode that is reverse-biased breaks down and conducts through the other diode, holding the total voltage drop close to the zener voltage of the reverse-biased diode. Zeners D_1–D_4 may be replaced by parallel diodes connected to "limiting voltage" sources (Figure 3.23b) in the reverse-biased configurations, but this will result in lower impedances, which may interfere with circuit performance. Choose zener breakdown voltages at least half a volt below the voltage limit desired; high reverse impedances are necessary.

The circuits of Figure 3.24 illustrate the use of voltage feedback, usually in order to maintain a high imput impedance. Note that the only load on V_i is the op amp input impedance, rather than a series resistor to a virtual ground or other reference point. The gain of the circuits is computed by assuming that the negative input voltage very nearly equals the positive input voltage V_i.

Thus, for Figure 3.24a, the net gain must be unity, because

$$V_o = V^- = V^+ = V_i. \tag{3.47}$$

The circuit of Figure 3.24b feeds back a fraction of the output voltage that is less than unity, thus the gain must be greater than unity:

$$V^- = (V_o/(R_1 + R_2)) \cdot R_2 = V^+ = V_i;$$

therefore,

$$V_0 = V_i(R_1 + R_2)/R_2. \tag{3.48}$$

This often is referred to as potentiometric feedback.

The circuit of Figure 3.24c may have more or less than unity gain, depending on whether the interposed gain element in the feedback loop has less or more than unity gain, respectively:

$$V^- = V_o R_f/R_i = V^+ = V_i;$$

therefore,

$$V_o = V_i R_i/R_f. \tag{3.49}$$

However, owing to additional phase lag in the feedback loop, extra precautions must often be taken to prevent instability. The technique usually has no advan-

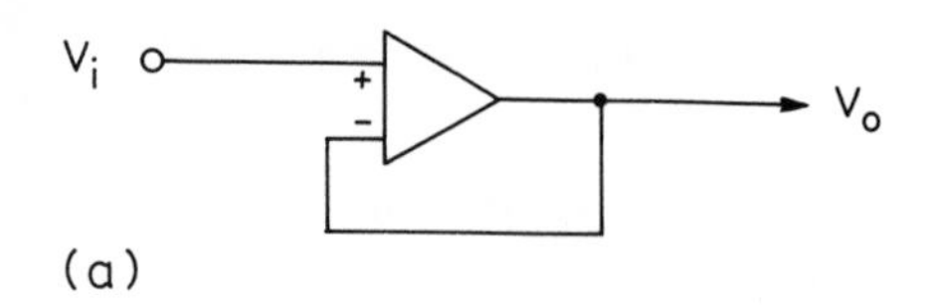

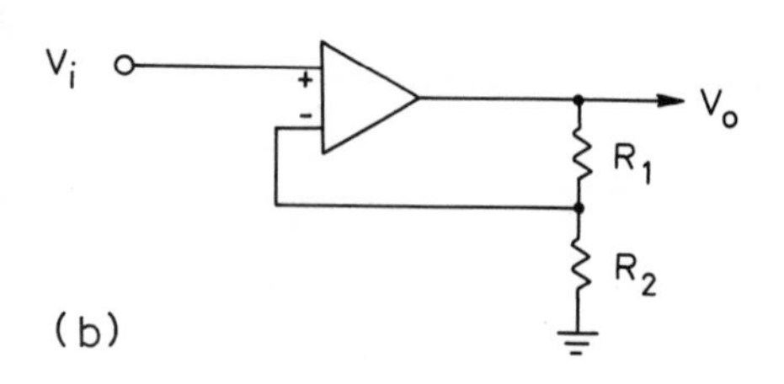

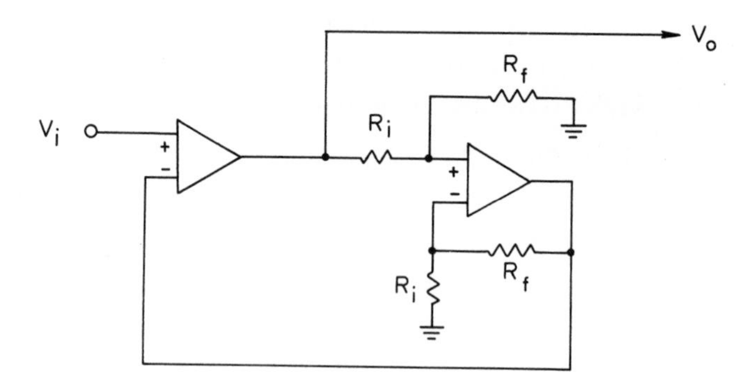

(c)

Figure 3.24
Voltage feedback, a method for noninverting amplification:
(a) unity gain follower, where $V_o = V_i$;
(b) potentiometric feedback, where

$$V_o = V_i \frac{(R_1 + R_2)}{R_2};$$

(c) interposed gain element in feedback loop, where

$$V_o = V_i \frac{R_i}{R_f}.$$

tage over a unity-gain configuration such as that of Figure 3.24a followed in series by a noninverting negative-feedback amplifier.

Conventional bipolar IC op amps generally have input impedances ranging from 10 kΩ to 10 MΩ. Recently introduced FET-input op amp hybrids can have input impedances as high as 10^{12} Ω. These are useful for such applications as microelectrode amplifiers, sample-and-hold circuits, and some types of filters. These applications are discussed in later chapters.

Before going on to consider device output modifications, we will examine a simple technique for limiting feedback current without resorting to high feedback resistances. Such a tactic is useful, because very high feedback resistances give rise to instabilities and noise problems. The circuit of Figure 3.25 illustrates the use of a "Tee" network to reduce feedback current without resorting to high feedback resistances. In fact, we can select the effective "R_o" (resistance to ground seen by the output) and "R_f" (V_o/I_f) to fit any value desired, by appropriate choice of components. There results not only a decrease in noise and an increase in stability but also a decrease in the effect of stray capacitance.

We can calculate the "effective" output, input, and feedback resistances (all three are, of course, the same in a simple resistive-feedback circuit utilizing a single resistor):

$$R_o = R_2 + \frac{1}{\dfrac{1}{R_1} + \dfrac{1}{R_3}} = \frac{R_1 R_3}{R_1 + R_3} + R_2 = \frac{R_1 R_2 + R_2 R_3 + R_1 R_3}{R_1 + R_3}.$$

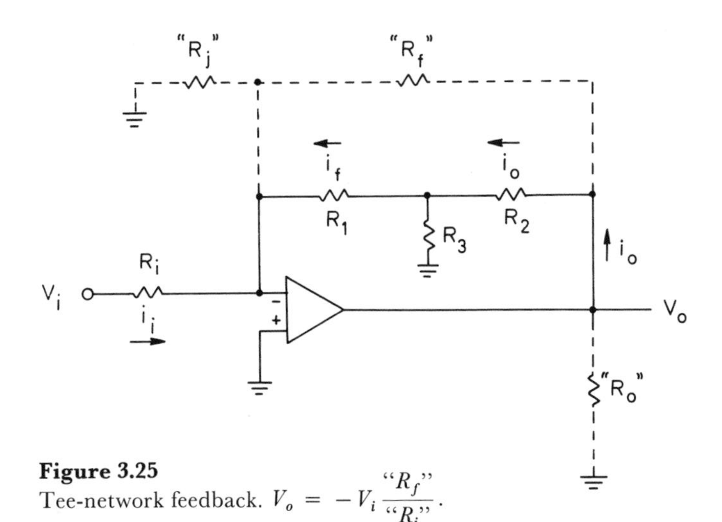

Figure 3.25
Tee-network feedback. $V_o = -V_i \dfrac{\text{"}R_f\text{"}}{\text{"}R_i\text{"}}$.

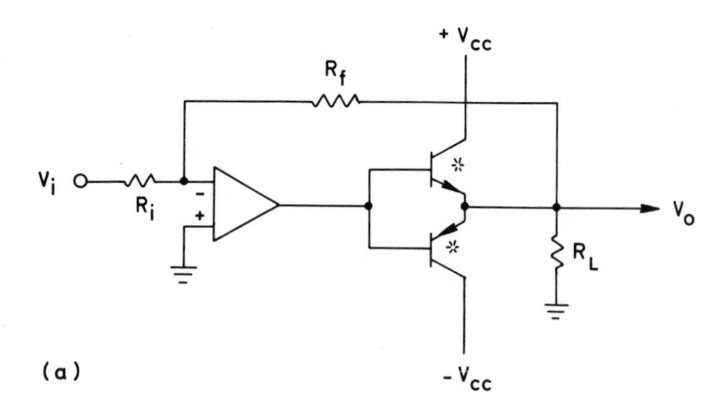

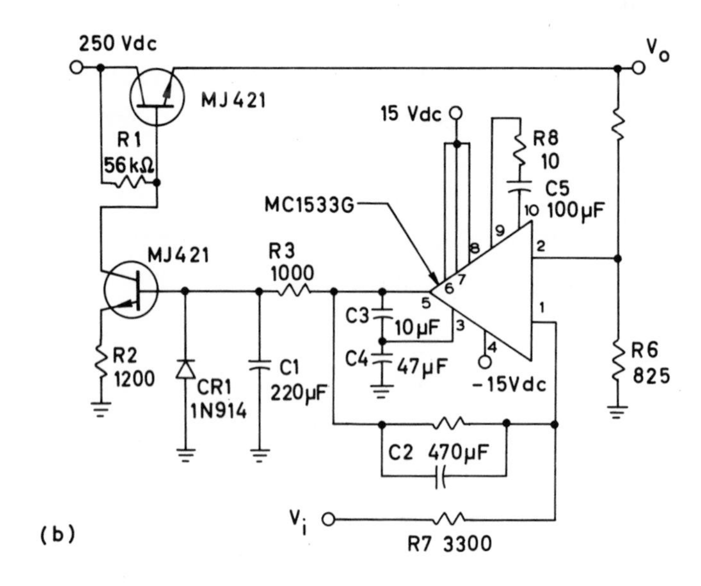

Figure 3.26
(a) Current booster. $V_o = -V_i \frac{R_f}{R_i}$. Use heat sinks (*) and power transistors if necessary. (b) Voltage-boost circuit (from "IC amp with 200 V output uses few components," 1971, by Robert Oswald, *Electronic Design 19*, 17: 82. Used with permission of *Electronic Design*.).

Assuming zero output impedance of the amplifier itself, we have

$$R_j = R_1 + \frac{1}{\frac{1}{R_2} + \frac{1}{R_3}} = \frac{R_2R_3}{R_2 + R_3} + R_1 = \frac{R_1R_2 + R_1R_3 + R_2R_3}{R_2 + R_3}.$$

We know $I_o = V_o/R_o$; therefore,

$$I_f = \frac{V_1}{R_1} = \frac{V_o - (I_oR_2)}{R_1} = \frac{V_o - \dfrac{V_oR_2(R_1 + R_3)}{R_1R_2 + R_2R_3 + R_1R_3}}{R_1}$$

$$R_f = \frac{V_o}{I_f} = \frac{R_1}{1 - \dfrac{R_2(R_1 + R_3)}{R_1R_2 + R_2R_3 + R_1R_3}}$$

$$= \frac{R_1}{\dfrac{R_1R_2 + R_2R_3 + R_1R_3 - R_1R_2 - R_2R_3}{R_1R_2 + R_2R_3 + R_1R_3}}$$

$$= \frac{R_1R_2 + R_2R_3 + R_1R_3}{R_3};$$

for values of

$R_1 = 2\ \mathrm{k}\Omega$,
$R_2 = 2\ \mathrm{k}\Omega$,
$R_3 = 10\ \mathrm{k}\Omega$,

we obtain

$R_o \cong 2\ \mathrm{k}\Omega$
$R_j \cong 2\ \mathrm{k}\Omega$
$R_f \cong 400\ \mathrm{k}\Omega$.

Low R_o and R_j ensure low noise and good stability, and R_f provides a low feedback current for high gain operation.

Figure 3.26a illustrates current boosting of an op amp output. Although there is a dead zone in which the output of the op amp will not cause either emitter follower to conduct, this is compensated for by bringing the feedback from the output of the entire circuit rather than from the output of the op amp. The resulting "crossover distortion" is insignificant for most applications and is roughly inversely proportional to the ratio of circuit gain to amplifier gain—that is, for a given circuit gain, distortion is minimized by using the highest open-loop op amp gain *m* possible. Bandwidth is slightly reduced.

Voltage-boosting is much more difficult to accomplish; the simplest solution is to use a high-voltage op amp in the first place. However, there is an ingenious and inexpensive method, developed by Robert Oswald (1971), using a high-voltage regulator as an amplifier. These devices are generally used as voltage regulators in power supplies, but they are essentially op amps. Figure 3.26b illustrates this application. Normally the input would be a reference voltage, and the amplifier output would be the regulated supply voltage. The gain of this amplifier configuration is $(R_5 + R_6)/R_6$.

Some op amps tend to become unstable and oscillate if they are connected to loads with too much capacitance to ground. Properly terminating their outputs with series resistors is often adequate; otherwise, it will be necessary to lower the output impedance with a current-boost stage, adding a series resistor *outside* the feedback loop for termination.

Bound operation (Figure 3.27) is a mode of operation wherein the output voltage limits are held lower than the gain times the input voltage limits. Although this can be accomplished by clipping at the input, we can look upon the bound operation as more of a circuit protection, preventing the amplifier from having to work too hard pushing large amounts of current through a feedback resistor to maintain zero input differential current. In essence, the pairs of zener diodes (zener breakdown voltage chosen according to desired limits) conduct only when the desired bounds are exceeded. The normal feedback path is the only one that is significant below the bounds (the resistive path must be a few orders of magnitude more conductive than the diode in this state), and the diode path carries part of the current above the bounds, allowing much greater feedback current with an insignificant increase in output voltage.

In some applications, for example, in bench design work, it is wise to protect the op amp from the ill effects of short circuiting the output. The simplest technique is to put a fuse on the output, rated below the output current limits of the op amp. For many circuits, this will be adequate, because some can operate in the shorted mode for a few seconds. Some op amps are internally protected against

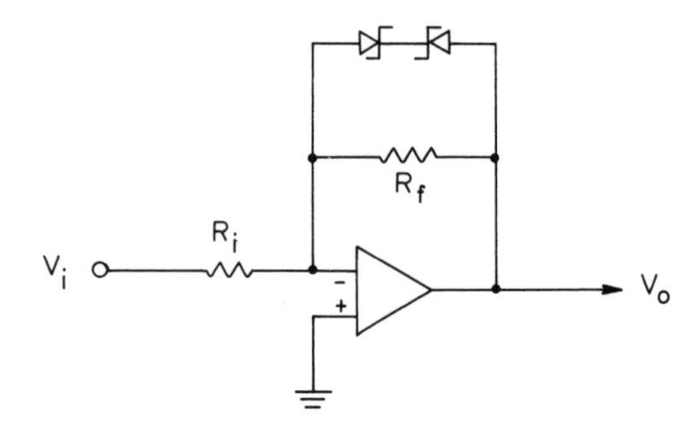

Figure 3.27
Bound operation of op amp.

shorting output to ground for indefinite periods. But for some amplifiers, there would be a risk of irreversible damage to the circuit even before a fuse could blow. A simple approach is to use an output resistor in series with the output, such that the short circuit current will still be less than the tolerable limits. If this solution is not acceptable because of requirements for low output impedance, the current-boost configuration can be used, with cheap transistors in transistor sockets. For a few cents each, transistors can be found that will serve as solid-state "fuses." Chapter 11 discusses a means of dynamically limiting output current.

We must protect large circuits built out of op amp building blocks from the effects of component breakdown: Even semiconductors "go bad" in the best-designed circuits. The power to the circuit should be fused at slightly more than the estimated maximum current drain.

Also, since the power lines have a finite time constant, the power supply regulator cannot totally prevent transients from occurring in the power leads to one circuit as a result of current surges in another circuit. To prevent this, "decouple" each circuit card from the others by connecting a 0.001–0.2 μF capacitor between each supply voltage and ground, at each point where power is introduced into the card. In some applications it is best to decouple the power leads right at each op amp socket. Where very small signals are processed, on-board IC voltage regulators may be required. Decoupling and regulation are discussed in detail in Chapters 6 and 11.

3.5 Operational Amplifier Performance Specifications

Selecting an operational amplifier, or any other analog device, requires an intelligent examination of data sheet specifications. We will review the specifications that are most commonly provided for such devices, in order to give some feeling for the properties which must be taken into account in the process of selection. Some of these parameters have been defined elsewhere, but they are provided here in order to assemble all the op amp specifications in one convenient list:

1. *Input Resistance and Capacitance.* These are the resistance and capacitance presented by either input to a signal, with the other input grounded. Differential measures may also be provided, representing the series resistance or capacitance across the two inputs. Resistance is usually measured with a low-frequency ac signal, to avoid effects of input dc offset. The ideal op amp has infinite input resistance and zero input capacitance.

2. *Input Offset Voltage.* This is the dc voltage that must be applied differentially to the amplifier inputs to produce a zero output voltage. It can vary with tem-

perature and time, and these variations are often specified. Variations in supply voltage, and in some applications, source and feedback resistances, may also affect this figure. The ideal op amp offset voltage is zero.

3. *Input Offset Current.* This is the differential input dc current required to produce a zero output voltage. It is affected by the same factors as the input offset voltage. Ideal op amps have no offset current. Many op amps come with offset adjust input pins, whereby the offset voltage and current can be trimmed to very low values with a potentiometer whose end terminals are tied to these pins and whose wiper is tied to one of the supply voltages. These are convenient in that the offset inputs do not affect input parameters or gain, and often trimming results in better temperature dependence of dc offset voltage.

4. *Input Offset Drift.* This is the average drift of dc offset, with time or temperature. Both are zero in an ideal op amp.

5. *Input Bias Current.* Whereas the last three specifications refer to differential dc voltage or current, input bias current is the average of the two input currents required to bring the output to zero volts. This average is essentially the *common-mode* dc offset current. It is zero in an ideal op amp. It may be affected by supply voltages or temperature, and it may drift with time.

6. *Input Voltage Range.* Input voltages outside this range will cause improper operation of the op amp, which may range from increased nonlinearity to clipping. Single-ended (one input grounded) and differential figures may be separately specified. The ideal op amp has no input voltage limit. This specification may be affected by temperature, and is usually related to supply voltage.

7. *Transfer Characteristics.* This is most commonly represented as a plot of open-loop gain m versus frequency f where gain is in dB, and frequency is also plotted on a logarithmic scale. The designer must select an op amp which has the desired gain capability over the frequency band of interest keeping in mind the effect of gain margin on gain error (see closed-loop gain error, below). For high-gain, high-frequency applications, it is often necessary to use an op amp with external frequency compensation. One problem with such devices is the common requirement for different compensation networks when the device is operated with different closed-loop gains. A novel way of avoiding this problem is applied in the high-gain amplifier of Chapter 9. Different compensation networks also cause different open-loop transfer characteristics. The transfer characteristic may also be affected by temperature and supply voltages. Some data sheets indicate the nature of these variations. The ideal operational amplifier model, used for many of the derivations in this chapter, assumes an infinite gain at all frequencies.

8. *Maximum Output Swing.* This is the output parameter corresponding to input

voltage range: Beyond this range, the op amp will operate improperly, or the op amp is simply incapable of exceeding this range. An ideal op amp has infinite output swing.

9. *Large-Signal Voltage Gain.* Operating open-loop, this is the maximum output voltage swing divided by the change in differential input voltage required to produce it. It may be affected by supply voltage, temperature, and frequency. Like any other frequency-dependent variable, it may be affected by changes in the compensation network. Usually the specification refers to a low frequency, where the value is maximum. Ideal op amps have infinite large-signal voltage gain.

10. *Closed-Loop Gain Error.* This is the deviation of the closed-loop gain, using a specified input and feedback network, from the gain predicted by assuming infinite open-loop gain. It is defined as

$$\text{error} = \frac{m'_{\text{theoretical}} - m'_{\text{actual}}}{m'_{\text{theoretical}}} \times 100 \text{ percent.}$$

The error can be approximated if m is known, by

$$\frac{m'}{m} \times 100 \text{ percent} = \frac{1}{\text{gain margin}} \times 100 \text{ percent.}$$

This variable is only specified for situations where other nonidealities are not limiting, such as slew rate and component tolerance. All factors which affect m will affect this specification. Ideal op amps have no closed-loop gain error.

11. *Common-Mode Rejection Ratio* (CMRR). This is the ratio of the input voltage range to the maximum change of input offset voltage over this range and is affected by anything that influences these variables, as well as frequency. This term is often used to describe the inverse of the open-loop gain for a common-mode signal (the common-mode signal is the average of the two input signals). The open-loop gain for such a signal should be the same as the ratio of the common-mode signal to a differential signal that would produce the same output. Since any measure of CMRR is a ratio, it can be expressed in dB. CMRR is a meaningful specification for any device with a differential input. It is infinite in the ideal op amp.

12. *Supply Voltage Rejection Ratio* (SVRR). This is the ratio of a change in supply voltage to the change in input offset voltage that would result in the same output swing. Note that, although this parameter is relatively independent of loop configuration, the actual dependence of output on supply voltage is not. The variable is affected by temperature and frequency of supply voltage fluctuation. An ideal op amp would have infinite SVRR.

13. *Equivalent Input Ripple Voltage.* This is another way of expressing SVRR, that is, the input differential signal amplitude which produces the same output ripple as a given supply ripple. This may be expressed in microvolts at the input per volt at the supply, or as microvolts of equivalent input ripple, assuming 1 V supply ripple. Equivalent ripple for an ideal op amp is zero.

14. *Rise Time.* This is the time the output takes to rise to a new value, in response to a step voltage change at the input. It is usually specified as the time between arrival at the output of 10% of the total output step and 90% of the output shift. Since this is usually the portion of the output step with the highest derivative, the time from baseline to plateau may be significantly longer. Rise time from 10% to 90% is about 4 $RC = 4\tau$ for passive networks, and this sometimes holds for active devices, where $\tau = 1/f_0, f_0$ being the 3 dB frequency of the transfer function. Rise times are sometimes specified separately for large and small steps, or for negative and positive derivatives. Ideal op amps have zero rise times.

15. *Overshoot.* As implied by the term, this is the degree to which the response to a step overshoots the plateau at the output, usually expressed as percent of output step size. It is zero for an ideal op amp.

16. *Settling Time.* This is the time, measured from the beginning of an input voltage step, after which the output will never deviate more than a specified amount from the theoretical plateau value. This implies that the error value must be larger than the error of the final steady-state plateau. If the output "rings" (rises to a damped oscillation around the plateau value), the settling time refers to that time at which the last oscillation, which exceeds the $\pm$ error margins, reenters the permissible boundaries. The error is usually specified as the percentage of the actual output voltage plateau, and is therefore not a function of step size in contrast to rise time. It is calculated for worst-case conditions of step size and final plateau voltage, at specified temperature, source impedance, and load impedance. Settling time is also a useful concept for analog switches, where the time is measured from the onset of the control pulse (see Chapter 5 for a description of analog switches). Ideal settling time is of course zero.

17. *Linearity.* This is a worst-case figure for deviation of the device from a fixed ratio of output to input voltage, over the maximum operating range, under open-loop conditions (in the case of a feedback device such as an op amp). It is usually specified for a given temperature and frequency range.

18. *Distortion.* There are two types of distortion: *harmonic distortion*, where the output signal is entirely derived from the input signal, but it is not a faithful reproduction of the expected output (neglecting phase lags or linear attenuation of

frequency components), and *intermodulation distortion*, derived from some signal other than the input, such as interference from another signal channel in a multichannel device. Both types of distortion are usually expressed as the amount of power contained in frequencies other than the test input sine wave frequency. Harmonic distortion consists of energy contained entirely in harmonics of the input sine wave. If all other inputs in a multichannel device are limited to frequencies that are not harmonics of the input sine wave, intermodulation distortion is in frequencies other than harmonics of the input sine wave, namely, harmonics of the frequencies present in the other channels. Both are expressed as a percent of the output power at the desired frequency, or as number of dB down of the desired output frequency. They may be combined, as the total power at *all* frequencies other than the desired one. An ideal device has no distortion.

19. *Output Resistance.* Expressed in ohms, this is the resistance presented by the output when an external voltage source is connected, and when the output without any load is zero. Ideal op amps have zero output impedance; that is, they are perfect voltage sources.

Noise is essentially everything in a signal that isn't supposed to be there. This includes pickup and distortion, but noise specifications for operational amplifiers are generally restricted to *random* noise, that is, noise having no relation to input or interference signals and showing no sign of periodicity. Such noise is generated for the most part at the molecular level, due to random thermal agitation of charge carriers or other random effects. Statistical mechanics has provided means for predicting certain properties that, on the average, are observed in random noise:

(a) *Zero serial correlation.* Knowledge of the voltage at one point in time does not provide knowledge of voltage at any later time, except where there is an upper frequency cutoff, in which case serial correlation diminishes to 0 with time.

(b) *Additivity of noise power.* If two random noise signals are added, then *on the average*, the output power at any frequency is equal to the sum of the powers at that frequency in the two noise inputs, and the output is random.

(c) *Any linear transformation* of a random noise produces a random noise.

Gaussian noise has the following additional properties:

(d) *Normal voltage distribution.* The probability distribution of the voltage over a large number of equally spaced sampling intervals is a normal distribution with zero mean, and the standard deviation is equal to the rms voltage. There is no theoretical peak voltage, although the probability that the voltage will be below a certain value at any time can be computed from the rms voltage, using the equation for the normal distribution. Thus the absolute voltage is

$$\text{less than} \left\{ \begin{array}{ll} \text{rms} \times 2, & 68\% \\ \text{rms} \times 4, & 96\% \\ \text{rms} \times 5, & 99\% \\ \text{rms} \times 6, & 99.9\% \\ \text{rms} \times 8, & 99.99\% \end{array} \right\} \text{of the time.}$$

White noise has the following additional property:

(e) *Flat power spectrum.* The power contained in any frequency component is, on the average, the same as the power in any other frequency component. If band-pass filtering is applied, the output power spectrum is flat for that portion of the spectrum over which the filter transfer function is flat.

Thermal, or "Johnson," noise is Gaussian noise generated by thermal agitation of charge carriers in resistors. The formula predicting the rms noise voltage E_J generated in a resistor with no load is

$$E_J = \sqrt{Rkt\,\Delta f} \cong 7.4 \times 10^{-12}\sqrt{Rt\,\Delta f}, \tag{3.50}$$

where R = resistance of the thermal noise source, k = Boltzman's constant, t = temperature in degrees K (= 273 + °C), and Δf = bandwidth, dc excluded. For most well-designed devices, including op amps, most of the noise generated internal to the device, as seen at the output, is that generated at the input stage. Therefore noise is usually that measured at the output, referred back to the input.

20. *Input Noise Voltage.* This is the rms narrow-band voltage measured at the output, divided by the gain. This usually consists of white noise and so-called pink $1/f$ or "flicker" noise. The frequency components of the latter have power contents proportional to $1/f$, exclusive of very low frequencies. The major components are relatively low frequencies, however, as is suggested by the proportionality of power to the reciprocal of frequency. The noise is random, even though it

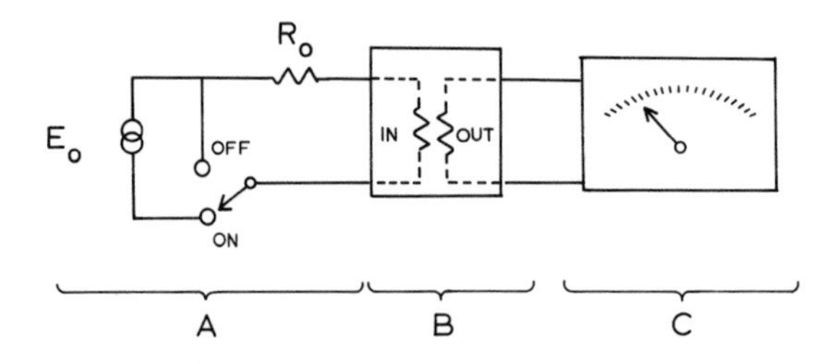

Figure 3.28
Model for derivation of noise figure. *A* is signal generator, *B* is 4-terminal linear device, *C* is rms meter.

is not white. The rms voltage of bandpass white noise is proportional to the square root of the bandwidth, and the rms voltage of $1/f$ noise is proportional to the log of the ratio of upper bandpass limit to lower bandpass limit. That is, for white noise we know that the power is the same at each frequency, so the rms bandpass voltage, which is proportional to the square root of the bandpass power, must be

$$\text{white rms} = \sqrt{\int_a^b K\,df} = k\sqrt{b - a}.$$

Flicker noise rms voltage must be

$$\text{flicker rms} = \sqrt{\int_a^b \frac{K}{f}\,df} = k\sqrt{\log \frac{b}{a}}.$$

Since the powers of these two random components must be additive,

$$\text{rms}_{\text{total}} = \sqrt{(\text{rms}_{\text{flicker}})^2 + (\text{rms}_{\text{white}})^2}. \tag{3.51}$$

Op amp specifications for noise are usually expressed as rms volts per $\sqrt{\text{Hz}}$ or mean square volts per Hz. When flicker noise is significant, two or three different values may be given for different frequency bands. Some specifications indicate equivalent input noise as a function of temperature, source resistance, or frequency.

The input resistance that would produce the calculated input rms noise voltage over a specified bandwidth can be calculated using Equation 3.50. This is sometimes referred to as the equivalent input noise resistance.

The following discussion of noise figure F is based on the treatment by Goldman (1967). If a signal source is coupled to an amplifier whose output is subjected to appropriate measurements, the system as a whole is amenable to description in terms of certain standard specifications which describe the relations of signal and noise amplitudes. Consider for example the circuit of Figure 3.28, consisting of a signal source with output rms voltage E_o and output resistance R_o; a four-terminal input/output device; and an rms meter. We can define the *signal-to-noise ratio*, sometimes called the *noise rating*, of this system as the ratio of rms signal voltage to rms noise voltage, determined by the rms meter reading with E_o on and off:

$$\begin{aligned} S/N &= \frac{\text{rms signal voltage}}{\text{rms noise voltage}} \\ &= \frac{(\text{rms meter reading with signal on}) - (\text{reading with signal off})}{(\text{rms meter reading with signal off})} \end{aligned} \tag{3.52}$$

The signal is turned off by bypassing the generator of E.

Other common S/N ratios are (a) ratio of peak-to-peak voltages and (b) ratio of signal power to noise power. The rms voltage and power ratios may be expressed in decibels, or the noise may be specified as number of decibels below the signal level.

The maximum power that can be delivered by the signal generator is

$$S_g = \frac{E_o^2}{4R_o} \tag{3.53}$$

if the output impedance of the source is perfectly matched with the input impedance of the 4-terminal network. Commonly, S_g is referred to as *available signal power*. The available power at the output of the 4-terminal device is called the *available output power*

$$S = \frac{E^2}{R}, \tag{3.54}$$

where S = output power, E = output rms voltage, and R = output impedance.

We can now define *available power gain* G as

$$G = \frac{S}{S_g}. \tag{3.55}$$

Generally, G is defined as the ratio S/S_g for the middle of the 4-terminal network's pass band.

If G_f is the available power gain of the network for frequency f, the *effective bandwidth* B is

$$B = \frac{1}{G}\int G_f\, df. \tag{3.56}$$

The noise power generated within R_o in the frequency interval df is

$$\frac{E_n^2}{4R_o} = \frac{4ktR_o\, df}{4R_o} = kt\, df. \tag{3.57}$$

If the device has no power gain, but is merely an impedance transformer with input impedance R_o and output impedance R, output power equals input power. If the network has power gain, the anticipated output noise power, neglecting internally generated noise, would be $ktBG$.

We can therefore define the ideal *available input noise power* N_g as

$$N_g = ktB, \tag{3.58}$$

obtained by dividing the ideal output noise power $ktBG$ by the gain G. Since the network is not ideal, it will have an available *output noise power* N such that

$$N > N_g G,$$

although the difference may be unmeasureable in some instances.

21. *Noise Figure.* A common specification for amplifiers is called the *noise figure* F defined as

$$F = \frac{\text{available input signal power/ideal available input noise power}}{\text{available output signal power/available output noise power}}$$

$$= \frac{S_g/ktB}{S/N} = \frac{N}{GktB}. \tag{3.59}$$

Inspection will reveal that this is the ratio of ideal input signal-to-noise ratio to actual output signal to noise ratio. This is equivalent to the ratio of the actual available output noise power to the available output noise power of an ideal network having the same gain characteristic. The noise figure of a network that generates no noise of its own is therefore $F = 1$, and of course the component of the noise figure of a real network due to noise generated within the network must be $F - 1$.

Generally, measurement of noise figure does not follow this idealized procedure. Usually only approximate impedance matching is used, on the grounds that signal and noise are equally mismatched. Reactive components may cause a differential mismatch of signal and noise at different frequencies, due to different frequency composition of the two inputs E_o^2 and E_n^2. This can be circumvented by using a bandpass white noise as E_o^2, since E_o^2 and E_n^2 will then both have the same frequency components. The signal generator used for such measurements is therefore commonly a white noise generator.

22. *Tangential Noise.* If a variable-amplitude square wave is summed with noise of smaller amplitude, and an oscilloscope sweep is allowed to free run, the display will consist of two bands across the screen, with noise superimposed on each band. If the square wave is adjusted to that amplitude at which the two bands of noise begin to merge on the oscilloscope trace, the amplitude of the square wave is equal to the so-called tangential noise. This is a convenient, easy measure of the voltage resolution of which the system is capable; furthermore, it is roughly equal to twice the rms noise, providing a crude measure of the rms noise level if an rms meter is not available.

Finally, two other parameters are often specified for op amps:

23. *Power Consumption.* This is the maximum power consumed by the op amp *with no load*, at a specified combination of supply voltages and temperature.

ABSOLUTE MAXIMUM RATINGS

Supply Voltage	±22 V
Internal Power Dissipation	500 mW
Differential Input Voltage	±30 V
Input Voltage	±15 V
Voltage between Offset Null and V−	±0.5 V
Storage Temperature Range	−65°C to +150°C
Operating Temperature Range	−55°C to +125°C
Lead Temperature (Soldering, 60 sec)	300°C
Output Short-Circuit Duration	Indefinite

CONNECTION DIAGRAM
(TOP VIEW)

OFFSET NULL 1, INVERTING INPUT 2, NON-INVERTING INPUT 3, V− 4, OFFSET NULL 5, OUTPUT 6, V+ 7, NC 8

NOTE: PIN 4 CONNECTED TO CASE

ELECTRICAL CHARACTERISTICS ($V_S = \pm 15$ V, $T_A = 25°C$ unless otherwise specified)

PARAMETER	CONDITIONS	MIN.	TYP.	MAX.	UNITS
Input Offset Voltage	$R_S \leq 10$ kΩ		2.0	6.0	mV
Input Offset Current			30	200	nA
Input Bias Current			200	500	nA
Input Resistance		0.3	1.0		MΩ
Large-Signal Voltage Gain	$R_L \geq 2$ kΩ, $V_{out} = \pm 10$ V	20,000	100,000		
Output Voltage Swing	$R_L \geq 10$ kΩ	±12	±14		V
	$R_L \geq 2$ kΩ	±10	±13		V
Input Voltage Range		±12	±13		V
Common Mode Rejection Ratio	$R_S \leq 10$ kΩ	70	90		dB
Supply Voltage Rejection Ratio	$R_S \leq 10$ kΩ		30	150	μV/V
Power Consumption			50	85	mW
Transient Response (unity gain)	$V_{in} = 20$ mV, $R_L = 2$ kΩ $C_L \leq 100$ pF				
Risetime			0.3		μs
Overshoot			5.0		%
Slew Rate (unity gain)	$R_L \geq 2$ kΩ		0.5		V/μs
The following specifications apply for $0°C \leq T_A \leq +70°C$:					
Input Offset Voltage	$R_S \leq 10$ kΩ			7.5	mV
Input Offset Current				300	nA
Input Bias Current				800	nA
Large-Signal Voltage Gain	$R_L \geq 2$ kΩ, $V_{out} = \pm 10$ V	15,000			
Output Voltage Swing	$R_L \geq 2$ kΩ	±10			V

VOLTAGE OFFSET NULL CIRCUIT

μA741, 10kΩ, V−

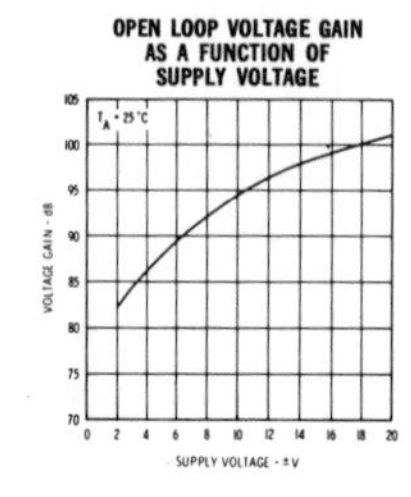

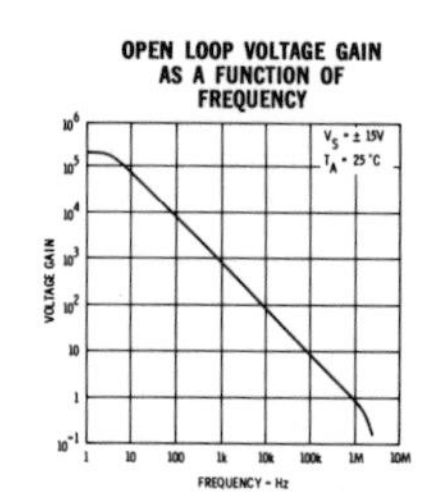

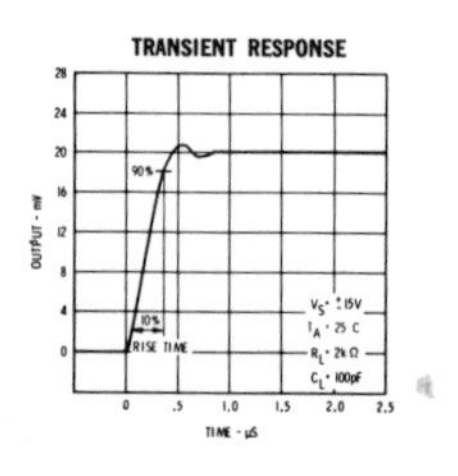

Figure 3.29
Data sheet information for 741 op amp (from *Semiconductor Integrated Circuits Data Catalog, 1970*, by Fairchild Semiconductor. Used with permission of Fairchild Camera and Instrument Corporation.).

24. *Absolute Maximum Ratings.* These are the maximum values of certain operating conditions, beyond which the device may be permanently damaged. They may include the input voltage (differential and single-ended), supply voltages, output short-circuit duration, and temperature.

Data sheet information for the 741 op amp, the most commonly used op amp in this book, is reproduced in Figure 3.29. This information is reproduced by permission of Fairchild Semiconductor.

Selected References

Eimbinder, J. 1969. *Designing with Linear Integrated Circuits.* New York: John Wiley & Sons.

Fairchild Semiconductor. 1970. *Semiconductor Integrated Circuits Data Catalog, 1970.* Mountain View, Calif.: Fairchild Camera and Instrument Corporation.

Goldman, Sanford. 1967. *Frequency Analysis, Modulation and Noise.* New York: Dover Publications.

Morrison, Ralph. 1970. *DC Amplifiers in Instrumentation.* New York: Wiley-Interscience.

Oswald, Robert. 1971. IC amp with 200 V output uses few components. *Electronic Design, 19,* 17: 82.

Philbrick/Nexus Research. 1968. *Application Manual for Operational Amplifiers.* Dedham, Mass.: Philbrick/Nexus.

4 DIGITAL LOGIC

Paul B. Brown

4.1 Analog *vs.* Digital Signals; Positive Feedback

A device that has a finite number of discrete stable output states is often used to implement computing functions, with the output used to represent numerical values. Because of this application, circuits having discrete stable states are called *digital* circuits. A digital circuit that has only two stable states is called a *binary* circuit; these are the ones most generally used in digital computation, because the two states can correspond to saturation and cutoff in a transistor.

An example of such a device is the positive-feedback op amp configuration of Figure 4.1a. The input-output function is illustrated in Figure 4.1b. The output of such a circuit is shown in 4.1e, for the sinusoidal input of Figure 4.1c. The output of a negative-feedback circuit like that of Figure 3.1 is given for comparison in Figure 4.1d. The only possible output states of the positive feedback circuit are $\pm V_{max}$ (except during the rapid transitions from one state to the other). Note also that the input states between the output voltage transitions cannot uniquely determine the value of the output, because there are two possible output values for any input voltage within that range. Such a dual-valued, input-output relation, which is a function of the existing state of the output (that is, the point of entry to the dual-valued region), is termed *hysteresis* and is a property of positive-feedback devices.

Theoretically, if an ideal op amp output were initially zero and the differential

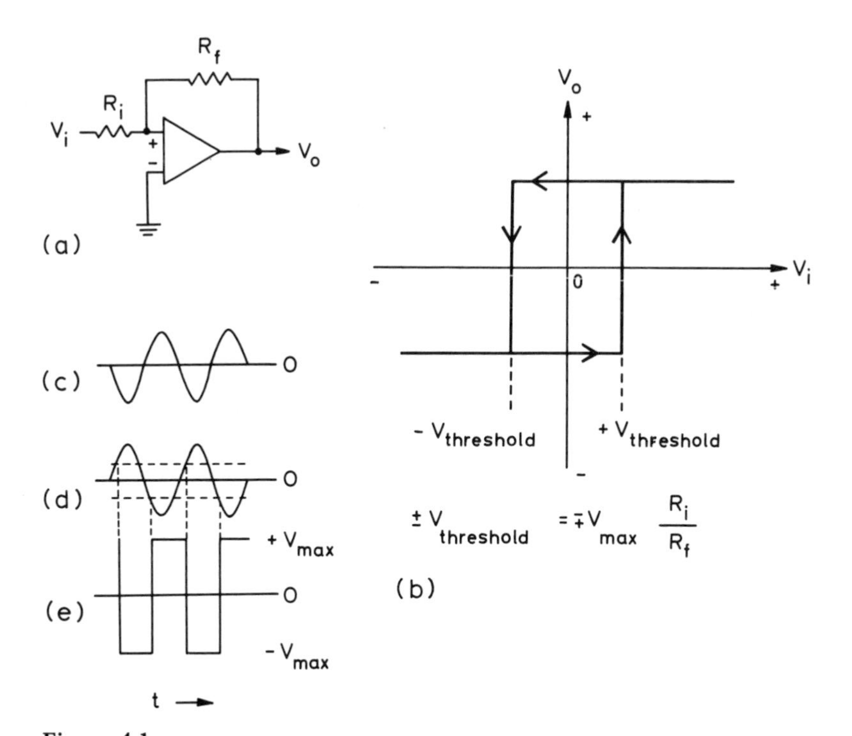

Figure 4.1
Positive feedback configuration: (a) generalized schematic; (b) input-output characteristic; (c) input sine wave; (d) output of negative feedback circuit of Figure 4.1, where $R_f = R_i$; (e) output of positive feedback circuit in part (a) of this figure, where

$R_f = \frac{1}{2}R_i$.

input voltage (in this case V_i) were also zero, the output would be stable at zero volts, because the feedback would be zero, and the amplifier would see a zero differential input. However, small deviations from ideality, such as input offset voltage or thermal noise, would tend to cause the amplifier output to drift away from zero. Once this drift had begun, it would be fed back to the noninverting input via the feedback resistor. This would then be amplified, driving the output voltage farther away from zero, *in the same direction.* This enlarged voltage difference would be fed back and further enlarged, in a self-regenerative loop that would force the amplifier voltage to one output voltage extreme or the other. Hence the zero voltage output, which would logically result from a zero input voltage, constitutes a *metastable* state, because any slight deviation would be regeneratively amplified. In the negative feedback configuration, any small deviation would be compensated by the negative feedback, to pull the output back to zero. In contrast, the two voltage extremes of the positive feedback configuration are truly stable output states for the device.

We specify that the circuit is *binary* (and hence digital), because it has only two stable output voltage states. However, the output frequency or pulse duration may be continuously variable (analog). Such a distinction is analogous to the distinction between all-or-nothing action potential voltage and continuously variable action potential frequency or interval in neural coding.

We have noted that returning the input voltage V_i to zero does not suffice to bring the differential input voltage to zero, because of the positive feedback. This means that we must actually exceed a *threshold* of opposite polarity before the device will switch to the other extreme. This process, whereby a simple return of the input voltage to zero is not adequate to bring the output voltage back to zero, is described by saying the amplifier "latches." This is reflected in the input-output curve of the device by the hysteresis portion of the function (Figure 4.1b).

The threshold for switching is

$$\pm V_{\text{threshold}} = \mp V_{\text{max}} \frac{R_i}{R_f} \tag{4.1}$$

where $V_{\text{threshold}}$ is defined as the voltage V_i needed to make the output transition to the opposite extreme.

A general form of the equation is the equation for the positive feedback adder-subtracter, illustrated in Figure 4.2,

$$\left(\sum_{i=a}^{n} \frac{V_i}{R_i} - \sum_{j=p}^{t} \frac{V_j}{R_j} \right)_{\text{threshold}} = \frac{-V_o}{R_f}, \tag{4.2}$$

provided that

$$\sum_{i=a}^{n} \frac{1}{R_i} = \sum_{j=p}^{t} \frac{1}{R_j}, \tag{4.3}$$

where $V_o = \pm V_{\text{max}}$, and where R_f is an *adder* term (R_i) instead of a subtracter term, because we now use positive feedback instead of negative feedback.

The equations for an adder-subtracter network are entirely analogous to those used for negative feedback, keeping in mind the fact that Equation 4.2 specifies a *threshold* voltage, and the right-hand term can have only one of two values,

$$\mp \frac{V_{\text{max}}}{R_f}.$$

Binary devices are used for most digital logic electronics, for two major reasons: (1) they are easily constructed, because the outputs of the devices need only occupy the two voltage extremes and not intermediate voltages (that is, they can be

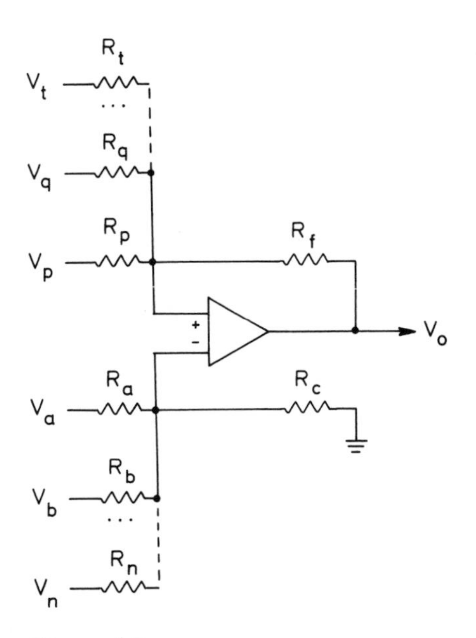

Figure 4.2
Generalized positive feedback adder-subtracter.

$$\left(\pm \sum_{i=a}^{n} \frac{V_i}{R_i} - \sum_{j=p}^{t} \frac{V_j}{R_j}\right)_{\text{threshold}} = \frac{\mp V_{\text{max}}}{R_f},$$

provided that:

$$\sum_{i=a}^{n} \frac{1}{R_i} = \sum_{j=p}^{t} \frac{1}{R_j},$$

where R_f is an *adder* input.

driven to saturation or cutoff, which are easily obtained in comparison with intermediate states), and (2) the two states can be used to represent the two possible states of classical two-valued logic: "true" and "false."

4.2 Principles of Binary Logic

Classically, logic has been a technique for determining the truth or falsity of propositions, given the truth or falsity of related propositions. For example, if the statement, "apples are red," and the statement, "lemons are yellow," are both true, then the statement, "apples are red and lemons are yellow," is also true. This can be represented symbolically:

let A mean "apples are red"
let B mean "lemons are yellow"
let C mean "apples are red and lemons are yellow"
let $\wedge$ mean AND
let $=$ mean "is logically equivalent to."

Table 4.1
Truth table defining logical equivalence.

p	q	$p = q$
True	True	True
True	False	False
False	True	False
False	False	True

Table 4.2
Truth table defining logical AND.

p	q	$p \wedge q$
True	True	True
True	False	False
False	True	False
False	False	False

Then, the equation

$$A \wedge B = C$$

is a symbolic representation of the facts that "apples are red" *and* "lemons are yellow" *is equivalent to* "apples are red and lemons are yellow." The entities A, B, and C (propositions, in classical logic) are called *elements*. The entity *AND* is a *relation*. The relation of logical equivalence can itself be defined by stating that the two sides of a logical equation are equivalent if, for any combination of assumed truth or falsity of the elements (propositions such as A or B), the right side is true if and only if the left side is true, and the right side is false only if the left side is false. We can define the equivalence relation with the "truth table" of Table 4.1.

We can use a truth table (Table 4.2) to define unambiguously the relation "AND" as well.

An unambiguous definition of a relation requires that we define the *resultant* truth value for all possible combinations of the related elements. For a *dyadic* relation (one that relates two elements), there are four possible combinations. In general, we must define the resultant truth value of 2^n different combinations of the truth values of the elements, where n is the number of independent elements in the relation. Thus, for a *monadic* relation, which has only one argument (an argument is an element in a relation), there are only two possible combinations of the truth values of the elements: This is illustrated with the defining truth table

(Table 4.3) for logical inversion INV (represented by a bar before the inverted element).

Note that the definitions of AND and INV correspond very closely to the meanings ascribed to them in everyday usage. There is one more relation (Table 4.4) that we will find useful, which is also similar to that of everyday English usage, OR($\vee$).

This relation corresponds to the "inclusive or" of everyday usage, often expressed as "and/or," and must not be confused with the "exclusive or" (EOR, $\oplus$), which would be false if both elements were true (top line of truth table, Table 4.4).

We can represent each of these relations in several ways, symbolically. Some of the other commonly used representations of AND, OR, and INV are listed in Table 4.5.

Table 4.3
Truth table defining logical INV.

p	$-p$
True	False
False	True

Table 4.4
Truth table defining logical OR.

p	q	$p \vee q$
True	True	True
True	False	True
False	True	True
False	False	False

Table 4.5
Alternative representations of AND, OR, and INV.

p AND q	p OR q	INV p
$p \wedge q$	$p \vee q$	$-p$
$p \cap q$	$p \cup q$	$\bar{p}$
$p \cdot q$	$p + q$	$\tilde{p}$
$p \times q$	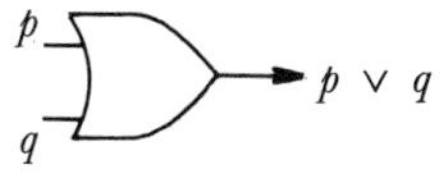	$\sim p$
pq		$\dot{p}$
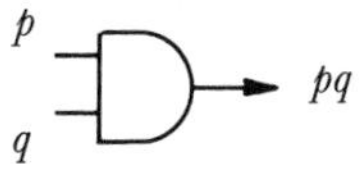		not p
		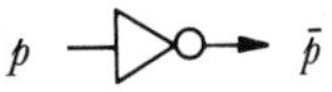

Table 4.6
Truth tables defining NAND and NOR.

p	q	p NAND q	p NOR q
1	1	0	0
0	1	1	0
1	0	1	0
0	0	1	1

Table 4.7
Alternative representations of NAND and NOR.

p NAND q	p NOR q
$p \overline{\wedge} q$	$p \overline{\vee} q$
$p \overline{\cap} q$	$p \overline{\cup} q$
$\overline{(p \cdot q)}$	$\overline{(p + q)}$
$\overline{(p \times q)}$	
$\overline{(pq)}$	
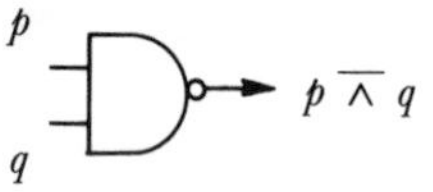 p, q → $p \overline{\wedge} q$	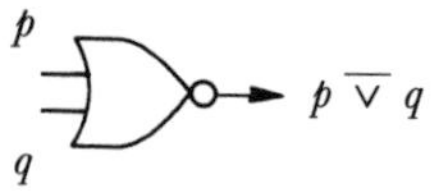 p, q → $p \overline{\vee} q$

We can represent true and false as T and F, + and −, 1 and 0, yes and no, affirmative and negative, up and down, right and left, on and off, in and out, clockwise and counterclockwise, −12 V and 0 V, +5 V and 0 V, and so forth. In the discussions that follow, we will usually use the notation 1 and 0, except where we discuss signals in logic circuits, when we will occasionally refer to the actual voltage levels corresponding to true and false, or refer to a 1 as "on" and a 0 as "off." The use of 1 and 0 will have a further utility in the discussion of binary arithmetic and its implementation.

Transistor-Transistor Logic (TTL) implementation of binary logic most commonly uses three basic logical operations: NAND, NOR, and the familiar INV. The truth tables in Tables 4.6 and 4.7 for NAND and NOR are presented. Note that the operations produce the inverse of AND and OR, respectively. The names are simply contractions of *N*ot *AND* and *N*ot *OR*.

It is possible to group expressions: $(A \overline{\wedge} B) \overline{\vee} (C \overline{\wedge} D)$ means "the quantity $(A \overline{\wedge} B)$ $\overline{\vee}$ the quantity $(C \overline{\wedge} D)$." We can also nest parentheses, as in algebra.

We can substitute logically equivalent terms for each other: Given $B = C$, the terms $(A \wedge B)$ and $(A \wedge C)$ can be freely interchanged in logical expressions.

Thus, for example,

$-[(A \wedge B) \vee D] = -[(A \wedge C) \vee D].$

We now state some theorems of logic that the logical designer will find useful. Two are illustrated with truth tables.

Law of Identity: $A = A$ (4.4)

Laws of Tautology (Table 4.8): $A \wedge A = A$ (4.5a)

$A \vee A = A$ (4.5b)

All three Expressions 4.4, 4.5a, and 4.5b are identical; therefore they are always identical, because A is always either 0 or 1.

Commutative Laws (Table 4.9): $A \wedge B = B \wedge A$ (4.6a)

$A \vee B = B \vee A$ (4.6b)

Distributive Laws: $A \wedge (B \vee C) = (A \wedge B) \vee (A \wedge C)$ (4.7a)

$A \vee (B \wedge C) = (A \vee B) \wedge (A \vee C)$ (4.7b)

Law of Double Negation: $-(-A) = A$ (4.8)

Laws of Absorption: $A \wedge (A \vee B) = A$ (4.9a)

$A \vee (A \wedge B) = A$ (4.9b)

Table 4.8
Truth table proving
A ∧ A = A ∨ A = A.

A	$A \vee A$	$A \wedge A$
1	1	1
0	0	0

Table 4.9
Truth table proving commutative laws.

A	B	$A \wedge B$	$B \wedge A$	$A \vee B$	$B \vee A$
1	1	1	1	1	1
0	1	0	0	1	1
1	0	0	0	1	1
0	0	0	0	0	0
		identical		identical	

Associative Laws: $A \wedge (B \wedge C) = (A \wedge B) \wedge C$ (4.10a)

$$A \vee (B \vee C) = (A \vee B) \vee C \qquad (4.10b)$$

Some other useful relations are:

$$A \wedge 1 = A \qquad A \vee 1 = 1 \qquad (4.11a,b)$$

$$A \wedge 0 = 0 \qquad A \vee 0 = A \qquad (4.12a,b)$$

$$A \wedge \bar{A} = 0 \qquad A \vee \bar{A} = 1 \qquad (4.13a,b)$$

$$(A = -B) = (-B = A) = (-A = B) = (B = -A) \qquad (4.14)$$

$$(A \wedge B) \vee (A \wedge \bar{B}) = A \qquad (4.15)$$

$$(A \vee B) \wedge (A \vee \bar{B}) = A \qquad (4.16)$$

$$\sim(A \wedge B) = \bar{A} \vee \bar{B} \qquad (4.17)$$

$$\sim(A \vee B) = \bar{A} \wedge \bar{B} \qquad (4.18)$$

Equations 4.17 and 4.18 (De Morgan's theorem) are of particular interest: They state that given INV and AND, we can get OR; or given INV and OR, we can get AND.

We can derive INV, AND, OR, NAND, and NOR, just using NAND and NOR:

$$\sim A = A \barwedge A = A \overline{\vee} A \qquad (4.19)$$

$$A \wedge B = (A \overline{\vee} A) \overline{\vee} (B \overline{\vee} B) = (A \barwedge B) \barwedge 1 \qquad (4.20)$$

$$A \vee B = (A \barwedge A) \barwedge (B \barwedge B) = (A \overline{\vee} B) \overline{\vee} 0 \qquad (4.21)$$

$$A \barwedge B = ((A \overline{\vee} A) \overline{\vee} (B \overline{\vee} B)) \overline{\vee} 0 \qquad (4.22)$$

$$A \overline{\vee} B = ((A \barwedge A) \barwedge (B \barwedge B)) \barwedge 1 \qquad (4.23)$$

We cannot derive the "two-argument" operators AND, OR, NAND, or NOR from a "one-argument" operator like INV, for the simple reason that there is no way to relate two variables (A and B) with a one-argument operator like INV.

4.3 Hardware Logic Implementation: AND, OR, INV, NAND, NOR

The digital circuits we consider in this book are all binary circuits. That is, their outputs can only assume two possible states with respect to voltage: 1 (or "on," "affirmative," "up," "positive," or "true") or 0 (or "off," "negative," "down," "ground," or "false"). As implied by the choice "positive-ground," the 1 state is represented in most circuits in this book by a positive voltage, and the 0 state is represented as ground potential. In fact, we can define 1 and 0 by an input-output function, as in Figure 4.3.

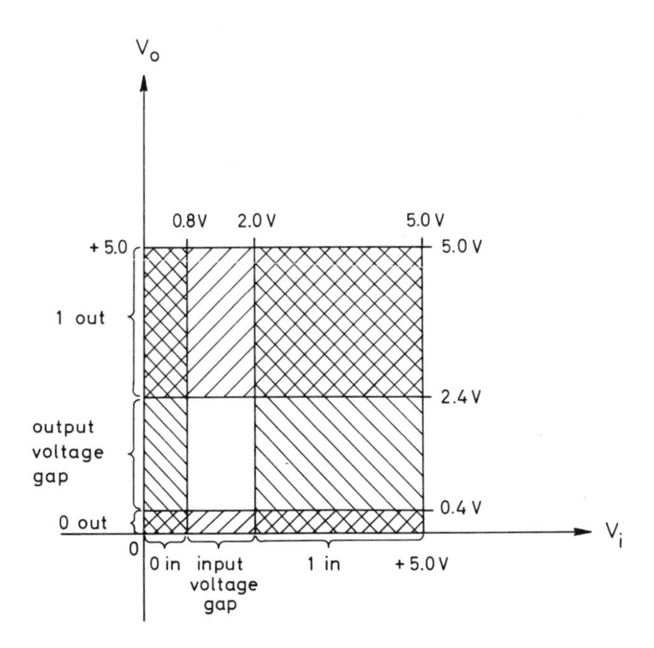

Figure 4.3
Input-output relation for 7400 series TTL.

Note that the 1 state (or 1 level, as it is often called) is any voltage within a certain *range* of voltages. Also note that this is true of the 0 state, for a lower set of voltages. There is a gap between the two voltages; for the device to have an unambiguous output when used to provide an input for a similar device, the output voltage of the "transmitter" device must never lie within the input gap of the "receiver" device except during transitions from one state to the other. To ensure that outputs may be used as inputs to other devices, the 1 and 0 output ranges are narrower than the corresponding input ranges and are completely included by the latter. Also, the output gap is wider than the input gap and completely includes it. The device is said to be a "positive logic" device: This means simply that the 1 voltage is more positive than the 0 voltage (although they may both be negative, both positive, or any other combination that fits the definition).

The 1-level and 0-level can be illustrated schematically, as is done in Figure 4.4a. We always use these symbols to indicate steady levels. Signals that are potentially variable are not indicated as levels, as shown in Figure 4.4b.

In general, for the device illustrated, a "0 level" is obtained by tying the desired point to ground. A "1 level" is obtained by tying the point to +5 V (supply voltage) through a 1 kΩ resistor, or if the supply is very well regulated, directly to

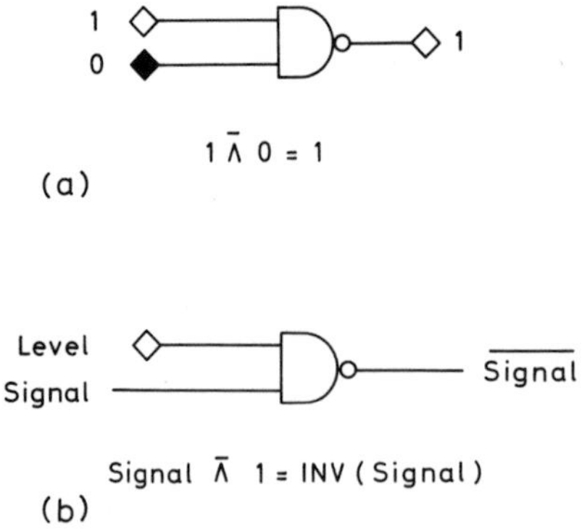

1
0
1
$1 \bar{\wedge} 0 = 1$
(a)

Level
Signal
$\overline{\text{Signal}}$
Signal $\bar{\wedge}$ 1 = INV (Signal)
(b)

Figure 4.4
Symbols for 1 and 0 levels: (a) Schematic representation of logic levels; (b) representation of signals *vs.* levels.

+5 V. The 1 kΩ resistor is intended to protect the device against overvoltage transients when the power supply is turned on.

The input-output relation of Figure 4.3 is specifically one for a 7400 series TTL (Transistor-Transistor Logic) device. These devices are used for almost all digital designs in this book. This series, now manufactured by several companies, is relatively cheap, fast, noise-immune, and small and consists of a large variety of different logical circuits. These IC devices are available as Flat Packs or Dual Inline Packages (DIPs) with four or more pins. They require only a single supply voltage ($V_{CC} = +5$ V). They are compatible with many other logic series, including all TTL and DTL (Diode-Transistor Logic) devices. In addition, many hybrid (analog-digital) devices such as differential comparators and analog switches are designed to be TTL compatible. Circuits are available to interface TTL to other logic series that are not TTL compatible, such as Metal-Oxide-Semiconductor (MOS) devices.

Figure 4.5 illustrates TTL implementation of AND, INV, NAND, and NOR. These are schematics for 7400 series devices. All illustrations of 7400 series TTL devices are based on data sheets for Texas Instruments devices; material is reprinted from these data sheets with the kind permission of Texas Instruments.

The AND gate of Figure 4.5a consists of an input transistor, three inverting and level-shifting transistors, and two output transistors. The input multiple-emitter transistor will conduct if either emitter is low (0 level), since the base is held in a forward-biased state relative to about 0.8 V. The collector voltage therefore can be represented as

$$V_{C_1} = -(\bar{A} \vee \bar{B}) = \bar{A} \mathbin{\overline{\vee}} \bar{B} = A \wedge B.$$

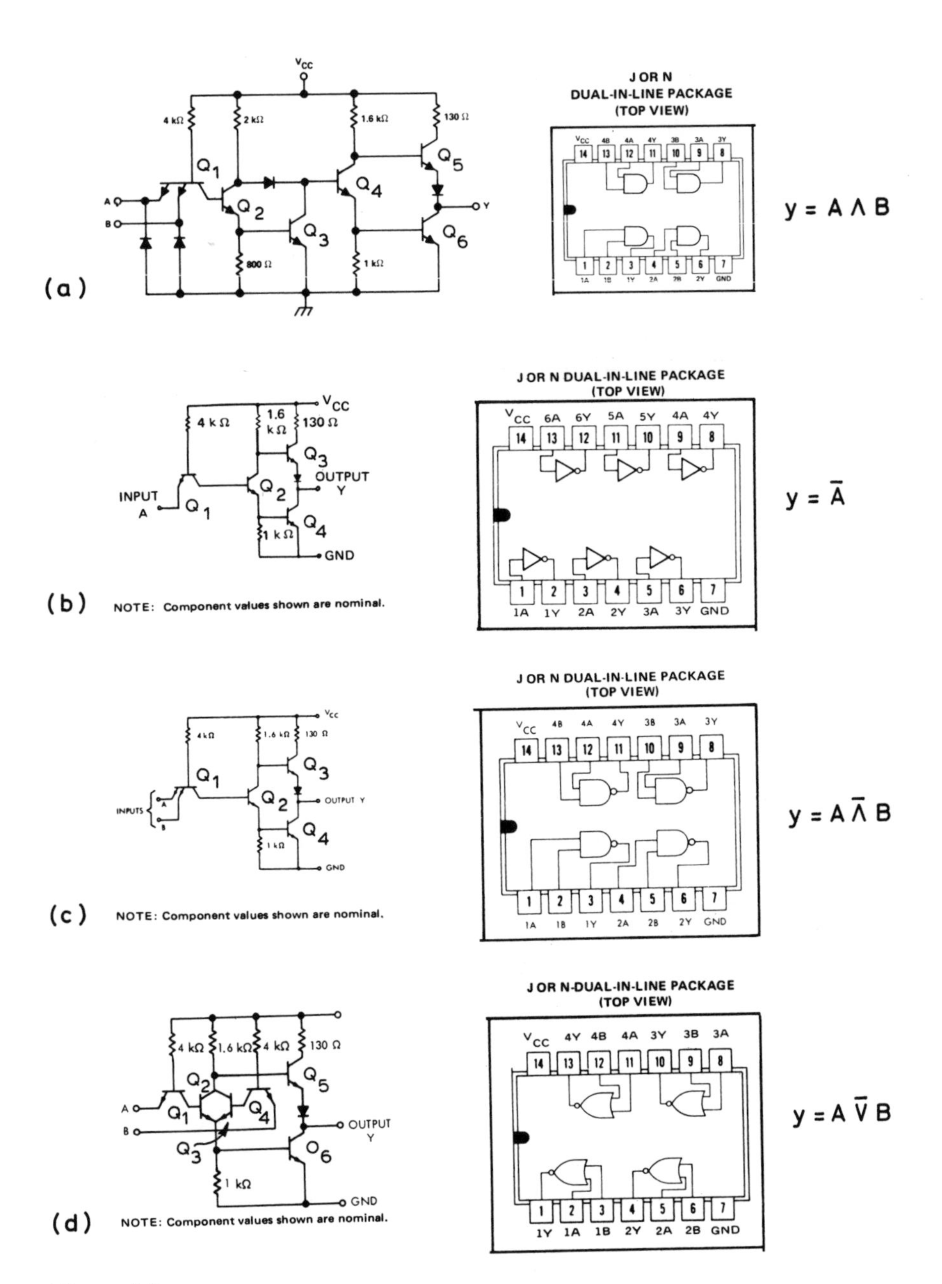

Figure 4.5
TTL implementation of (a) SN7408N AND; (b) SN7404N INV; (c) SN7400N NAND; (d) SN7402N NOR (from *The Integrated Circuits Catalog for Design Engineering, Catalog CC-401*, 1971, by Texas Instruments. Used by permission of Texas Instruments).

Transistor Q_1 provides the base bias voltage for Q_2, which in conjunction with Q_3 provides an inverted (relative to V_{C_1}) base bias for transistor Q_4. Therefore, Q_4 conducts whenever the collector of Q_1 is low. When Q_4 conducts, Q_6 conducts, providing a low-impedance path from the output to ground, and Q_5 is turned off, presenting a high impedance from the output to V_{CC}. This "totem pole" output stage therefore has a low impedance to ground when the Q_1 collector voltage is low.

Transistor Q_5 conducts and Q_6 is turned off when the collector of Q_1 is high, presenting a high-impedance path to ground, and a low-impedance path to +5 V at the output. Thus, the totem-pole configuration provides us with a low-impedance output for either logical level. This permits higher speed operation, independence of output loading, and better noise immunity. Thus,

$$V_o = Y = V_{C_1} = A \wedge B.$$

The inverter of Figure 4.5b consists of a noninverting transistor input (Q_1 conducts when $A = 0$, therefore $V_{C_1} = A$), which drives Q_2 (which therefore conducts when $V_{C_1} = 1$), which then drives the totem-pole output. The output therefore is simply the inverse of the input, because the only inversion occurs at Q_2.

The NAND gate (Figure 4.5c) is a simplification of the AND gate. The double-emitter transistor Q_1 performs the AND operation, which is inverted by Q_2, Q_3, and Q_4 to provide $A \overline{\wedge} B$ at the output. The saving of two transistors results in less circuit complexity, lower cost, and lower power consumption. The NAND gate is therefore more commonly used than the AND gate.

The NOR gate (Figure 4.5d) consists of two noninverting input transistors used to drive the bases of two transistors whose collectors and emitters are connected in parallel. If either of the parallel transistors conducts, their common collector voltage is low relative to that voltage obtained when they do not conduct. Therefore the common collector voltage is $-(A \vee B)$. The common collector and common emitter voltages of the parallel pair are used to drive the totem-pole output stage, giving the NOR function: $Y = A \overline{\vee} B$.

The two-input devices are called *gates*, because the level on one input can determine whether or not changes at the other input will be reflected as changes in the output state. One input is said to "gate" the other; the gate is either "open" or "closed." The use of these three devices as enable-disable gates is illustrated in Figure 4.6.

Figure 4.7 provides pin configurations for other gates that we will commonly use: three-input and eight-input NAND gates, and the four-input NAND buffer. They allow the NANDing of multiple inputs with a single gate. In general, the

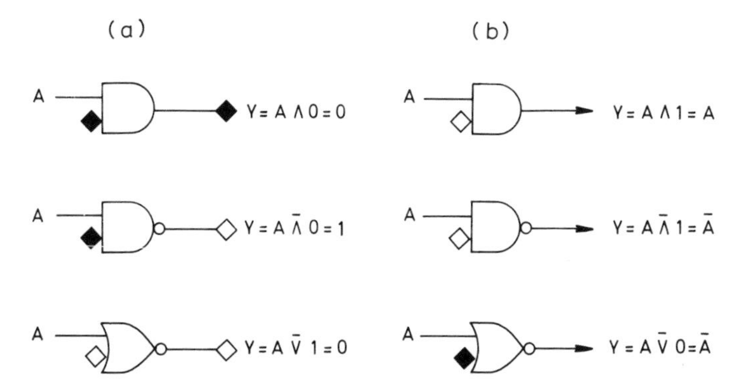

Figure 4.6
Use of AND, NAND, and NOR gates as inhibit (enable-disable) gates: (a) disabled; (b) enabled.

7400 series devices can be used to drive 10 "unit loads" (generally, a unit load is the emitter of a single forward-biased TTL input transistor) without exceeding their output capability. The NAND buffer, SN7440N, can drive as many as 30 such loads. Most TTL inputs are single unit loads, but a few (which will be pointed out when encountered) consist of two or more transistors in parallel, and therefore constitute more than one unit load. The number of unit loads which a TTL device can drive is called its *fanout*.

There are older design schemes such as Diode-Transistor Logic (DTL), Resistor-Transistor Logic (RTL), and Diode-Capacitor-Transistor Logic (DCTL) that implement logical functions. The TTL type is presently the most advantageous in terms of speed, noise immunity, cost, and variety of available logic devices. All of these types use saturating logic; that is, they drive their internal transistors to saturation and cutoff for the two logic levels. This results in simple biasing and wide tolerance on the internal resistors but also higher power consumption and lower speed than the more sophisticated Current-Mode Logic (CML) that does not rely on driving the transistors to saturation and cutoff. The gains achieved by using CML are not enough at present to outweigh the advantages of TTL, in most biological instrumentation.

4.4 Multivibrators, Flipflops, and Counters

We will have occasion to use devices whose outputs are not only a function of input levels but also a function of input *transitions* (changes from one input state to the other).

The SET-RESET flipflop or *R-S* flipflop (Figure 4.8a) has two outputs, which we shall call Q and $-Q$. When we refer to "the output," and don't specify Q or $-Q$, we will be referring to Q. Note that in the *R-S* flipflop of Figure 4.8a with no

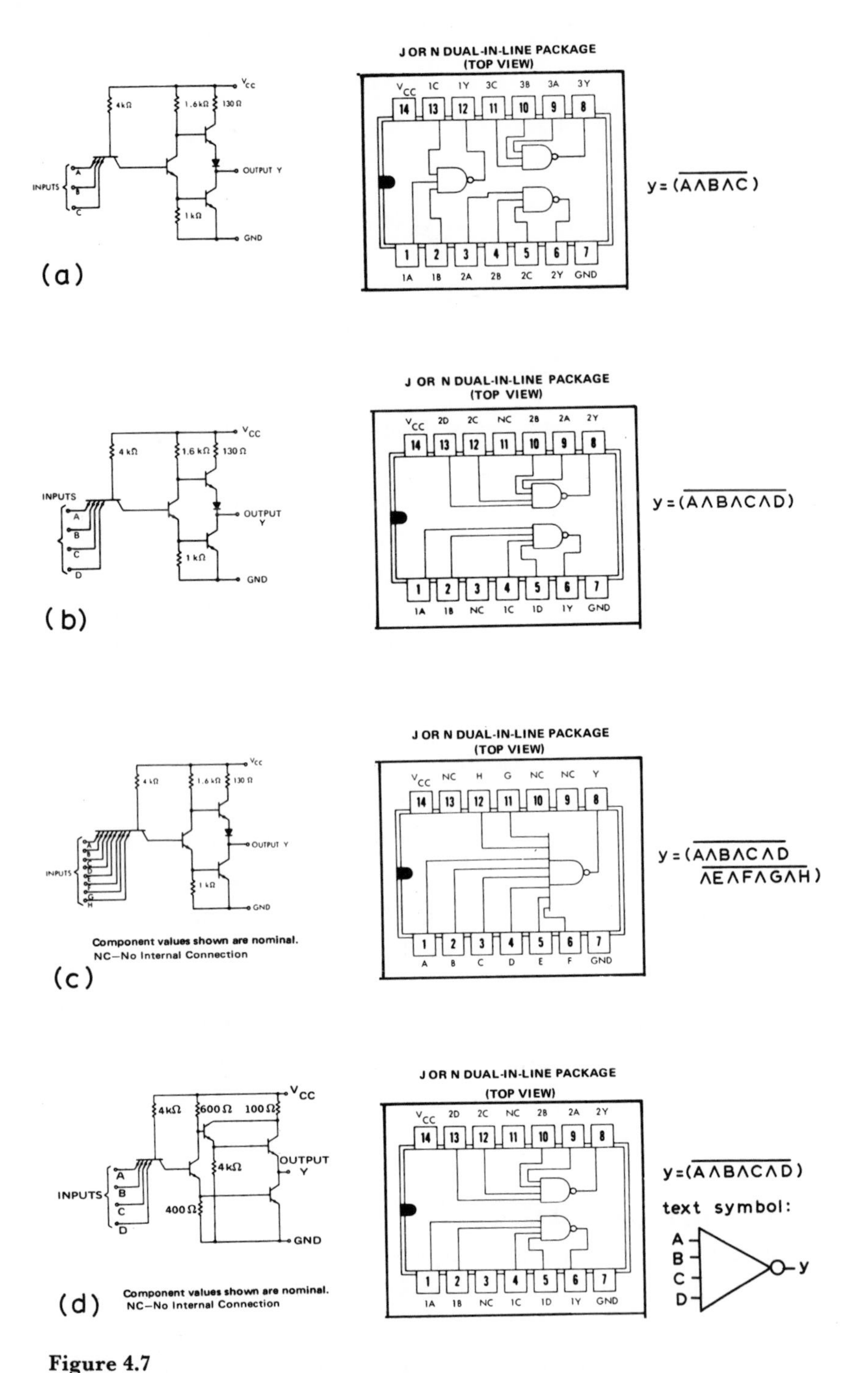

Figure 4.7
Multiple-input NAND gates and NAND buffer: (a) SN7401N triple 3-input NAND; (b) SN7420N dual 4-input NAND; (c) SN7430N 8-input NAND; (d) SN7440N dual 4-input NAND buffer (from *The Integrated Circuits Catalog for Design Engineers, Catalog CC-401*, 1971, by Texas Instruments. Used with permission of Texas Instruments).

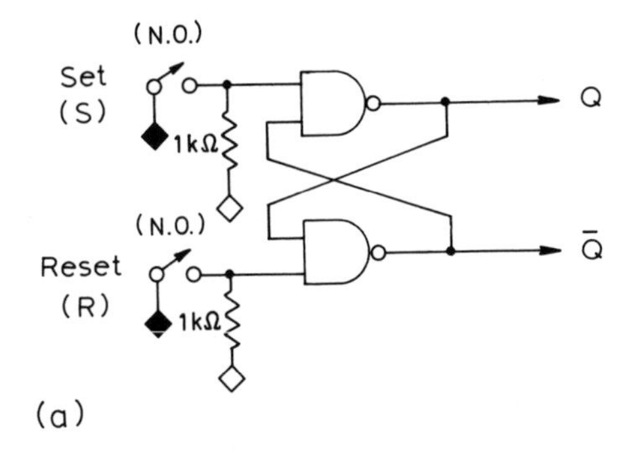

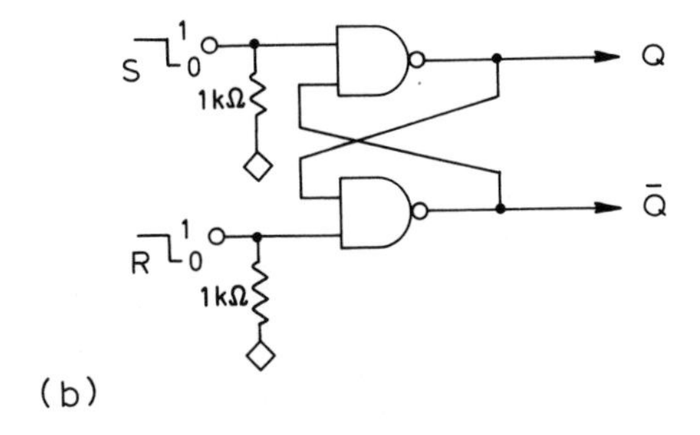

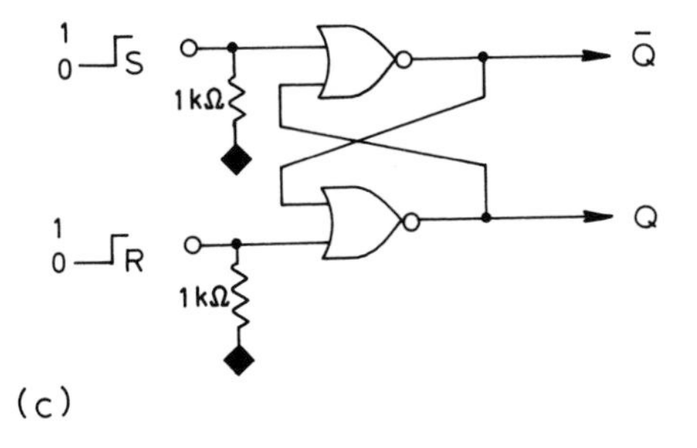

Figure 4.8
R-S flipflops: (a) manual triggering; (b) negative-edge triggering; (c) positive-edge triggering.

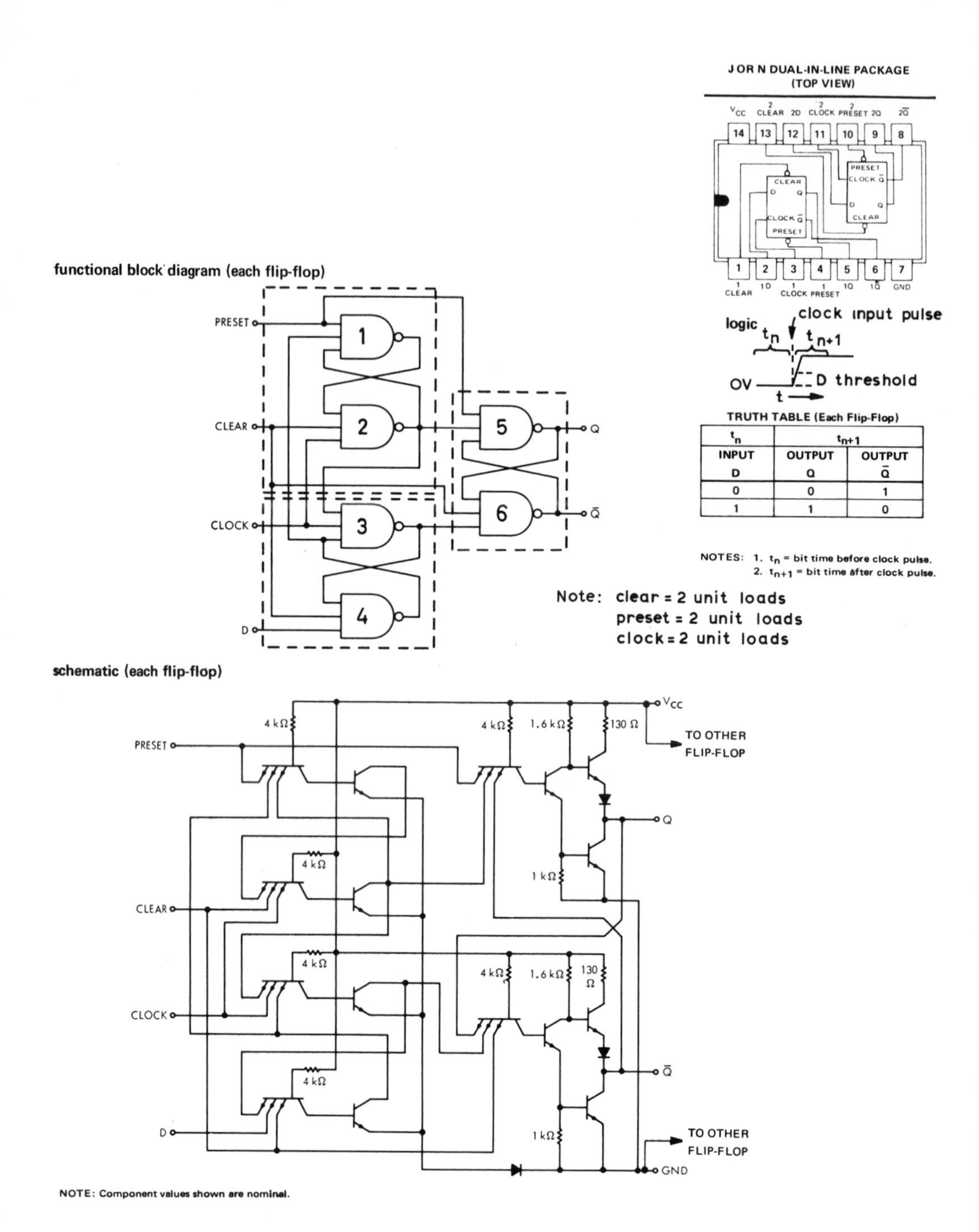

t_n	t_{n+1}	
INPUT D	OUTPUT Q	OUTPUT $\bar{Q}$
0	0	1
1	1	0

Figure 4.9
D-Type flipflop SN7474N (from *The Integrated Circuits Catalog for Design Engineers, Catalog CC-401*, 1971, by Texas Instruments. Used with permission of Texas Instruments).

inputs, if Q is on, it holds $-Q$ off. In turn $-Q$ holds Q on. If Q is off, it holds $-Q$ on, which in turn holds Q off.

If the "set" (S) pushbutton switch (normally open) is depressed, the corresponding input to the NAND gate goes on—this forces Q on, shutting $-Q$ off. This is a stable state, until "reset" (R) is pressed, regardless of further activity at the S button.

If both buttons are pressed, both Q and $-Q$ go on. As soon as one button is released, the corresponding gate output goes off and the other stays on (e.g., if S is released, Q goes off and $-Q$ stays on).

Note that this is a positive-feedback configuration. If we did the same with an op amp, we would have the condition illustrated in Figure 4.2, where we decided that the device had only two possible output states; the positive-feedback op amp configuration is in fact a SET-RESET flipflop with one input, and three input states: "set" ($V_i < V^-_{\mathrm{threshold}}$), "neutral" ($V^+_{\mathrm{threshold}} > V_i > V^-_{\mathrm{threshold}}$), and "reset" ($V_i > V^+_{\mathrm{threshold}}$).

We can use electrical inputs instead of pushbuttons, as illustrated in Figure 4.8b. The inputs are also tied to logical 1 through 1 kΩ resistors to allow either input to be disconnected without affecting operation of the other input. These "quiescent" input voltages are overridden by TTL outputs connected to the inputs. In Figure 4.8b a negative transition (from 1 to 0) electrical input to either input sets the corresponding output. However, we will often prefer a circuit where a positive transition (from 0 to 1) causes the device to switch. In Figure 4.8c, Q and $-Q$ are reversed. The reader can verify that a positive transition to the R input (in the absence of a positive level at the S input) causes the corresponding gate to go to 0, and vice versa.

A more complicated device is the D-type flipflop (Figure 4.9). The 3-input NAND gates configure 3 flipflops, enclosed in dashed lines. They can be distinguished by their positive-feedback configurations.

Operationally a D flipflop can be described as a device whose output (Q) is a function of the D-input, clear and preset inputs, and the "clock" (C) input. If either clear or preset is at ground (0), the output is held cleared or set, respectively, and will continue in that state after removal of the set or clear ground level until C goes positive. At that time, the value at D is "strobed" onto the output and stays there at least until the next positive C transition or until clear or preset is grounded. If the output was already at the value of D, it remains unchanged. Clear and preset 0 levels predominate over any combination of C, D, and previous output state. Clear and preset 1 levels allow the output to be completely determined by D, C, and the previous state.

description

These J-K flip-flops are based on the master-slave principle and each has AND gate inputs for entry into the master section which are controlled by the clock pulse. The clock pulse also regulates the state of the coupling transistors which connect the master and slave sections. The sequence of operation is as follows:

1. Isolate slave from master
2. Enter information from AND gate inputs to master
3. Disable AND gate inputs
4. Transfer information from master to slave.

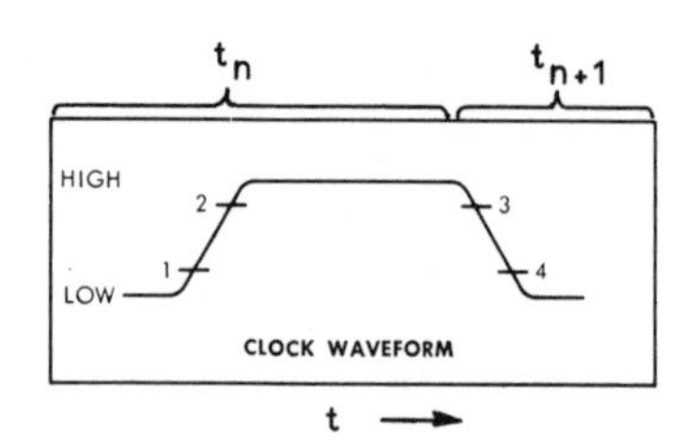

functional block diagram (each flip-flop)

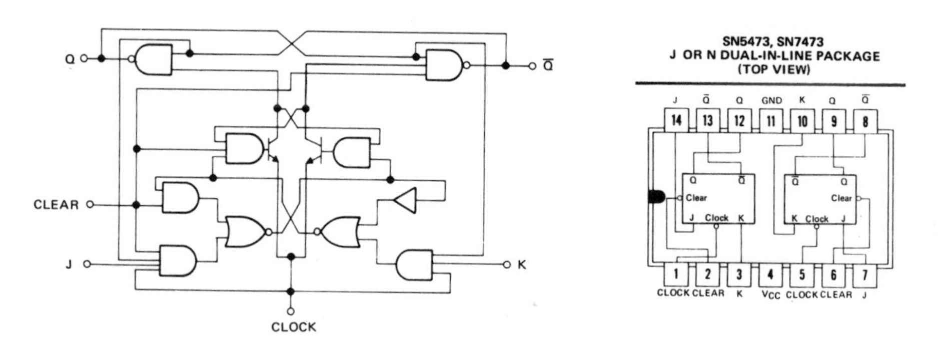

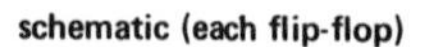

schematic (each flip-flop)

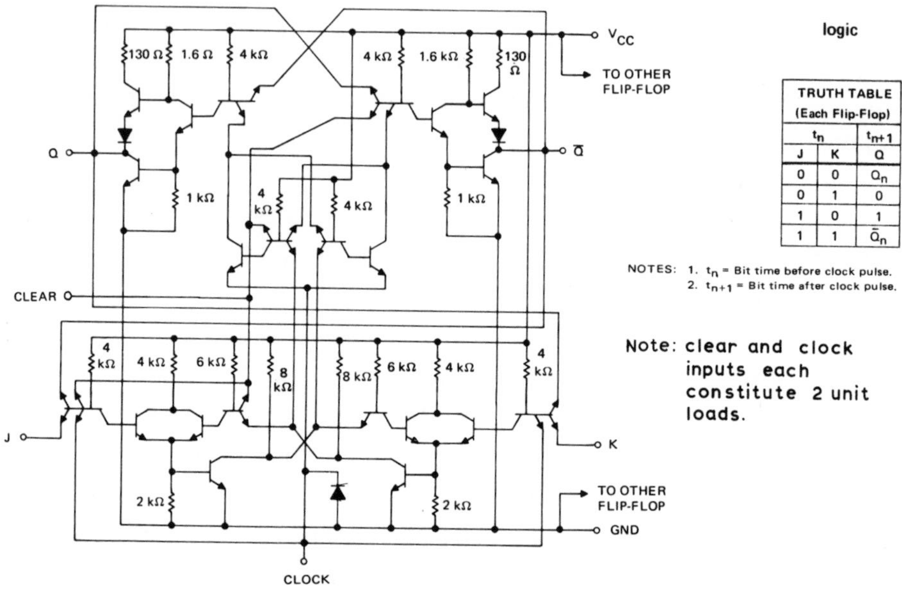

TRUTH TABLE (Each Flip-Flop)		
t_n		t_{n+1}
J	K	Q
0	0	Q_n
0	1	0
1	0	1
1	1	$\bar{Q}_n$

NOTES: 1. t_n = Bit time before clock pulse.
2. t_{n+1} = Bit time after clock pulse.

NOTE: Component values shown are nominal.

Figure 4.10
J-K Master-Slave flipflop SN7473N (from *The Integrated Circuits Catalog for Design Engineers, Catalog CC-401*, 1971, by Texas Instruments. Used with permission of Texas Instruments).

Assume the following initial condition:

Clear = 1
Preset = 1
Clock = 0
D = 1

(Note that the preset and clock inputs are tied to two emitters: They therefore constitute *two unit loads* each. The clear input is tied to three emitters, and constitutes *three unit loads*.)

From these, we may deduce immediately that some gates must have an output value of 1: gates 2 and 3, because the clock input is zero. Then gate 4 must have an output of 0, because all of its inputs are 1. Therefore, gate 1 has a 1 output, because the input from 4 is 0. Under these circumstances, we cannot predict the values of 5 and 6, because we know only that each has two inputs valued "1." We *do* know, however, that one must be on and the other must be off because of the feedback between them.

Now let C change from 0 to 1. Gate 2 becomes 0, forcing gate 5 to a value of 1 (if it isn't 1 already). This forces gate 6 to a zero, if it isn't already. Gates 1, 3, and 4 remain unchanged. Now bring C back to zero. Gate 2 becomes a 1; gate 3 remains a 1 (so gate 4 remains a zero); gate 1 remains unchanged, because C went to 0 before 4 went to 1, and gate 1 thus never has all three inputs positive. Now 5 and 6 both have two 1s at their inputs, but the feedback holds them in the states of 1 and 0, respectively.

Now change D to 0, then 4 becomes a 1. Gate 3 remains 1, because $C = 0$. If C were a 1 when D went to 0, then 3 would still remain unchanged because in that case gate 2 was 0. Gate 1 goes to 0 (if C were 1, gate 1 would remain a 1, because of the input from 2). We can now specify the output of 2: If C is 0, it is forced to remain 1. If C is 1, 2 becomes 0, which has no effect on gates receiving inputs from 2, because they are all 1: gates 1, 3, and 5. Thus, the output remains the same if D is changed, regardless of the state of C.

With D in the 0 state, 5 will switch to 0 on the next positive C transition. We will not prove this here.

Of course, we have not analyzed the response to all possible input combinations (for example, we have not demonstrated that preset and clear predominate over other inputs when either is grounded), but rather than perform a more extensive analysis, we will go on to a third type of flipflop, the J-K flipflop (Figure 4.10).

This flipflop operates in two cycles. On a positive clock transition, the inputs from J and K are sampled, and on a negative clock transition the values are used

Table 4.10
Behavior of *J-K* flipflop.

J	K	New value of Q
0	1	0
0	0	no change, regardless of old value of Q
1	0	1
1	1	reverses state, regardless of old value of Q

to determine the output, in the following manner:

Clear positive causes Q to go to 0.

Clear grounded allows output to be determined as in Table 4.10.

The reversal of output state in the last line of the truth table (Table 4.10) is called "toggling." Note that the strobing of inputs to output occurs in four stages, as described in Figure 4.10. Essentially, the next value of the output is determined by J and K during a positive clock transition; during the negative clock transition, the outputs assume that value. The clear and clock inputs both constitute two unit loads.

The two-transition clocking requirement is often referred to as "two-phased" operation.

The master-slave *R-S* flipflop (Figure 4.11) is similar to the *J-K* flipflop in that there is an input flipflop which is set on the leading edge of the clock pulse and gated onto the output on the trailing edge of the clock pulse. The logical design, pin configuration, and operating characteristics of the SN74L71N are illustrated in Figure 4.11. The "L" within the device number indicates that it is a low-power device, with a lower fanout and lower input load factors. There is no *R-S* flipflop available in the standard-power 7400 series or the high-power 74H series.

The *R-S* flipflops are an example of one type of *multivibrator*. The general configuration of a multivibrator is illustrated in Figure 4.12. The nature of the multivibrator (MVB) operation is determined by the types of feedthrough and feedback elements and the gates. Three general types are possible: (1) the bistable MVB, which has two stable output states like the *R-S* flipflop; (2) the monostable MVB, which, upon the arrival of an appropriate "trigger" at the input, produces a finite-duration level-change at the output—a pulse—after which it returns to its original state, regardless of whether or not the input has returned to the original state; and (3) the astable MVB, which alternates between the two possible output states regardless of external conditions. The monostable MVB, or "one-shot," as it is frequently called, will be considered here, and the astable MVB will be examined briefly in the next chapter.

functional block diagram

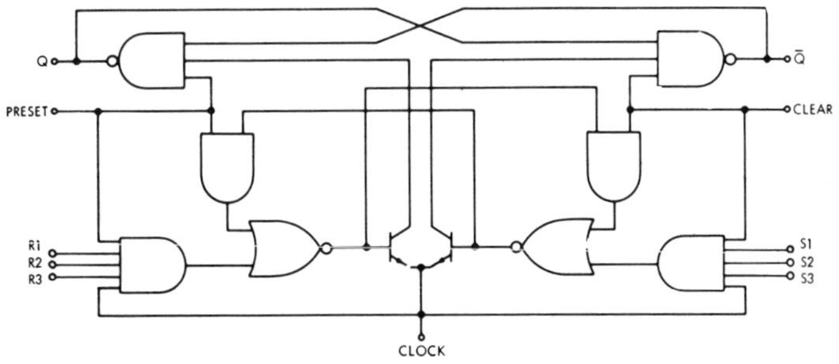

JOR N
DUAL-IN-LINE PACKAGE (TOP VIEW)

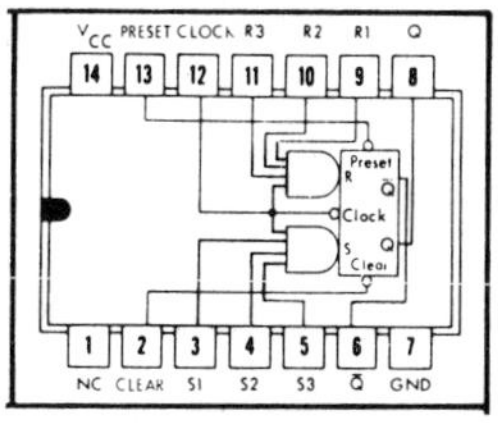

positive logic
Low input to preset sets Q to logical 1
Low input to clear sets Q to logical 0
Preset and clear are independent of clock

schematic

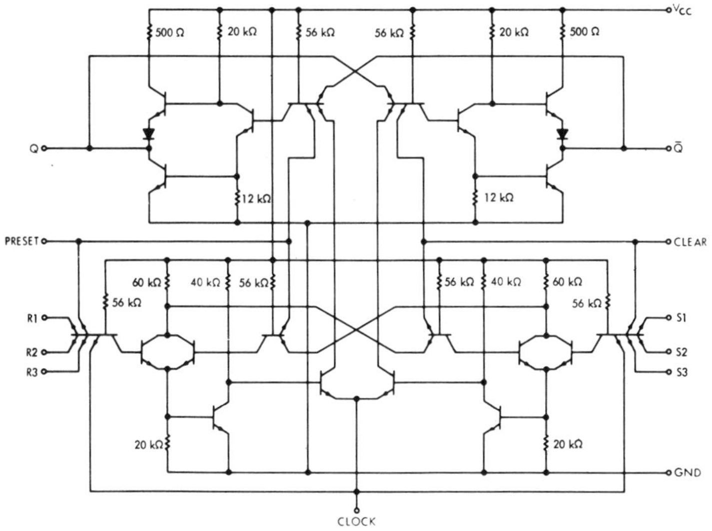

Loading factors:
R1, R2, R3, S1, S2, S3 : 0.25 unit load each
clock, preset, clear : 0.50 unit load each

Fan-out for Q or $\bar{Q}$: 1.25

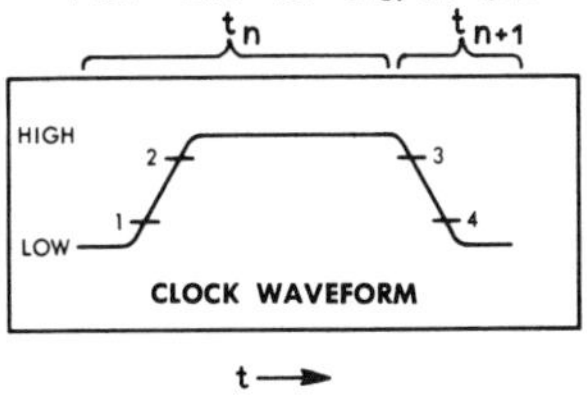

description

These R-S flip-flop circuits are based on the master-slave principle. The AND gate inputs for entry into the master section are controlled by the clock pulse. The clock pulse also regulates the state of the coupling transistors which connect the master and slave sections. The sequence of operation is as follows:

1. Isolate slave from master
2. Enter information from AND gate inputs to master
3. Disable AND gate inputs
4. Transfer information from master to slave.

CLOCK WAVEFORM

logic

TRUTH TABLE

t_n		t_{n+1}
R	S	Q
0	0	Q_n
0	1	1
1	0	0
1	1	Indeterminate

NOTES: 1. R = R1 • R2 • R3
2. S = S1 • S2 • S3
3. t_n = Bit time before clock pulse.
4. t_{n+1} = Bit time after clock pulse.
5. NC — No internal connection.

Figure 4.11
SN74L71N Master-Slave *R-S* flipflop (from *The Integrated Circuits Catalog for Design Engineers, Catalog CC-401*, 1971, by Texas Instruments. Used with permission of Texas Instruments).

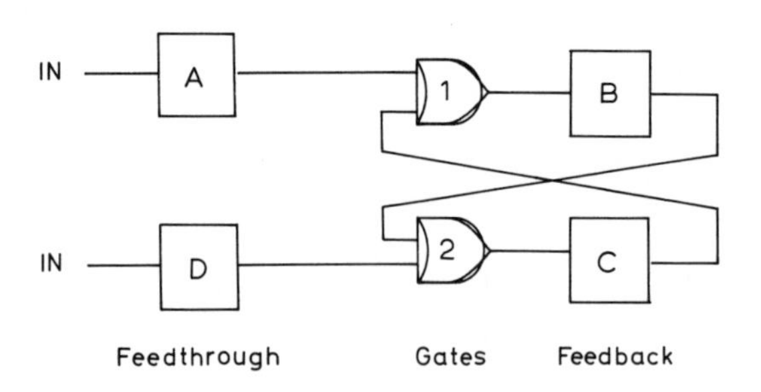

Figure 4.12
Generalized multivibrator.

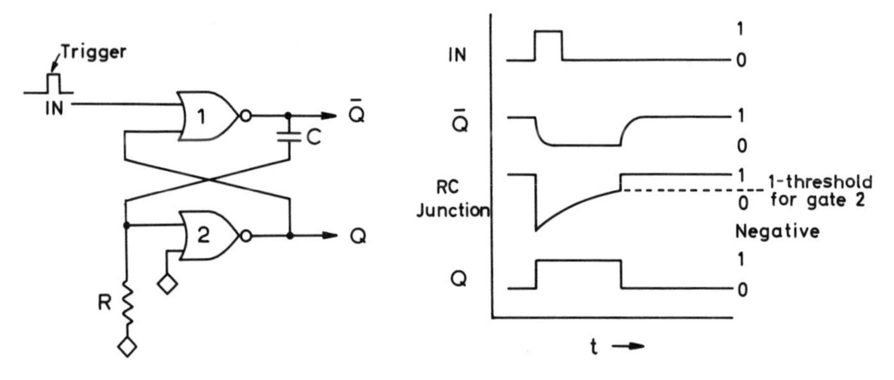

Figure 4.13
Monostable multivibrator.

A simple monostable design is illustrated in Figure 4.13.

The stable state is one in which the Q output is 0, and $-Q = 1$, since both inputs to 2 are 0 and the inputs to 1 are therefore 0 and 1. When a 1 appears at IN, $-Q$ goes to 0 and capacitor C is grounded by $-Q$. As C discharges its positive charge through $-Q$, the voltage on the RC junction goes negative, to a voltage equal to and opposite that of the original positive voltage. This negative voltage on the junction between R and C then exponentially rises toward the original positive voltage, until it reaches the logical 1 threshold for gate 2. The output of 2, meanwhile, goes positive as soon as the capacitor begins to discharge and stays positive as long as the voltage at the RC junction remains below its threshold. When the threshold is attained, the output of 2 goes back to 0.

As soon as 2 goes positive, the feedback connection to 1 ensures that $-Q$ stays at 0 *even if the input pulse returns to ground.* This means that the output pulse width is not affected by a shorter input pulse. If the input pulse is longer than the output pulse, however, the $-Q$ output will not return to 1 at the end of the Q pulse; however, the Q pulse width will be unaffected by virtue of the fact that the capacitor still discharges to ground and remains discharged until the IN pulse is turned off. Hence the output at Q is theoretically totally independent of the duration of the IN pulse. It is also of finite duration, because the threshold of 2 must eventually be reached at the RC input of 2. This implies that the device has only one truly stable state, to which it will always return if removed from that state, namely, with output $Q = 0$—hence the term "monostable."

There is one aspect of the input which is of importance to the performance of the device as seen at the output: the interval between positive transitions. If the capacitor has not had time to attain full charge by the time that the next positive input transition occurs, the output pulse width will suffer degradation (it will be shortened), or if the discharge is not sufficient to pull the RC input of 2 below threshold, there will be no second output pulse at all. For this reason, it is often advisable to capacitor couple the input, to limit the duration of the input pulse to the minimum necessary for stable operation. Then, even if the input pulse lasts almost until the beginning of the next input pulse, the capacitor has time to recharge—assuming that the interval between positive transitions is adequate for recharging the capacitor.

This dependence on the interval between input transitions is often expressed as "duty cycle," the maximum

$$D = \frac{T}{t} \tag{4.24}$$

where D = duty cycle, T = interval between triggers, and t = pulse output duration. The maximum duty cycle of the circuit described above is about 50%.

For pulses of short duration (less than 1 msec), this circuit is quite adequate. The R and C should be adjusted not only for the proper pulse duration (not to be confused with the time constant, RC) but also the net impedance of the RC path should be picked to lie halfway between the point where the input to 2 changes too little to produce an output, and the point where the device "hangs" in the on state.

We can vary the duration of the pulse continuously by using variable R and/or C, within the limits of impedance required for proper operation. However, unless one actually switches in different values of C for a "decade multiplier" and carefully selects a potentiometer value that will give the proper range for each decade, the device will have a limited range of durations with just a potentiometer: say, a range of 1–20. However, trimming capacitors or pots are useful for trimming the duration of the output pulse.

One can now buy integrated circuit one shots (another name for a monostable MVB) with excellent performance specifications, including large duty cycle and

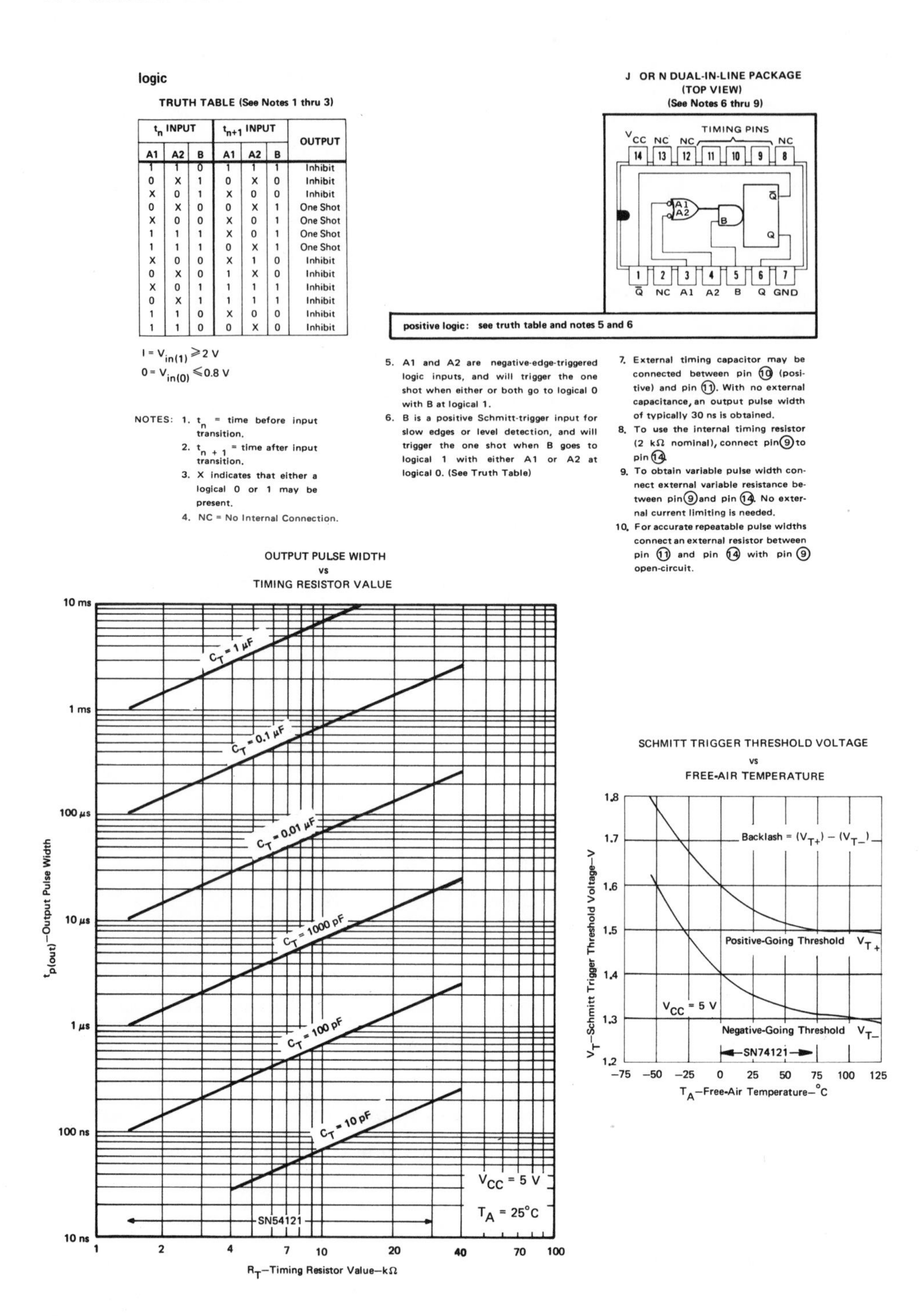

logic

TRUTH TABLE (See Notes 1 thru 3)

t_n INPUT			t_{n+1} INPUT			OUTPUT
A1	A2	B	A1	A2	B	
1	1	0	1	1	1	Inhibit
0	X	1	0	X	0	Inhibit
X	0	1	X	0	0	Inhibit
0	X	0	0	X	1	One Shot
X	0	0	X	0	1	One Shot
1	1	1	X	0	1	One Shot
1	1	1	0	X	1	One Shot
X	0	0	X	1	0	Inhibit
0	X	0	1	X	0	Inhibit
X	0	1	1	1	1	Inhibit
0	X	1	1	1	1	Inhibit
1	1	0	X	0	0	Inhibit
1	1	0	0	X	0	Inhibit

$1 = V_{in(1)} \geqslant 2$ V
$0 = V_{in(0)} \leqslant 0.8$ V

NOTES:
1. t_n = time before input transition.
2. t_{n+1} = time after input transition.
3. X indicates that either a logical 0 or 1 may be present.
4. NC = No Internal Connection.

J OR N DUAL-IN-LINE PACKAGE (TOP VIEW) (See Notes 6 thru 9)

positive logic: see truth table and notes 5 and 6

5. A1 and A2 are negative-edge-triggered logic inputs, and will trigger the one shot when either or both go to logical 0 with B at logical 1.
6. B is a positive Schmitt-trigger input for slow edges or level detection, and will trigger the one shot when B goes to logical 1 with either A1 or A2 at logical 0. (See Truth Table)
7. External timing capacitor may be connected between pin (10) (positive) and pin (11). With no external capacitance, an output pulse width of typically 30 ns is obtained.
8. To use the internal timing resistor (2 kΩ nominal), connect pin (9) to pin (14).
9. To obtain variable pulse width connect external variable resistance between pin (9) and pin (14). No external current limiting is needed.
10. For accurate repeatable pulse widths connect an external resistor between pin (11) and pin (14) with pin (9) open-circuit.

OUTPUT PULSE WIDTH vs TIMING RESISTOR VALUE

SCHMITT TRIGGER THRESHOLD VOLTAGE vs FREE-AIR TEMPERATURE

Figure 4.14
SN74121N monostable multivibrator (from *The Integrated Circuits Catalog for Design Engineers, Catalog CC-401*, 1971, by Texas Instruments. Used with permission of Texas Instruments).

excellent stability. The SN74121N (Figure 4.14) can produce pulses at TTL level with durations of 40 nsec up to 40 sec, controllable by external timing resistors and capacitors, with a duty cycle of 90%. The *B* input is a positive feedback threshold detector similar to that of Figure 4.1, which is TTL compatible. Generally such circuits are cheaper than the cost of labor involved in constructing a monostable from discrete components or smaller scale ICs.

The retriggerable monostables of Figure 4.15, the SN74122N and SN74123N, are specially designed devices which have a 100% duty cycle. In fact, if a "retrigger" occurs during the output pulse, the output duration is timed from the arrival of the new trigger level. Furthermore, a "clear" pulse terminates the output pulse, if the clear arrives when the output is on. The availability of multiple inputs for leading and trailing edge triggering is an added convenience. A 4-input capability is offered in the SN74122N, and two generators are included in one package in the SN74123N. Note that the timing characteristics are different from those of the SN74121N.

4.5 Registers and Binary Arithmetic

It may have occurred to the reader that the bistable MVB is a form of "memory," in that the output state is a function of a past input state. Indeed such devices are often used for just such a purpose, and some manufacturers are even producing multibit memories based on Large Scale Integration (LSI) implementation using these logic circuits. These devices presently are used for small special-purpose computers, electronic calculators, and the like. They also make excellent "scratchpad memories," and they may prove useful for "programming" stimulation sequences in the laboratory, or in other processes that might be amenable to such approaches.

There is a very useful class of devices that commonly use flipflops for memory purposes: These are multiflipflop devices called "registers," of which counters are an example. Figure 4.16a illustrates the use of *J-K* flipflops in a binary counter; in this application, each flipflop output represents a *b*inary dig*it*, or "bit," for short, in a multibit number.

Such a counter provides us with a good introduction to binary arithmetic. First, observe the functioning of the circuit: The clear line resets all "digits" to 0. If we keep in mind the fact that the *T* input requires a positive-negative *pair* (a complete "cycle") of transitions, it is clear that each "higher" digit is set to 1 only when the preceding digit goes to zero. The sequence of events therefore looks like that depicted in Table 4.11.

The 1 output flips once per input cycle; the 10 output flips once per 1 cycle or

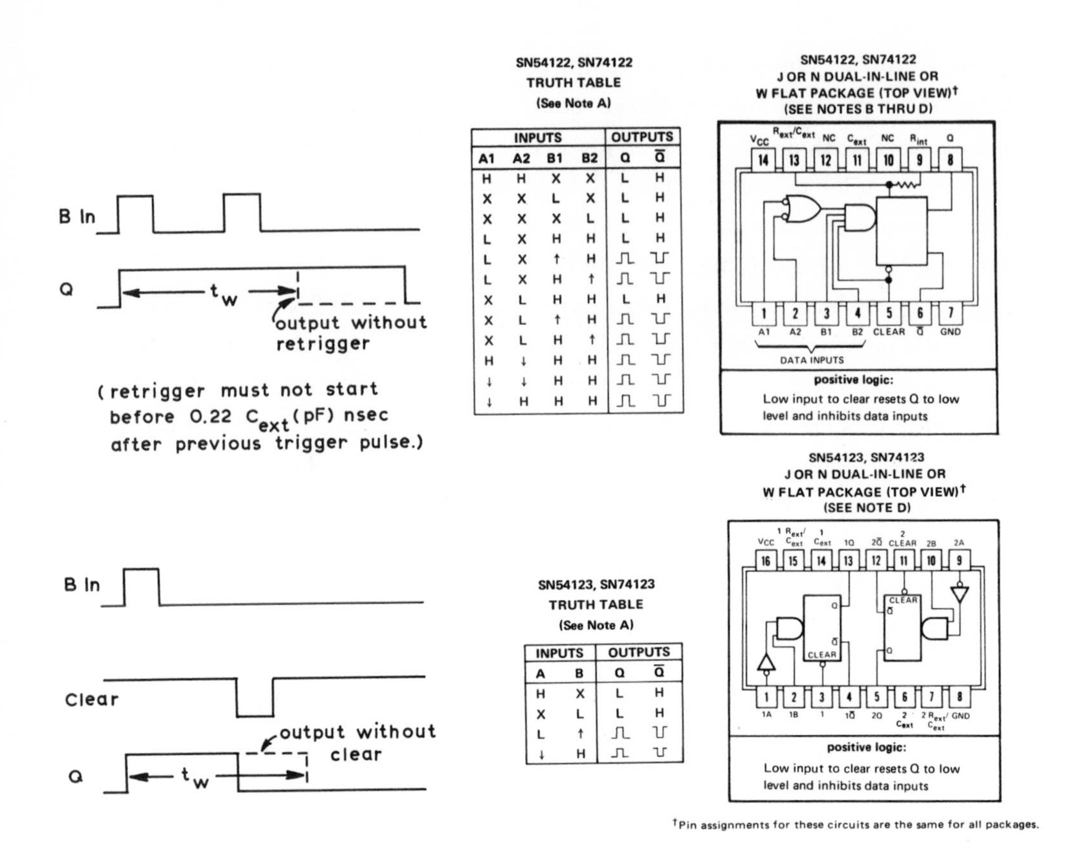

SN54122, SN74122
TRUTH TABLE
(See Note A)

INPUTS				OUTPUTS	
A1	A2	B1	B2	Q	$\overline{Q}$
H	H	X	X	L	H
X	X	L	X	L	H
X	X	X	L	L	H
L	X	H	H	L	H
L	X	↑	H	⊓	⊔
L	X	H	↑	⊓	⊔
X	L	H	H	L	H
X	L	↑	H	⊓	⊔
X	L	H	↑	⊓	⊔
H	↓	H	H	⊓	⊔
↓	↓	H	H	⊓	⊔
↓	H	H	H	⊓	⊔

SN54123, SN74123
TRUTH TABLE
(See Note A)

INPUTS		OUTPUTS	
A	B	Q	$\overline{Q}$
H	X	L	H
X	L	L	H
L	↑	⊓	⊔
↓	H	⊓	⊔

NOTES: A. H = high level (steady state), L = low level (steady state), ↑ = transition from low to high level, ↓ = transition from high to low level, ⊓ = one high-level pulse, ⊔ = one low-level pulse, X = irrelevant (any input, including transitions).
B. NC = No internal connection.
C. To use the internal timing resistor of SN54122/SN74122 (10 kΩ nominal), connect R_{int} to V_{CC}.
D. An external timing capacitor may be connected between C_{ext} and R_{ext}/C_{ext} (positive).

fan-out : 20 when output high, 10 when output low
inputs: data inputs = 1 unit load each
clear inputs = 2 unit loads each
timing resistor range : 5 - 25 kΩ
timing capaciter range: no limits

Figure 4.15
SN7400N series retriggerable monostables: SN74122N and SN74123N (from *The Integrated Circuits Catalog for Design Engineers*, *Catalog CC-401*, 1971, by Texas Instruments. Used with permission of Texas Instruments).

The output pulse is primarily a function of the external capacitor and resistor. For $C_{ext} > 1000$ pF, the output pulse width (t_W) is defined as:

$$t_W = 0.32\, R_T C_{ext} \left(1 + \frac{0.7}{R_T}\right)$$

where

R_T is in kΩ (either internal or external timing resistor)
C_{ext} is in pF
t_W is in ns

For pulse widths when $C_{ext} \leqslant 1000$ pF, see curve below.

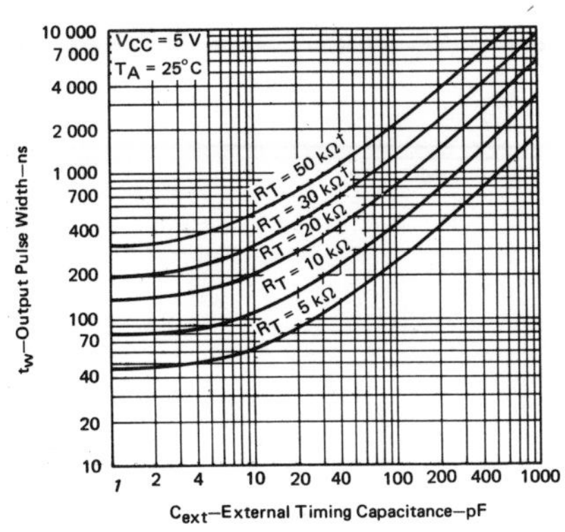

†These values of resistance exceed the maximums recommended for use over the full temperature range of the SN54122 and SN54123.

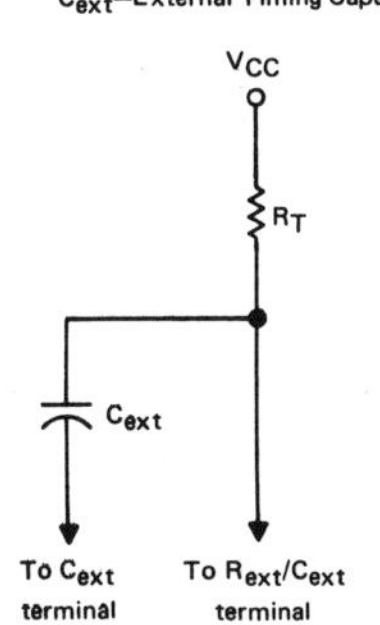

TIMING COMPONENT CONNECTIONS WHEN $C_{ext} \leqslant 1000$ pF

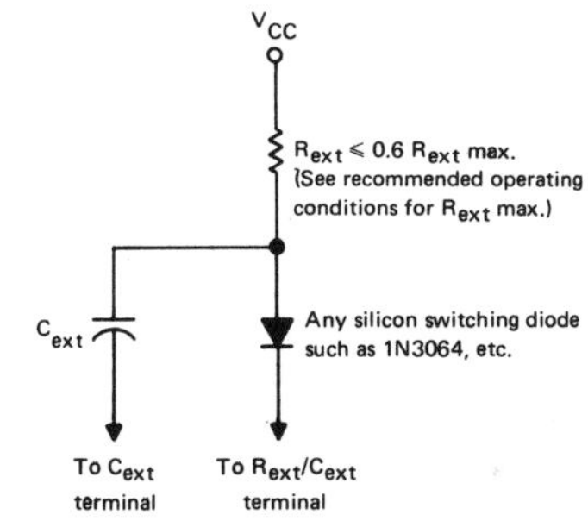

TIMING COMPONENT CONNECTIONS WHEN $C_{ext} > 1000$ pF AND CLEAR IS USED

To prevent reverse voltage across C_{ext}, it is recommended that the method shown in Figure D be employed when using electrolytic capacitors and in applications utilizing the clear function. In all applications using the diode, the pulse width is:

$$t_W = 0.28\, R_{ext} C_{ext} \left(1 + \frac{0.7}{R_{ext}}\right)$$

where

R_{ext} is in kΩ
C_{ext} is in pF
t_W is in ns

Figure 4.15 (continued)

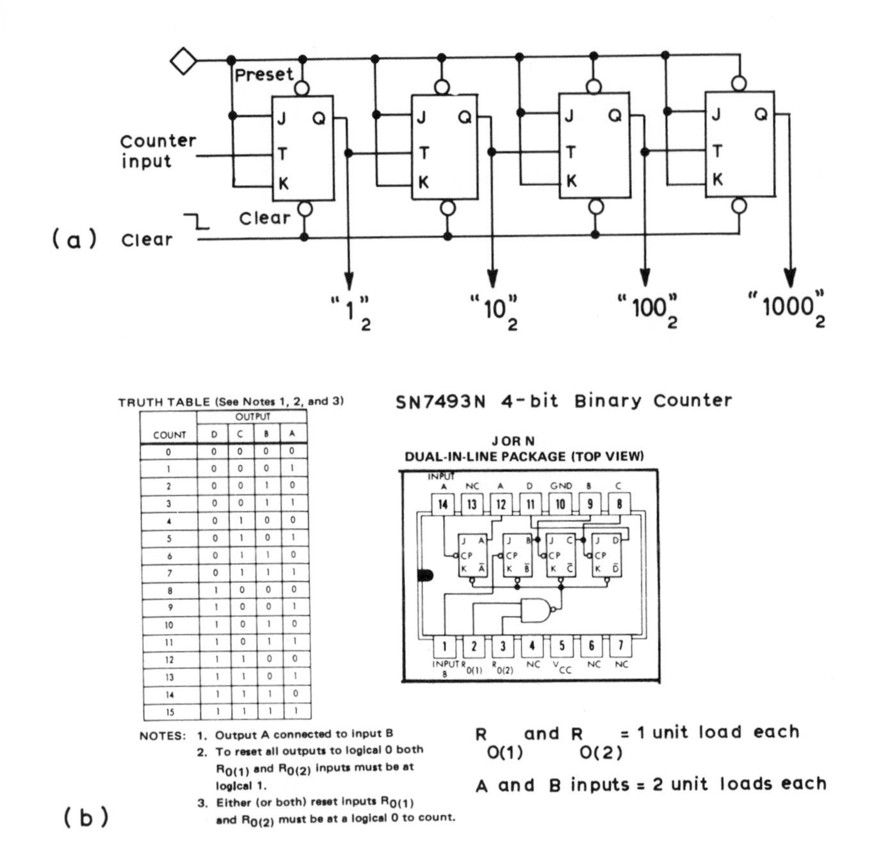

TRUTH TABLE (See Notes 1, 2, and 3)

COUNT	OUTPUT D	C	B	A
0	0	0	0	0
1	0	0	0	1
2	0	0	1	0
3	0	0	1	1
4	0	1	0	0
5	0	1	0	1
6	0	1	1	0
7	0	1	1	1
8	1	0	0	0
9	1	0	0	1
10	1	0	1	0
11	1	0	1	1
12	1	1	0	0
13	1	1	0	1
14	1	1	1	0
15	1	1	1	1

Figure 4.16
Four-bit binary counters. (a) Constructed from flipflops; (b) SN7493N (from *The Integrated Circuits Catalog for Design Engineers, Catalog CC-401*, 1971, by Texas Instruments. Used with permission of Texas Instruments).

once every 2 input cycles; the 100 output flips once per 10 cycle, or once every 4 input cycles. The general pattern is that each "higher" (or "more significant") bit represents a count twice as high as the preceding ("less significant") bit. It is a general rule that in any number system, regardless of base n (number of possible values for a digit: in decimal, $n = 10$; in binary, $n = 2$) we can represent any integer by a sufficiently long string of digits, where each digit of successively higher significance represents the face value of the digit times the base n raised to a successively higher integral power, starting with the zeroth power of n in the rightmost position. For example,

$$93874 = (9 \times 10^4) + (3 \times 10^3) + (8 \times 10^2) + (7 \times 10^1) + (4 \times 10^0)$$

We will refer to the *rightmost digit* in any string of digits as the first digit; and proceeding to the left, we shall call them the 2nd, 3rd, 4th digits, and so forth.

Table 4.11
Bit pattern at input and outputs of a 4-bit binary counter.

Count in	"1000"	"100"	"10"	"1"	Input cycle number
1	0	0	0	0	1
0	0	0	0	1	1
1	0	0	0	1	2
0	0	0	1	0	2
1	0	0	1	0	3
0	0	0	1	1	3
1	0	0	1	1	4
0	0	1	0	0	4
1	0	1	0	0	5
0	0	1	0	1	5
1	0	1	0	1	6
0	0	1	1	0	6
1	0	1	1	0	7
0	0	1	1	1	7
1	0	1	1	1	8
0	1	0	0	0	8
1	1	0	0	0	9
0	1	0	0	1	9
1	1	0	0	1	10
0	1	0	1	0	10
1	1	0	1	0	11
0	1	0	1	1	11
1	1	0	1	1	12
0	1	1	0	0	12
1	1	1	0	0	13
0	1	1	0	1	13
1	1	1	0	1	14
0	1	1	1	0	14
1	1	1	1	0	15
0	1	1	1	1	15

Preset and clear = 0.
Count enable = 1.
Count is cleared to 0000 before enabling count.

The requirements for representing all possible integers of values between 0 and 15 are met by the counter of Figure 4.16a: Each integer is represented by a unique pattern of bits, and each pattern of bits corresponds to a unique integer.

The states of the input and output bits of the counter are represented in Table 4.11. As the input alternates (each positive-negative pair of transitions is a count "cycle"), the output increments through successively higher values. Note, as in decimal counting, that the lowest-order digit counts from minimum to maximum (in decimal, 0–9; in binary, 0–1). Then it cycles back to zero and a one is "carried" (added) to the next more significant digit. A carry "ripples" to the left until it is carried into a bit which goes from 0 to 1 on the carry. Each digit behaves in the same fashion, incrementing with each carry from the preceding digit. The input, or counter signal, can be considered a carry into the first digit.

We can write an addition and subtraction table for binary arithmetic starting with the knowledge that each table is a 2 × 2 matrix (since the arguments—addend, augend, subtrahend, or minuend—must be binary, or two valued, and the relations diagrammed are dyadic). Addition of zero in any number system results in a sum that is equal to the original augend. Addition of 1 is equivalent to incrementing a count. These two facts cover all possible additions and result in the addition table of Table 4.12a. The subtraction table of Table 4.12b is derived from the addition table.

The addition and subtraction of signed numbers is accomplished as it is in decimal arithmetic, using the binary addition and subtraction tables and the customary sign conventions.

Larger numbers are treated as in any other number system, by carrying (addition) and borrowing (subtraction). The following examples of binary addition and subtraction should suffice to illustrate the similarity:

	Addition			*Subtraction*	
(+)	111 1 ←	carries	(−)	111 1 ←	borrows
	1101011	addend	Subtrahend	11000101	
	+1011010	augend	minuend	−1011010	
	11000101	sum	difference	1101011	

(Proceed from right to left as in decimal addition and subtraction.)

It is obvious that a method is needed for representing negative numbers in binary logic circuits. Since there are twice as many signed numbers as positive numbers (not counting zero) within a given magnitude range, a signed binary number must be one digit longer if we plan to represent the sign as a binary bit.

Table 4.12
Binary addition and subtraction.

(a) Addition

Addend		0	1
		Sum	
Augend	**0**	0	1
	1	1	10

(b) Subtraction

Subtrahend		0	1	10
		Difference		
Minuend	**0**	0	1	10
	1	−1	0	1
	10	−10	−1	0

Table 4.13
Representation of negative binary numbers.

Positive binary	Positive decimal	Negative one's complement	Negative two's complement	Negative decimal
0:000	+0	1111	0000	−0
0:001	+1	1110	1111	−1
0:010	+2	1101	1110	−2
0:011	+3	1100	1101	−3
0:100	+4	1011	1100	−4
0:101	+5	1010	1011	−5
0:110	+6	1001	1010	−6
0:111	+7	1000	1001	−7
sign : magnitude				

Although we could use any of a multitude of possible methods to represent negative numbers, we will examine here only the two most popular: two's complement representation and one's complement representation.

Both representation systems utilize the leftmost bit of a binary register as the sign bit. This bit does not contribute to the magnitude of the number. Although the rest of the number could be left unchanged, the *one's complement* system uses a bit-by-bit *complementation* (inversion) of the bit logical values. The resulting number is essentially the product of the original number times −1. However, when adding a negative number to a positive number, the resulting value is always 1 less than the true sum. Therefore, the *two's complement* (negative number) of a positive number is derived by complementing the number as in one's complement arithmetic and *incrementing by one*. Table 4.13 gives the one's and two's complements of all positive four bit signed binary numbers, and their decimal equivalents.

By using negative two's complement numbers, we can perform subtraction with the same logic circuits as we use for addition, keeping in mind the necessity for detecting add and subtract *overflows* (resulting number too large for the number of bits available) and ensuring that the sign of the resultant is correct.

A multiplication table for binary arithmetic is derived from the fact that the product of any number times one is the original number (multiplicand), and any number times zero is zero. Division by one results in a quotient which is equal to the dividend, and division by zero is undefined. Multiplication tables for single-digit multiplication and division are given in Table 4.14, and examples of multiple-digit multiplication and division are

```
    101                              100
  × 101                      101) 11000
  -----                           ------
    101  (101 × 1)               - 10100
   000   (101 × 00)              -------
 + 101   (101 × 100)                 100
 ------                            - 000
  11001                            -----
                                     100
                                   - 000
                                   -----
                                     100 remainder
```

The conventions for determining the sign of a product or quotient in signed multiplication or division are identical to those of decimal multiplication and division of signed numbers.

We can combine successive groups of bits as digits of a higher-base number system to conveniently represent the content of a binary register. For example, it is common to represent binary numbers as *octal* numbers (radix = 8), because three binary bits can represent the values from 0 to 7. The radix is written as a

Table 4.14
Binary multiplication and division.

(a) Multiplication:

		Product	
Multiplicand		**0**	**1**
Multiplier	**0**	0	0
	1	0	1

(b) Division:

		Quotient	
Dividend		**0**	**1**
Divisor	**0**	*	*
	1	0	1

* undefined: x/0

Table 4.15
Examples of equivalent representations of numbers in decimal, octal, and binary.

Decimal	Octal	Binary
0	0	0
1	1	1
2	2	10
3	3	11
4	4	100
5	5	101
6	6	110
7	7	111
8	10	1000
9	11	1001
10	12	1010
11	13	1011
12	14	1100
13	15	1101
14	16	1110
15	17	1111
16	20	10000
25	31	11001
32	40	100000
144	220	10010000
256	400	100000000
1024	2000	10000000000

subscript, for example,

$$111100001010_2 = 7412_8 = 3850_{10}$$

Some examples of decimal numbers and their representations in binary and octal are given in Table 4.15.

Table 4.16 gives addition and multiplication tables for octal numbers. Conversion rules for going from one number system to another can best be described by separately specifying methods for converting to a higher or a lower radix.

To go from a lower radix to a higher one, divide the "source" number by the radix of the desired "resultant" number, as represented in the source number system (it will always be represented by more than one digit in the source system), using source arithmetic rules. The remainder, after converting to the resultant equivalent, will be the least significant digit of the resultant number. Divide the quotient obtained from the first division by the resultant radix, as before. The new remainder is the second least significant digit of the resultant number. Continue

Table 4.16
Octal addition and multiplication.

(a) Octal addition

	0	1	2	3	4	5	6	7
0	0	1	2	3	4	5	6	7
1	1	2	3	4	5	6	7	10
2	2	3	4	5	6	7	10	11
3	3	4	5	6	7	10	11	12
4	4	5	6	7	10	11	12	13
5	5	6	7	10	11	12	13	14
6	6	7	10	11	12	13	14	15
7	7	10	11	12	13	14	15	16

(b) Octal multiplication

	0	1	2	3	4	5	6	7
0	0	0	0	0	0	0	0	0
1	0	1	2	3	4	5	6	7
2	0	2	4	6	10	12	14	16
3	0	3	6	11	14	17	22	25
4	0	4	10	14	20	24	30	34
5	0	5	12	17	24	31	36	43
6	0	6	14	22	30	36	44	52
7	0	7	16	25	34	43	52	61

dividing the quotients of the successive divisions with the resultant radix, saving remainders as successively more significant digits. When the quotient is zero, the remainder is the most significant digit, and the conversion is complete. For example,

Convert 1234_8 *to decimal.*

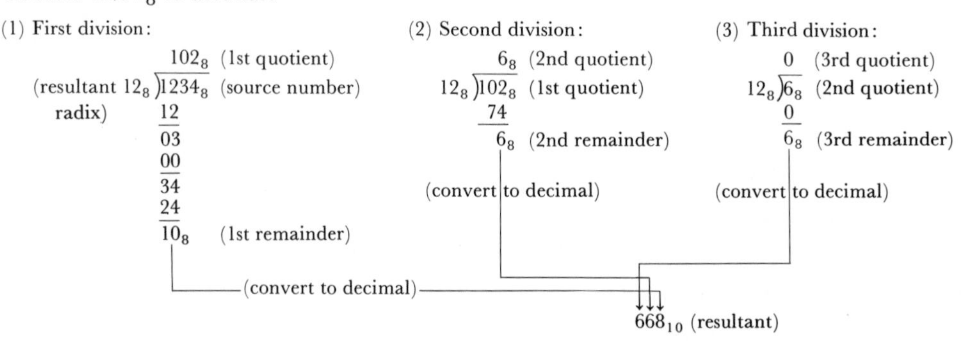

To go from a higher number base system to a lower one, the same method can be used, but inconvenient carries are sometimes generated in the remainders, which are not always single digits after conversion to the resultant system. Instead, it is easier to treat each digit as follows: For the mth digit of the source number (radix $= n$) whose face value is $r_m \times n^{m-1}$, multiply r_m (converted to the resultant system) by n^{m-1}, using resultant system arithmetic. Total all the digits that have been converted in this way to obtain the resultant number, for example:

Convert 668_{10} *to octal.*

$$
\begin{array}{llllll}
\text{1st digit:} & 8_{10} = 8_{10} \times 10^0_{10} & = & 10_8 \times 12^0_8 & = & 10_8 \\
\text{2nd digit:} & 60_{10} = 6_{10} \times 10^1_{10} & = & 6_8 \times 12^1_8 & = & 74_8 \\
\text{3rd digit:} & 600_{10} = 6_{10} \times 10^2_{10} & = & 6_8 \times 12^2_8 & = & 1130_8 \\
 & & & & \text{Total} & 1234_8 = \text{resultant number}
\end{array}
$$

The reader can verify, on closer examination, that the two methods are simply different ways of doing the same thing.

Fractions are represented in all number systems in the same way: as a numerator over a denominator. To convert from one system to another, simply convert the numerator and denominator separately:

$$\left(\frac{19}{17}\right)_{10} = \left(\frac{23}{21}\right)_8 = \left(\frac{10011}{10001}\right)_2.$$

A fraction that is reduced in one number system will be reduced in all other systems.

To represent fractions with digital logic, we must use the equivalent of a decimal point (a binary point). The portion of the number to the left of the point is treated like any other whole number and is converted by using the rules already prescribed. For the portion to the right of the point, use a variation of the second rule prescribed above. Every integer r_m to the right of the point is the face value r of the integer times the corresponding negative power of the radix, n^{-m}, and the entire portion to the left of the point is therefore the sum of all the integers, as in the second method above. Therefore, to convert to a new radix, compute the value of each integer in the new system and find the total, using the resultant arithmetic rules; for example:

(a) *Convert* 0.1234_{10} *to octal.*

$$
\begin{array}{lllll}
0.1_{10} & = 1 \times 10^{-1}_{10} = 1 \times 12^{-1}_8 = & 12_8 \overline{)1.00000_8} & = & 0.06315_8 \\
0.02_{10} & = 2 \times 10^{-2}_{10} = 2 \times 12^{-2}_8 = & 144_8 \overline{)2.00000_8} & = & 0.01217_8 \\
0.003_{10} & = 3 \times 10^{-3}_{10} = 3 \times 12^{-3}_8 = & 1750_8 \overline{)3.00000_8} & = & 0.00142_8 \\
0.0004_{10} & = 4 \times 10^{-4}_{10} = 4 \times 12^{-4}_8 = & 23420_8 \overline{)4.00000_8} & = & 0.00016_8 \\
 & & & & 0.07714_8 \\
 & & \text{rounded off:} & & 0.0772_8
\end{array}
$$

Table 4.17
Input and output bit patterns of a 2-digit BCD counter.

Cycle	Input	A_1 (LSB_1)	B_1	C_1	D_1 (MSB_1)	A_2 (LSB_2)	B_2	C_2	D_2 (MSB_2)
1	0	0	0	0	0	0	0	0	0
1	1	0	0	0	0	0	0	0	0
2	0	1	0	0	0	0	0	0	0
2	1	1	0	0	0	0	0	0	0
3	0	0	1	0	0	0	0	0	0
3	1	0	1	0	0	0	0	0	0
4	0	1	1	0	0	0	0	0	0
4	1	1	1	0	0	0	0	0	0
5	0	0	0	1	0	0	0	0	0
5	1	0	0	1	0	0	0	0	0
6	0	1	0	1	0	0	0	0	0
6	1	1	0	1	0	0	0	0	0
7	0	0	1	1	0	0	0	0	0
7	1	0	1	1	0	0	0	0	0
8	0	1	1	1	0	0	0	0	0
8	1	1	1	1	0	0	0	0	0
9	0	0	0	0	1	0	0	0	0
9	1	0	0	0	1	0	0	0	0
10	0	1	0	0	1	0	0	0	0
10	1	1	0	0	1	0	0	0	0
11	0	0	0	0	0	1	0	0	0
11	1	0	0	0	0	1	0	0	0
12	0	1	0	0	0	1	0	0	0
12	1	1	0	0	0	1	0	0	0
13	0	0	1	0	0	1	0	0	0
13	1	0	1	0	0	1	0	0	0
14	0	1	1	0	0	1	0	0	0
14	1	1	1	0	0	1	0	0	0
15	0	0	0	1	0	1	0	0	0
15	1	0	0	1	0	1	0	0	0
16	0	1	0	1	0	1	0	0	0
16	1	1	0	1	0	1	0	0	0
17	0	0	1	1	0	1	0	0	0
17	1	0	1	1	0	1	0	0	0
18	0	1	1	1	0	1	0	0	0
18	1	1	1	1	0	1	0	0	0
19	0	0	0	0	1	1	0	0	0
19	1	0	0	0	1	1	0	0	0
20	0	1	0	0	1	1	0	0	0
20	1	1	0	0	1	1	0	0	0
21	0	0	0	0	0	0	1	0	0

(b) *Convert* 0.0772_8 *to decimal.*

$$
\begin{array}{llllll}
0.0_8 & = 0 \times 10_8^{-1} & = 0 \times 8_{10}^{-1} & = 8_{10} & \overline{)0.00000_{10}} & = 0.00000_{10} \\
0.07_8 & = 7 \times 10_8^{-2} & = 7 \times 8_{10}^{-2} & = 64_{10} & \overline{)7.00000_{10}} & = 0.10906_{10} \\
0.007_8 & = 7 \times 10_8^{-3} & = 7 \times 8_{10}^{-3} & = 512_{10} & \overline{)7.00000_{10}} & = 0.01369_{10} \\
0.0002_8 & = 2 \times 10_8^{-4} & = 2 \times 8_{10}^{-4} & = 4096_{10} & \overline{)2.00000_{10}} & = \underline{0.00049_{10}} \\
 & & & & & 0.12324_{10} \\
 & & & & \text{rounded off:} & 0.123_{10}
\end{array}
$$

Before going on to examine the implementation of binary arithmetic in digital logic systems, let us examine one other of the many different systems for representing numbers with binary levels. This is the BCD, or Binary Coded Decimal system. Each BCD "digit" consists of four binary subdigits used to represent a decimal digit. The four binary bits of a BCD counter cycle upward from zero to nine on negative clock transitions exactly as they would in the binary system. However, when the value is incremented from nine, the number goes to zero, and there is a "carry" to the next BCD digit. The subdigits within each BCD digit (the binary bits) are labeled *A*, *B*, *C*, *D*, from least significant ("1") to most significant ("8"). Table 4.17 illustrates the states of *A*–*D* for a 2-digit BCD counter, where D_1 provides the input for the second bit.

One design for a BCD counter, the SN7490N, is shown in Figure 4.17. The device actually consists of two counters: a scale-of-two counter consisting of a single flipflop, like a single bit in a binary counter; and a scale-of-five counter internally wired to reset on the increment from a count of four.

Figure 4.18 presents a more detailed schematic of the internal wiring of the device, and timing diagrams indicate the status of bits *A*–*D* in the count-to-ten configuration (output of bit *A* drives bits *B*–*D*) as well as the very useful symmetrical-divide-by-ten configuration (output of bit *D* drives bit *A*).

The count-to-ten configuration output represents, in BCD code, the number of input cycles which have been completed (that is, number of positive-negative transition pairs, *modulo* the counter's maximum value, since the counter was last reset). A multidigit count is obtained by feeding the *D* output of the *n*th BCD digit (counter) to the *A* input of the $(n + 1)$th BCD digit. The *A* input to the first BCD counter is the signal to be counted.

The divide-by-ten configuration uses the scale-of-five counter to drive the scale-of-two counter. If a square wave of fixed frequency is fed to the *BD* input, the *D* output will transition at regular intervals, once each five input cycles. The *D* output negative transition (at the end of each five cycles) causes the *A* output to toggle. Since the *A* output toggles once every five input cycles, the *A* output will be a square wave whose frequency is exactly one-tenth that of the input (two toggles per output cycle).

logic

TRUTH TABLES

BCD COUNT SEQUENCE
(See Note 1)

COUNT	OUTPUT D	C	B	A
0	0	0	0	0
1	0	0	0	1
2	0	0	1	0
3	0	0	1	1
4	0	1	0	0
5	0	1	0	1
6	0	1	1	0
7	0	1	1	1
8	1	0	0	0
9	1	0	0	1

RESET/COUNT (See Note 2)

RESET INPUTS $R_{0(1)}$	$R_{0(2)}$	$R_{9(1)}$	$R_{9(2)}$	OUTPUT D C B A
1	1	0	X	0 0 0 0
1	1	X	0	0 0 0 0
X	X	1	1	1 0 0 1
X	0	X	0	COUNT
0	X	0	X	COUNT
0	X	X	0	COUNT
X	0	0	X	COUNT

NC—No Internal Connection

NOTES: 1. Output A connected to input BD for BCD count.
2. X indicates that either a logical 1 or a logical 0 may be present.

J OR N
DUAL-IN-LINE PACKAGE (TOP VIEW)

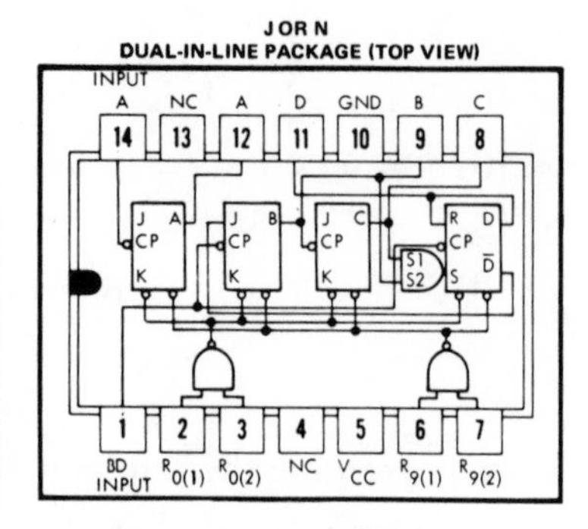

$R_{0(1)}, R_{0(2)}, R_{9(1)}, R_{9(2)}$ inputs =
1 unit load each

BD input = 4 unit loads
A input = 2 unit loads

1. When used as a binary coded decimal decade counter, the BD input must be externally connected to the A output. The A input receives the incoming count, and a count sequence is obtained in accordance with the BCD count sequence truth table shown above. In addition to a conventional zero reset, inputs are provided to reset a BCD count for nine's complement decimal applications.

2. If a symmetrical divide-by-ten count is desired for frequency synthesizers or other applications requiring division of a binary count by a power of ten, the D output must be externally connected to the A input. The input count is then applied at the BD input and a divide-by-ten square wave is obtained at output A.

3. For operation as a divide-by-two counter and a divide-by-five counter, no external interconnections are required. Flip-flop A is used as a binary element for the divide-by-two function. The BD input is used to obtain binary divide-by-five operation at the B, C, and D outputs. In this mode, the two counters operate independently; however, all four flip-flops are reset simultaneously.

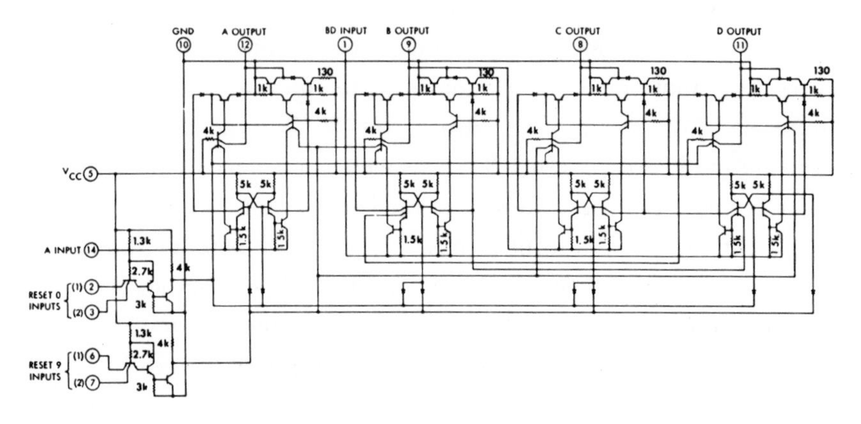

Figure 4.17
SN7490N decade counter (from *The Integrated Circuits Catalog for Design Engineers, Catalog CC-401*, 1971, by Texas Instruments. Used with the permission of Texas Instruments).

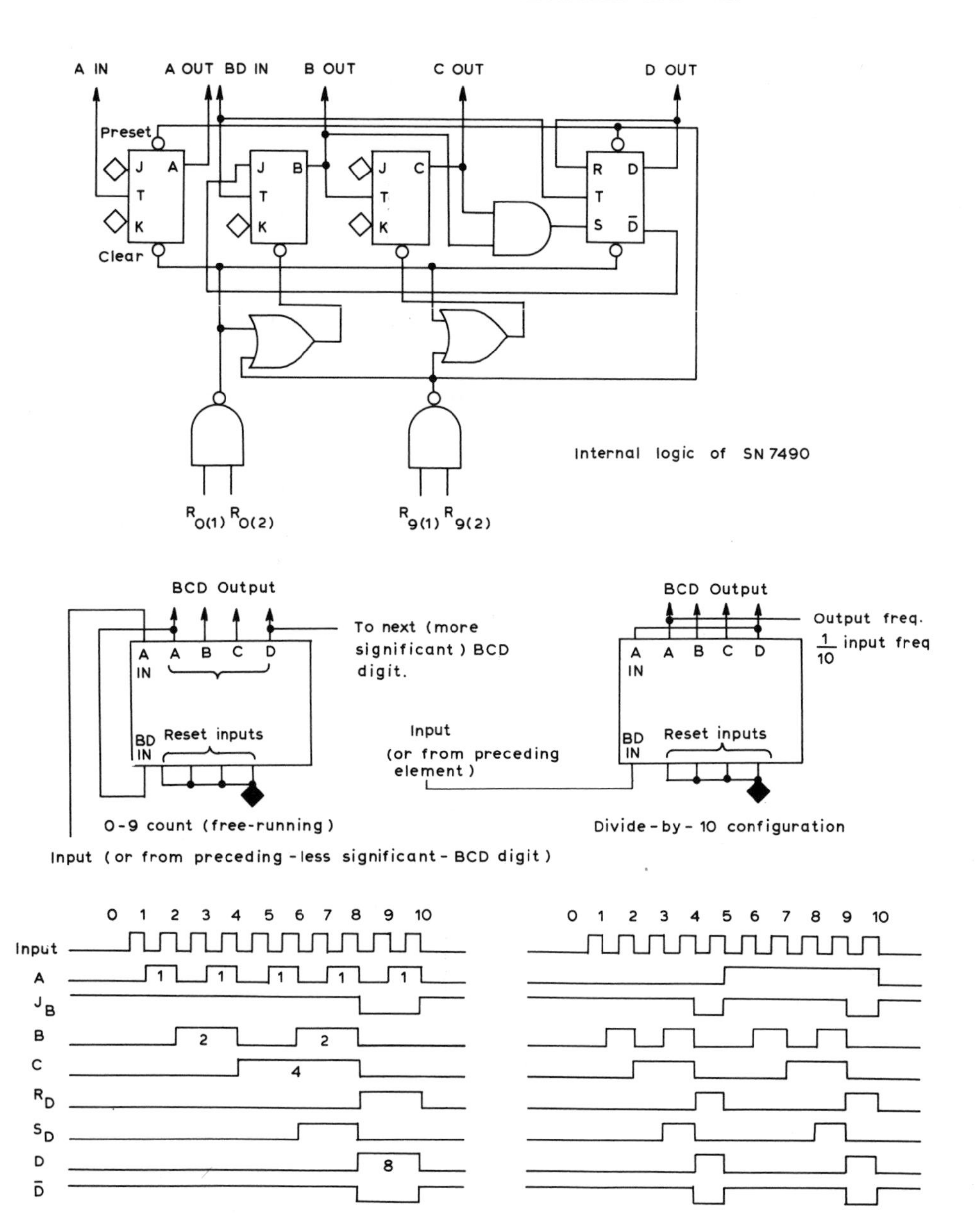

Figure 4.18
Operation of SN7490N.

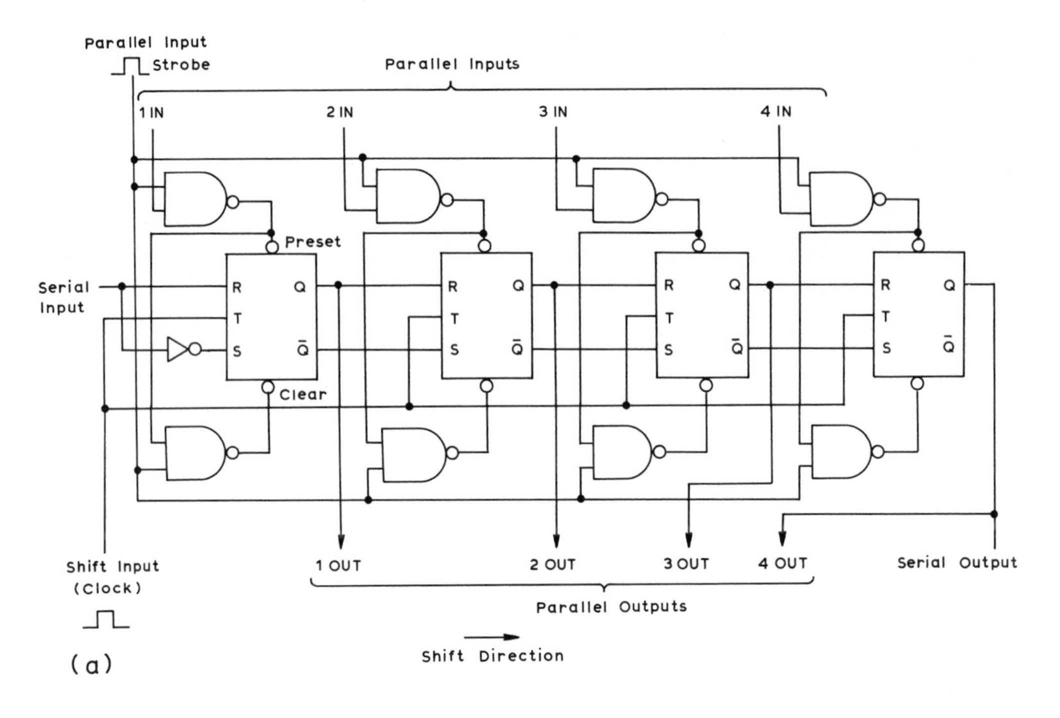

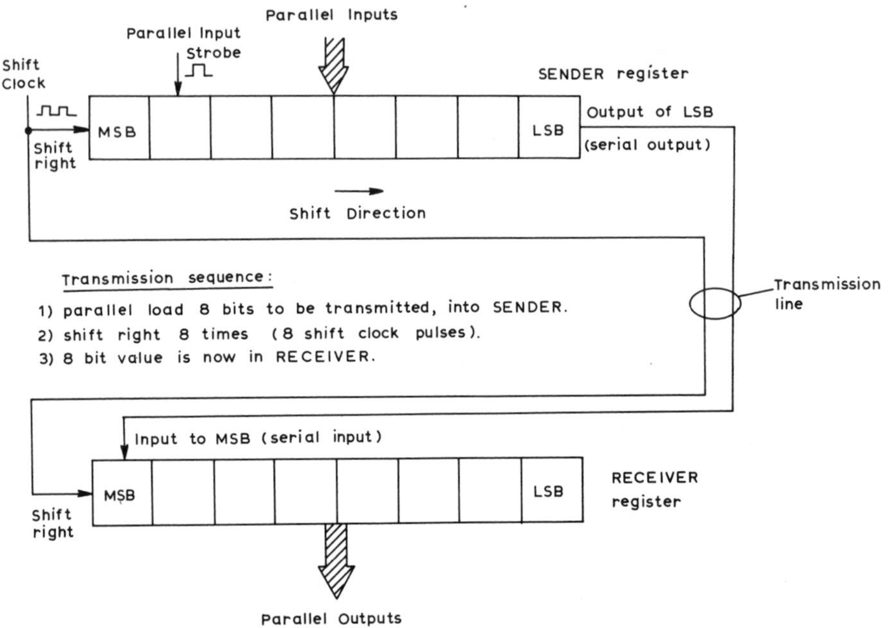

Figure 4.19
Shift registers: (a) parallel-input, serial-input, parallel-output, serial-output, 4-bit right-shift registers; (b) 8-bit serial transmitter and receiver.

Although there are arithmetic elements that directly handle BCD numbers, we will not consider them. We will only describe the simplest binary arithmetic elements.

A device that is essential in some types of arithmetic operations is the *shift register* (Figure 4.19), consisting of a string of flipflops whose states can be determined either by the values of a corresponding set of external inputs ("parallel loading" of values); or the value of each flipflop output can be determined by the value of the flipflop to the "left" or "right," with the only external input coming to the flipflop at the left or right end of the chain ("serial loading" of values).

In the former mode of operation, the values are "strobed" into the register simultaneously, by forcing the flipflops to assume the values of the parallel inputs via the preset and clear inputs of the flipflops. In the serial mode of operation, the current values of the flipflops are *shifted* one bit on the occurrence of a clock cycle. The requirement for two clock transitions per shift is often referred to as "two-phased shifting." The example of Figure 4.19a is a right-shift register; that is, the shift input clock causes a flipflop to assume the value of the flipflop to the left of it, via the *R-S* inputs and the clock input of each flipflop. The leftmost flipflop is the "serial input" for the register. There is no flipflop to the left of it, but the first input can be tied to some external signal source. If the clock is synchronized to the external serial input in such a way as to occur once for each new "state" of the time-varying serial input, the n shift register outputs will reflect the n successive states occupied by the input at the time of the n most recent clock cycles. This process is referred to as serial-to-parallel conversion and can be used to receive a multibit value transmitted serially via a two-wire transmission line, where one wire carries the serial bits and the other channel transmits the shift pulses.

Similarly, we can load the flipflop with one operation, strobing all n values in simultaneously through the parallel inputs. Then, we can sequentially output the n bits, least significant first, by performing n shifts and reading the output before each shift. This technique, called parallel-to-serial conversion, can be used to set up the serial outputs to a two-channel transmission line; one channel carries the output of the least significant bit of the "sender" shift register, and the other channel carries the clock. The same clock signal that is used to shift the "sender" shift register can be used to shift the "receiver" shift register. Such a transmission system is illustrated in Figure 4.19b. The entire system is thus a 16-bit shift register. The eight most significant bits are parallel-loaded, eight shifts take place, and the original eight bits are now in the eight least significant locations. The upper and lower eight bits are connected via the transmission line.

Figure 4.20 illustrates some of the many integrated circuit shift registers available. These designs trade versatility for small size: Because there is a limited number

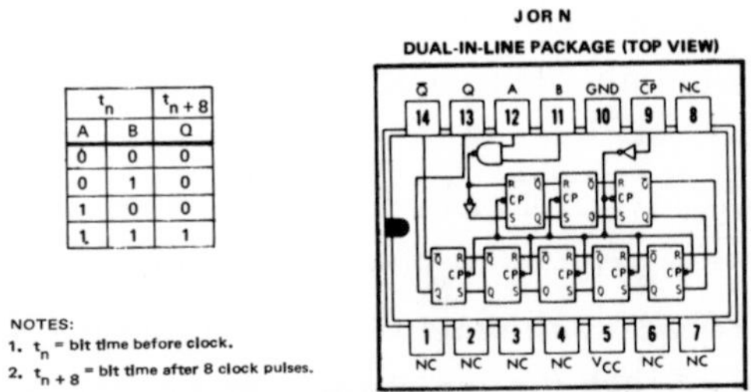

t_n		t_{n+8}
A	B	Q
0	0	0
0	1	0
1	0	0
1	1	1

NOTES:
1. t_n = bit time before clock.
2. t_{n+8} = bit time after 8 clock pulses.

Single-rail data and input control are gated through inputs A and B and an internal inverter to form the complementary inputs to the first bit of the shift register. Drive for the internal common clock line is provided by an inverting clock driver. Each of the inputs (A, B, and $\overline{CP}$) appear as only one TTL input load.

(a) The clock pulse inverter/driver causes these circuits to shift information to the output on the positive edge of an input clock pulse, thus enabling the shift-register to be fully compatible with other edge-triggered synchronous functions.

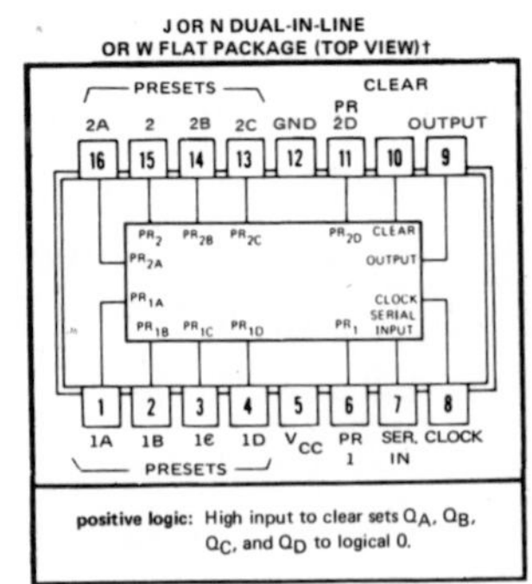

All flip-flops are simultaneously set to the logical 0 state by applying a logical 1 voltage to the clear input. This condition may be applied independent of the state of the clock input, but not independent of state of the preset input. Preset input is independent of the clock and clear states.

The flip-flops are simultaneously set to the logical 1 state from either of two preset input sources. Preset inputs 1A through 1D are activated during the time that a positive pulse is applied to preset 1 if preset 2 is at a logical 0 level. When the logic levels at preset 1 and preset 2 are reversed, preset inputs 2A through 2D are active.

Transfer of information to the outputs occurs when the clock input goes from a logical 0 to a logical 1. Since the flip-flops are R-S master-slave circuits, the proper information must appear at the R-S inputs of each flip-flop prior to the rising edge of the clock input waveform. The serial input provides this information for the first flip-flop. The outputs of the subsequent flip-flops provide information for the remaining R-S Inputs. The clear input, preset 1, and preset 2 must be at a logical 0 when clocking occurs.

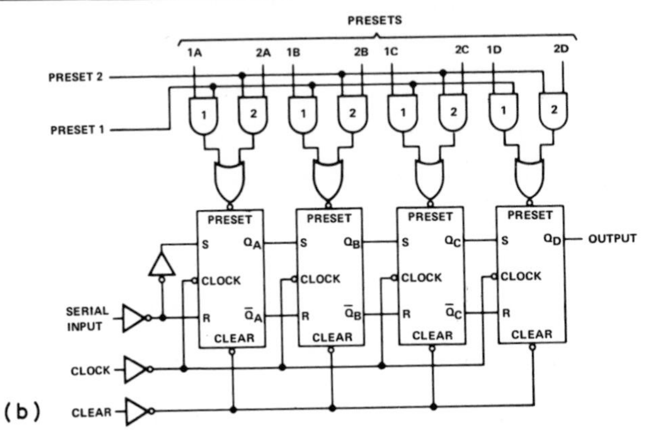

Preset 1, Preset 2 = 2 loads each
All other inputs = 1 load each

Figure 4.20
Some SN7400N series shift registers: (a) SN7491AN 8-bit serial-in, serial-out shift register; (b) SN7494N parallel-in, parallel-out shift register; (c) SN7496N parallel-in, parallel-out, 5-bit shift register; (d) SN7495AN 4-bit parallel-in, parallel-out, right-left shift register (from *The Integrated Circuits Catalog for Design Engineers, Catalog CC-401*, 1971, by Texas Instruments. Used with permission of Texas Instruments).

All flip-flops are simultaneously set to the logical 0 state by applying a logical 0 voltage to the clear input. This condition may be applied independent of the state of the clock input.

The flip-flops may be independently set to the logical 1 state by applying a logical 1 to both the preset input of the specific flip-flop and the common preset input. The preset-enable input is provided to allow flexibility of either setting each flip-flop independently or setting two or more flip-flops simultaneously. Preset is also independent of the state of the clock input or clear input.

Transfer of information to the output pins occurs when the clock input goes from a logical 0 to a logical 1 . Since the flip-flops are R-S master-slave circuits, the proper information must appear at the R-S inputs of each flip-flop prior to the rising edge of the clock input voltage waveform. The serial input provides this information to the first flip-flop, while the outputs of the subsequent flip-flops provide information for the remaining R-S inputs. The clear input must be at a logical 1 and the preset input must be at a logical 0 when clocking occurs.

J OR N
DUAL-IN-LINE PACKAGE (TOP VIEW)

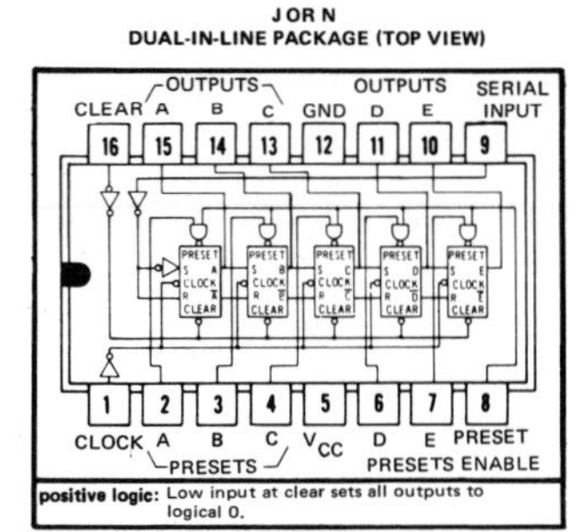

Preset input = 5 unit loads
All other inputs = 1 unit load each

(c)

When a logical 0 level is applied to the mode control input, the number-1 AND gates are enabled and the number-2 AND gates are inhibited. In this mode the output of each flip-flop is coupled to the R-S inputs of the succeeding flip-flop and right-shift operation is performed by clocking at the clock 1 input. In this mode, serial data is entered at the serial input. Clock 2 and parallel inputs A through D are inhibited by the number-2 AND gates.

When a logical 1 level is applied to the mode control input, the number-1 AND gates are inhibited (decoupling the outputs from the succeeding R-S inputs to prevent right-shift) and the number-2 AND gates are enabled to allow entry of data through parallel inputs A through D and clock 2. This mode permits parallel loading of the register, or with external interconnection, shift-left operation. In this mode, shift-left can be accomplished by connecting the output of each flip-flop to the parallel input of the previous flip-flop (Q_D to input C, and etc.), and serial data is entered at input D.

J OR N
DUAL-IN-LINE PACKAGE (TOP VIEW)

V_{CC} OUTPUTS Q_A Q_B Q_C Q_D CLOCK 1 R-SHIFT CLOCK 2 L-SHIFT
14 13 12 11 10 9 8
1 2 3 4 5 6 7
SERIAL INPUT A B C D INPUTS MODE CONTROL GND

positive logic
Mode control = 0 for right shift
Mode control = 1 for left shift or parallel load

Mode control input = 2 unit loads
All other inputs = 1 unit load each

Clocking for the shift register is accomplished through the AND-OR gate E which permits separate clock sources to be used for the shift-right and shift-left modes. If both modes can be clocked from the same source, the clock input may be applied commonly to clock 1 and clock 2. Information must be present at the R-S inputs of the master-slave flip-flops prior to clocking. Transfer of information to the output pins occurs when the clock input goes from a logical 1 to a logical 0.

(d)

Figure 4.20 (continued)

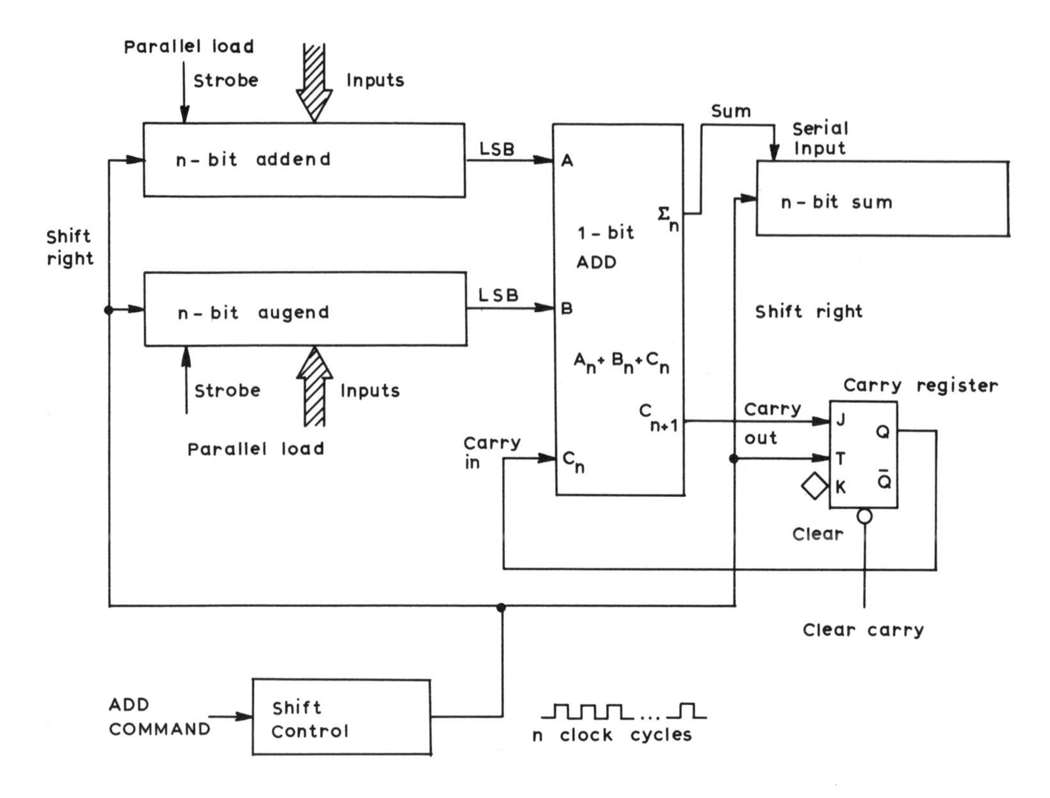

Figure 4.21
Serial addition.

of pins to the integrated circuit, some shift registers sacrifice parallel output for number of bits; others may sacrifice number of bits for parallel outputs; still others may require more complex logical control signals but can provide shifting in either direction.

Another application for shift registers is illustrated in Figure 4.21: serial addition of two n-bit signed numbers. The device uses three n-bit shift registers, a two-bit shift register (a single master-slave flipflop will do) and a two-input adder circuit to perform the addition of two n-bit signed numbers. The shift control indicated in the figure consists of a device that generates $n + 1$ clock pulses, initiated by an input ADD COMMAND signal. It is assumed that the addend and augend have been loaded and the carry register cleared before the ADD COMMAND is given.

The output of the adder circuit is defined by the truth table (Table 4.18). Note that the sum output D is equivalent to the least significant of two bits resulting from a one-bit addition of two numbers and a carry in C_n, and the carry output C_{n+1} is equivalent to the most significant bit of such an addition. The outputs thus defined are the result of adding the nth bit of the augend and the nth bit of

Table 4.18
Input and output bit patterns for a binary adder.

A_n Addend	B_n Augend	C_n Carry in	$D_r(\Sigma_n)$ Sum	C_{n+1} Carry out
0	0	0	0	0
0	0	1	1	0
0	1	0	1	0
0	1	1	0	1
1	0	0	1	0
1	0	1	0	1
1	1	0	0	1
1	1	1	1	1

the addend, along with the carry from the $(n - 1)$th addition C_n. For the least significant bit, there is of course no carry in, and the C_1 is therefore zero. For this reason, the carry shift register must be cleared before the initiation of addition (it could be cleared at the same time that the addend and augend are loaded). The sum register need never be cleared because the content is entirely determined by the most recent n-bit addition, regardless of its previous value. As each addend-augend pair appears in the inputs of the adder, along with the carry from the previous add, the sum output of the adder assumes the value D and is fed to the serial input (MSB) of the sum register. When the next shift occurs, the sum is shifted right, and the new MSB is loaded. After n shifts, all n addend-augend-carry triplets have been added, and the corresponding sums serially loaded into the sum register. If the sum is larger than n bits ("add overflow"), the output of the carry shift register will be one.

A logic circuit that performs the one-bit add is illustrated in Figure 4.22.

Serial addition of multibit numbers is slower than parallel addition but uses less hardware. The latter is diagrammed in Figure 4.23. In the parallel adder, the addend, augend, and sum registers are not shifted. Rather, a separate adder is used to add each pair of bits and the carry from the next lower-order addition simultaneously. Although more logic circuitry is required, the addition occurs just as fast as the carries can "ripple" from the lowest-order adder to the output of the highest-order adder (that is, in the "worst case," $111\ldots111_2 + 111\ldots111_2$) rather than the length of time required to perform n shifts. Options exist for "look-ahead," wherein faster addition is made possible. Figure 4.24 illustrates the SN7483N, a four-bit binary parallel adder. By stringing the carry output to the carry input of another adder, four more bits of higher significance can be introduced. Hence, as many bits as desired can be obtained.

$$C_{n+1} = (A_n \wedge B_n) \vee (B_n \wedge C_n) \vee (A_n \wedge C_n) = (A_n \overline{\wedge} B_n) \overline{\wedge} (A_n \overline{\wedge} C_n) \overline{\wedge} (B_n \overline{\wedge} C_n)$$

$$\Sigma_n = ((A_n \vee B_n \vee C_n) \wedge \overline{C_{n+1}}) \vee (A_n \wedge B_n \wedge C_n) = ((\overline{A_n} \overline{\wedge} \overline{B_n} \overline{\wedge} \overline{C_n}) \overline{\wedge} \overline{C_{n+1}}) \overline{\wedge} (A_n \overline{\wedge} B_n \overline{\wedge} C_n)$$

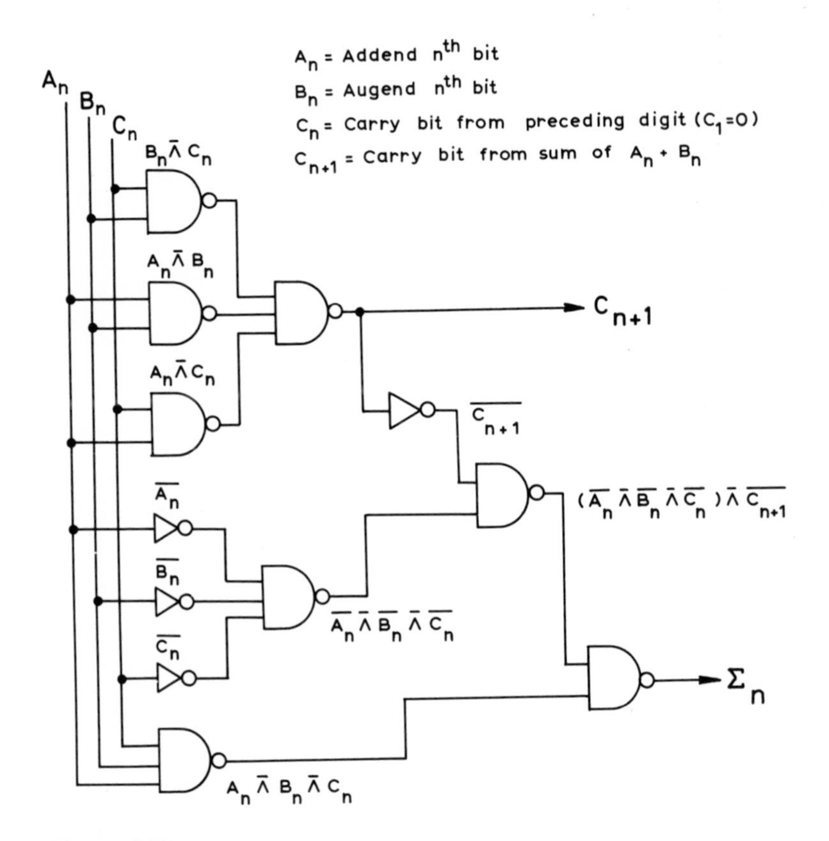

Figure 4.22
One-bit adder:

$$C_{n+1} = (A \wedge B) \vee (B \wedge C_n) \vee (A \wedge C_n) = (A \overline{\wedge} B) \overline{\wedge} (A \overline{\wedge} C_n) \overline{\wedge} (B \overline{\wedge} C_n)$$

$$\Sigma_n = ((A \vee B \vee C_n) \wedge \bar{C}_{n+1}) \vee (A \wedge B \wedge C_n) = ((\bar{A} \overline{\wedge} \bar{B} \overline{\wedge} \bar{C}) \overline{\wedge} \bar{C}_{n+1}) \overline{\wedge} (A \overline{\wedge} B \overline{\wedge} C),$$

where A_n = addend, nth bit

B_n = augend, nth bit

C_n = carry bit from preceding bit, $(n-1)$st bit

$C_1 = 0$

C_{n+1} = carry bit from nth sum $A_n + B_n$

Σ_n = sum bit from nth sum $A_n + B_n$.

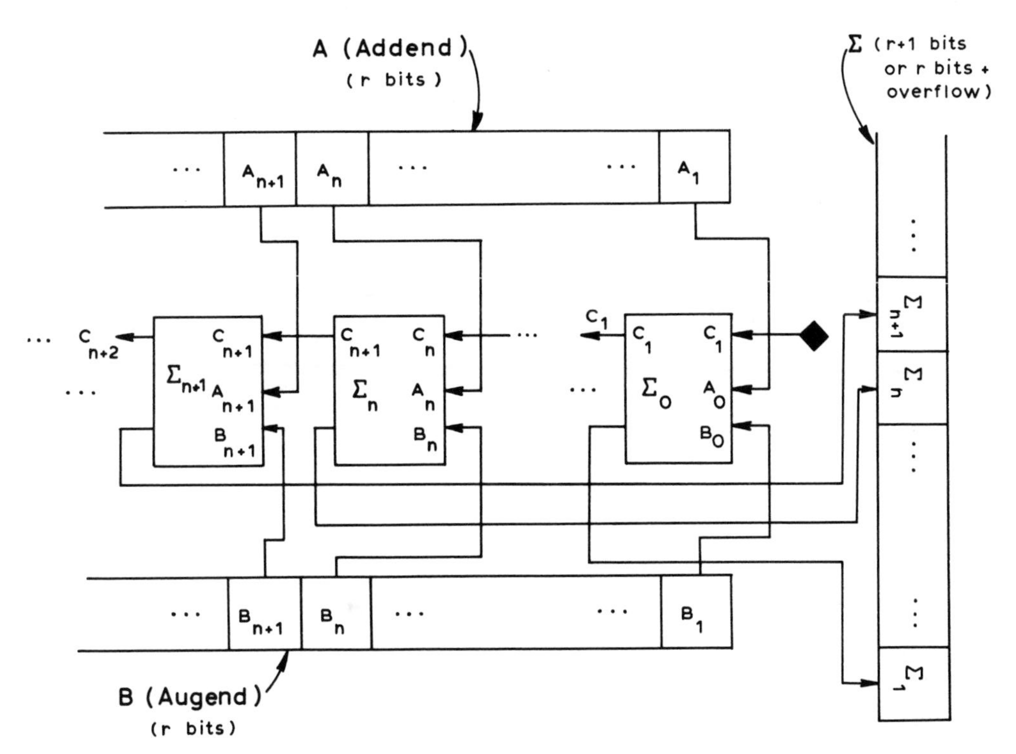

Figure 4.23
Multibit parallel adder.

logic

INPUT				OUTPUT					
				WHEN $C_0 = 0$ / WHEN $C_2 = 0$			WHEN $C_0 = 1$ / WHEN $C_2 = 1$		
A_1 / A_3	B_1 / B_3	A_2 / A_4	B_2 / B_4	Σ_1 / Σ_3	Σ_2 / Σ_4	C_2 / C_4	Σ_1 / Σ_3	Σ_2 / Σ_4	C_2 / C_4
0	0	0	0	0	0	0	1	0	0
1	0	0	0	1	0	0	0	1	0
0	1	0	0	1	0	0	0	1	0
1	1	0	0	0	1	0	1	1	0
0	0	1	0	0	1	0	1	1	0
1	0	1	0	1	1	0	0	0	1
0	1	1	0	1	1	0	0	0	1
1	1	1	0	0	0	1	1	0	1
0	0	0	1	0	1	0	1	1	0
1	0	0	1	1	1	0	0	0	1
0	1	0	1	1	1	0	0	0	1
1	1	0	1	0	0	1	1	0	1
0	0	1	1	0	0	1	1	0	1
1	0	1	1	1	0	1	0	1	1
0	1	1	1	1	0	1	0	1	1
1	1	1	1	0	1	1	1	1	1

NOTE 1: Input conditions at A_1, A_2, B_1, B_2, and C_0 are used to determine outputs Σ_1 and Σ_2, and the value of the internal carry C_2. The values at C_2, A_3, B_3, A_4, and B_4, are then used to determine outputs Σ_3, Σ_4, and C_4.

J OR N DUAL-IN-LINE
OR W FLAT PACKAGE (TOP VIEW)†

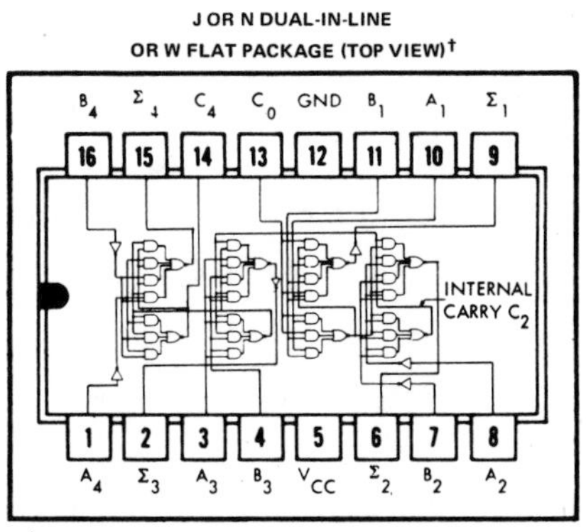

†Pin assignments for these circuits are the same for all packages.

Figure 4.24
SN7843N 4-bit binary adder (from *The Integrated Circuits Catalog for Design Engineers, Catalog CC-401*, 1971, by Texas Instruments. Used with permission of Texas Instruments).

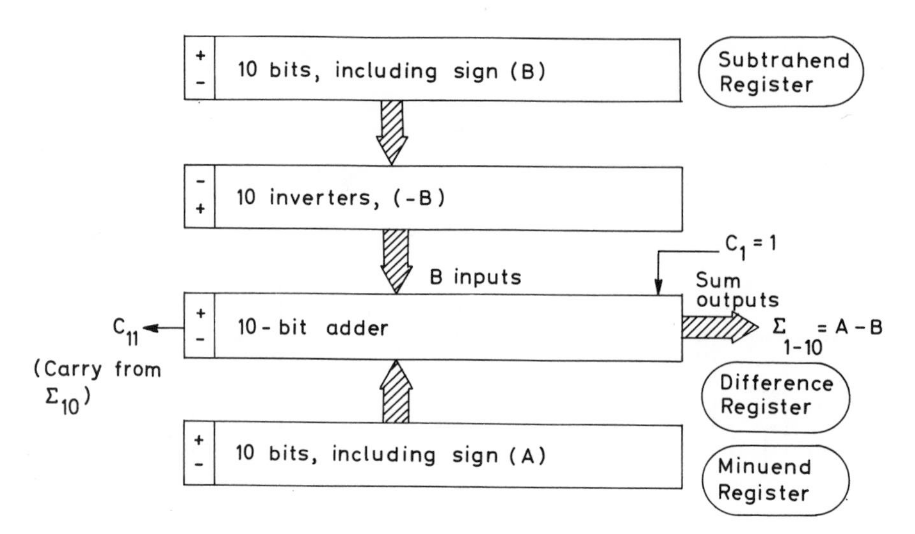

Figure 4.25
Multibit subtracter.

Subtraction is accomplished by adding the two's complement of the subtrahend to the minuend. A block diagram is used to illustrate this process in Figure 4.25. The ten-bit subtrahend, including sign, is inverted by ten inverters. These provide one input of a two-input ten-bit parallel adder. The lowest-order carry in, C_1 in, is a one, because the two's complement is the inverse of the subtrahend, *incremented by one.* The output of the adder is the difference, with correct sign.

We have managed to add and subtract signed numbers without mentioning what becomes of the sign bits. The reader can verify that, except in the case in which the resultant number is too large to fit in the $n - 1$ bits allotted to the "magnitude" portion of the number, the sign of the resultant is the correct sign if the sign bits are treated as the most significant bits of unsigned numbers and are added or subtracted along with the rest. Under certain circumstances, however, the resultant will be too large, and the sign and the sum will both be incorrect.

This could be avoided by having the sum register (or difference register) one bit larger than the input registers, but this is impractical in most situations, because the sum may be an intermediate value that will be used for a later addition or subtraction. Therefore, most adder and subtracter hardware devices have an output register that is the same size as the input registers with the addition of an overflow register, which indicates whether or not the output number is correct. If the overflow register output (OVF) is zero, no overflow has occurred and the sum or difference is correct. If OVF = 1, however, overflow has occurred and the result is incorrect and should be indicated by the hardware.

Table 4.19 specifies the conditions under which an add or subtract overflow occurs, when the inputs to the operation are two signed r-bit numbers. All possible output conditions of the critical bits are illustrated, for all possible input sign combinations. Figure 4.26 illustrates logic circuitry used to generate OVF, the overflow indicator "flag."

Positive multiplication is accomplished much as it is in the process of multidigit multiplication using pencil and paper. The process consists of multiplying each bit of the n-bit positive multiplicand, first by the least significant bit of the multiplier. This multiplication is accomplished by an AND; the input/output truth tables of AND and binary multiplication are equivalent. This is stored as the n least significant bits of the product. Then the multiplication is repeated, using the next more significant bit of the multiplier this time and multiplying the resulting number by ten in the number system used, which in any number system is the same as shifting the number one place to the left, and filling the vacated bit (LSB) with zero. This is then added to the stored number, and the sum replaces the stored number. The multiplication, shift left, addition, and store operation is repeated once for each bit of the multiplier.

We can simplify the process (Figure 4.27) by the following method: Perform the multiplication of the multiplicand by the LSB, and parallel load the result into the *highest*-order $n + 1$ bits of the product register. Now shift the multiplier and the product right. The new LSB is multiplied (ANDed) with the multiplicand (which was not shifted), and the sum of this AND output and the highest order $n + 1$ bits of the shifted product register is obtained. Actually, this sum occurred in the first operation and will occur in all subsequent operations; therefore, the product register must be cleared before the multiplication is initiated (for example, when the multiplier and multiplicand are loaded), so that the output of the AND operation is summed with zero the first time. The output of the parallel adder is then parallel-loaded into the first $n + 1$ bits of the product register. The product and multiplier are once again shifted, and the operation repeated. The cycle (AND, ADD, shift, parallel-load) is repeated n times, ending with the nth parallel load of the product register.

Division is accomplished by performing a series of trial subtractions of the divisor from the dividend. A $2n$-bit dividend and an n-bit divisor are used, resulting in an n-bit quotient and an n-bit remainder. If the divisor is too small or the dividend too large, the quotient size is not large enough to hold the correct quotient, and "divide overflow" is said to occur.

The scheme for division of a 20-bit positive dividend by a 10-bit positive divisor is illustrated in Figure 4.28. The divisor is subtracted from the ten most significant

Table 4.19
Detection of overflow in signed and unsigned addition and subtraction.

$$\pm A\begin{Bmatrix}\text{augend}\\ \text{minuend}\end{Bmatrix} \pm \left(\pm B\begin{Bmatrix}\text{addend}\\ \text{subtrahend}\end{Bmatrix}\right)$$

signed addition and subtraction: r bits + sign
unsigned addition: $r + 1$ bits

Addition	Given:			Resulting in:		Overflow bit $(A + B)$	
	A_r	B_r	C_r	Σ_r	C_{r+1}	Signed addition	Unsigned addition
Definitions:							
C_r = carry from	0	0	0	0	0	0	0
$(r-1)$th adder	0	0	1	1	0	1	0
A_r = rth augend bit	0	1	0	1	0	0	0
B_r = rth addend bit	0	1	1	0	1 $(C_1 = 0)$	0	1
Σ_r = sum output of	1	0	0	1	0	0	0
rth adder	1	0	1	0	1	0	1
C_{r+1} = carry output	1	1	0	0	1	1	1
of rth adder	1	1	1	1	1	1	1

Therefore, for unsigned addition: $\mathrm{OVF}^+ = C_{r+1}$,
and for signed addition: $\mathrm{OVF}^+ = (S_A \wedge S_B \wedge C_{r+1}) \vee (\bar{S}_A \wedge \bar{S}_B \wedge C_{r+1})$
$= (S_A \mathbin{\overline{\wedge}} S_B \mathbin{\overline{\wedge}} C_{r+1}) \mathbin{\overline{\wedge}} (\bar{S}_A \mathbin{\overline{\wedge}} \bar{S}_B \mathbin{\overline{\wedge}} C_{r+1})$,
where S_A = sign of A, and S_B = sign of B.

Subtraction	Given:			Resulting in:		Overflow bit $(A - B)$	
	A_r	B_r	C_r	Σ_r	C_{r+1}	Signed	Unsigned
Definitions:							
C_r = carry from	0	1	0	0	0	0	1
$(r-1)$th adder	0	1	1	1	0	1	1
A_r = rth augend bit	0	0	0	1	0	0	1
B_r = rth subtrahend bit	0	0	1	0	1	0	0
Σ_r = rth difference bit	1	1	0	1	0 $(C_1 = 1)$	0	1
	1	1	1	0	1	0	0
C_{r+1} = carry output	1	0	0	0	1	1	0
of rth adder	1	0	1	1	1	1	0

Therefore, for unsigned subtraction: $\mathrm{OVF}^- = \mathrm{OVF}^+ = C_{r+1}$,
and for signed subtraction, $\mathrm{OVF}^- = \mathrm{OVF}^+ = (S_A \wedge S_B \wedge C_{r+1}) \vee (\bar{S}_A \wedge \bar{S}_B \wedge C_{r+1})$
$= (S_A \mathbin{\overline{\wedge}} S_B \mathbin{\overline{\wedge}} C_{r+1}) \mathbin{\overline{\wedge}} (\bar{S}_A \mathbin{\overline{\wedge}} \bar{S}_B \mathbin{\overline{\wedge}} C_{r+1})$,
where S_A = sign of A, and S_B = sign of B.

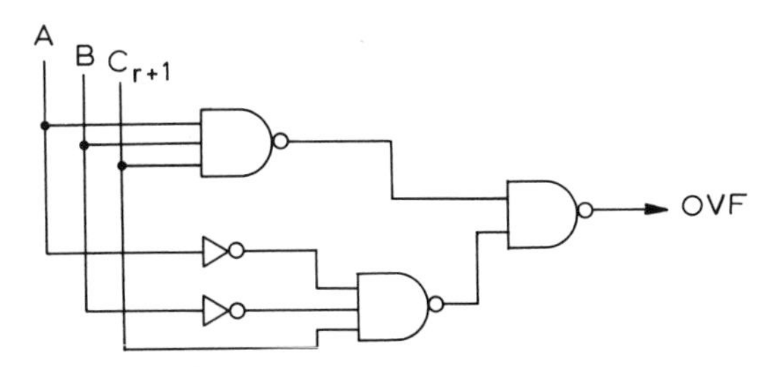

Figure 4.26
Overflow detection for signed addition and subtraction.
Unsigned addition: $C_{r+1} \rightarrow$ OVF.
Unsigned subtraction: $C_{r+1} \rightarrow$ OVF.

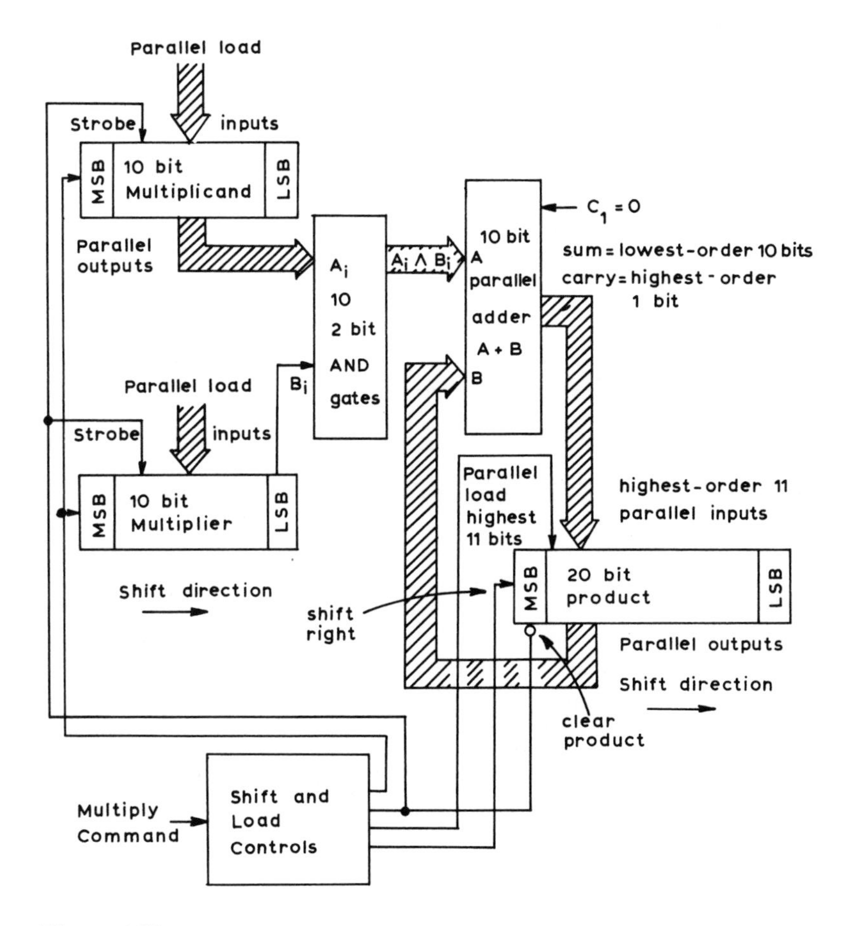

Figure 4.27
Ten-bit positive multiplication. Sequence of operation:
(1) Load multiplier and multiplicand; clear product.
(2) Parallel load the highest order 11 bits of product, from the 10 sum bits and carry of the parallel adder.
(3) Shift right the multiplier and product.
(4) Repeat steps 2 and 3 nine more times. 20-bit positive product is left in the product register.

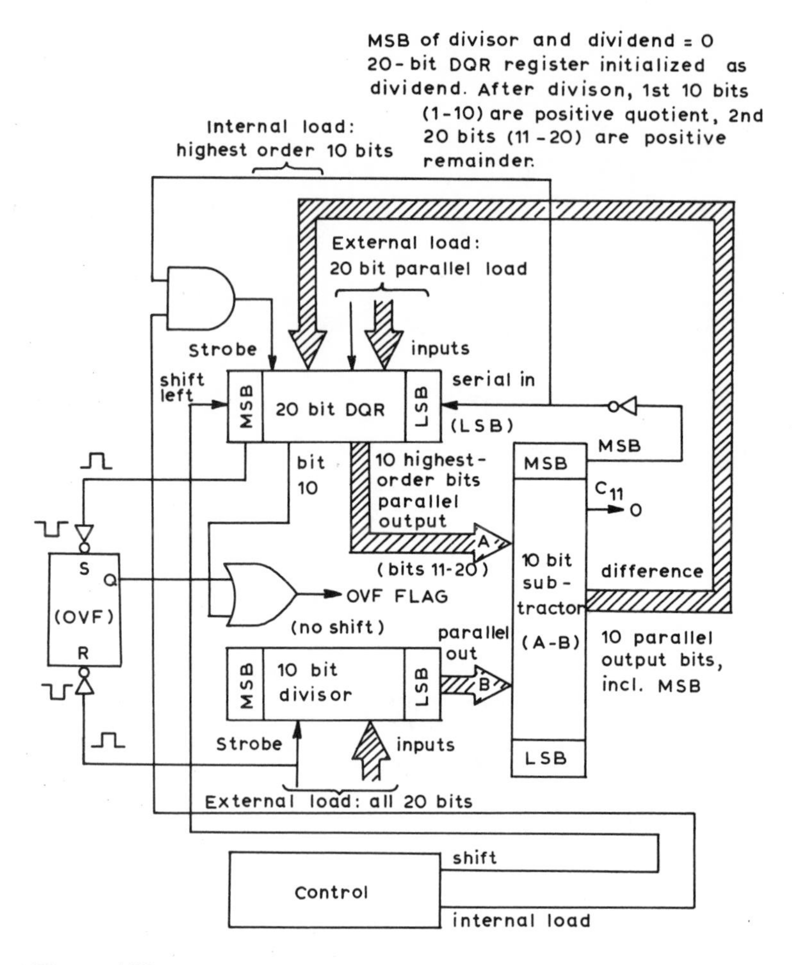

Figure 4.28
Division of 20-bit positive number by 10-bit positive number:
(1) Parallel load (external load) 20-bit DQR with dividend, and parallel load (external load) 10-bit divisor. Clear OVF FF.
(2) Subtract divisor from DQR's 10 most significant bits. If difference is positive (MSB of difference = 0), feed a 1 to the serial input (LSB) of the DQR, and enable strobe for internal load. If MSB of difference is 1 (negative difference), feed a 0 to the serial input of the DQR, and disable the strobe for internal load.
(3) Internal load: load difference into the 10 most significant bits of the DQR, if the strobe is enabled.
(4) Shift DQR 1 place left.
(5) Repeat steps 2–4 nine more times.
(6) After last left shift, the positive quotient is in the 10 lowest-order bits of the DQR, and the positive remainder is in the highest-order 10 bits of the DQR, *if* the OVF FLAG is off. If OVF FLAG is on, the MSB of the DQR was on at some time and divide overflow occurred or the quotient is negative (bit 10 of DQR = 1).

bits of the dividend. If the difference is positive, the most significant bit of the desired quotient must be one. If the difference is negative, the MSB of the quotient is zero. The difference is parallel-loaded into the ten most significant bits of the dividend if the quotient bit is one, and the dividend is left unchanged if the quotient bit is zero. This is analogous to the long-hand method of long division.

When the ten most significant bits of the dividend have been adjusted according to the value of the obtained MSB of the quotient, the quotient bit is fed to the *serial* input of the dividend register (the LSB) and a shift left is performed. The 10th bit of the quotient is now the first bit of the "dividend" register and no longer contains the dividend at the end of the division, but rather the remainder (in bits 20–11) and the quotient (in bits 10–1). We will therefore refer to this register from this point on as the DRQ register, for Dividend-Remainder-Quotient.

After this first shift, the ten most significant bits of the "new" dividend are in the ten most significant bits of the DRQ. After performing another trial subtraction and adjustment of the dividend value, the second most significant bit of the quotient (one if the difference is positive, zero if the difference is negative) is once again inserted via the serial input during the second shift left. The subtraction-adjustment-shift process is repeated nine more times, for a total of eleven times. The entire ten-bit quotient has been shifted into bits 1–10 of the DRQ in the correct order. The number remaining in the upper half of the DRQ (bits 11–20) is the remainder.

We have just described an ideal case, where no divide overflow occurs. In what situation does overflow occur? The answer is immediately apparent: when the quotient obtained from the first or the second subtraction is one. Our overflow detector, then, is a pair of flipflops, one of which "enables" the other during the first two shifts, and the other of which is set if either of the first two bits shifted out of the MSB of the DRQ is one.

Having devised methods for multiplying and dividing unsigned (positive) numbers, it remains only to consider means of determining the sign of the resultant of such an operation when signed numbers are used, and to devise a means of generating a correct product, quotient, or remainder when various sign combinations are input to the device. Although there are designs for directly multiplying or dividing the signed inputs, we will rely on the much simpler method of dividing or multiplying the absolute values of the arguments and correcting the sign of the resultants when necessary.

Figure 4.29 illustrates a simple gating circuit used to determine the sign of the resultants, given the signs of the arguments, for multiplication and division. Note the definition of EOR, Exclusive OR, which is identical to addition modulo 2,

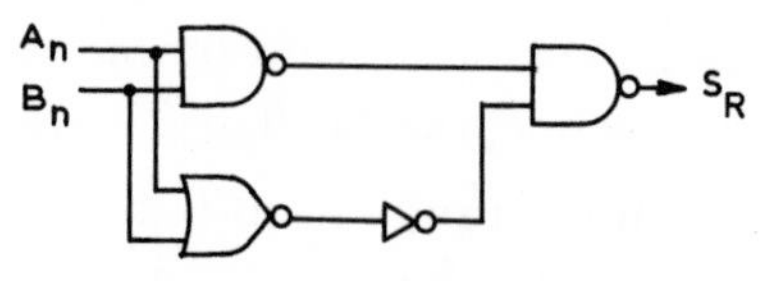

(a) $S_R = (A \wedge B) \vee \overline{(A \vee B)} = (A \bar{\wedge} B) \bar{\wedge} (A \vee B) = A \oplus B$

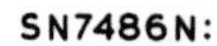

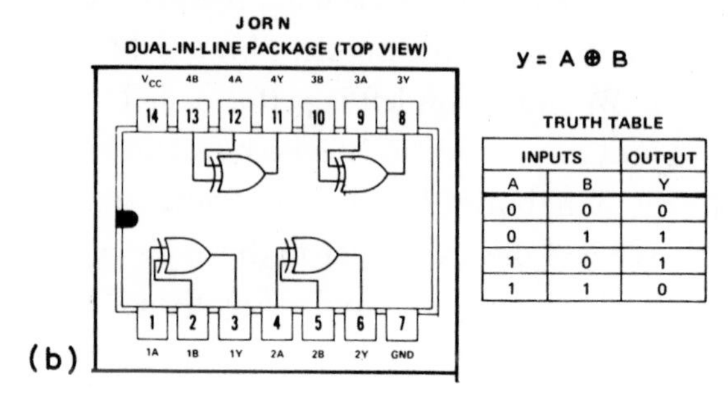

INPUTS		OUTPUT
A	B	Y
0	0	0
0	1	1
1	0	1
1	1	0

(b)

Figure 4.29
Generation of resultant sign from signs of the arguments in multiplication and division: (a) Exclusive OR built from NAND, INV, and NOR; (b) SN7486N Exclusive OR gates (from *The Integrated Circuits Catalog for Design Engineers, Catalog CC-401*, 1971, by Texas Instruments. Used with permission of Texas Instruments).'

Table 4.20
Determination of the sign of a product or quotient, given the signs of the arguments.

A	B	C
0	0	0
0	1	1
1	0	1
1	1	0

$C(A \times B) = C(A \div B)$

$$S_R = (S_A \wedge S_B) \vee \overline{(S_A \vee S_B)} = (S_A \bar{\wedge} S_B) \bar{\wedge} (S_A \vee S_B)$$
$$= S_A \oplus S_B = S_A \text{ EOR } S_B$$

S_A = sign of multiplicand or dividend
S_B = sign of multiplier or divisor
S_R = sign of product, or quotient and remainder

1 = negative, 0 = positive } sign bit convention

in Table 4.20. Figures 4.30 and 4.31 illustrate the use of adders and gates to obtain the absolute values of the arguments (prior to multiplication or division) and the value of the resultants (product, quotient, sign) after multiplication or division. The strategy, then, is to use the MSBs of the arguments to determine the sign (S_R in the figures) of the resultant; perform the multiply or divide operation after converting both arguments to their absolute values; and correct the sign of the resultant(s) according to the value of S_R.

Digital ICs that perform very rapid multiplication became available as this book was going to press. For example, the Advanced Micro Devices Am 2505 can produce the quantity $S = XY + K$, where each number is a signed binary (two's complement) number. The number of binary bits can be expanded by using several ICs, in order to process any word length. Two eight-bit signed numbers can be multiplied in 135 nsec.

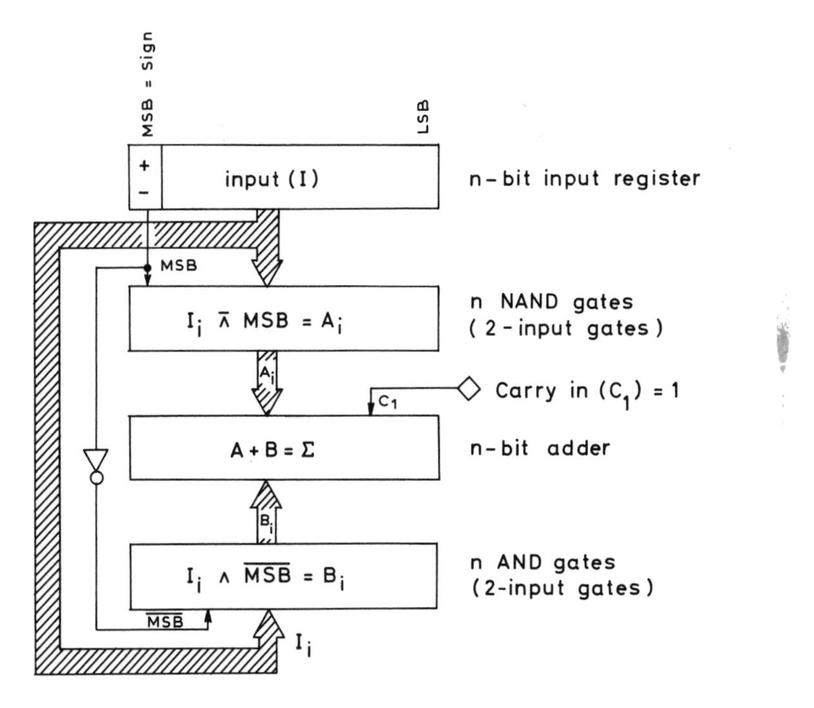

Figure 4.30
Absolute-value circuit.

Σ (output of adder) $= |I|$

I	MSB	$\overline{\text{MSB}}$	$I_i \,\overline{\wedge}\, \text{MSB} = A_i$	$I_i \wedge \overline{\text{MSB}} = B_i$	$A + B\,(+C_1) = \Sigma$
+	0	1	all 1s: $A_i = 1$	$B_i = I_i$	$-1 + I + 1 = I(+)$
−	1	0	complement: $A_i = \bar{I}_i$	$B_i = 0$	$\bar{I} + 0 + 1 = -I\,(+)$

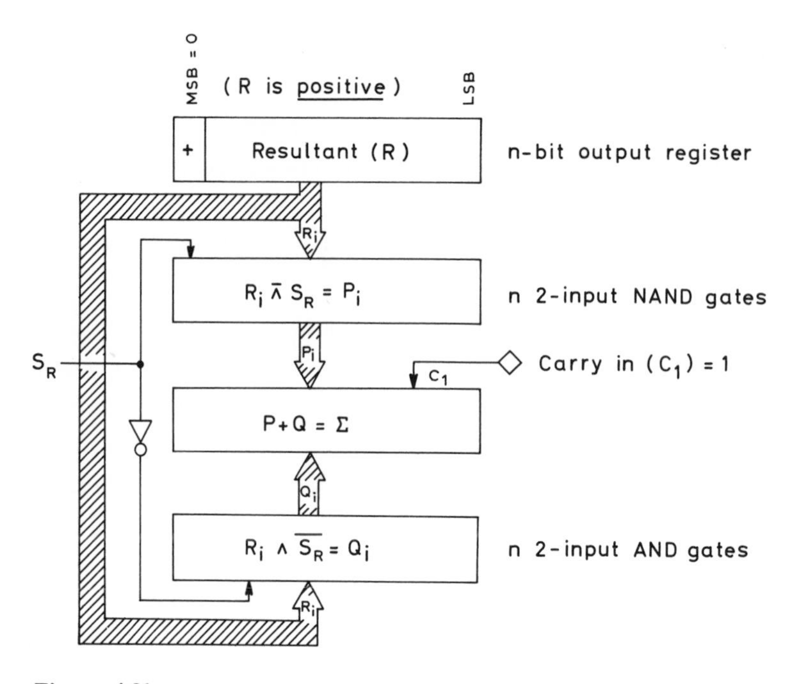

Figure 4.31
Sign correction of resultant from multiplication and division. Resultant sign $S_R = S_A + S_B$ = sign of argument A EOR sign of argument B. Σ (output of adder) = output with corrected sign.

Correct R	S_R	$\bar{S}_R$	$R_i \overline{\wedge} S_R = P_i$	$R_i \wedge \bar{S}_R = Q_i$	$P + Q\ (+C_1) = \Sigma$
+	0	1	all 1s: $P_i = 1$	$Q_i = R$	$-1 + R + 1 = R\ (+)$
−	1	0	complement: $P_i = \bar{R}_i$	$Q_i = 0$	$\bar{R} + 0 + 1 = -R\ (-)$

4.6 Parity Generation

When a number is stored or transmitted, it is useful to devise a simple means of determining whether the transfer was correct. If we assume errors occur rarely enough so one-bit errors are much more probable than two-bit errors, we can generate an additional bit, called a parity bit, which when added modulo 2 to each of the other bits in succession always totals one, or alternatively, always zero. The former system is called *odd parity* and the latter *even parity*. We can generate an even parity bit by successive addition of all the data bits modulo 2; when the parity bit is added to all the data bits modulo 2, the sum is always zero. To generate odd parity simply add 1 modulo 2 to the even parity result, or invert the even parity result:

$$\text{Even parity} = \left(\sum_{i=0}^{n} a_i\right) \text{modulo } 2. \qquad (4.25a)$$

$$\text{Odd parity} = \left(1 + \sum_{i=0}^{n} a_i\right) \text{modulo } 2 = \left(-\sum_{i=0}^{n} a_i\right) \text{modulo } 2. \qquad (4.25b)$$

$C_{even} = A \oplus B$

$C_{odd} = \overline{A \oplus B}$

A
B
($\frac{1}{4}$ SN7486N)
C_{odd}
C_{even}

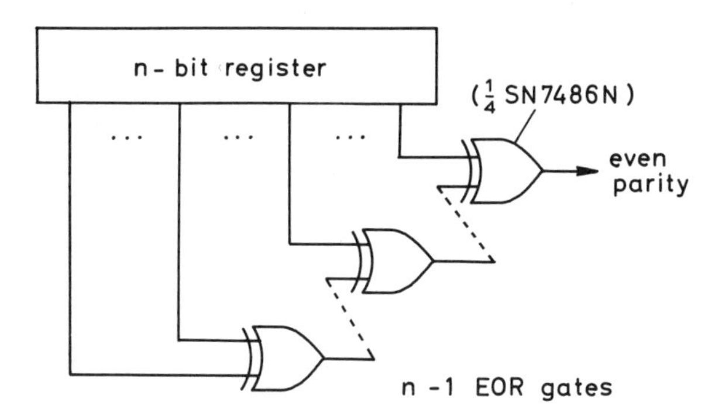

Figure 4.32
Parity generation:

A	B	C_{even}	C_{odd}
1	1	0	1
0	1	1	0
1	0	1	0
0	0	0	1

Definitions:
A = 1-bit variable
B = 1-bit variable
C = 1-bit variable, determined by A and B, such that:
$C_{even} = [10 - (A + B)]$ modulo 10_2
$C_{odd} = [11 - (A + B)]$ modulo 10_2

Addition modulo 2 is the same as the Exclusive OR (EOR) operation. The diagrams of Figure 4.32 indicate the use of EOR to generate parity bits. Many computer memories have a parity bit associated with each multibit word. The parity bit is generated and stored whenever the word is stored. When the word is retrieved, if the sum of the parity bit and the n bits of the word is the wrong value, a parity check alarm is initiated.

In transmission of strings of words, each word usually has a parity bit, and the last word is a set of bits such that the sum of ith bits of all words, modulo 2, is used to generate the ith bit of the last word, called the Longitudinal Parity Check Character (LPCC), in either even or odd parity. The receiver device keeps a running sum, modulo 2, of each bit, and after adding the LPCC, should consist of all 1s (odd) or all 0s (even), depending on the type of parity used.

Parity checking depends on there being only one incorrect bit in a word; if an even number of bits were incorrect, no error would be detected. This is not a serious limitation; because if two errors can occur, one error can usually occur

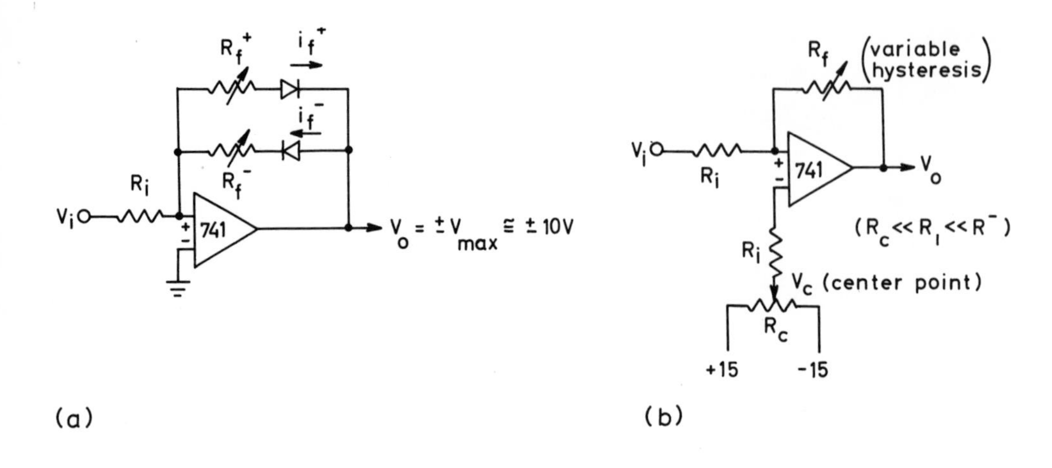

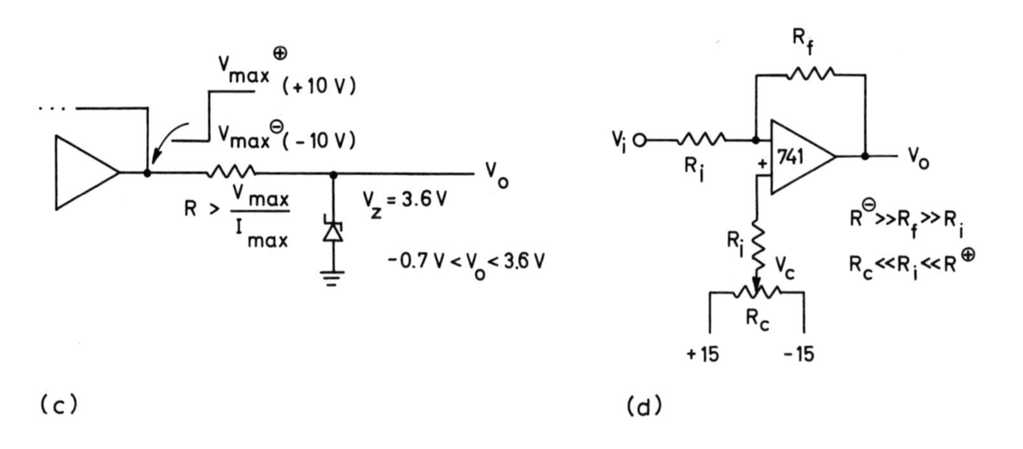

Figure 4.33
Positive feedback level-detection: (a) level detector with separate adjustments for positive and negative thresholds; (b) level detector with separate adjustments of "center point" and hysteresis; (c) TTL-compatible output configuration; (d) negative feedback level detection.

even more often, and parity violations will be detected the majority of the time. Obviously, if parity errors occur often, a hardware failure is occurring often enough to be detected, diagnosed, and corrected.

4.7 Level Detection

There are several methods of coding analog properties of signals, such as voltage, frequency, and phase, as digital numbers. We will discuss various analog to digital (A/D) and digital to analog (D/A) conversions in Chapter 10. However, in order to establish a technique that we will use in the generation of wave forms, we will consider one special form of A/D conversion here: *level detection*, often referred to as threshold detection, voltage comparison, or voltage discrimination.

The concept of a threshold device was introduced at the beginning of this chapter. The positive feedback configuration of Figure 4.1 is a dual threshold device. A more general form of such a device that might be used for level detection is that of Figure 4.33a where the threshold in each direction is independently variable. Another variation is presented in Figure 4.33b. An output configuration that confines the output voltage to the TTL range is illustrated in Figure 4.33c. The level detector of Figure 4.33a is adequate for low-frequency work. The circuit suffers from the disadvantage of never having zero hysteresis and a slight interaction of the two thresholds due to the nonideal behavior of the diodes. The thresholds for ideal circuit components are

$$V^{+}_{\text{threshold}} = -V^{-}_{\max}\frac{R_i}{R_f}, \tag{4.26a}$$

$$V^{-}_{\text{threshold}} = -V^{+}_{\max}\frac{R_i}{R_f}. \tag{4.26b}$$

Keep in mind the fact that the positive input is not a virtual ground, and that feedback voltage may therefore interact with V_i if the output impedance of the V_i source is not at least a couple of orders of magnitude lower than R_i. An input stage consisting of a unity-gain follower can be used to circumvent this problem.

The circuit of Figure 4.33a has an additional disadvantage. The positive threshold can never be a negative level and the negative threshold can never be a positive level. Figure 4.33b uses a different approach, which consists of using an adjustable comparison voltage V_C for the negative input. The thresholds of this device are

$$V^{+}_{\text{threshold}} = -V^{-}_{\max}\frac{R_i}{R_f} - V_C, \tag{4.27a}$$

$$V^{-}_{\text{threshold}} = -V^{+}_{\max}\frac{R_i}{R_f} - V_C. \tag{4.27b}$$

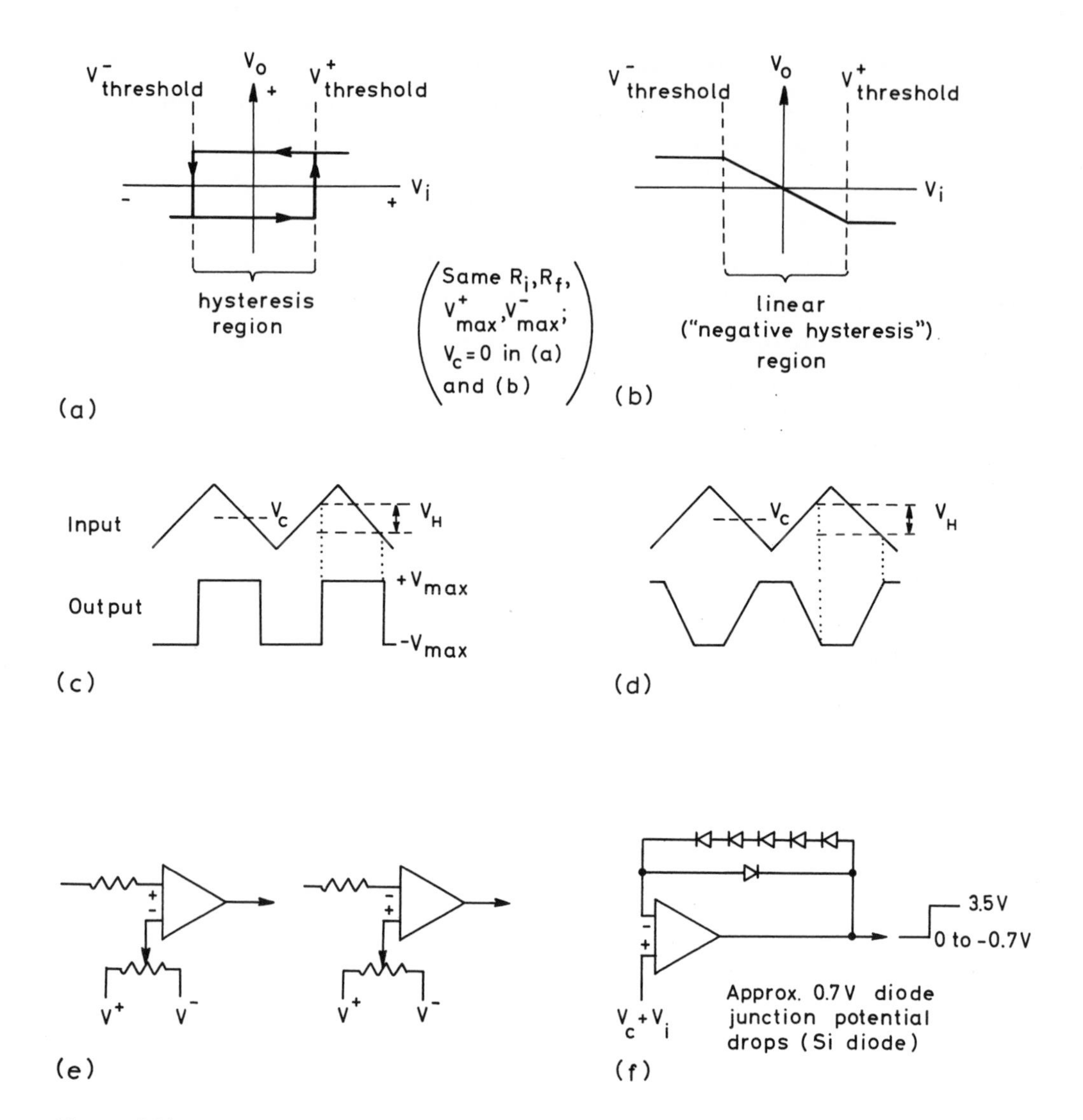

Figure 4.34
Input-output relations for positive and negative feedback discriminators, and alternative configurations: (a) positive feedback I/O relation; (b) negative feedback I/O relation; (c) sample input and output waveforms for positive feedback; (d) sample waveforms for negative feedback; (e) special-case positive and negative feedback level detectors: $R_f = \infty$, therefore gain is limited to open-loop gain m. Hysteresis is virtually zero; (f) alternative method for TTL-compatible output, used with level detectors of (e).

This can be rearranged to express the "center point" voltage V_{CP} and "hysteresis" V_H:

$$V_{CP} = -V_C, \tag{4.28a}$$

$$V_H = (-V^-_{\max} - V^+_{\max}) \frac{R_i}{R_f}. \tag{4.28b}$$

Therefore, as R_i/R_f approaches 0, then V_H approaches 0 as well.

Here V_{CP} is independent of R_f, because there is no voltage divider between V_C and the inverting input (except the one composed of R_i and the inverting input impedance: hence keep R_i less than $R^-/100$, where R^- is the inverting input impedance).

The output circuit of Figure 4.33c converts the ± 10 V output of the 741 to a TTL-compatible voltage range: R is added to prevent overloading the output, and the 3 V zener restricts V_o to the range 0 to 3 V. Figure 4.33d illustrates another form of level detector, consisting of a high-gain negative feedback configuration.

Compare the positive and negative feedback devices (Figure 4.34). The negative feedback device displays what might be considered a "negative hysteresis." That is, when the input voltage is more positive than the positive boundary the output voltage is $V^+_{\max}$ with positive feedback and $V^-_{\max}$ with negative feedback; when the input voltage is more negative than the negative hysteresis boundary, the output voltage is $V^-_{\max}$ with the positive feedback and $V^+_{\max}$ with the negative feedback. Behavior within the hysteresis region is also different: The positive feedback output voltage regeneratively traverses the region once it is entered, and the negative feedback output voltage is inversely proportional to the input voltage. If we define $V^+_{\text{threshold}}$ as the voltage which must be crossed in order to move V_o away from $V^{\mp}_{\max}$, given $V_o = V^{\mp}_{\max}$ initially, Equations 4.27 and 4.28 apply equally well for both positive and negative feedback. Note, however, that for a given threshold voltage the input is travelling in opposite directions with the two circuits: V_i is the same sign as V_o in the positive feedback case and increasing in magnitude; V_i is the opposite sign and decreasing in magnitude in the negative feedback case. The output of positive and negative feedback discriminators is illustrated for triangle wave input and $V_C = 0$ in Figure 4.34c, d. Variants on the positive and negative feedback configurations, having very high gain and high input impedance, are illustrated in Figure 4.34e. A simple method for obtaining TTL compatibility is illustrated in 4.34f, where diodes limit the output voltage range, and the input consists of V_i added to the comparison voltage V_C.

Figure 4.35 illustrates the characteristics of a commercially available level detector, the 710. It is essentially a high-gain op amp with TTL-compatible output.

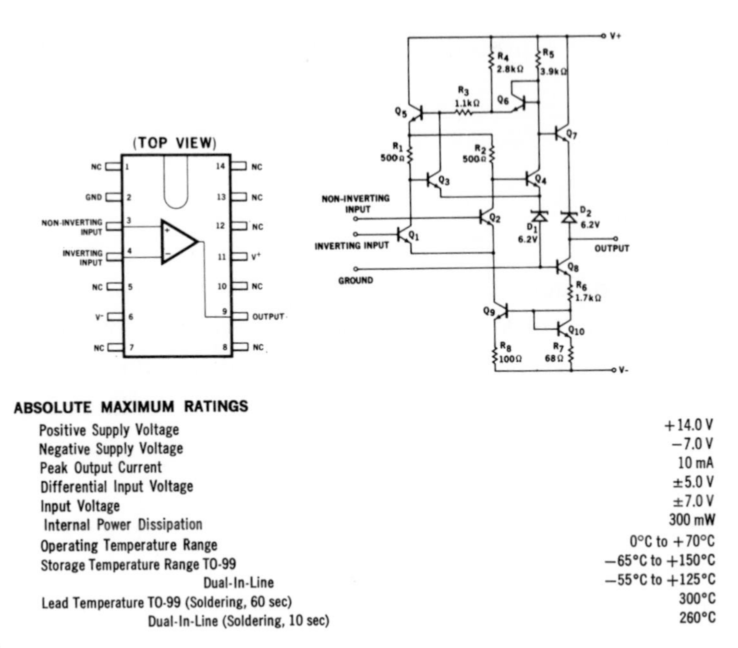

ABSOLUTE MAXIMUM RATINGS

Positive Supply Voltage	+14.0 V
Negative Supply Voltage	−7.0 V
Peak Output Current	10 mA
Differential Input Voltage	±5.0 V
Input Voltage	±7.0 V
Internal Power Dissipation	300 mW
Operating Temperature Range	0°C to +70°C
Storage Temperature Range TO-99	−65°C to +150°C
Dual-In-Line	−55°C to +125°C
Lead Temperature TO-99 (Soldering, 60 sec)	300°C
Dual-In-Line (Soldering, 10 sec)	260°C

ELECTRICAL CHARACTERISTICS ($T_A = 25°C$, $V^+ = 12.0V$, $V^- = -6.0V$ unless otherwise specified)

PARAMETER (see definitions)	CONDITIONS (Note 3)	MIN.	TYP.	MAX.	UNITS
Input Offset Voltage	$R_s \leq 200\Omega$		1.6	5.0	mV
Input Offset Current			1.8	5.0	μA
Input Bias Current			16	25	μA
Voltage Gain		1000	1500		
Output Resistance			200		Ω
Output Sink Current	$\Delta V_{in} \geq 5$ mV, $V_{out} = 0$	1.6	2.5		mA
Response Time (Note 2)			40		ns

The following specifications apply for $0°C \leq T_A \leq +70°C$:

PARAMETER	CONDITIONS	MIN.	TYP.	MAX.	UNITS
Input Offset Voltage	$R_s \leq 200\Omega$			6.5	mV
Average Temperature Coefficient of Input Offset Voltage	$R_s = 50\Omega$, $T_A = 0°C$ to $T_A = +70°C$		5.0	20	μV/°C
Input Offset Current				7.5	μA
Average Temperature Coefficient of Input Offset Current	$T_A = 25°C$ to $T_A = +70°C$ $T_A = 25°C$ to $T_A = 0°C$		15 24	50 100	nA/°C nA/°C
Input Bias Current	$T_A = 0°C$		25	40	μA
Input Voltage Range	$V^- = -7.0V$	±5.0			V
Common Mode Rejection Ratio	$R_s \leq 200\Omega$	70	98		dB
Differential Input Voltage Range		±5.0			V
Voltage Gain		800			
Positive Output Level	$\Delta V_{in} \geq 5$ mV, $0 \leq I_{out} \leq 5.0$ mA	2.5	3.2	4.0	V
Negative Output Level	$\Delta V_{in} \geq 5$ mV	−1.0	−0.5	0	V
Output Sink Current	$\Delta V_{in} \geq 5$ mV, $V_{out} = 0$	0.5			mA
Positive Supply Current	$V_{out} \leq 0$		5.2	9.0	mA
Negative Supply Current			4.6	7.0	mA
Power Consumption			90	150	mW

Figure 4.35
710C voltage comparator (from *Semiconductor Integrated Circuit Data Catalog, 1970*, by Fairchild Semiconductor. Used with the permission of Fairchild Camera and Instrument Corporation).

J OR N DUAL-IN-LINE OR
W FLAT PACKAGES (TOP VIEW)†

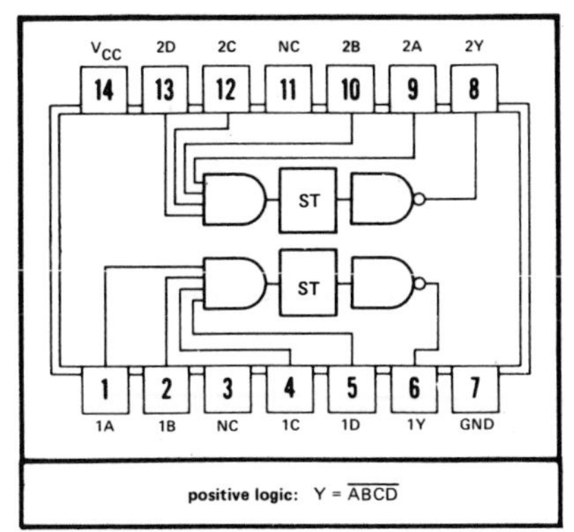

NC—No internal connection.
†Pin assignments for these circuits are the same for all packages.

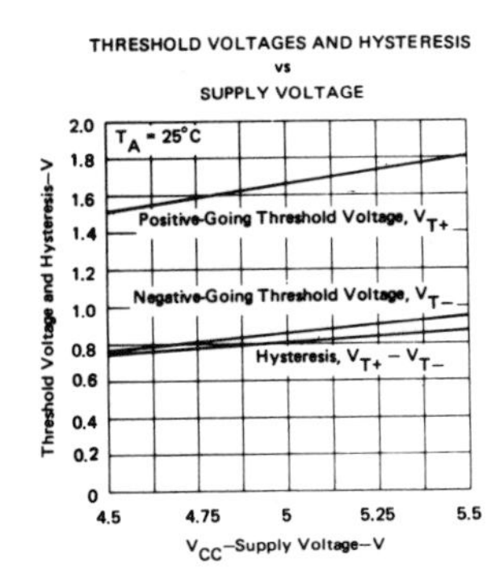

Figure 4.36
SN7413N Schmitt Trigger NAND gate (from *The Integrated Circuits Catalog for Design Engineers, Catalog CC-401, 1971,* by Texas Instruments. Used with the permission of Texas Instruments).

The device is a "negative hysteresis" device. The circuit suffers from the disadvantage of requiring +12 and −6 V supply voltages. Data sheet information was provided by Fairchild Semiconductor.

Figure 4.36 illustrates a "Schmitt trigger" (positive feedback) input NAND gate, the SN7413N. The device suffers from a restricted input range; but if it is preceded by an op amp with variable polarity, level, and gain, it is possible to use it as a flexible discriminator with TTL output, triggering on positive or negative slopes and with positive or negative thresholds. It requires only a +5 V supply.

The reader is referred back to Figure 4.14 for a description of the input characteristics of another Schmitt trigger: the *B* input of the SN74121N multivibrator. This device produces an output pulse whose duration is independent of the duration during which the input threshold is exceeded, in contrast with the 710 and SN7413N.

4.8 Construction with TTL ICs

In order to obtain trouble-free operation of TTL circuits, observe the following rules:

1. Power supply ripple $\leqq 5\%$.
2. Power supply regulation to $\leqq \pm 5\%$.
3. *RF* bypass the primary of the power supply.
4. For every 5 to 10 IC cans, decouple with 0.01–0.1 μF. Good decoupling is especially important for flipflops and one-shots.
5. A ground plane is desirable, especially for a large number of ICs on a single board. If no ground plane is available, use a wide bus around the edges of the board. Return both ends of the bus to ground.
6. All pulse widths must exceed 25 nsec for 54/74 TTL.
7. Tie all unused inputs to ground or +5 V, or parallel to another input, even if they appear irrelevant. Tie the input to that level which will have no effect on circuit operation.
8. Ground the inputs of unused gates for lowest power drain.
9. The inputs and outputs of gates or buffers in the same IC package may be paralleled to increase fanout. Resulting fanout is the total of the fanouts of all gates thus paralleled.
10. For transmission lines shorter than 10 inches, use a single conductor. For 10 to 20 inches use a ground plane as well. For more than 20 inches use a twisted pair or coaxial cable, preferably with 100 Ω characteristic impedance. Twisted pairs can be made from #26 to #28 wire with thin insulation and about 30 twists per foot. Ground returns should be carried through at both ends. Use 500–1000 Ω resistive pullup (shunt) at receiving end of long cable for increased noise margin and improved rise times. Reverse terminate at the driving end with 27–47 Ω in series to prevent negative overshoot. Drive only one line with only one gate. Receive only one line with only one gate. Generally flipflops make poor line drivers, because they are prone to resetting through their outputs. Therefore buffer all flipflops and flipflop-output pulse generators with gates. Use 0.1 μF *RF* capacitors between V_{CC} and ground on the drivers and receivers. In noisy environments also decouple all flipflops and noise generators.

Transients on supply lines during turn on or turn off can demolish TTL circuits if they exceed maximum rated voltages. If there exists any danger of such transients, do not tie any inputs directly to V_{CC}; instead, tie them to V_{CC} through a 1 kΩ resistor. As many as ten unit loads can be tied to a single 1 kΩ resistor. If inputs are from external devices and may or may not be tied to a TTL output at different times during normal operation, tie the input through a resistor to ground or V_{CC} for maintaining desired quiescent voltage in the absence of external input. Use a resistance equivalent to $n(1\ k\Omega)$ resistors in parallel where n = number of unit loads. Thus, for 1 unit load, use 1 kΩ; for two unit loads, use 500 Ω, and so forth.

Selected References

Fairchild Semiconductor. 1970. *Semiconductor Integrated Circuit Data Catalog, 1970.* Mountain View, Calif.: Fairchild Camera and Instrument Corporation.

Kintner, Paul M. 1968. *Electronic Digital Techniques.* New York: McGraw-Hill Book Co.

Texas Instruments. 1971. *The Integrated Circuits Catalog for Design Engineers, Catalog CC-401.* Dallas: Texas Instruments.

5 WAVE-FORM GENERATION

Paul B. Brown

Much neurophysiological research relies on the use of quantitative, repeatable stimulation by natural activation of sensory receptors or direct electrical stimulation of nervous tissue. In order to produce such stimuli with precise control of the various stimulus parameters, an electrical wave form is usually used to drive a transducer, providing a corresponding wave form of acoustic pressure, light intensity, electric current, mechanical displacement, or the like.

This chapter examines various techniques for generating electrical wave forms, and Chapter 8 reviews some of the methods used to produce stimuli, using these wave forms to drive appropriate transducers.

The wave-form generators discussed here were state-of-the-art at the time they were designed, but the reader should keep abreast of wave-form generator modules that are appearing on the market. Rapid advances are being made, particularly in digital wave-form generation.

5.1 Switching Techniques

It is frequently necessary to switch current paths of signals under electronic control. In the past, such switching was usually accomplished with electromechanical relays. Such devices operate at low speed, produce electrical and magnetic field transients, suffer from interaction of switching voltage and switched voltage, and often produce contact "bounce" artifacts. Since they are mechanical devices with moving parts, they are subject to periodic breakdown. The audible noise accompanying switch action is a disadvantage in many applications, especially in sensory and behavioral studies. For these reasons, such devices should be used only for low-speed or high-current applications. Solid-state devices exist that can perform nearly all the functions of electromechanical relays.

We have already discussed a form of digital switch, the gate. A logic level is passed or not passed through a gate, depending on the state of the other gate input(s). Figure 5.1 illustrates the use of a set of gates and a flipflop for controlling the passage of a number of signals through independent channels. External control of the switch is accomplished here by manual or electrical means.

In data transmission and processing, it may be necessary for many signals to share a common transmission line or device. Such sharing is called *multiplexing*. Figure 5.2 illustrates a simple form of multiplexing of digital signals. The address inputs enable the gate that is selected according to the digital code in the two address lines. The output is equivalent to the input of the selected channel. The minimum number of bits needed to specify the address is the smallest integer n, satisfying the equation

$$n = \log_2 a \quad (5.1)$$

where n = number of bits, and a = number of addresses. Unused addresses can generate 0s or 1s as desired.

Analog switching is more difficult to accomplish. The most successful method now in use employs a MOSFET in a series, shunt, or series-shunt mode (Figure 5.3).

The series switching device passes the input voltage to the output when the MOSFET resistance is much lower than the shunting resistance to ground. When the MOSFET is not conducting the input voltage faces a very high resistance to the output and the output is essentially zero volts. We are, in essence, varying the value of one resistance in a voltage divider, such that it is either several orders of magnitude greater than the other, or several orders of magnitude less. The junction is therefore very nearly at the voltage of one input terminal V_i or the other (ground), depending on the ratio of the resistances.

The shunt switch operates by varying the other resistor in the divider. The MOSFET presents a low resistance from ground to the output when it conducts, shunting the output voltage to ground. When it is not conducting, the shunting effect is lost, and the output voltage is essentially the same as the input.

The series-shunt switch requires two switching voltages, such that the series MOSFET conducts when the shunt MOSFET is off, and vice versa. This results in a great improvement in the ratio of R_{series}/R_{shunt}.

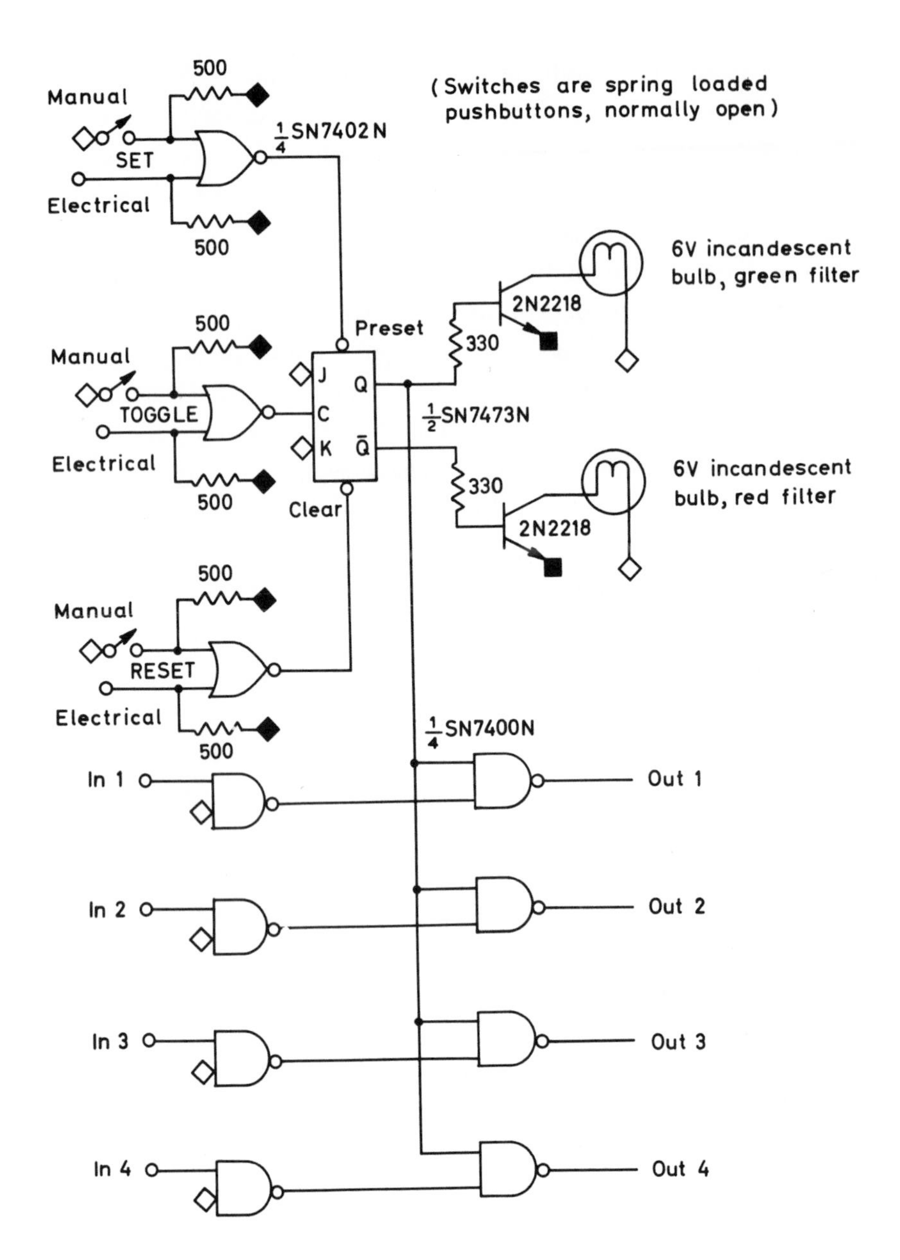

Figure 5.1
Flipflop-gate combination for parallel gating of TTL signals.

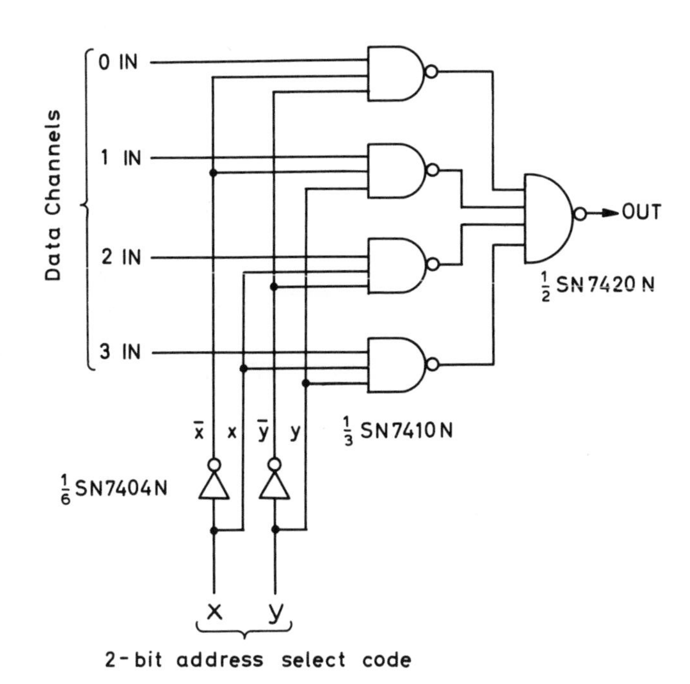

Figure 5.2
Four-channel digital multiplexer.

Address code X Y	Selected data channel number	Gating structure
0 0	0	$\bar{X} \wedge \bar{Y} \wedge$ (0 IN)
0 1	1	$\bar{X} \wedge Y \wedge$ (1 IN)
1 0	2	$X \wedge \bar{Y} \wedge$ (2 IN)
1 1	3	$X \wedge Y \wedge$ (3 IN)

$$\begin{aligned}\text{output} &= (\bar{X} \wedge \bar{Y} \wedge (0\text{ IN})) \vee (\bar{X} \wedge Y \wedge (1\text{ IN})) \vee (X \wedge \bar{Y} \wedge (2\text{ IN})) \vee (X \wedge Y \wedge (3\text{ IN}))\\ &= (\bar{X} \overline{\wedge} \bar{Y} \overline{\wedge} (0\text{ IN})) \overline{\wedge} (\bar{X} \overline{\wedge} Y \overline{\wedge} (1\text{ IN})) \overline{\wedge} (X \overline{\wedge} \bar{Y} \overline{\wedge} (2\text{ IN})) \overline{\wedge} (X \overline{\wedge} Y \overline{\wedge} (3\text{ IN}))\end{aligned}$$

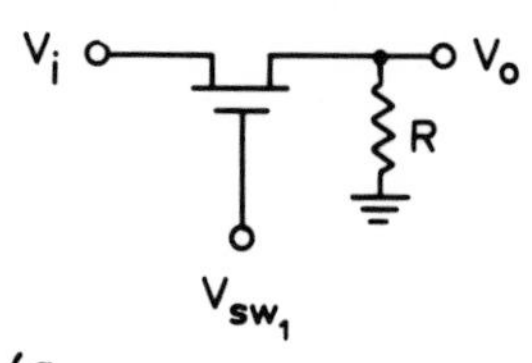

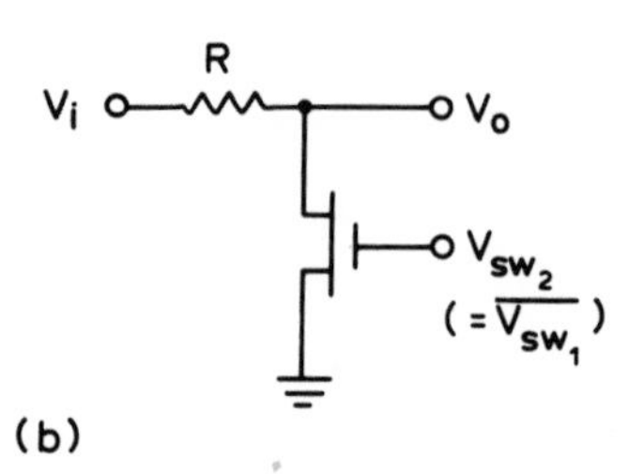

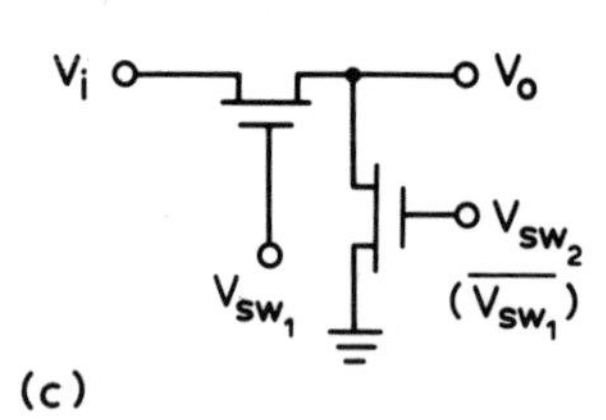

Figure 5.3
MOSFET analog switches: (a) series switch; (b) shunt switch; (c) series-shunt switch.

The output voltage for each configuration is

$$V_{\text{series}} = \frac{V_{\text{i}} R_{\text{fixed}}}{R_{\text{MOSFET}} + R_{\text{fixed}}}, \tag{5.2}$$

$$V_{\text{shunt}} = \frac{V_{\text{i}} R_{\text{MOSFET}}}{R_{\text{MOSFET}} + R_{\text{fixed}}}, \tag{5.3}$$

and

$$V_{\text{series—shunt}} = \frac{V_{\text{i}} R_{\text{shunt}}}{R_{\text{series}} + R_{\text{shunt}}}. \tag{5.4}$$

As R_{fixed} is varied, the ratio of $V_{\text{on}}/V_{\text{off}}$ and the value of V_{on} change systematically, in series and shunt modes:

$$\lim_{R_{\text{fixed}} \to \infty} \left(\frac{V_{\text{on}}}{V_{\text{off}}}\right)_{\text{series}} = 1, \tag{5.5a}$$

$$\lim_{R_{\text{fixed}}\to\infty}\left(\frac{V_{\text{on}}}{V_{\text{off}}}\right)_{\text{shunt}} = \frac{R_{\text{MOSFET(min)}}}{R_{\text{MOSFET(max)}}}, \tag{5.5b}$$

$$\lim_{R_{\text{fixed}}\to\infty} V_{\text{series}} = V_i \text{ (both on and off)}, \tag{5.5c}$$

$$\lim_{R_{\text{fixed}}\to\infty} V_{\text{shunt}} = 0 \text{ (both on and off)}, \tag{5.5d}$$

$$\lim_{R_{\text{fixed}}\to 0}\left(\frac{V_{\text{on}}}{V_{\text{off}}}\right)_{\text{series}} = \frac{R_{\text{MOSFET(max)}}}{R_{\text{MOSFET(min)}}}, \tag{5.5e}$$

$$\lim_{R_{\text{fixed}}\to 0}\left(\frac{V_{\text{on}}}{V_{\text{off}}}\right)_{\text{shunt}} = 1, \tag{5.5f}$$

$$\lim_{R_{\text{fixed}}\to 0} V_{\text{series}} = 0 \text{ (both on and off)}, \tag{5.5g}$$

$$\lim_{R_{\text{fixed}}\to 0} V_{\text{shunt}} = V_{\text{i}} \text{ (both on and off)}. \tag{5.5h}$$

These derivations depend on the assumption of a zero source impedance and infinite load impedance. Regardless of the fact that we recommend IC analog switches for all our applications rather than MOSFETs, because they approach the behavior of ideal MOSFETs, the necessity of trading off $(V_{\text{on}}/V_{\text{off}})$ against

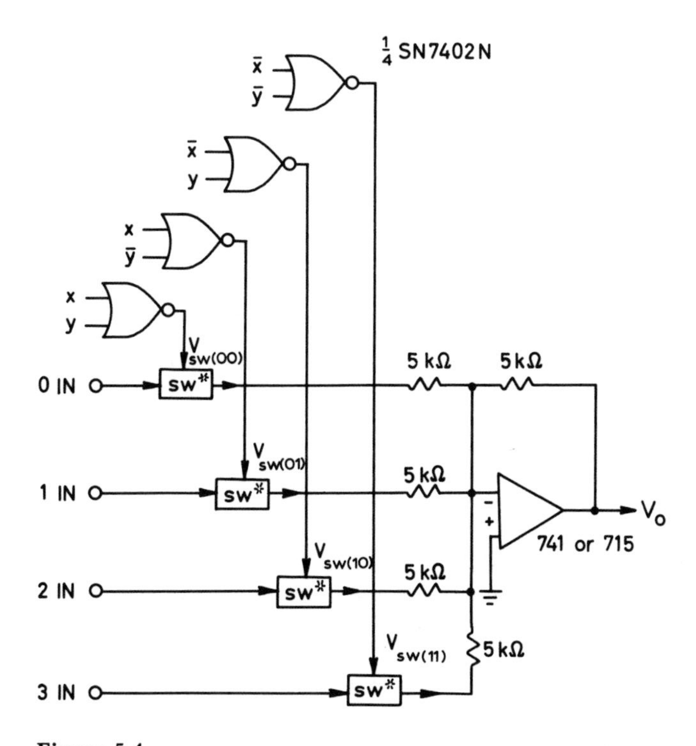

Figure 5.4
Analog multiplexer (output inverted). *TTL-compatible switch, such as Fairchild SH3001 4-channel analog switch (supply requirements: +10 V, −20 V).

voltage attenuation must be taken into account in all designs using analog switches in series or shunt modes. Since

$$\frac{V_{\text{on}}}{V_{\text{off}}} = \frac{R_{\text{MOSFET(max)}}}{R_{\text{MOSFET(min)}}} \tag{5.6}$$

for the series-shunt configuration, this is generally the configuration of choice for circuits requiring high $\frac{V_{\text{on}}}{V_{\text{off}}}$.

Analog multiplexing is accomplished with the circuit of Figure 5.4. In this case, the one switch that is conducting is the one that provides the lowest input resistance. The summing circuit will produce a weighted sum of voltages, with the selected input voltage being weighted much more heavily than the others. Shunt or series-shunt configurations may also be used for the switching sections.

Several integrated circuits are on the market now that accomplish digital and analog switching and multiplexing. We will use these circuits, because they are generally as economical as anything that could be built from discrete components and are small, reliable, and easy to use.

5.2 Oscillators

Oscillators are positive-feedback devices which, through the interposition of a delay element in the feedback circuit, cycle periodically through a sequence of voltages. The shape of the wave form is determined by the type of network and, sometimes, by subsequent processing with op amps or nonlinear transconductors.

5.2.1 Square-Wave Generator

One type of oscillator that has already been mentioned is the astable multivibrator, which is a form of square-wave generator. Its main characteristics are that it possesses only two stable output voltages and that it undergoes periodic rapid transitions, from one voltage state to the other. The durations of these states determine the frequency of oscillation.

A simple astable multivibrator constructed with an op amp is shown in Figure 5.5. The device has a frequency of oscillation that is continuously variable, determined by the feedback potentiometer and the decade capacitors. The positive feedback from the output forces the device to clip at one voltage extreme or the other, say ± 10 to ± 14 V for the 741 op amp, depending on supply voltage. The negative feedback current charges the capacitor until the voltage exceeds the positive feedback voltage at V^+. The rate of charging is determined by RC. When the negative input voltage exceeds threshold for the device (Equation 4.1), the output goes toward zero. The positive feedback ensures that once this swing begins,

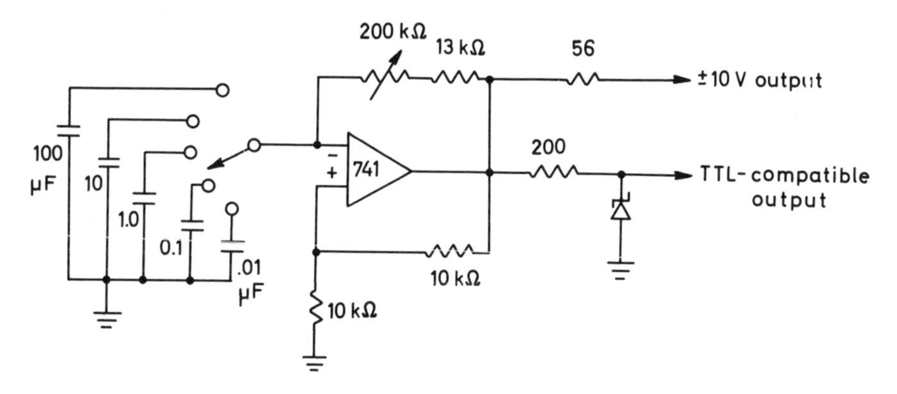

Figure 5.5
Analog-controlled square-wave oscillator.

the voltage is regeneratively driven to the opposite limit. The sequence then repeats, with voltage going the other way. Frequency is varied by changing *R* or *C*. The fixed 13 kΩ series resistor prevents a zero *R*. Square waves of frequencies up to about 1 kHz can be obtained with the 741 in this configuration. For higher frequency limits, use an operational amplifier with higher frequency cutoff, such as the 715, which is described later, or use two op amps, where one generates a sine wave (see below) and the other amplifies it at such a high gain that a square wave results due to clipping.

The output circuit shows a simple technique for achieving TTL compatibility. The resistor limits the load on the op amp to a minimum of 200 Ω, and the zener diode restricts the output voltage to a range of approximately 0–4 V. For symmetrical square-wave output of about ±10 V, remove the output circuit.

For precise control of square-wave oscillator frequency, a quartz crystal may be used in the feedback circuit. The resonant frequency is determined by the thickness of the crystal, which is cut to precise dimensions. By cutting in the right plane, temperature effects are minimized. The accuracy and stability of the crystal frequency is generally better than 0.1% and with careful design and temperature control, it can reach a few parts per million. A simple crystal oscillator is illustrated in Figure 5.6. In this oscillator, the crystal acts as a series-resonant device; in some circuits, parallel-resonant crystals are used. Generally, crystals are used for frequencies above 10 kHz, and timing is accomplished by a trimmer capacitor in parallel with the crystal for small frequency changes, or by switching in different crystals for large changes (more than 1%).

The frequency of a square wave can be controlled digitally. The technique consists of dividing a high frequency by a single-integer division factor, as schematized in Figure 5.7. The output flipflop converts the preset counter output, which

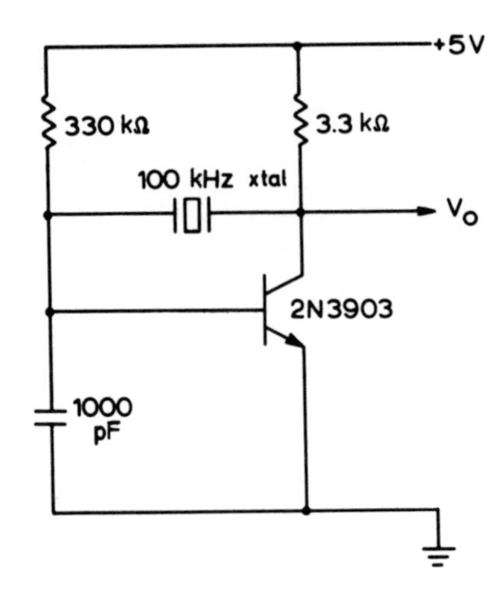

Figure 5.6
Crystal-controlled oscillator.

is in the form of pulses, to a symmetrical square wave. The output frequency in this example is limited to integral submultiples of 5 MHz (the output flipflop forces a twofold frequency division). The most obvious advantage of such a device is the high degree of frequency accuracy provided by the crystal oscillator. Also, by using several square-wave generators driven by the same crystal oscillator, fixed and controllable phase relations among outputs are possible. In generating sine waves and pulse trains for two-point stimulation procedures, this can be a very useful feature.

The preset counter used for the square-wave generator is a free-running counter that cycles up through zero, *modulo* the preset count. The divider section allows successive frequency division by factors of 10 and can be extended as many decades as desired, using the SN7490N decade counters in the symmetrical divide-by-10 configuration. The decade period multiplier selector switch allows choice of the frequency divide factor. The preset count SN7490N is in the 0–9 count configuration.

The BCD selector switch is a specially designed switch (several varieties are available, including rotary and thumb-wheel types) which connects the switch wiper to all those output bits which should be on when the desired count is reached. The diodes ensure that, if any of the selected output bits is zero, the wiper of the switch will be at a zero level. The wiper voltage will be positive (ON) only when all the bits are on: it performs a selective AND. The positive output, inverted by the INV, and slowed by the 2700 pF capacitor (to allow time for the flipflop to

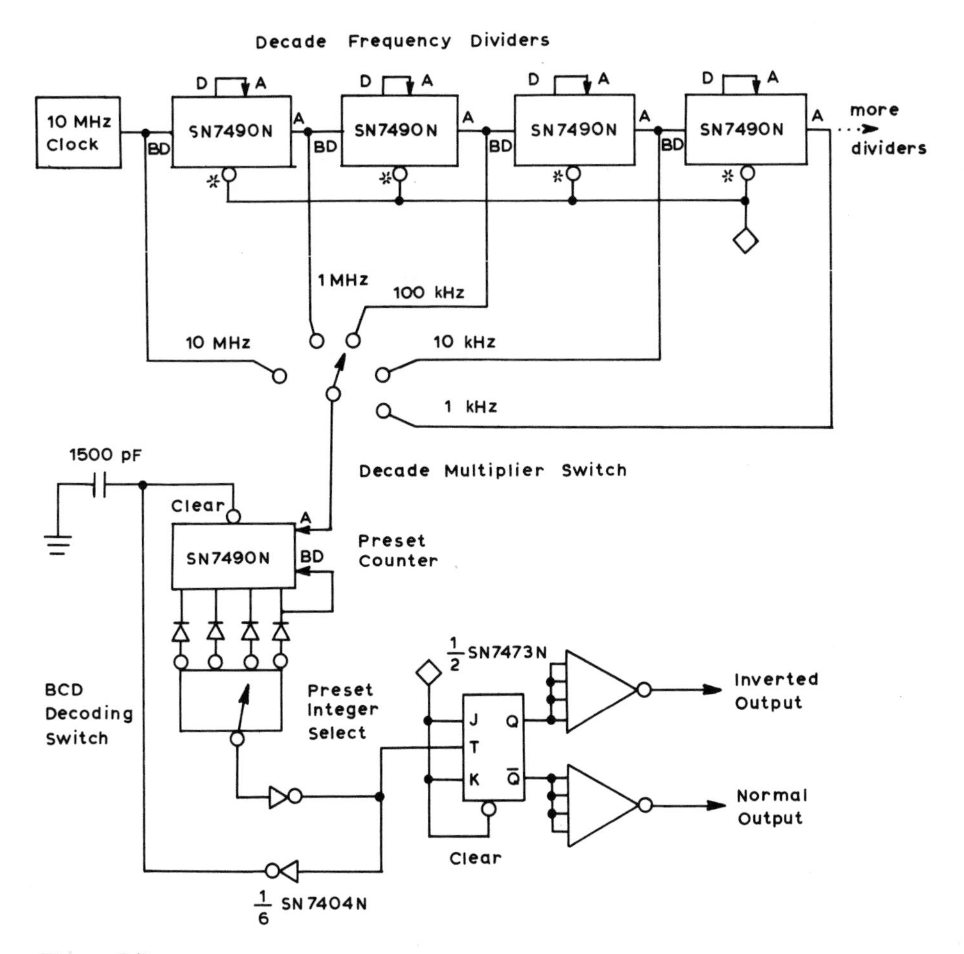

Figure 5.7
Digitally controlled square-wave oscillator.
* Both $R(0)$ and both $R(9)$ inputs (4 inputs per counter) are grounded.
** Both $R(9)$ inputs are grounded, and one $R(0)$ input is tied to logical 1.

$$\text{frequency} = \frac{5 \text{ MHz}}{\text{Integer} \times \text{Multiplier}}.$$

settle) feeds back to clear the timer. The timer then counts from zero to the preset count again. The flipflop outputs are buffered to prevent resetting by transmission line noise.

Multidigit precision of the preset count is easily obtained by using a modification that will be discussed later in this chapter (triggerable digital pulse generator, Figures 5.16 and 5.17).

This method does not provide any frequencies other than integral submultiples of the clock frequency, so choice of clock frequency is important. Other, much more sophisticated methods can generate any frequency that is a rational fraction of the clock frequency $f\frac{p}{q}$, where f is the clock frequency, and p is an integer smaller than the integer q. These are presently too expensive for inclusion here.

5.2.2 Triangle-Wave Generator

An analog-controlled triangle-wave (serrasoidal wave) generator is illustrated in Figure 5.8. The first op amp (A_1) forms a bistable multivibrator, whose output state is determined by an input-output relation similar to that of Figure 4.1, as specified in Equation 4.1. The output levels of A_1 are determined by A and B,

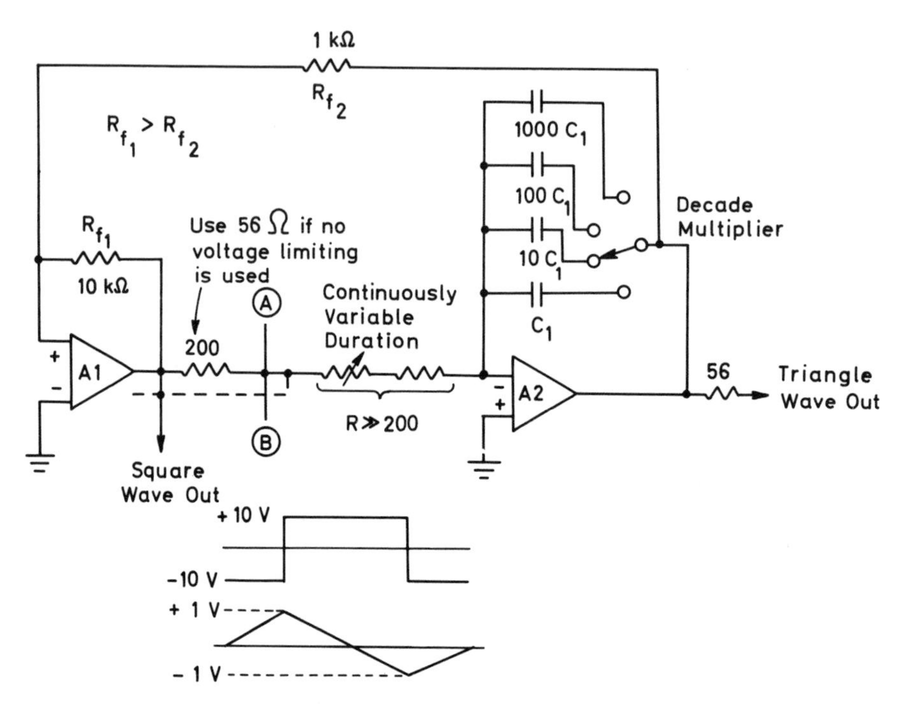

Figure 5.8
Analog-controlled triangle-wave oscillator.

$A1 = A2 = 741$ or equivalent.

which may be level-clamping devices, or the wave form may simply be limited by the upper and lower dynamic limits of the amplifier, which for the 741 are symmetrical with symmetrical supply voltage. This output is used to drive amplifier A_2, which integrates the steady input voltage and produces a ramp whose constant slope is determined by R and C as well as the input voltage. If the voltage limits are controlled independently, different slopes can be obtained on the rising and falling edges of the triangle wave, although it will still be symmetrical about zero. Whenever the output of A_2 reaches the threshold of A_1, then A_1 switches to the opposite extreme of its output range, and the triangle-wave output proceeds in the opposite direction, as illustrated in Figure 5.8. Note the phase relation between the two outputs. If a square wave is desired that switches on the zero crossings of the triangle wave, use a high-speed differential comparator such as the 710 to detect the zero crossings of the triangle wave.

The variable resistor R provides continuous variation of the slopes of the triangle; a decade switch with capacitances that are spaced by factors of 10 will provide decade selection of frequency range. The variable resistor R should be composed of a potentiometer and a series resistor that is less than one-tenth and more than one one-hundredth of the maximum value of the potentiometer (for example, use a 100 kΩ potentiometer and a fixed 5 kΩ series resistor) in order to obtain overlapping ranges. Since the slope is determined by RC, the frequency is also determined by RC, because the threshold of the A_1 amplifier is specified entirely by the value

$$(\pm V_{\max}) \cdot \frac{R_{f2}}{R_{f1}},$$

as indicated in Equation 4.1. The maximum values of the triangle output voltage can be determined by this relation. Asymmetry of the triangle wave about the zero voltage can be obtained by shifting the threshold of A_1 by a constant, by injecting a weighted bias via the summing junction of A_1. Alternatively, asymmetrical voltage limits on the output of A_1 will have the same effect, or R_{f2} may consist of two different-valued resistors in parallel, each of which has a series diode facing in opposite directions.

The 741 will provide accurate triangle waves up to 100/sec. For higher frequencies, use an amplifier such as the 715, discussed below.

The digitally controlled triangle-wave generator (Figure 5.9) operates on a principle that is essentially the same as that used for the analog-controlled device. It consists of an operational amplifier that integrates a positive voltage for the descending ramp, and a negative voltage for the ascending ramp. The circuit

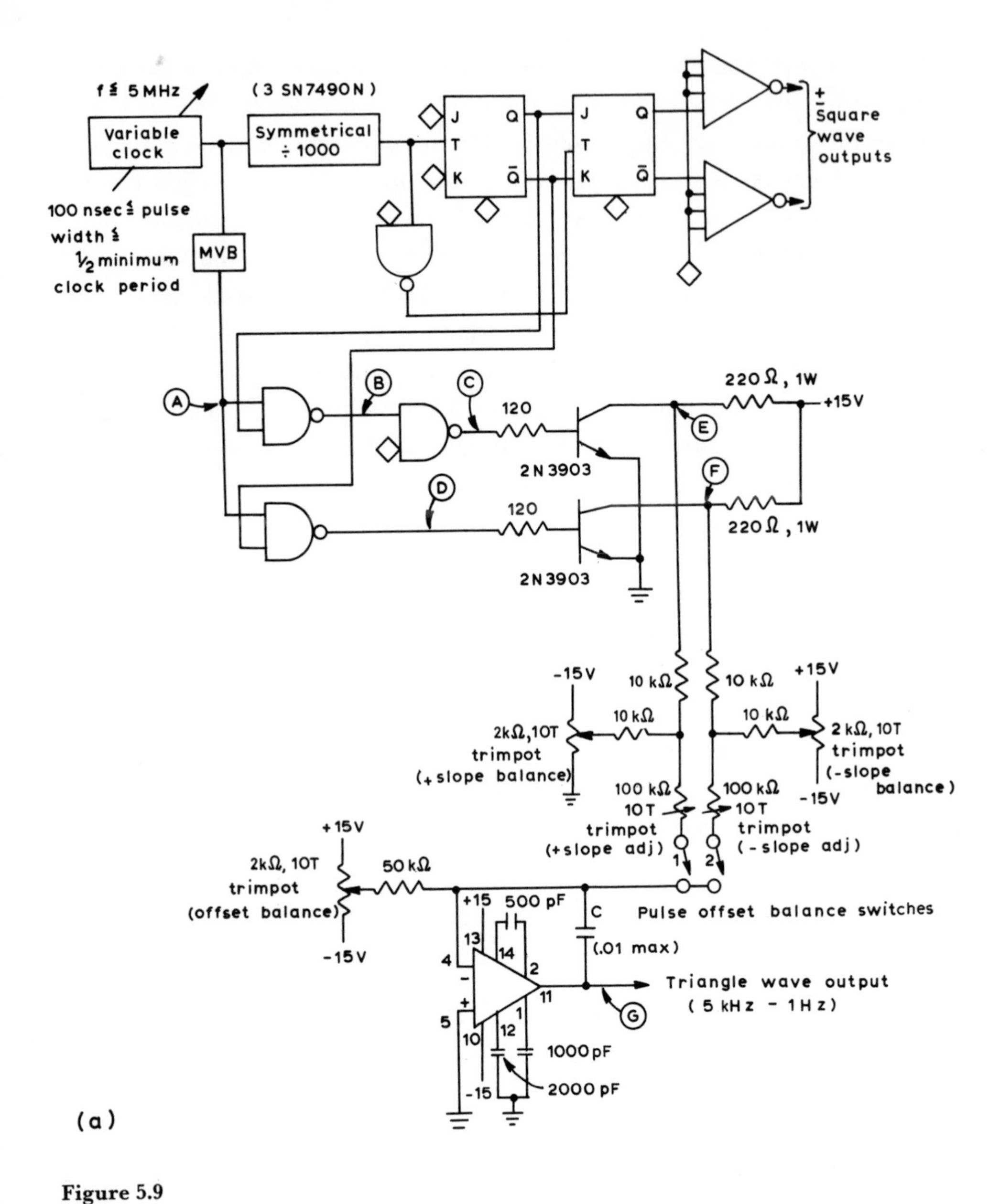

Figure 5.9
(a) Digitally controlled triangle-wave oscillator; (b) 715 op amp specifications (from *Semiconductor Integrated Circuits Data Catalog, 1970*, by Fairchild Semiconductor. Used with permission of Fairchild Camera and Instrument Corporation.); (c) wave forms within digital triangle-wave generator (number of pulses per half-cycle reduced to 10 for clarity).

ELECTRICAL CHARACTERISTICS ($V_S = \pm 15$ V, $T_A = 25°C$ unless otherwise specified)

PARAMETER	CONDITIONS	MIN.	TYP.	MAX	UNITS
Input Offset Voltage	$R_S \leq 10$ kΩ		2.0	5.0	mV
Input Offset Current			70	250	nA
Input Bias Current			400	750	nA
Input Resistance			1.0		MΩ
Input Voltage Range		±10	±12		Volts
Large Signal Voltage Gain	$R_L \geq 2$ kΩ, $V_{out} = \pm 10$ V	15,000	30,000		
Output Resistance			75		Ω
Supply Current			5.5	7.0	mA
Power Consumption			165	210	mW
Acquisition Time (Unity Gain)	$V_{out} = +5$ V		800		ns
Settling Time (Unity Gain)			300		ns
Transient Response (Unity Gain)	$V_{in} = 400$ mV				
Risetime			30	60	ns
Overshoot			25	40	%
Slew Rate	Av = 100		70		V/μs
	Av = 10		38		V/μs
	Av = 1 (non-inverting)	15	18		V/μs
	Av = 1 (inverting)		100		V/μs
The following apply for $-55°C \leq T_A \leq +125°C$:					
Input Offset Voltage	$R_S \leq 10$ kΩ			7.5	mV
Input Offset Current	$T_A = +125°C$			250	nA
	$T_A = -55°C$			800	nA
Input Bias Current	$T_A = +125°C$			750	nA
	$T_A = -55°C$			4.0	μA
Common Mode Rejection Ratio	$R_S \leq 10$ kΩ	74	92		dB
Supply Voltage Rejection Ratio	$R_S \leq 10$ kΩ		45	300	μV/V
Large Signal Voltage Gain	$R_L \geq 2$ kΩ, $V_{out} = \pm 10$ V	10,000			
Output Voltage Swing	$R_L \geq 2$ kΩ	±10	±13		V

NOTES:

(1) Rating applies for case temperatures to +125°C, derate linearly at 6.5 mW/°C for ambient temperatures above +75°C.

(2) For supply voltages less than ±15 V, the absolute maximum input voltage is equal to the supply voltage.

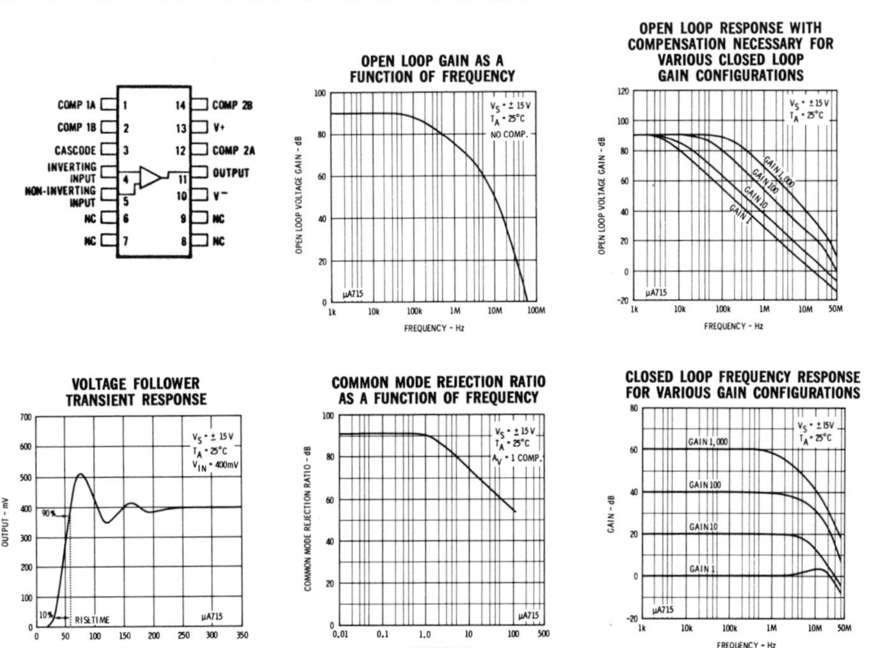

Figure 5.9 (continued)

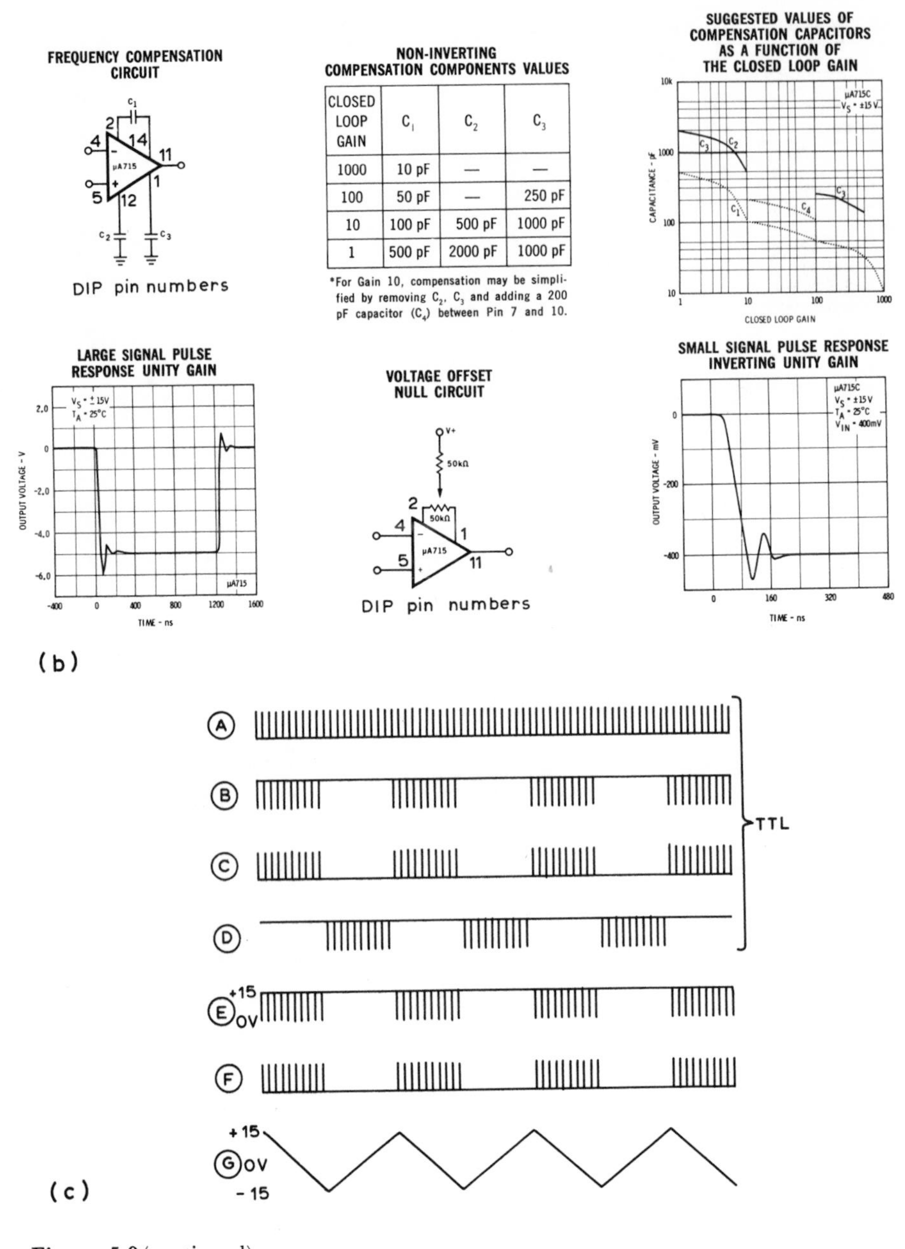

CLOSED LOOP GAIN	C_1	C_2	C_3
1000	10 pF	—	—
100	50 pF	—	250 pF
10	100 pF	500 pF	1000 pF
1	500 pF	2000 pF	1000 pF

Figure 5.9 (continued)

differs in that the voltages to be integrated are pulses of opposite polarity rather than steady levels. The ramp rate is determined by the pulse frequency.

In fine structure, the ramps actually consist of small staircase "steps," but because 1000 steps per ramp are used, it is essentially linear. If even greater linearity is desired, a larger number of pulses may be used to synthesize the ramps. Since the upper limit on TTL logic frequencies at present is under 100 MHz, the upper frequency limit of the resulting triangle wave is under 100 kHz: practically speaking, about 5 kHz. The frequency limit of the output can be raised by sacrificing linearity, that is, by decreasing the number of pulses per ramp. For many purposes, 100 steps would provide adequate linearity and would increase maximum output triangle frequency to 50 kHz.

A variable frequency TTL-compatible clock, which may be either digital or analog design, is used to control the frequency of the clock pulses. The clock also feeds a symmetrical divide-by-1000 counter, which is simply three SN7490s in the symmetrical divide-by-10 mode connected in series. The output of the frequency divider is fed to a steering flipflop that switches on each negative transition of the divided clock frequency. The steering flipflop in turn guides the transitions of another *J-K* flipflop that is driven by the inverted output of the frequency divider. This flipflop changes state at times halfway between transitions of the steering flipflop and provides a square-wave output which goes ON on the positive zero crossing of the triangle wave, and OFF at the negative zero crossing.

The steering flipflop outputs are also used to guide the pulses of the multivibrator through steering gates. The gated pulses are used to drive bases of transistors to provide well-saturated 15 V on- and off-pulses. These two trains are biased for zero baselines and summed at the inverting input of an integrator.

Although fewer trim pots could be used, three separate bias controls and a switch are included in the circuit for ease of drift compensation. Unless the baseline current into the summing junction is very nearly zero between pulses, the dc current will cause a "drift" of the integrator output that would be independent of the clock frequency, resulting in severe distortion of the output at certain frequencies. To adjust slopes of pulses and input offset compensation, proceed as follows:

1. Open both pulse offset balance switches and adjust the offset balance trim pot for minimum drift of the integrator (that is, maximum time for the integrator to drift from one voltage extreme to the other). This maneuver compensates for input offset of the operational amplifier.

2. Close pulse offset balance switch 1 and with the +SLOPE adj. trim pot adjusted for minimum resistance, adjust the +SLOPE balance trim pot for minimum drift of the integrator, with the input clock off. This zeros the baseline for

the negative-going pulses, allowing later adjustment of pulse height without re-adjustment of offset.

3. Open pulse offset balance switch 1 and close pulse offset balance switch 2. Adjust the −SLOPE balance trim pot (with the −SLOPE adj. trim pot set to minimum resistance) for minimum integrator drift.

4. Close both offset balance switches. If the offset balance adjustments have been made carefully, it should now be possible to adjust the + and −SLOPE adjust trim pots, with the clock frequency on, for symmetrical rising and falling triangle wave slopes. In order to prevent a dc offset on the output, adjust total triangle-wave output so the peaks exactly reach the output voltage limits, with minimal clipping. The output frequency should be completely controllable by the input clock frequency with no distortion of wave form. If supply regulation is good, this balancing procedure will never need repeating, except for very low frequencies, where even small offsets due to thermal drift may produce asymmetrical slopes.

With 100 nsec pulses, and $C = 0.01\ \mu F$, frequencies of 1 Hz to 5 kHz can be obtained. Remember that the effect of input offset is minimized by using as large a value of C as possible and as wide a pulse as possible. Faster triangle waves can be obtained by using fewer pulses per ramp. Thus, a 50 kHz upper output frequency limit is possible using ÷100 network rather than ÷1000, with consequent loss of smoothness of the staircase wave form.

For very low frequency applications, the integrator drift can be a serious problem. In these applications, the integrator can be replaced by an up/down binary counter, used to count the input clock pulses. The output bits of the counter are then used to drive a digital-to-analog converter (see Chapter 10 for a description of digital-to-analog conversion), with no drift. Such a circuit is presently more expensive, especially if high-speed D/A conversion is necessary (for example, for conversion times of less than 100 μsec). However, for very slow triangle waves, it is the only practical digital method, and 8-bit converters (256 steps) are now very inexpensive. If individual control of ascending and descending ramp rates is desired, use separate clocks, multivibrators, and counters for the 1 pulses and 0 pulses.

The op amp power supply must be well regulated (0.1%) and the op amp should be a low-drift, low-noise, high-frequency amplifier with symmetrical output voltage limits and minimal distortion up to those limits. The 715 op amp (data sheet information, courtesy Fairchild Semiconductor, is provided in Figure 5.9b) is used in the illustrated circuit.

5.2.3 Sawtooth Oscillator

Analog and digital versions of sawtooth oscillators are illustrated in Figures 5.10 and 5.11. The analog-controlled sawtooth generator produces the positive-going

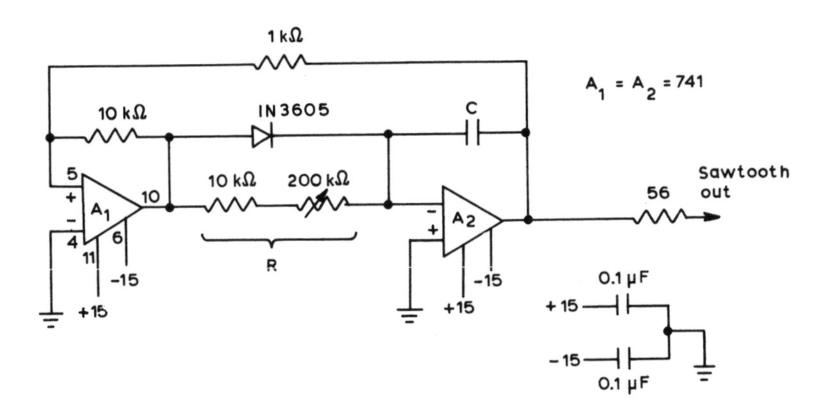

Figure 5.10
Analog-controlled sawtooth oscillator.

ramp in the same way as the triangle-wave generator. However, the negative-going ramp has a very fast slope, because the positive input voltage to A_2 is fed directly through the diode, bypassing the 10 kΩ to 200 kΩ resistor and providing a very low time constant. The positive-going ramp rate is controlled by RC, since the diode does not conduct the negative output of A_1 to the virtual-ground negative input of A_2.

The sawtooth wave form is generally used to sweep a recording device such as an oscilloscope or an X-Y recorder across the X-axis, varying position of the light spot or plotter pen linearly as a function of time.

The digitally controlled sawtooth generator produces a waveform by integrating a preset number of pulses. The slope of the sawtooth is controlled by varying the pulse frequency. A variable clock drives a monostable multivibrator to provide variable pulse frequency and uniform pulse duration. The monostable drives an op amp, which produces well-saturated pulses on a baseline that is biased with a resistive mixer to zero volts. The positive pulses from the op amp are integrated by an op amp integrator to produce a negative-going ramp. The R and C are selected to give the ramp amplitude that is desired. After 1000 pulses, the divide-by-1000 frequency divider triggers a pulse generator to reset the integrator to zero volts. The reset is accomplished by simultaneously shorting the capacitor and decoupling the input pulses. This results in a unity-gain follower with grounded input, giving a good zero-volt output. An SPST switch can be used to just short the capacitor if off-voltage need not be so accurate. This results in an inverting amplifier with very low gain and hence very low off-voltage. The switch used, the SH3002, is a relatively expensive device, and can be replaced by any of several cheaper analog switches which have become available since this circuit was designed.

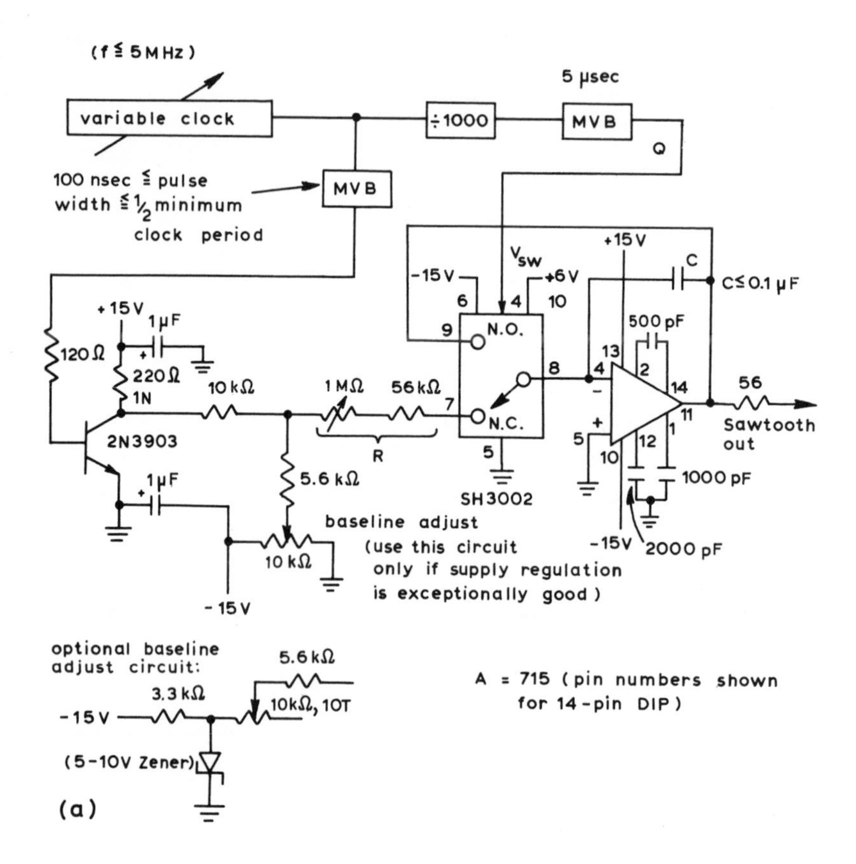

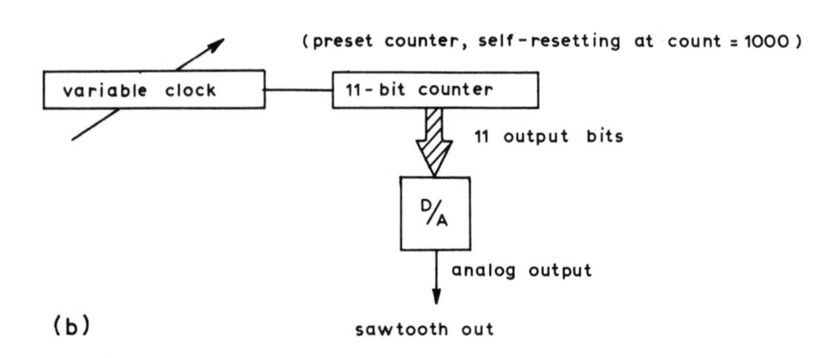

Figure 5.11
Digitally controlled sawtooth oscillator: (a) integrator method; (b) D/A converter method; (c) SH3002 analog switch characteristics (from *Semiconductor Integrated Circuits Data Catalog, 1970*, by Fairchild Semiconductor. Used with permission of Fairchild Camera and Instrument Corporation.).

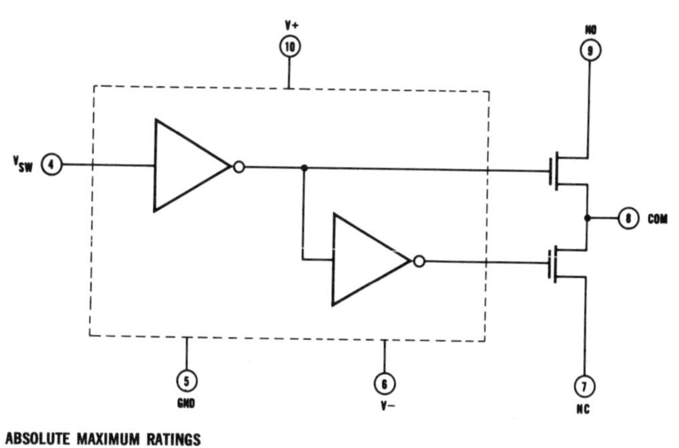

PHYSICAL DIMENSIONS
(in accordance with JEDEC TO-100)

.370 .335
.335 .305
.040 MAX.
.185 .165
10 LEADS .019 .016 DIA.
.040 MAX.
.500 MIN.
.230 TP
.115 TP
Bottom view:
36°
.034 .028
.045 .029

NOTES:
All dimensions in inches
Leads are gold-plated Kovar
Package weight is 1.02 grams

PART NO. HAG30021XX

ABSOLUTE MAXIMUM RATINGS

Maximum Temperatures

Storage Temperature	−65°C to +150°C
Operating Temperature	−55°C to +125°C

Maximum Power Dissipation

at 25°C Case	500 mW
at 25°C Ambient	350 mW

Maximum Voltages and Current

V_{in} (Pins 1, 2, 8 & 9)	±10 V
V_{out} (Pins 3 & 7)	±10 V
V^+ (Pin 10)	+11 V
V^- (Pin 6)	−22 V
I_{in}, I_{out}	100 mA
V_{switch} (Pin 4)	±6 V

SYMBOL	CHARACTERISTIC	MIN.	TYP.	MAX.	UNITS	TEST CONDITIONS
V_{SWH}	High Switch Drive Voltage	1.9			V	$T_A = 25°C$
V_{SWH}	High Switch Drive Voltage	2.2			V	$T_A = -55°C$
V_{SWH}	High Switch Drive Voltage	1.6			V	$T_A = 125°C$
V_{SWL}	Low Switch Drive Voltage			1.1	V	$T_A = 25°C$
V_{SWL}	Low Switch Drive Voltage			1.5	V	$T_A = -55°C$
V_{SWL}	Low Switch Drive Voltage			0.5	V	$T_A = 125°C$
I_{SWH}	High Switch Input Current			2.5	μA	$V_{SW} = 5.0$ V, $V_{10} = 10$ V, $V_6 = -22$ V
I_{SWL}	Low Switch Input Current			−1.5	mA	$V_{SW} = 0$ V, $V_{10} = 11$ V, $V_6 = -20$ V
R_{ON}/CHANNEL	Channel "On" Resistance		140	200	Ω	$V_8 =$ GND, I_7 or $I_9 = 100$ μA
I_{OFF}	Channel "Off" Leakage			25	nA	$V_8 = \pm 10$ V, $V_7 = \pm 10$ V, $V_9 = \pm 10$ V, $T_A = 25°C$
I_{OFF}	Channel "Off" Leakage			1.0	μA	$V_8 = \pm 10$ V, $V_7 = \pm 10$ V, $V_9 = \pm 10$ V, $T_A = 125°C$
V_{IN}	Analog Peak Signal Input			±10	V	
I_{10}	Positive Supply Current			8.0	mA	$V_{SW} = 4.0$ V, $V_{10} = 11$ V, $V_6 = -22$ V
I_{10}	Positive Supply Current			8.0	mA	$V_{SW} = 0$ V, $V_{10} = 11$ V, $V_6 = -22$ V
I_6	Negative Supply Current			6.5	mA	$V_{SW} = 4.0$ V, $V_{10} = 11$ V, $V_6 = -22$ V
t_{on+}	Turn-on Time (Pin 9)		75	150	ns	
t_{off+}	Turn-off Time (Pin 7)		575	650	ns	
t_{on-}	Turn-on Time (Pin 9)		75	160	ns	
t_{off-}	Turn-off Time (Pin 7)		260	340	ns	
t_{off+}	Turn-off Time (Pin 9)		1.6	1.9	μs	
t_{on+}	Turn-on Time (Pin 7)		1.35	2.0	μs	
t_{off-}	Turn-off Time (Pin 9)		1.5	1.7	μs	
t_{on-}	Turn-on Time (Pin 7)		1.6	2.5	μs	

(c)

Figure 5.11 (continued)

The SH3002 will operate properly in this circuit with a $+V_{CC}$ of +6 V, a $-V_{CC}$ of −12 V (same as $-V_{CC}$ for the op amp) and TTL switching voltage. The device characteristics are illustrated in Figure 5.11b, courtesy Fairchild Semiconductor.

Figure 5.11c illustrates a very simple method of generating a digitally controlled sawtooth, which is more expensive but avoids the disadvantages of using an integrator. An 11-bit counter cycles from zero to maximum and then resets (external reset at 1000 can be used), and the output bits are converted directly to a proportional analog voltage. See Chapter 12 for a description of *D/A* conversion.

A level-shifting or inverting amplifier may be added if the baseline, polarity, or amplitude must be changed.

5.2.4 Sine Wave Oscillator

There are many designs available for the direct generation of sine waves. They are all dependent on the use of a tuned circuit in a feedback network. One such oscillator is the popular Wien bridge sine wave generator of Figure 5.12. The output is fed back through the *RC* network, producing a sinusoidal voltage variation. The conditions for stable oscillation are twofold: (1) The gain around the loop must be unity. If it were not, the amplitude of an oscillation would decrease to zero (overdamped condition) or increase to a clipped sine wave (underdamped oscillation), limited by the voltage limits of the circuit. The stable condition of unity gain is called the critically damped condition. (2) The phase shift around the loop must be zero. If it is not, the frequency will change in the proper direction to make it zero. When the circuit automatically compensates gain and phase to realize these conditions, a stable sinusoidal oscillation results; such a device is called a harmonic oscillator.

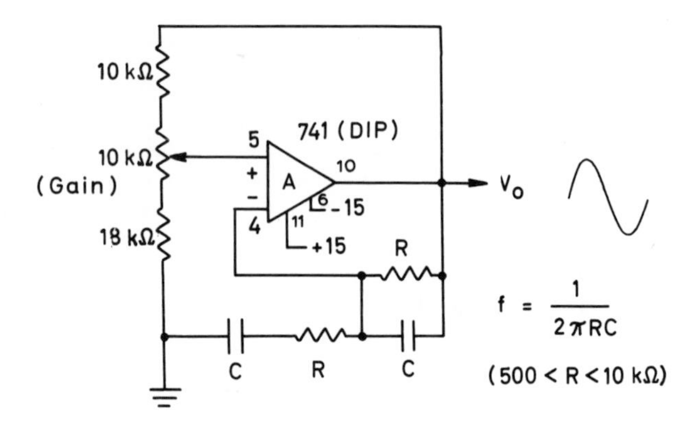

Figure 5.12
Wien bridge sine wave oscillator (after Figure 18.6, in *Designing with Linear Integrated Circuits*, 1969, by Jerry Eimbinder (ed.). Used with permission of John Wiley & Sons, Inc.).

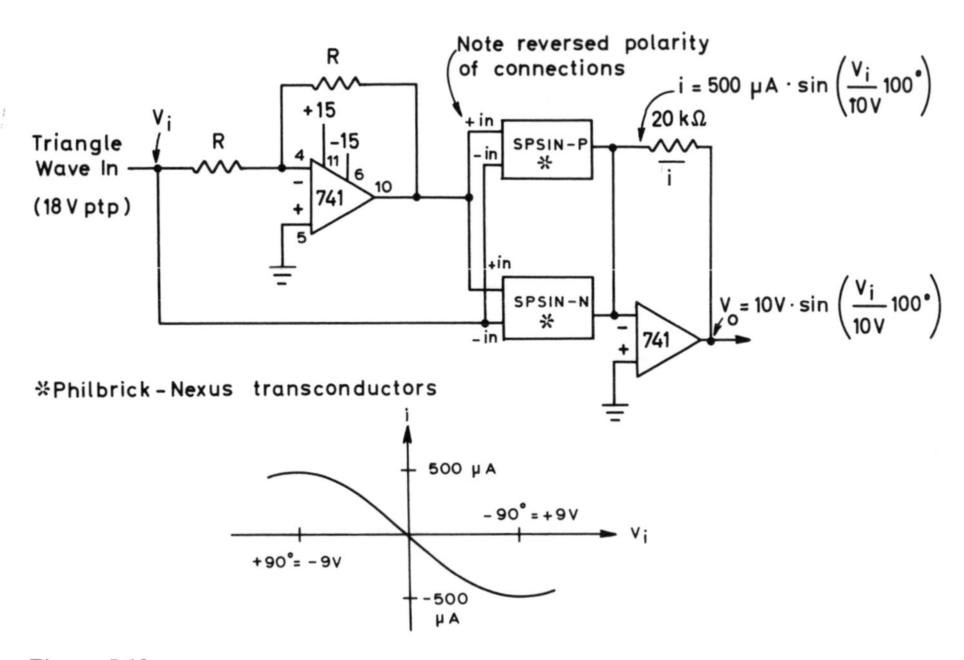

Figure 5.13
Triangle-sine wave conversion (after Figure 2.27, in *Application Manual for Operational Amplifiers*, 1968, by Philbrick/Nexus Research. Used with permission of Teledyne Philbrick.).

The output amplitude of the Wien bridge oscillator is to some extent a function of frequency, and gain must be adjusted manually. For very stable frequency and amplitude, the device should be temperature compensated or placed in a temperature controlled oven, and automatic gain control (described later in this chapter) should be added to produce an output that is of constant amplitude at all frequencies and temperatures.

Sine waves can also be synthesized by shaping the output of a triangle-wave generator, as illustrated in Figure 5.13. Since the nonlinear transconductors used rely on the input-output relation of Figure 5.13b, where ± 9 V $= \pm 90°$, the triangle wave must be exactly 18 V peak-to-peak and exactly centered around zero voltage. The digital triangle generator is the circuit of choice for precise control of frequency and phase, and the analog generator is recommended for continuous control of frequency. Harmonic distortion of digitally produced sine waves can be as low as 0.5%, adequate for most purposes: the total power contained in all the contaminating harmonics are 46 dB lower than the fundamental. Thus, for the low frequencies used in vestibular stimulation, a digital generator is useful; for auditory stimulation, at higher frequencies with lower harmonic distortion, the analog technique is sometimes preferable.

The transconductor of Figure 5.13 consists of resistor-diode pairs that lead the

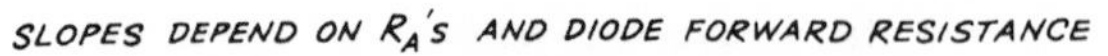

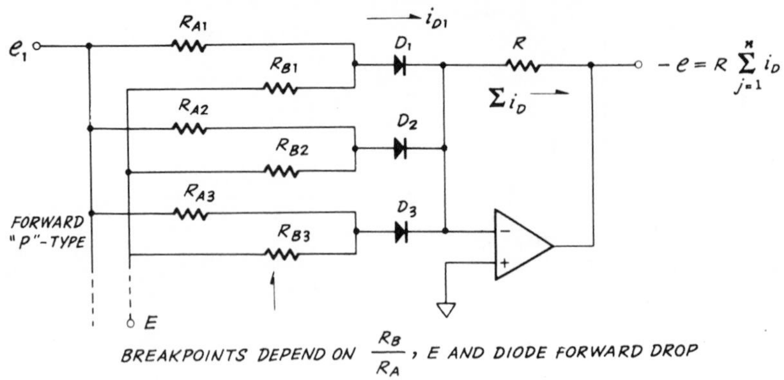

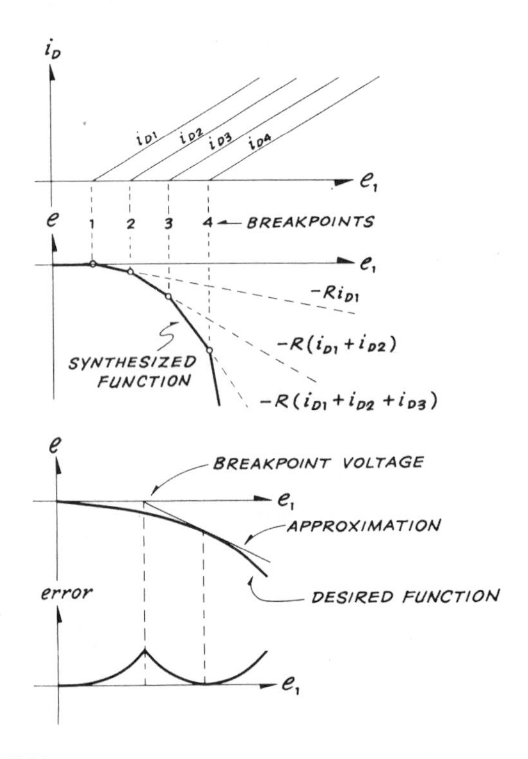

Figure 5.14
Nonlinear transconductor (from Figure 2.23, in *Application Manual for Operational Amplifiers*, 1968, by Philbrick/Nexus Research. Used with permission of Teledyne Philbrick.).

input voltage to a summing junction, producing a different gain for different portions of the input voltage range (Figure 5.14). Such transconductors can produce a large variety of input-output functions, such as trigonometric and log functions, determined by the values of the weighting resistors. The sine wave has a 0.1% error maximum, when the triangle wave is properly adjusted for amplitude and baseline. Greater accuracy is attained with more diode-resistor pairs.

Any wave form can be generated by converting a series of digital numbers with a *D/A* converter (see Chapter 10 for digital-to-analog conversion techniques). This can be accomplished with a digital computer, or by sequentially addressing a Read-Only-Memory (ROM) programmed for the proper number sequence. The Micro Networks Corporation MN350 is a module that contains a 128-word (8 bits per word) ROM and associated hardware, producing a sine wave output with a TTL clock input. The input frequency range is 0–1.2 MHz, and the output frequency range is 0–10 kHz. Output is accurate to 8 bits.

5.3 Triggerable Wave Forms

The oscillators discussed earlier will prove useful in several applications, but we will also occasionally need devices that will produce a voltage sequence upon external activation by a voltage "trigger," and that remain in a quiescent state between triggers. We will consider three types of triggerable wave forms: pulses, ramps, and triangle waves. These can be used to synthesize most other wave forms needed for neurophysiological studies.

All the triggerable circuits have six different modes of operation, modeled after the popular Tektronix 160 series wave-form generators. There are three free-running modes, including RECURRENT, MANUAL CONTINUOUS, and GATE. In these modes, under the proper circumstances, the interval between ON-transitions corresponds to the control setting and the OFF-duration is negligibly brief (approximately 5 μsec). There are also three "one-shot" modes, including MANUAL SINGLE, +TRIGGER, and −TRIGGER. In these modes the device produces a TTL pulse triggered (initiated) by a positive or negative TTL transition at one of the TRIGGER outputs, or by depressing the START push-button switch. These pulses are of the preselected duration and occur once for each trigger, unless a trigger occurs during an output wave form—such a trigger is ignored.

We will first describe the trigger section (Figure 5.15) used by all the triggerable devices.

The NORM IN (clamped at a quiescent 0 level when no external input is applied) is inverted by a NAND gate. The inverted NORM IN is NANDed with the INV

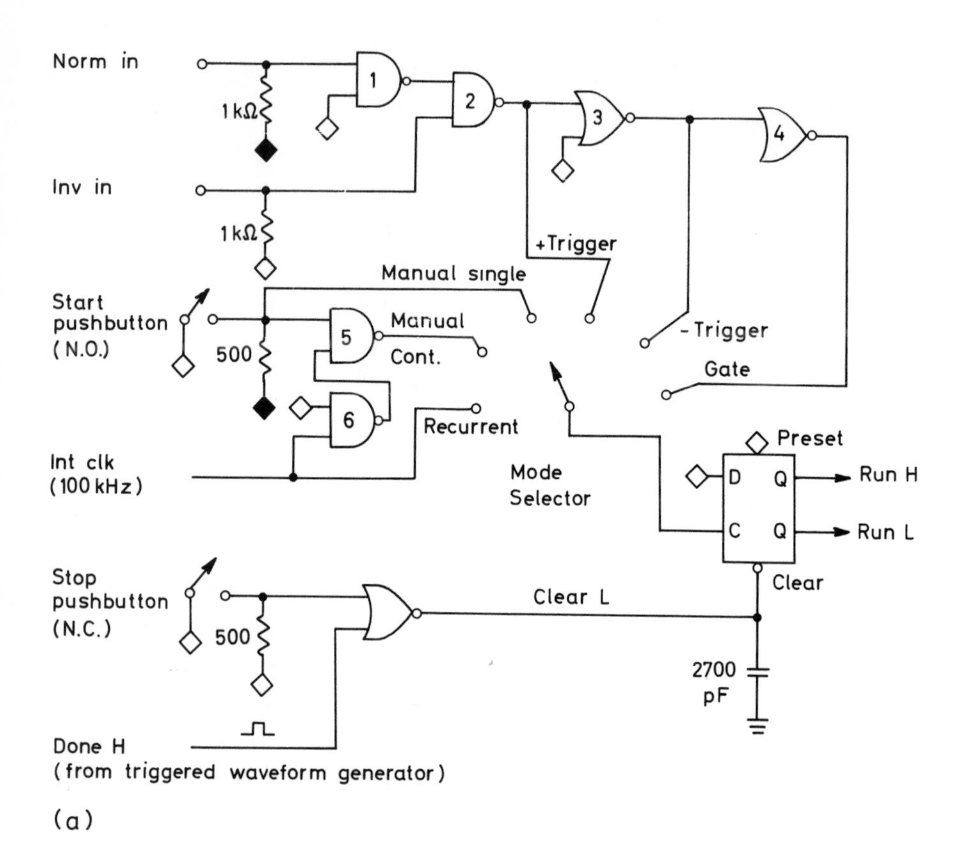

Figure 5.15
Trigger circuit for triggerable wave form generators: (a) schematic; (b) wave forms.

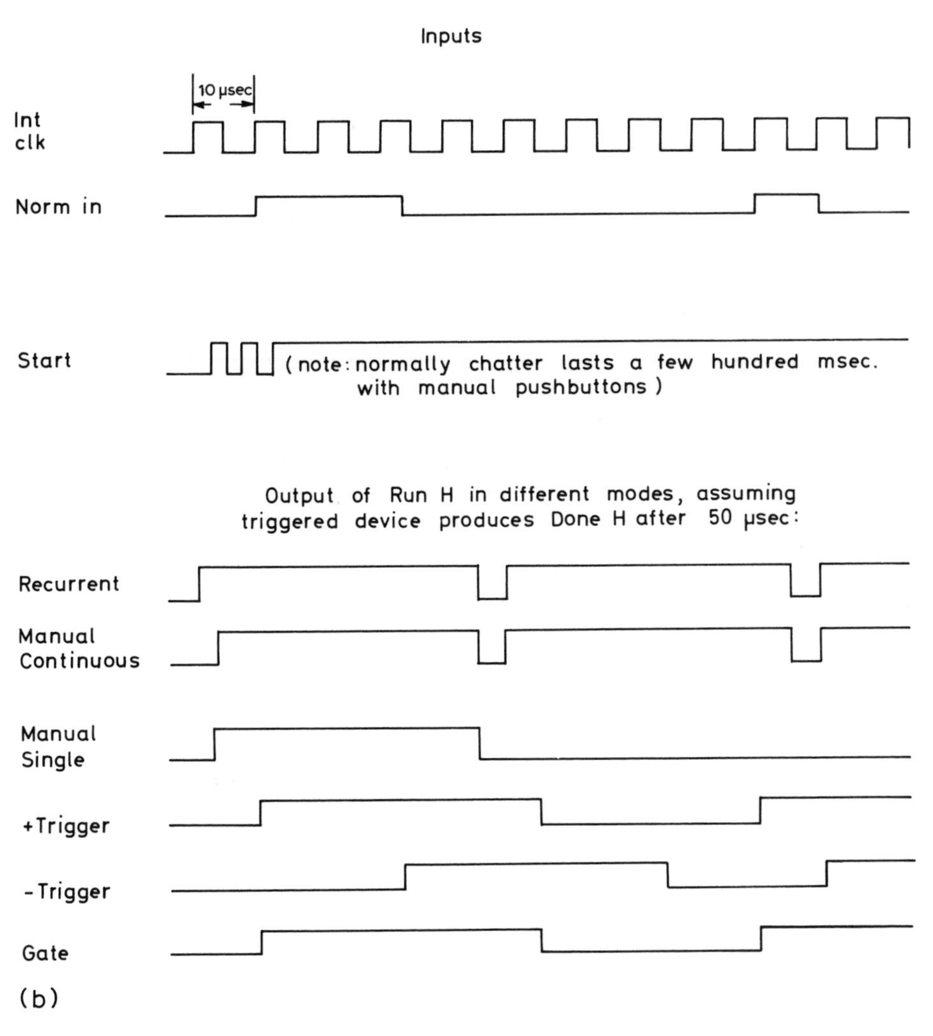

Figure 5.15 (continued)

IN (clamped at a logical 1 when no external input is applied). This provides the +TRIGGER input to the MODE SELECTOR switch. When the switch is in this position a positive NORM IN transition or a negative INV IN transition causes a positive transition to occur at the C-input of the RUN FLIPFLOP. This can only set the flipflop, since the D-input is tied to logical 1. This will occur only if the CLEAR input to the RUN FLIPFLOP is at a logical 1 at the time of the transition. By inverting the +TRIGGER level with a NOR gate we generate a −TRIGGER input to the MODE switch. This signal switches to a logical 1, whenever NORM IN goes off or INV IN goes on, and fires the device.

The −TRIGGER is NORed with the inverted 100 kHz clock to provide a positive C-transition on the first 100 kHz positive transition after (a) the CLEAR pulse goes off; (b) the STOP pushbutton is released; (c) the MODE switch is switched to GATE at a time when the RUN FLIPFLOP is off; all of these being effective only as long as NORM IN is on or INV IN is off. If the latter condition is not met, the NOR will not pass any transitions. If the GATE signal goes off during a wave form, the wave form is completed and the device returns to the quiescent state until the GATE signal goes on again. Therefore, there is a fourth condition when the NOR gate passes a positive transition to the C input of the RUN FLIPFLOP; (d) when the MODE switch is in the GATE position, the sawtooth is off, and on the first clock transition after the NORM IN goes on or INV IN goes off. As in any of the other modes, the positive transition can set the flipflop and initiate a wave form only if the STOP pushbutton is not depressed and the flipflop is not already on.

The RECURRENT position of the MODE switch passes the doubly inverted clock signal directly to the RUN FLIPFLOP, causing it to set on the first clock transition after it is cleared. The MANUAL CONTINUOUS signal is developed by gating the inverted CLEAR pulse with a NAND gate conditioned by the START pushbutton: the device free-runs in the RECURRENT mode, and free-runs in the MANUAL CONTINUOUS mode as long as the START pushbutton is depressed.

The MANUAL SINGLE mode allows one-shot triggering of the device each time the START pushbutton is depressed; note that, for very brief wave forms, switch contact "chatter" will probably cause multiple wave-form cycles.

To summarize, the trigger section provides a RUN H level upon appropriate trigger input or interval event. When one cycle of the triggered wave form has been completed, a DONE H pulse is returned to the trigger circuit to turn off RUN H. The trigger circuit is retriggerable as soon as the CLEAR input to the RUN FF goes off. A cycle can be aborted by depressing the STOP button. For a triggerable wave form generator to operate properly, it must return rapidly to its quiescent state as soon as RUN H goes off, and DONE H must go off as soon as the wave form generation section is retriggerable.

5.3.1 Pulses

Pulses of controllable width can be generated, using either analog or digital control of pulse width. Two such circuits are illustrated in Figures 5.16, 5.17, and 5.18.

The digital generator can also be used as a preset counter, producing ON and OFF TTL logic levels from the beginning of the count until the preset count is reached. Initiation of the count is controlled in the same manner as the initiation of a pulse or train of pulses.

The analog pulse generator is also used to produce a sawtooth. The device works by integrating a fixed voltage level until the sawtooth reaches the threshold of a device that then causes the sawtooth and pulse voltages to return rapidly to their quiescent states. Each cycle is initiated independently by RUN H and ends with the production of DONE H.

The digital generator (Figure 5.16) consists of a counter that counts either a 100 kHz clock frequency or an external TTL input (INT CLK and EXT CLK sources, respectively). The 100 kHz frequency is generated by a crystal-controlled clock oscillator like the one of Figure 5.2; all trigger and wave-form circuits that use a clock should use the same clock, for consistent phase relations. Since the counters are 7490s the count cycle is two-phased, with count transitions occurring on the negative transition of the clock or external input.

The output pulse is simply the output of the RUN FF, buffered with SN7440Ns to provide NORM OUT and INV OUT, which are on and off, respectively, during the timed duration. The RUN FF outputs are buffered with SN7440Ns in order to prevent resetting by transmission line noise. The output level and gain can be adjusted with an extra op amp (use a high-speed one, such as the 715). The NORM or INV output generally should be used to saturate a transistor or op amp if well-saturated on and off levels are desired, as for the application of Figure 5.22.

Setting the RUN FF has two effects: it turns on the slave output flipflop that drives the output buffers, and it enables all the counters.

All the counters but the preset-count counter are 7490s in the symmetrical divide-by-ten configuration, connected in series. The multiplier switch selects the output of one of the counters or the input to the first counter (the selected clock), providing a decade multiplier factor for the preset count. The CLOCK SELECT switch selects either the EXTERNAL CLOCK or the INTERNAL CLOCK (100 kHz). The former will produce an output pulse that goes on when the RUN FF is set

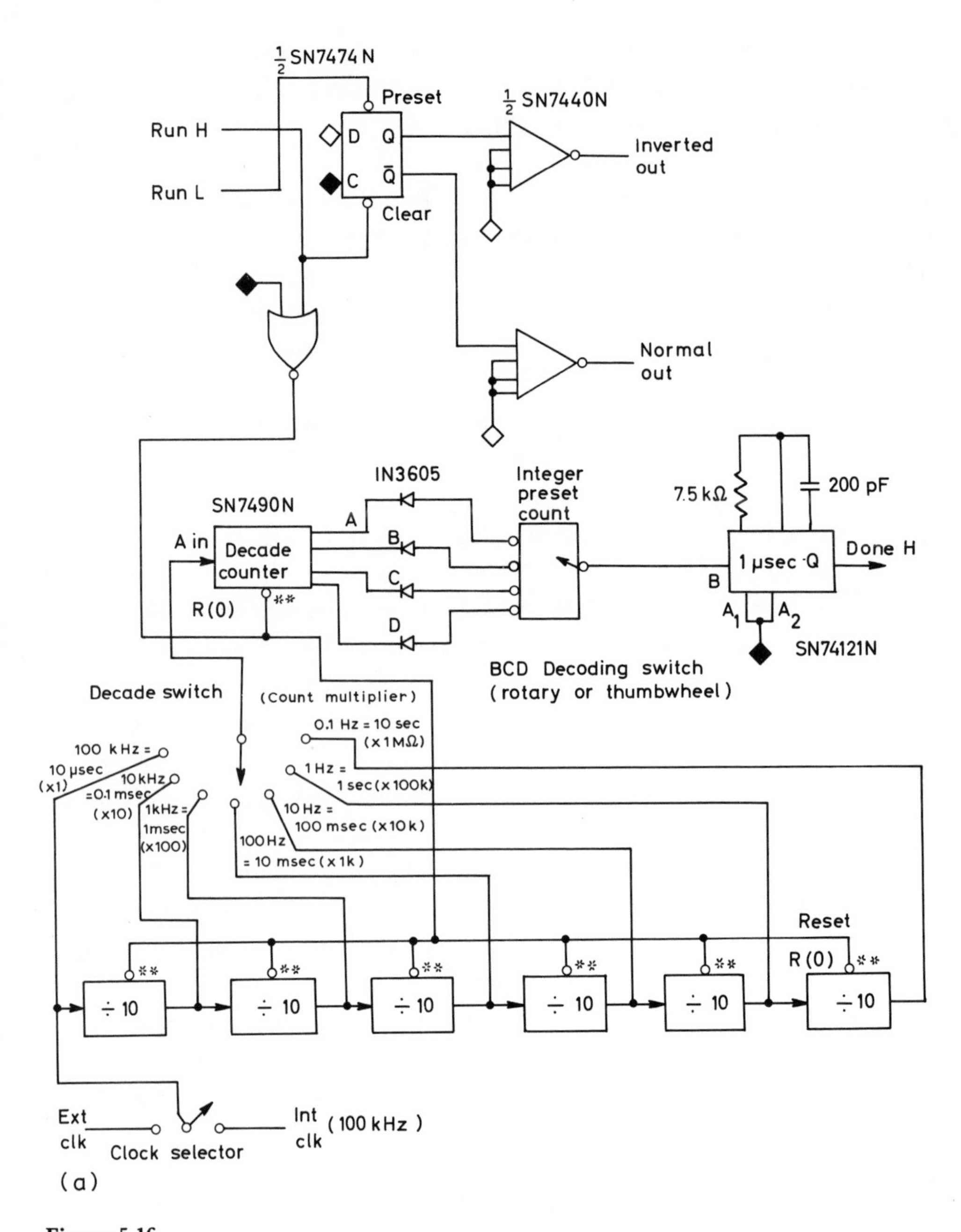

Figure 5.16

Triggerable digitally controlled preset counter-pulse generator: (a) schematic; (b) wave forms. * Tie unused $R(9)$s to 0; ** tie unused $R(0)$ to 1.

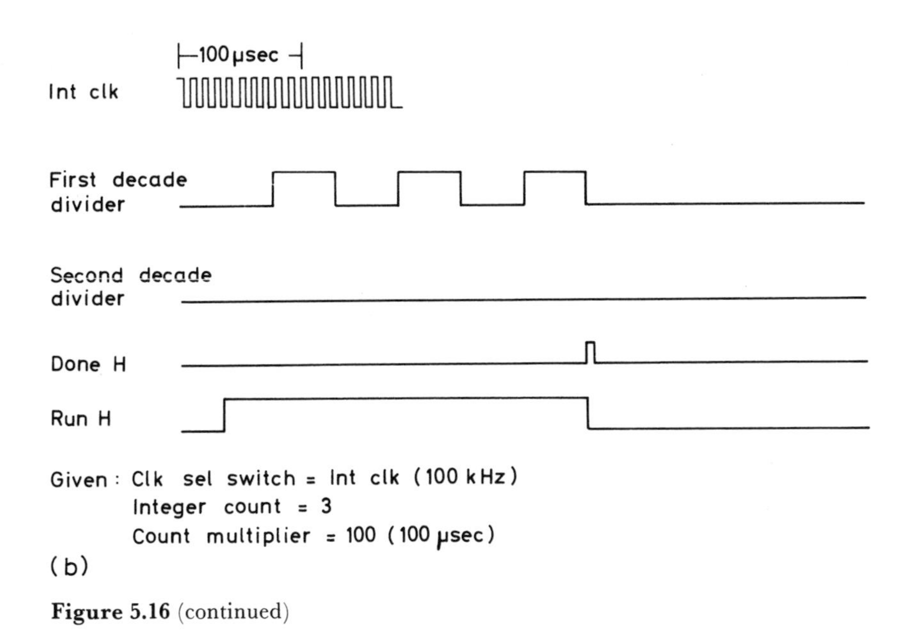

Figure 5.16 (continued)

and goes off when the PRESET COUNT ($\times$ MULTIPLIER) is reached. The corresponding pulse duration using the internal clock is (10 μsec) $\times$ (PRESET COUNT) $\times$ (MULTIPLIER).

The PRESET COUNT SN7490N is in the 0–9 count mode and starts off in the 0-count status, since the RUN FF holds it cleared to zero until the RUN FF is set. When the preset count is reached, the output of the BCD decoding switch goes positive. This triggers the 1 μsec DONE H pulse, which clears the RUN FF. This in turn feeds back to clear the counters. Note that because the counts increment on negative transitions of the selected clock, the RUN FF is cleared very soon after the negative clock transition, allowing a maximum of 5 μsec until the next positive transition to the RUN FF, in one of the three free-running modes (if the 100 kHz clock is selected).

A modification of the preset counter for three-digit precision is presented schematically in Figure 5.17. This modification can be used for any preset counter design and can be extended to any number of digits. The UNIT counter feeds the TEN counter, which in turn provides the input for the HUNDRED counter. Count outputs are buffered to the BCD selector switch in order to allow proper functioning of the devices. In the design of the single-digit preset counter the selected outputs are shorted to ground except when the count is attained. If the D-bit were selected in a multidigit counter, it could be shorted at the wrong time and would then incorrectly propagate the count to the next counter. The diode capacitances

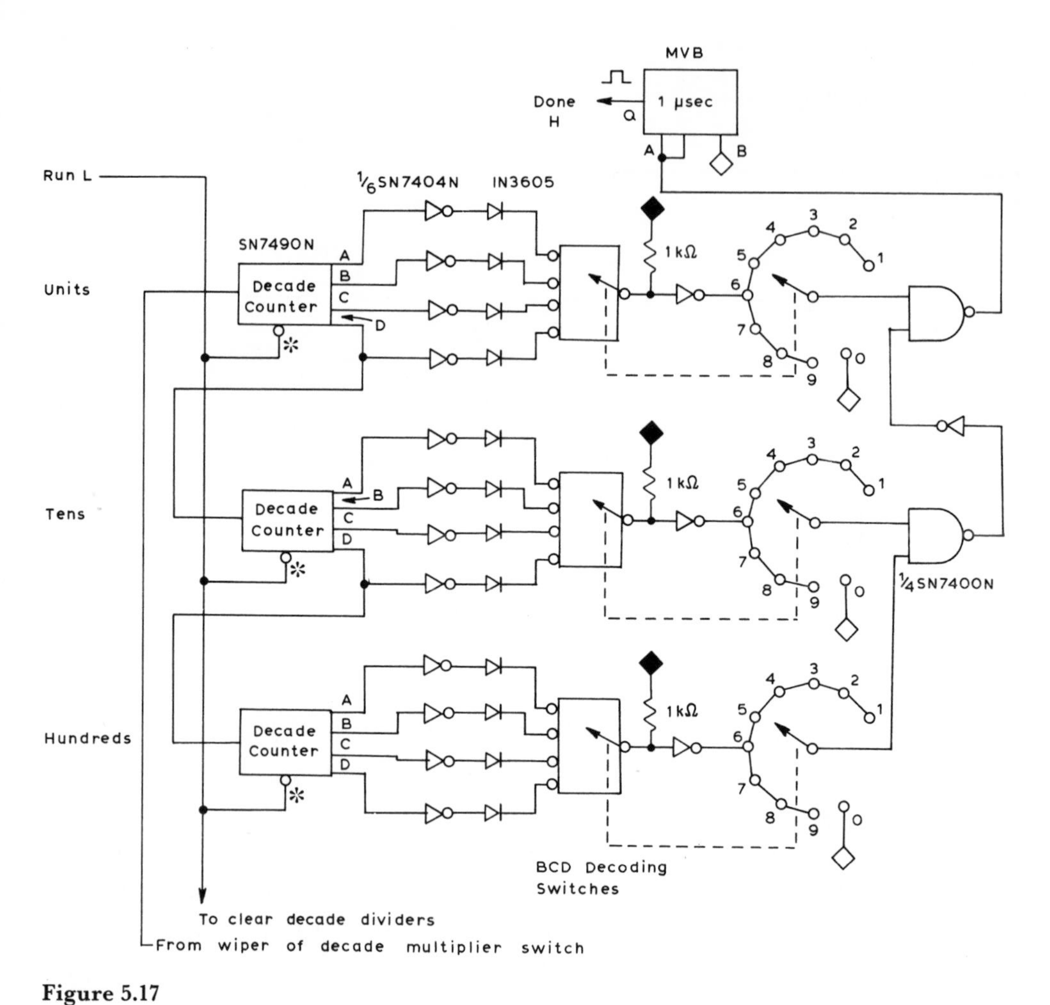

Figure 5.17
Modification of preset counter for 3-digit precision.
* Tie unused $R(9)$s to 0; tie single unused $R(0)$ to 1.

and asynchronous counter outputs are compensated for with the 2700 pF capacitors; otherwise, the UNIT section output may not have attained its new value by the time the TEN section has switched, and the TEN state may still appear to be in the old condition when the HUNDRED counter switches. This can give rise to incorrect counts.

When the HUNDRED count is attained, it enables the gate at the output of the TEN section—this output is disabled until that time. We know that the TEN count will be reached before the HUNDRED output level can go off again. When the TEN count is attained, the gated output level enables the output gate of the UNIT section, which was disabled until then. When the HUNDRED, TEN, and UNIT outputs are all on, the proper count has been attained, and the enabled output of the UNIT section passes through the NOR gate to clear the RUN FF. A zero count for any of the sections is attained by using a second wafer on the corresponding PRESET COUNT switch to switch a logical 1 to the output gate of that section instead of the counter output, when the zero count is selected. Then, as soon as the gate is enabled by the next higher-order section, the gate immediately passes a "count attained" level. If all three sections are set to a zero count, the RUN FF is held off by the logical 1 level into the CLEAR NOR gate.

The analog-controlled pulse generator (Figure 5.18) consists of two op amps that generate a positive-going sawtooth and a pulse. However, as in the digital device, the NORM and INV outputs are derived from the RUN H signal.

The RUN L 0-level drives an op amp to its negative voltage limit. This negative voltage is then fed to another op amp in the integrating configuration, through the variable resistance R. The parallel diode does not conduct to the virtual ground input of the second op amp when the output voltage of the first op amp is negative. The slope of the resulting positive-going ramp at the integrator output is determined by the continuously variable R and the decade-variable C. When the sawtooth voltage reaches the threshold of the differential comparator (zero volts in this case, although any voltage within the ± 10 V range would be adequate, as long as precautions are taken to ensure that the ± 5 V differential input limit of the comparator is not exceeded), the comparator output goes to a 1. This triggers a 1 μsec pulse, which is the DONE H pulse used to clear the RUN FLIPFLOP. The level at RUN L then pulls the first op amp back to the positive output voltage extreme. The positive output voltage of the first op amp is fed through the low-resistance path offered by the forward-biased diode, rapidly pulling the sawtooth level back to the negative extreme of the second op amp, since the effective R is now very small.

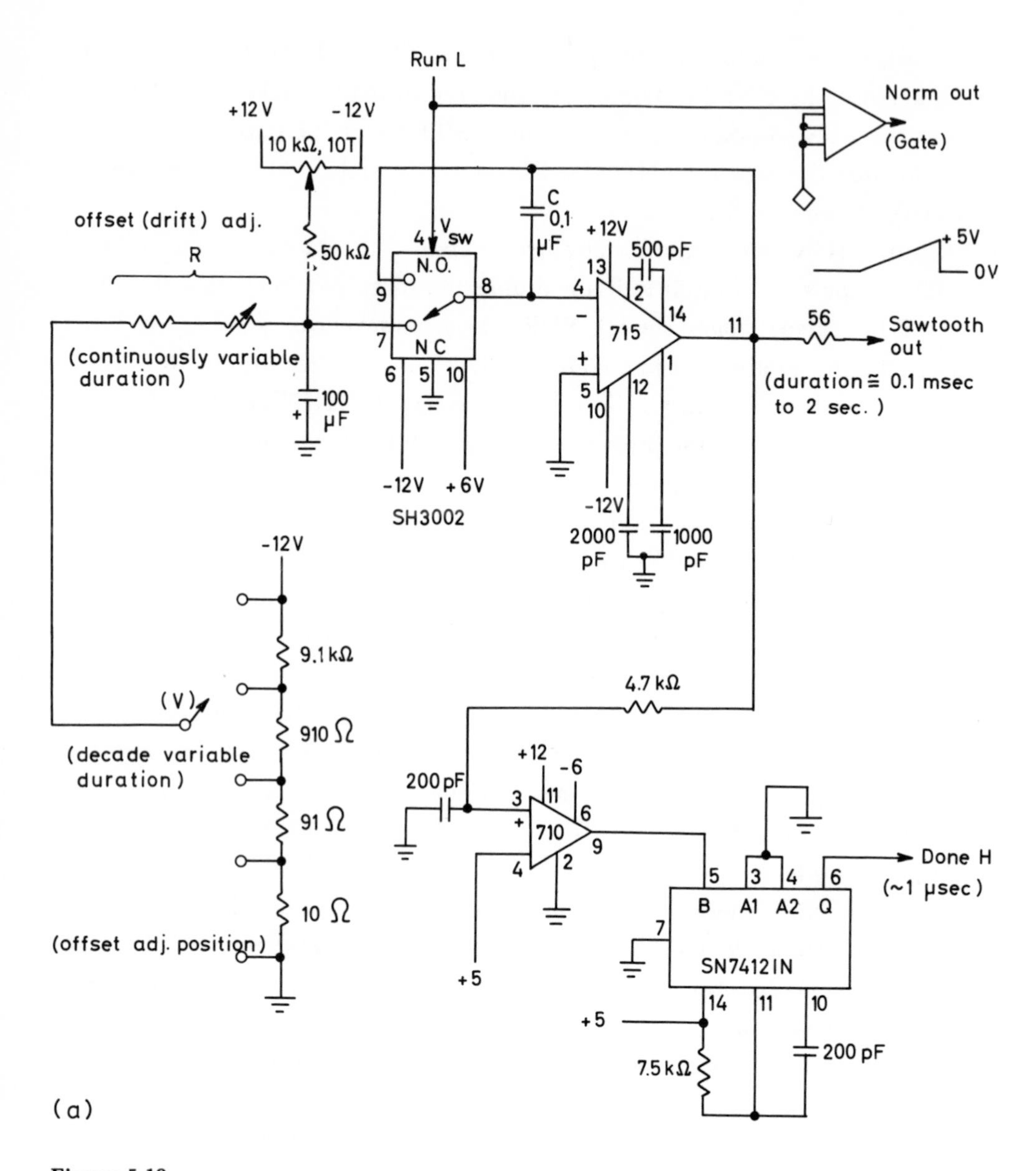

Figure 5.18
Triggerable analog-controlled sawtooth generator: (a) schematic; (b) wave forms.

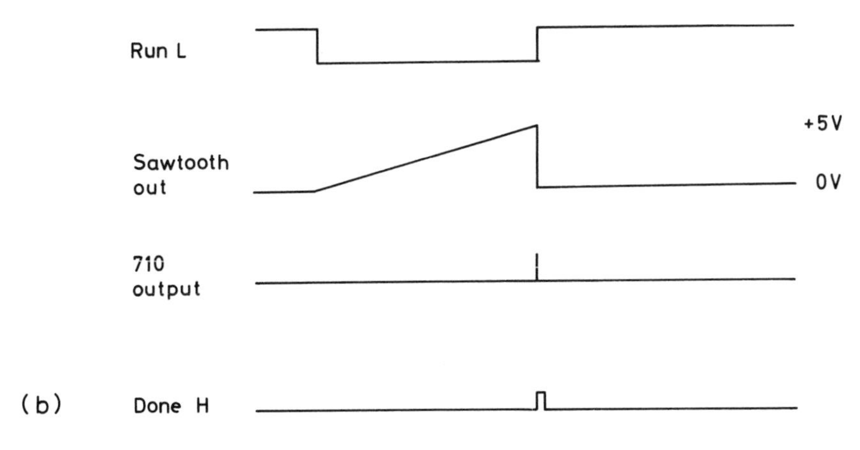

Figure 5.18 (continued)

The comparator may be replaced with another 715 in the positive-feedback configuration, in order to eliminate the need for any additional supply voltages. In that case, the output of the 715 should be clamped for TTL compatibility (see Figure 4.34 for an example of this technique).

5.3.2 Ramps

The analog-controlled sawtooth is generated with the circuit of Figure 5.18, as described in the previous section.

The digitally controlled triggerable sawtooth generator (Figure 5.19) integrates 1000 uniform clock pulses to produce a smooth ramp. The integration begins when RUN H goes on. When 1000 pulses have been integrated, the RUN FLIP-FLOP is cleared by a brief pulse, and the integrator output is forced to the quiescent negative voltage extreme.

Uniform pulses are generated at submultiples of the 10 MHz clock frequency with the familiar digital counter network. The minimum duration is thus 0.1 msec. To achieve shorter durations, use less than 1000 pulses to generate the ramp.

When RUN H goes on, the analog switch passes the mixed *drift adj.* and off-pulses to the inverting input of the integrator. If *drift adj.* is set to sum with the quiescent on-state of the 2N3903 inverting transistor for a zero net voltage, the drift of the integrator should be very slow. Very good supply regulation is necessary, however. The off-pulses result in positive staircase steps. Choose C such that the amplitude of the sawtooth is within the voltage limits of the op amp after 1000 pulses have been integrated, and drift caused by input offsets is minimum.

When 1000 pulses have been counted, the DONE H pulse clears the RUN H level. This results in the analog switch resetting the integrator.

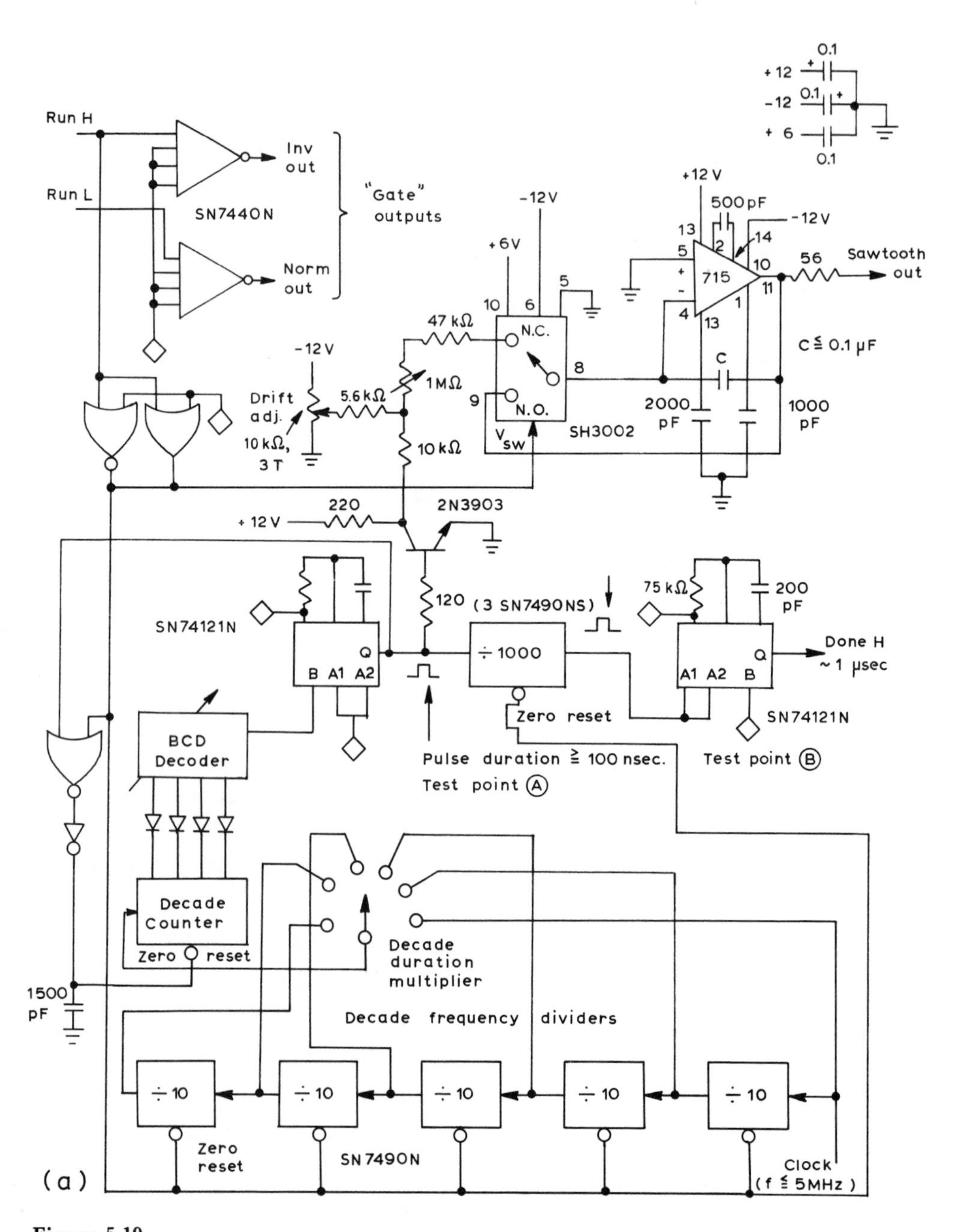

Figure 5.19
Digitally controlled triggerable sawtooth generator: (a) schematic; (b) wave forms; (c) delay registration technique for synchronizing 10 MHz and 100 kHz negative transitions.

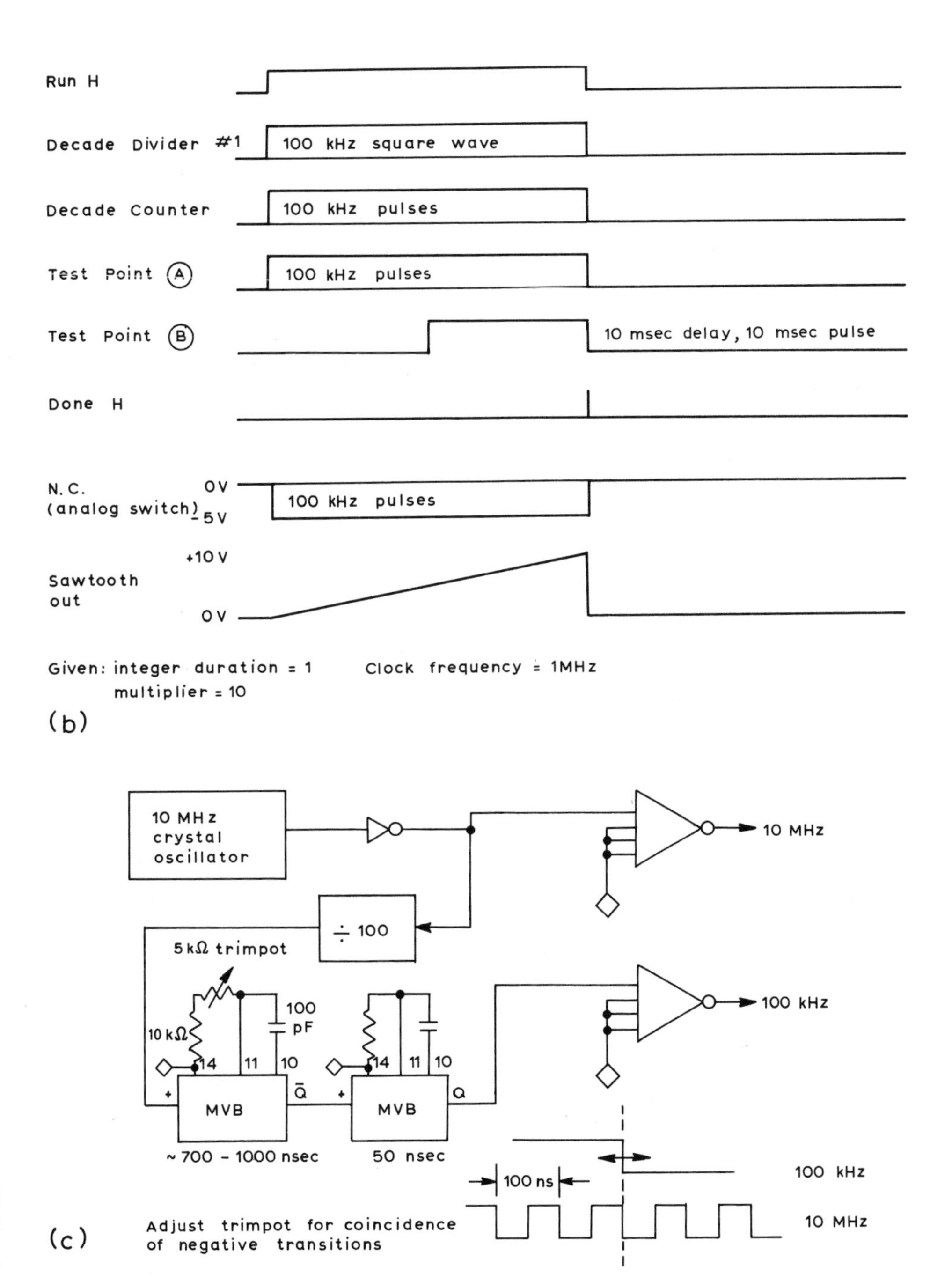

Figure 5.19 (continued)

If any digital sawtooth or serrasoid generators are contemplated, a single 10 MHz clock should be used to drive all of them. The 100 kHz clock for driving trigger circuits or the digital pulse generator should be derived from a ÷100 operation; the output of the second decade divider in the divider chain of either a digital sawtooth or a digital serrasoid generator could be used if properly buffered, and if it is not inverted. The circuit of Figure 5.19c is preferable, however, in that phase relations are more exactly preserved.

Instead of integrating pulses, we can feed the binary count value to an 11-bit D/A converter (see Chapter 10 for a discussion of digital-to-analog conversion), the output of which would be the desired sawtooth. In that case, synchronous up/down binary counters should be used instead of regular BCD counters. This solution is presently more expensive, but for very slow sawtooths, where drift of an integrator is too great, this is the only practical digital method.

In the free-running modes, the next positive transition comes on the next positive transition from the 100 kHz generator (a divide-by-100 pair of SN7490s which divides the 10 MHz clock frequency). It always occurs 5 μsec after the end of the sawtooth, because both sets of counters start counting at the same time and the sawtooth is always some integral multiple of 1000 oscillations in duration. There are exactly 10 100 kHz oscillations per 1000 10 MHz oscillations, and the negative transition of the tenth 100 kHz oscillation always must coincide with the negative transition of the 1000th 10 MHz cycle.

The analog switch chosen for this circuit, the SH3002, is relatively expensive. Since this circuit was designed, several less expensive switches have become available. In selecting a switch, keep the following requirements in mind:

1. Rise time $\leqq \frac{1}{10}$ settling time for clearing integrator.
2. $R_{on}C$ is time constant for integrator reset.
3. $R_{on} \ll R \ll R_{off}$.
4. Voltage extremes which can be passed by the switch must be greater than or equal to voltages fed to the switch inputs.
5. Switching control must be TTL-compatible.

The power requirements for the SH3002 constitute another disadvantage. Shortly before publication of this book, Harris Semiconductor released a 4-channel analog multiplexer with ± 15 V supply voltages and 8 MHz unity gain bandwidth (HA-2400) and Teledyne released a relay switch that derives its power from the TTL signal and analog voltage. These devices should be adequate replacements for the SH3002 in many applications.

5.3.3 Triangle Waves

The analog serrasoid (triangle wave) generator (Figure 5.20) produces a ramp from ground quiescent level to the positive peak, through zero to the negative

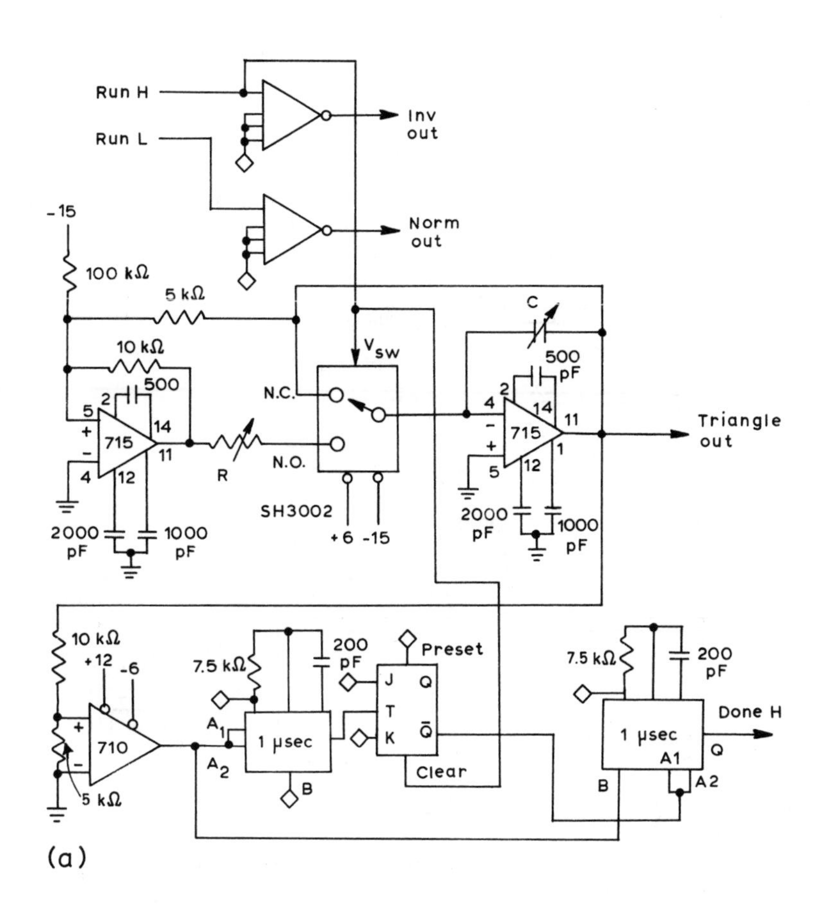

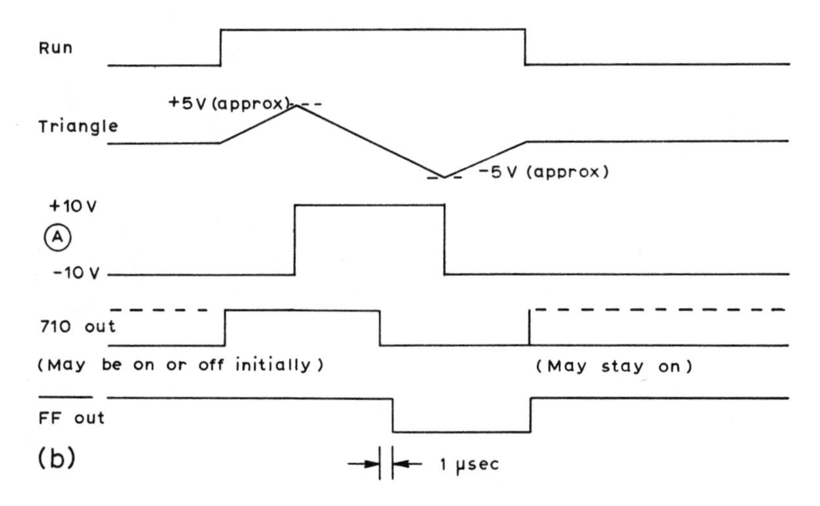

Figure 5.20
Triggerable analog-controlled serrasoid (triangle wave) generator: (a) schematic; (b) wave forms.

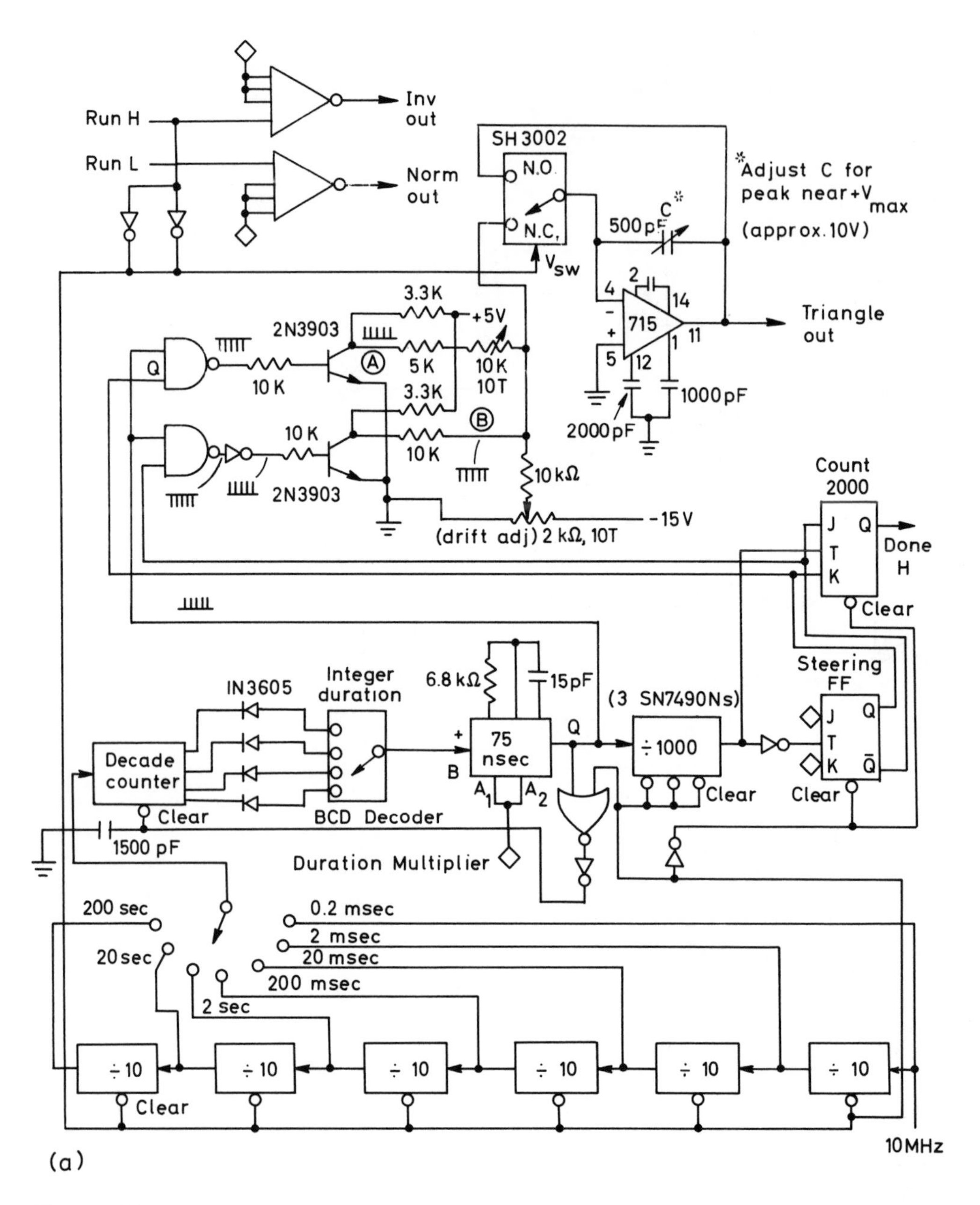

Figure 5.21
Digital triggerable serrasoid generator: (a) schematic; (b) wave forms.

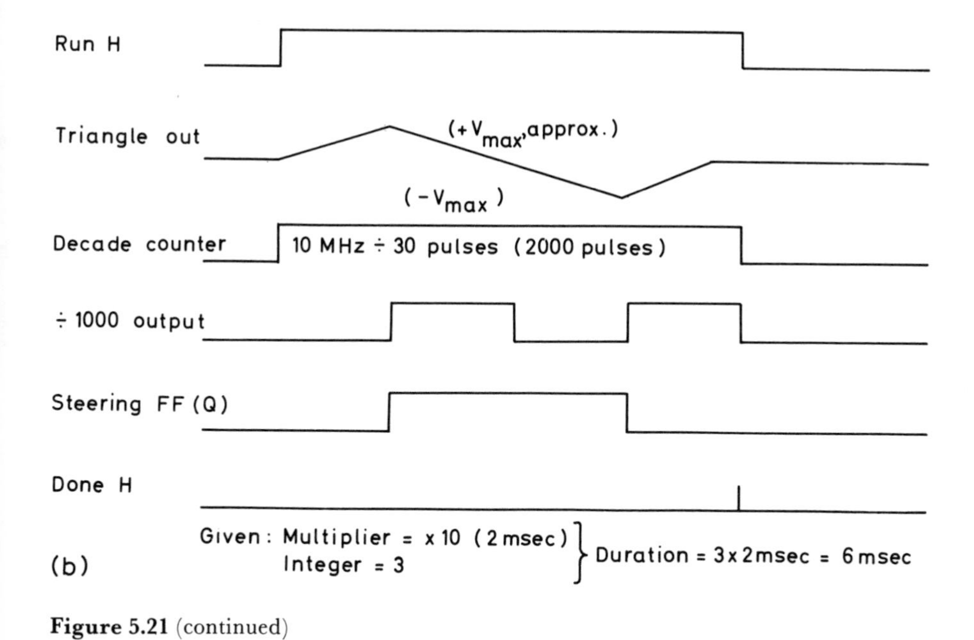

Figure 5.21 (continued)

peak, and back to the zero quiescent level. The ground level is attained and maintained with an analog SPDT switch, which disconnects the negative input and shunts the feedback capacitor, effectively making the integrator a unity-gain follower with grounded input.

The RUN H level flips the analog switch to the output of the first op amp, allowing the second op amp to integrate the initially negative voltage and go from ground to the positive voltage, which is the threshold for the first op amp to switch to its positive extreme. The second op amp then integrates the positive voltage, bringing the ramp back through zero to the negative threshold voltage of the first op amp, which then goes back to its negative extreme. The negative voltage is integrated to pull the ramp back up to ground. At that time, the differential comparator detects the zero crossing and turns off the RUN FF via a 1 μsec DONE H pulse. The D-flipflop inhibits the MVB until after the negative zero crossing, preventing spurious clearing on the initial takeoff from quiescent level. When RUN H goes off, the capacitor is discharged through the switch, and the output goes to ground.

The digital serrasoid generator (Figure 5.21) integrates positive pulses for the negative-going portion of the ramp and negative pulses for the positive slope. The $\div$1000 frequency divider starts with a zero output, switches on at 500, and flips back to zero at a count of 1000. The output switches again at counts of 1500 and 2000. The positive transitions, after inversion, cause the STEERING FF to switch to a 1 and then back to 0, at counts of 500 and 1500. The initial state of the STEERING FF is 0, because the 0 quiescent level of RUN H holds the STEERING FF off until the beginning of the count sequence. The positive and negative pulses are gated and amplified as in the digital triangle wave oscillator. An analog switch driven by the inverted Q output of the RUN FF holds the output at ground quiescent level between cycles.

Once again, a D/A converter can be used to generate the output wave form, if up-down binary counters are used.

5.4 Complex Wave Forms

With the few simple wave-form generators we have discussed, it is possible to synthesize a great variety of complicated voltage sequences. We will consider three such systems to illustrate some of the combinations that are possible. Any of the wave forms that we will synthesize with multiple devices could be generated with a single circuit, which would eliminate much redundancy and make maximum use of the entire circuit. The degree of modularity of a system design must be determined by the user's convenience. For example, if a trapezoidal wave form is the only one that will be used in the course of a few years' research, it is reasonable to build a trapezoid generator. If, on the other hand, a large number of different wave forms will be used, it is more efficient to design a few modular devices that can be combined in different ways to produce all the required voltage sequences. In most research laboratories, the latter alternative is preferable. Although some neurophysiologists are reluctant to operate the more complicated modular arrangement, anyone who can understand the design and build such a system will be able to operate it without any difficulty.

A system that produces two separately controllable trains of electrical pulses is illustrated in Figure 5.22. All of the generators are digital pulse generators.

The TRIAL counter (#1) counts an external clock, as a preset counter. Since it is in the MANUAL CONTINUOUS mode, when the START button is depressed, the output goes on, enabling the REP RATE generator (#2). The REP RATE generator free-runs as long as it is enabled, counting the internal 100 kHz clock. Generator #2 thus determines the repetition rate of the two pulse trains (and must therefore repeat at an interval greater than the duration of the two trains). Each repetition, or "trial," is counted by the TRIAL counter (#1), because the NORM OUT of #2 provides the EXT CLK source for #1. When the preset count of #1 is completed, its output goes off, and the REP RATE generator is no longer enabled, thus terminating the presentations of pulse trains until the START button of #1 is depressed again.

Not only is the NORM OUT of the REP RATE generator used to count trials, but it also triggers generator #3, DELAY. DELAY, fired on each positive transition of REP RATE, is used to trigger DUR1 (#4) and DUR2 (#5), which control the durations of the two trains. Either can be triggered on the leading or trailing edge of NORM OUT of #3, for immediate or delayed onset of the corresponding pulse train.

The DURATION generators independently gate the TRAIN RATE generators (#6, #7), which are in the gated mode and run recurrently as long as they are enabled by their corresponding DURATION generators. The DURATION generators may be used to control the number of pulses in each train by using them to count the pulses (EXT CLK), or they may control the absolute duration of the train by counting the internal clock. Similarly, the DELAY generator is fed an ORed output of the two TRAIN RATE generators (the INV OUTs of the two TRAIN RATE generators are NANDed) as an external clock, providing the opportunity to regulate the delay between the two pulse train onsets in terms of number of pulses instead of as absolute time. In this mode, it is necessary for at least one of the pulse trains to go on with no delay, and the first pulse train

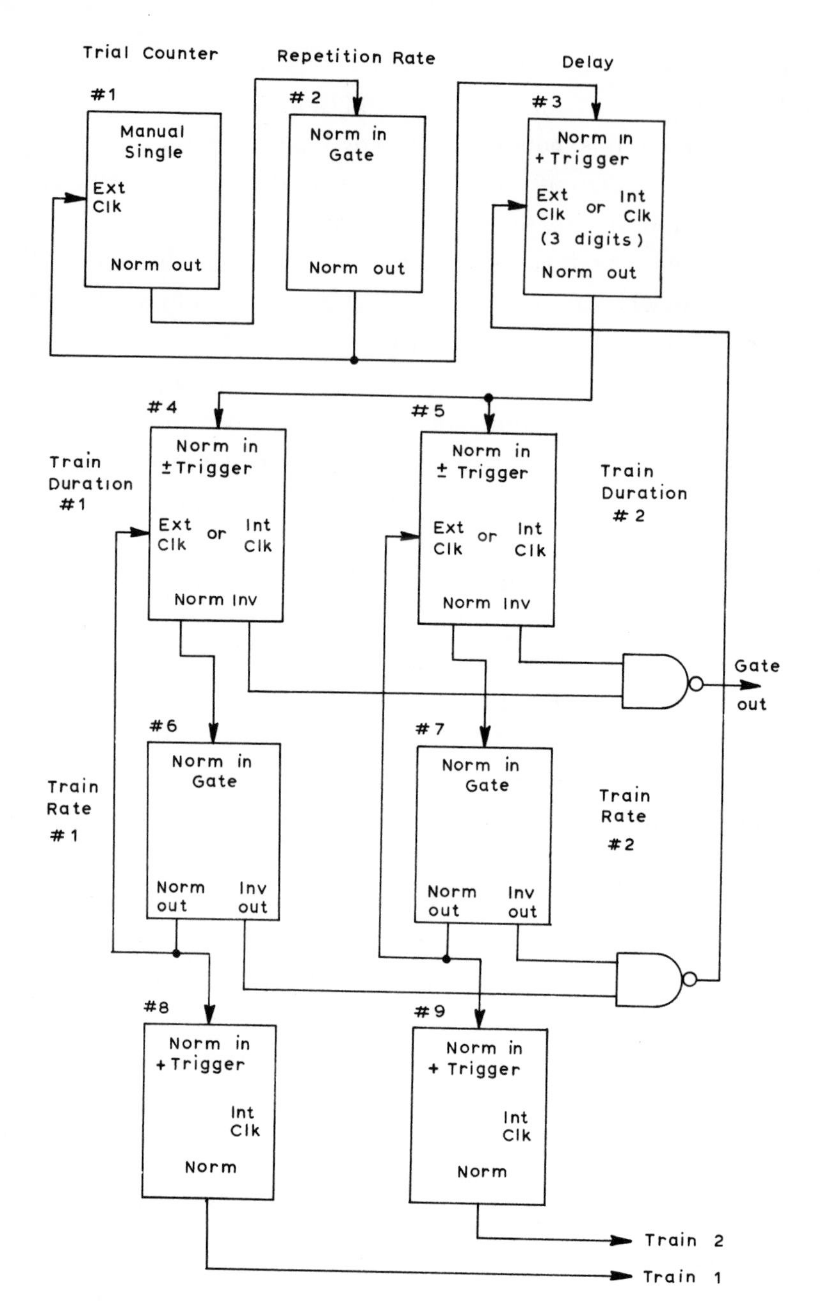

Figure 5.22
Configuration for two pulse trains. All pulse generators that are used as counters must be digital.

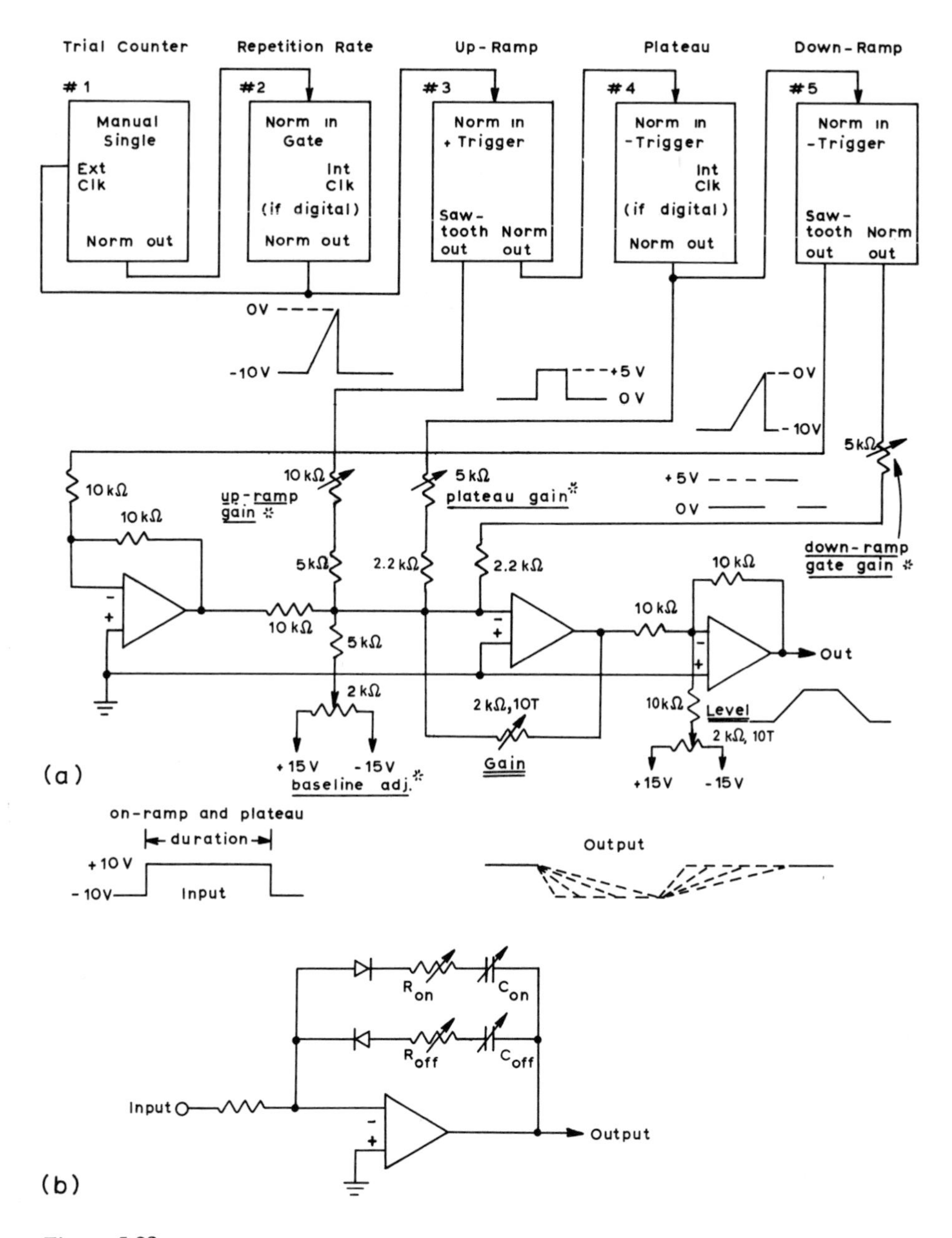

Figure 5.23
Synthesis of trapezoid wave form. (a) Using triggered wave forms.
#1: digital pulse generator.
#2: pulse generator with saturated output gate.
#3: sawtooth generator.
#4: pulse generator with saturated output gate.
#5: sawtooth generator with saturated output gate.
* screwdriver adjustments.
(b) Using a single input.
(Note: if ramp fails to reach maximum by end of INPUT duration, the plateau will be eliminated and the peak will be less than usual plateau amplitude.)

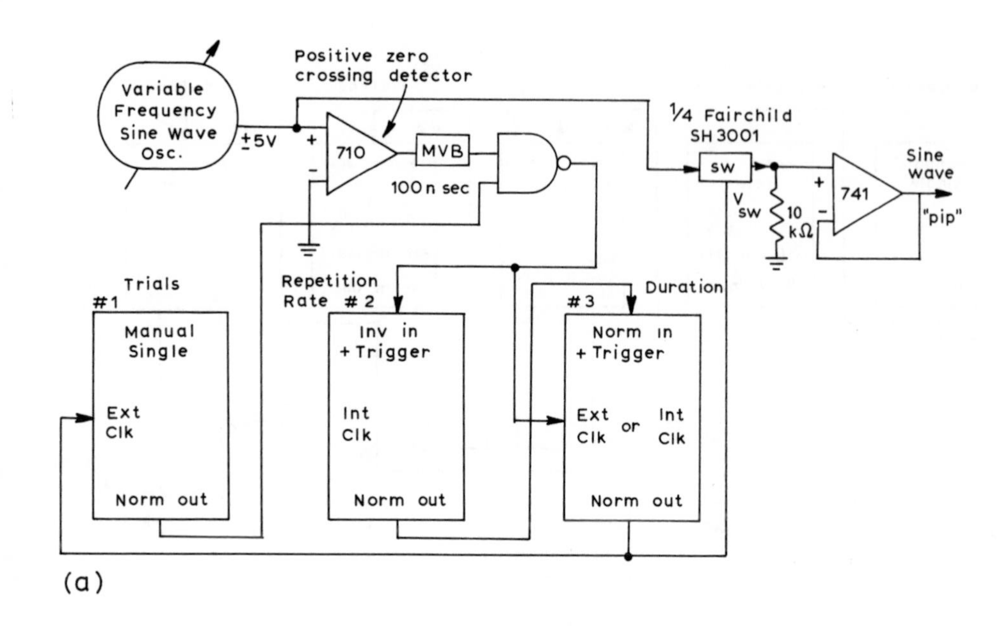

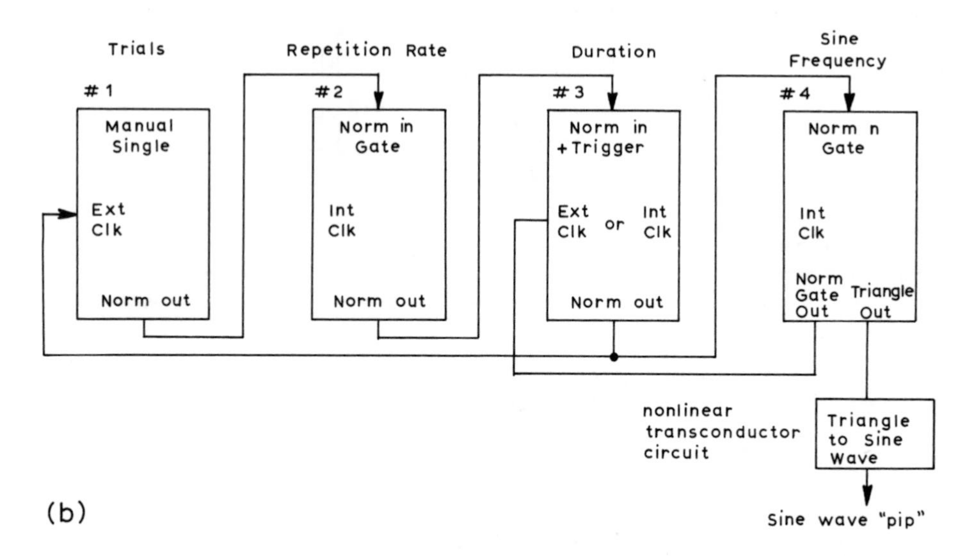

Figure 5.24
Two methods for producing sine wave "pips." (a) Analog switch technique.
#1 = digital pulse.
#2 = analog or digital pulse.
#3 = digital pulse.
(b) Triggerable serrasoid technique.
#1 = digital pulse.
#2 = digital or analog pulse.
#3 = digital pulse.
#4 = digital or analog serrasoid.

must consist of enough pulses to complete the count for DELAY, or the second train will not come on, and there will be no positive-going edge (because DELAY doesn't go off) to trigger either DURATION generator on the next trial.

The two TRAIN RATE generators trigger the two PULSE WIDTH generators (#8, #9), which provide independent control of the pulse durations in the two output trains. Pulse widths should be shorter than the intervals between pulses.

The INV OUTs of the DURATION generators are NANDed to provide an OR level indicating when either train is on, for recording a monitor of the stimulus duration or for triggering an oscilloscope.

A second simple system, this one for the generation of trapezoidal wave forms, is illustrated in Figure 5.23. In Figure 5.23a, operational amplifiers are used to combine triggered ramps and pulses, which are used to synthesize an up ramp, plateau, and down ramp. Since each triggers the next in the sequence, the durations of the three elements of the trapezoid are independently controlled. A bias level is used to adjust a zero baseline for the entire wave form, after which two more op amps provide separate control of amplitude and resting level. In Figure 5.22b, an alternate method for forming a trapezoid from a rectangular pulse is illustrated.

Figure 5.24 illustrates two methods for generating a sinusoidal "pip," which always starts at the positive zero crossing of the first cycle and ends with the positive zero crossing of the last cycle. Controls of sine wave frequency, number of trials, repetition rate, and "pip" duration are provided. To turn sine waves on and off slowly, thus preventing large-amplitude higher harmonics, the sine wave may be modulated with a trapezoid. Amplitude modulation is discussed in Section 5.5.

5.5 Amplitude and Frequency Modulation

When using oscillatory stimuli, it is often advantageous to have some means of varying the amplitude or frequency of the oscillation, under electrical control. Amplitude modulation (AM) and frequency modulation (FM) are the result of modulating one signal, the carrier (AM) or center frequency (FM), with another, the modulator. The carrier (or center frequency) is conventionally the higher of the two frequencies.

It is easy to comprehend AM and, with the advent of high-speed multipliers, to implement it. Figure 5.25 illustrates the use of an analog multiplier to produce an amplitude-modulated signal

$$V_o = V_A \times V_B. \tag{5.7}$$

Generally, the negative peak of the modulator is taken as zero gain, and the

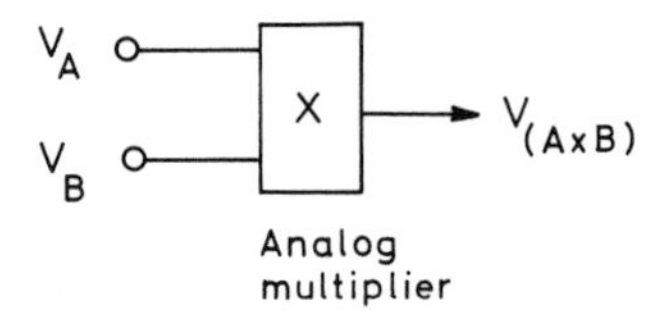

Figure 5.25
Analog multiplier used for amplitude modulation.

positive peak is used to produce maximum gain. This requires level shifting the input signal, which is symmetrical about zero, to produce a signal that has a minimum value of zero. After this shift, changes in the gain of V_A result in changes in the *percent modulation*, defined as the ratio

$$\% \text{ modulation} = \frac{V_o\ (\text{max}) - V_o\ (\text{min})}{V_o\ (\text{max})}, \tag{5.8}$$

where these voltages are ptp values.

The frequency spectrum of the output is easily predicted, if we recall that the product of two pure sine wave frequencies A and B consists of two new frequencies: $A - B$ and $A + B$. The two input frequencies are suppressed, if no dc component is present at either input. Such a modulator, used with two pure tone inputs, is called a *suppressed carrier* modulator (the modulating frequency is also suppressed), or a *balanced* modulator. If a dc level is present on either input, the output will contain the frequency from the other input. Thus, $(A + \text{dc}) \times B$ yields $A + B$, $B - A$, and B. If the dc offset is equal to the half-amplitude of A, that is, if A is always positive or zero, and reaches zero, we get a 100% modulation of B. On the other hand, it is crucial in the use of *balanced* modulation, to eliminate any dc bias, either within the modulator or at either of the inputs, which would permit the carrier or modulating frequency to come through to the output.

Balanced modulators are available that are specifically designed for suppressed-carried modulation.

Frequency modulation is as easily understood but less easily accomplished. The desired wave form is simply a sinusoidal (or other) oscillation whose frequency varies as a function of another signal. Generally the term FM is reserved for a sinusoidal wave form, and VCO (voltage-controlled oscillator) is a term used for any frequency-modulated wave form. However, this convention is by no means universal. One of many possible designs for a frequency modulator is illustrated in Figure 5.26. The device is the familiar triangle-wave generator with an interposed element between the square-wave op amp and the integrator. The interposed device is a means of varying the voltage V_x into the integrator as a function of another voltage V_3 the modulator. Since the frequency is directly proportional to the ramp velocity, which is in turn proportional to the voltage V_x for a given R and C, the interposed multiplier causes the frequency to be proportional to the modulator voltage V_3.

The output frequency is a linear function of the modulator voltage; that is, if the center frequency is 1 kHz (R and C adjusted for 1 kHz with $V_3 = 1$), then a V_3 modulator ramp going from +1.5 V to +0.5 V will produce an output frequency variation from 1.5 kHz to 500 Hz.

The triangular output of the frequency modulator can be shaped to produce a sine wave.

The device just described produces a linear variation of frequency with voltage. Thus, if the modulator were a triangle wave symmetrical about zero volts, the output would be a triangle wave whose frequency fluctuated as a linear function of time between limits that were equal numbers of Hz above and below the center frequency. It is occasionally advantageous to modulate the frequency as a function of the exponent or log of the input voltage. A simple technique for accomplishing

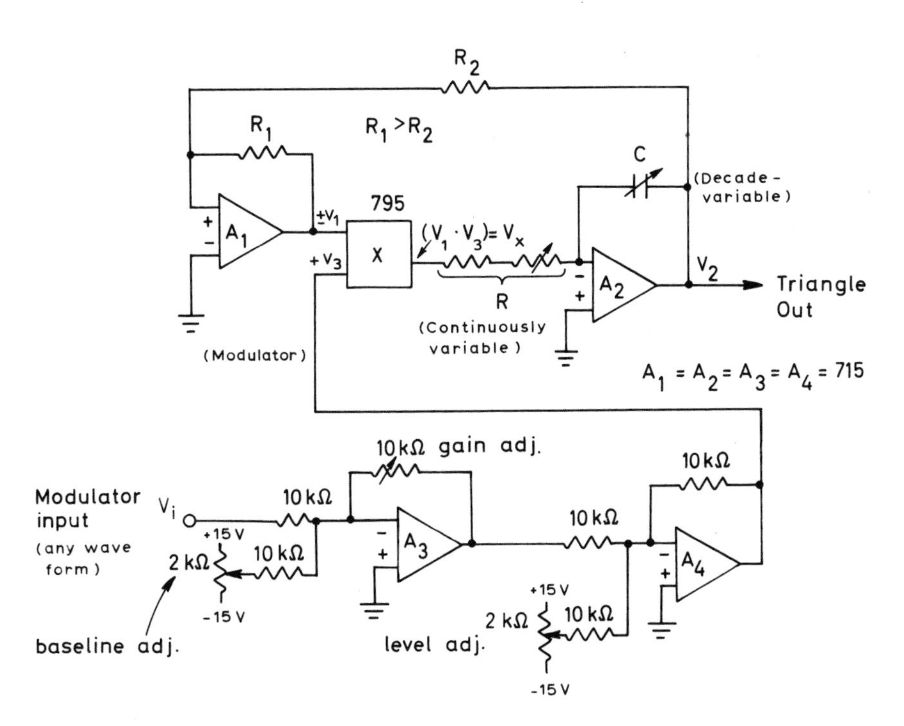

Figure 5.26
FM: linear modulation ($f_{out} = K_1 + K_2 V_i$). R and C adjust center frequency, which is also affected by level adj.

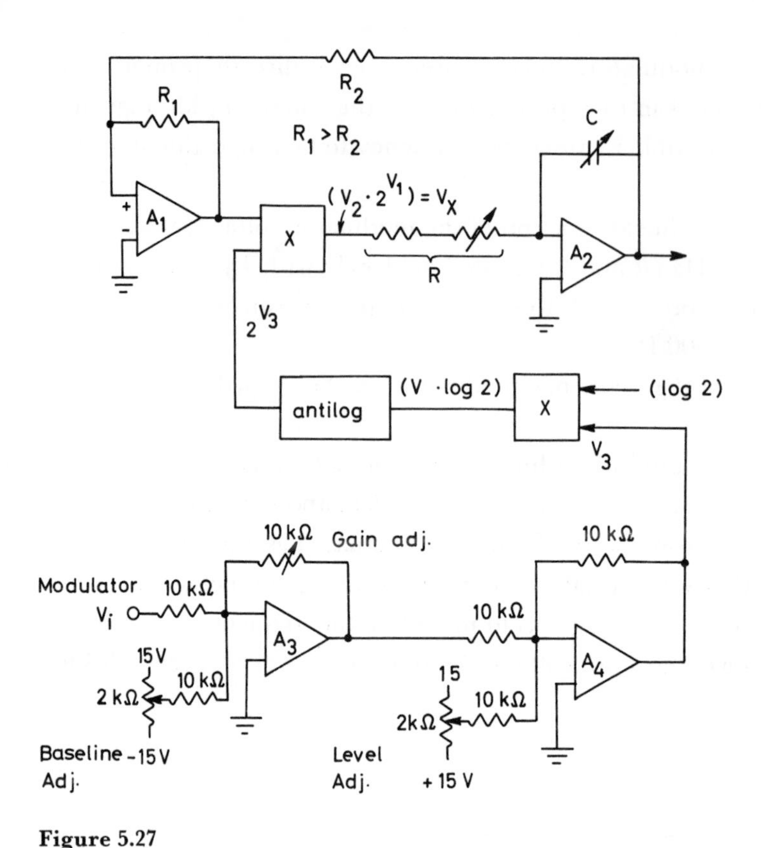

Figure 5.27
FM: exponential modulation $f_{\text{out}} = \text{C.F.} \cdot 2 \exp(K_1 + K_2 V_i)$. R and C adjust center frequency.

this is illustrated in Figure 5.27. The input voltage is used to produce a modulator voltage that is equal to the antilog of the input voltage

$$V_{\text{mod}} = 2^{V_3}. \tag{5.9}$$

The output frequency is thus proportional to the antilog of the input voltage. A modulator voltage varying from $+5$ V to -5 V would cause a frequency shift from 2 kHz to 500 Hz, if the center frequency is adjusted to 1 kHz with $V_3 = 0$ V. The *logarithm* of the frequency varies directly with the input voltage.

The voltage controlling the "gain" of the multiplier in an FM modulator should always be positive or zero, for output frequency to vary linearly with the gain. For negative voltages, the frequency varies directly as the absolute value of the voltage, and phase is reversed.

Frequency modulators can also be constructed in which, instead of varying the amplitude of the voltage level to be integrated, R or C is varied. For example, if we substitute a FET for R and use the gate voltage of the FET as a modulator, then R_{FET} varies as a function of the modulator voltage, causing a proportional variation of frequency.

Recently, some integrated circuits have been developed which can be used as voltage controlled oscillators (VCOs). The signetics SE556 and NE556 Function Generators are of particular interest in this regard. These devices have a tenfold voltage-controlled frequency modulation range, with range limits selected by external capacitors and resistors. With a fixed capacitor, a tenfold variation of frequency range can also be obtained by varying the resistor. Frequency stability is excellent (200 ppm/°C, 2%/volt supply) over a total range of approximately 5 Hz to 1 MHz. The outputs are a very linear (0.5% error) triangle wave, and a square wave with 50 μsec transition times.

5.6 Automatic Gain Control

The outputs of some devices tend to fluctuate in amplitude under varying conditions where they are supposed to remain constant in amplitude; for example, the output of the sine wave generator of Figure 5.12 varies slightly with changes in resonant frequency. It is, of course, inconvenient to have to adjust the amplitude with a variable gain control every time the frequency is changed: fortunately, there exist circuits, called Automatic Gain Controls (AGC), which can do it for us.

An AGC circuit is schematized in Figure 5.28. The device relies on the measurement of average power, which is used as a feedback to control the gain of a variable gain device; a simple four-quadrant multiplier in the divide configuration. Thus, the negative feedback principle is used to hold average power constant, rather than to hold voltage constant. This is achieved essentially by a power-to-voltage

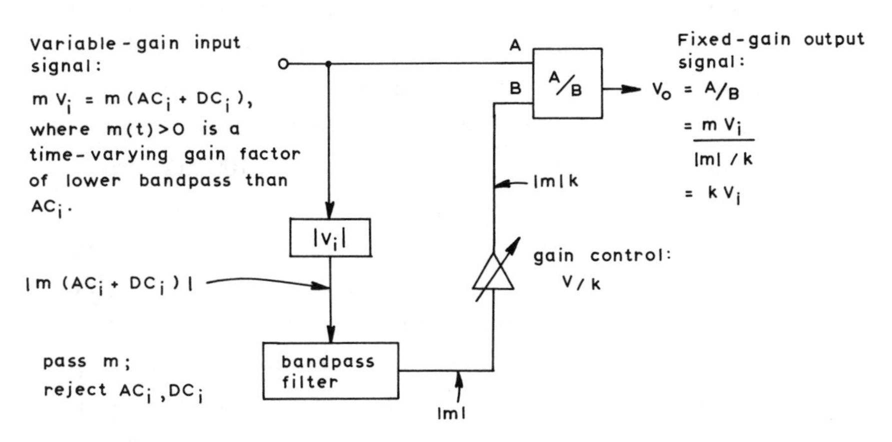

Figure 5.28
Automatic gain control (AGC).

conversion (low-pass filter, absolute value), feedback, and a voltage-controlled gain stage.

Automatic gain controls are commercially available as integrated circuits, generally for use in the audio, intermediate, or radio frequency ranges. Subaudio frequencies are more easily generated by digital techniques, which do not generally require any gain control.

5.7 Generation of White Noise

White noise is commonly employed by neurophysiologists to determine the transfer characteristics of receptors and central synaptic regions, or simply as a probe stimulus that will activate elements having a wide variety of frequency selectivities, as in the auditory system. In purely analog circuits, the following three criteria for the whiteness of noise are commonly used: (1) Gaussian distribution of voltage over time; (2) flat power spectrum within the desired frequency band; and (3) serial correlation that falls off rapidly on both sides of t_0 to a value near 0. Other properties, such as incoherence of phase relations among the various frequency components and lack of periodicity, among many others, are sometimes required, depending on the application.

Both digital and analog techniques are used to generate approximations to "perfect" white noise. Analog techniques rely on the amplification of naturally occurring electrical noise, such as thermal noise in large resistors, noise in vacuum-tube and semiconductor diodes, or the transformation of transduced random energy fluctuations such as radioactive emissions, into usable electrical noise. Analog noise generators are simple to construct and inexpensive, although care must be exercised to avoid resonance effects, pickup of interfering periodic signals such as line frequency, or other artifacts that introduce nonrandom elements into the signal. Tube and semiconductor diodes are commercially available which under appropriate conditions generate a very good approximation to white noise. Lodi Semiconductor and Solitron manufacture miniature noise generator modules that provide Gaussian noise over wide bands, at output levels of 100 mV and 1.5 V, respectively.

Digital techniques can give a very good approximation of white noise. One of the simplest methods consists of converting a table of numbers, computed with an appropriate algorithm and stored in some form of digital memory, into successive values of an analog electrical noise. An analogous but more economical technique uses a shift register and associated logic elements. The technique is derived from a treatment of the subject by Golomb in his book *Shift Register Sequences* (1967).

Consider the generalized shift register circuit with feedback, diagrammed in Figure 5.29: a serial-in, parallel-out right-shift register of length r is shifted right repeatedly, serially loading the leftmost bit with a 1 or 0, depending on the output of the feedback operator, which consists of an addition of a combination of some of the shift register parallel output bits, modulo 2.

Define the initial state of a, at time $t = 0$, to be a_0. Successive states $a_1, a_2, \ldots, a_n$ are generated with successive clock cycles at $t_1, t_2, \ldots, t_n$, at whatever intervals are desired, within the frequency limit of the shift register. The recursion formula representing the generation of a_n is

$$a_n = (c_1 a_{n-1} + c_2 a_{n-2} + c_3 a_{n-3} \cdots + c_r a_{n-r}) \text{ modulo } 2, \tag{5.11}$$

where the shift register serves as the memory of the previous r states of a, and a_{n-1} is the leftmost bit at time $n - 1$, when the next value of a (namely a_n) is generated by the feedback operator. The coefficients $c_1 \cdots c_r$ are 1s and 0s, and they are constant, for a given recursion formula.

Golomb proves that for a shift register of length r, it is possible to generate a string of "states" of the shift register, which we will simply consider binary numbers, which repeat only once every $2^r - 1$ time cycles. Because there are only 2^r possible numbers and 0 is necessarily excluded from any sequence of length greater than 1 (because only a 0 could generate a 0, and only a 0 could be generated by a 0), this is the longest possible sequence before a number occurs which has occurred already. As soon as an already encountered state is repeated, the sequence that follows it is the same as the sequence that followed the first occurrence of that number, because the device is entirely deterministic. We will call the number of states in a sequence before a number is repeated the *period* of the sequence. The period is *maximum* if it is $2^r - 1$. It should be noted that the period of a sequence is determined entirely by the recursion formula (Equation 5.11) and is not affected by the initial state (assuming a zero initial state is excluded).

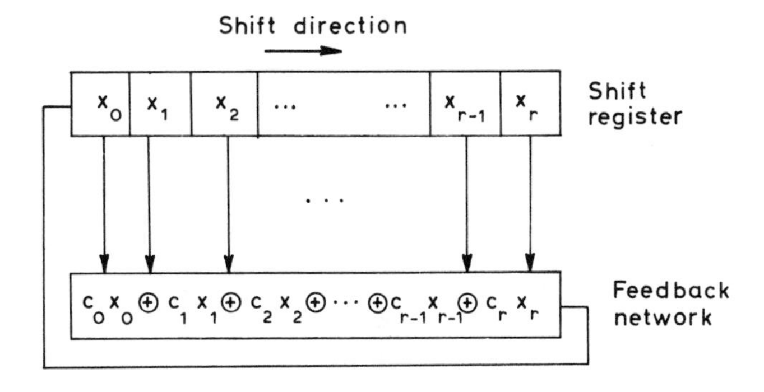

Figure 5.29
Generalized shift register pseudorandom interval generator with "linear" feedback.

Table 5.1

The first 23 numbers r, such that $2^r - 1$ is prime. (From Table III-1, p. 37, in *Shift Register Sequences*, Solomon Golomb. Copyright, 1967, by Holden-Day, Inc. Used with permission of Holden-Day, Inc.)

2	17	107	2203	9689
3	19	127	2281	9941
5	31	521	3217	11213
7	61	607	4253	
13	89	1279	4423	

The *characteristic polynomial* $f(x)$ is a convenient representation of the recurrence relation of Equation 5.11

$$f(x) = 1 - \sum_{i=1}^{r} c_i x^i, \qquad c_i = 1 \quad \text{or} \quad 0. \tag{5.12}$$

One necessary condition for a shift register sequence to be of maximum period is that the characteristic polynomial be irreducible (prime, incapable of factorization). However, this is not a sufficient condition: For some shift register lengths, there are irreducible polynomials that do not yield periods of maximum length. Fortunately, Golomb indicates that for all r such that $2^r - 1$ is prime, all irreducible polynomials of degree r (that is, containing a highest power term x^r) yield periods of maximum length. The first 23 integers r, satisfying this requirement, are listed in Table 5.1 (from Golomb). Table 5.2 (also from Golomb) lists all irreducible polynomials of degree 1–11, and the corresponding periods.

In the event that longer periods are required, the following technique, based on a more general method by Golomb, can be used to list all polynomials yielding maximum periods $2^r - 1$, or $r = 13$, 17, or 19 with the help of Table 5.2. All polynomials are represented as they are in Table 5.2, as

$$f(x) = \sum_{i=0}^{r} c_i 2^i.$$

A digital computer is required.

1. List all odd numbers from $2^{r-1} + 1$ through $2^r - 1$, because the required polynomials are known to be of degree r and even numbers always represent reducible polynomials.

2. If convenient, eliminate all numbers with an even number of 1-bits. Some digital computers have machine instructions that make this an easy task, and then step 3 can be performed on half as many numbers.

Table 5.2

All irreducible polynomials* of degree $\leqq 11$, and their shift register periods. (From Table III-5, pp. 62–65, in *Shift Register Sequences*, by Solomon Golomb. Copyright, 1967, by Holden-Day, Inc. Used with permission of Holden-Day, Inc.)

Degree (bold) and polynomial	Period	Degree (bold) and polynomial	Period	Degree (bold) and polynomial	Period
1		217	127	661	51
2		221	127	675	85
3	1	235	127	703	255
		247	127	717	255
2		253	127	727	17
7	3	271	127	735	85
		277	127	747	255
3		301	127	763	51
13	7	313	127	765	255
15	7	323	127	771	85
		325	127		
4		345	127	**9**	
23	15	357	127	1003	73
31	15	361	127	1021	511
37	5	367	127	1027	73
		375	127	1033	511
5				1041	511
45	31	**8**		1055	511
51	31	433	51	1063	511
57	31	435	255	1113	73
67	31	453	255	1137	511
73	31	455	255	1145	73
75	31	471	17	1151	511
		477	85	1157	511
6		515	255	1167	511
103	63	537	255	1175	511
111	9	543	255	1207	511
127	21	545	255	1225	511
133	63	551	255	1231	73
141	63	561	255	1243	511
147	63	567	85	1245	511
155	63	573	85	1257	511
163	63	607	255	1267	511
165	21	613	85	1275	511
		615	255	1317	511
7		637	51	1321	511
203	127	643	85	1333	511
211	127	651	255	1365	511

* If $f(x) = \sum_{i=0}^{n} c_i x^i$, the table entry is $\sum_{i=0}^{n} c_i 2^i$ written to base 8. Thus, $x^5 + x^3 + x^2 + x + 1$ becomes binary 101,111, which is octal "57."

Table 5.2 (continued)

Degree (bold) and polynomial	Period	Degree (bold) and polynomial	Period	Degree (bold) and polynomial	Period
1371	511	2231	341	3177	1023
1401	73	2251	33	3205	93
1423	511	2257	341	3211	1023
1425	511	2305	1023	3247	93
1437	511	2311	341	3255	341
1443	511	2327	1023	3265	1023
1461	511	2347	1023	3277	341
1473	511	2355	341	3301	1023
1511	73	2363	1023	3315	341
1517	511	2377	1023	3323	1023
1533	511	2413	93	3337	1023
1541	511	2415	1023	3367	341
1553	511	2431	1023	3375	1023
1555	511	2437	341	3417	341
1563	511	2443	1023	3421	341
1577	511	2461	1023	3427	1023
1605	511	2475	1023	3435	1023
1617	511	2503	1023	3441	1023
1641	73	2527	1023	3453	93
1665	511	2541	93	3465	341
1671	511	2547	341	3471	1023
1707	511	2553	1023	3507	1023
1713	511	2605	1023	3515	1023
1715	511	2617	1023	3525	1023
1725	511	2627	1023	3531	1023
1731	511	2633	341	3543	1023
1743	511	2641	1023	3573	341
1751	511	2653	341	3575	1023
1773	511	2671	341	3601	341
		2701	341	3607	341
10		2707	1023	3615	1023
2011	1023	2745	1023	3623	1023
2017	341	2767	1023	3651	341
2033	1023	2773	1023	3661	1023
2035	341	3023	1023	3705	341
2047	1023	3025	1023	3733	1023
2055	1023	3043	33	3753	341
2065	93	3045	1023	3763	1023
2107	341	3061	341	3771	1023
2123	341	3067	1023	3777	11
2143	341	3103	1023		
2145	1023	3117	1023	**11**	
2157	1023	3121	341	4005	2047
2201	1023	3133	1023	4027	2047
2213	1023	3171	1023	4053	2047

Table 5.2 (continued)

Degree (bold) and polynomial	Period	Degree (bold) and polynomial	Period	Degree (bold) and polynomial	Period
4055	2047	5025	2047	6013	2047
4107	2047	5051	2047	6015	2047
4143	2047	5111	2047	6031	2047
4145	2047	5141	2047	6037	2047
4161	2047	5155	2047	6061	89
4173	2047	5171	2047	6127	2047
4215	2047	5177	2047	6141	2047
4225	2047	5205	2047	6153	2047
4237	2047	5221	2047	6163	2047
4251	2047	5235	2047	6165	23
4261	2047	5247	2047	6205	2047
4303	89	5253	2047	6211	2047
4317	2047	5263	2047	6227	2047
4321	2047	5265	2047	6233	2047
4341	2047	5325	2047	6235	2047
4347	2047	5337	2047	6263	2047
4353	2047	5343	23	6277	2047
4365	2047	5351	2047	6307	2047
4415	2047	5357	2047	6315	2047
4423	2047	5361	2047	6323	2047
4445	2047	5373	2047	6325	2047
4451	2047	5403	2047	6343	2047
4467	89	5411	2047	6351	2047
4473	2047	5421	2047	6367	2047
4475	2047	5463	2047	6403	2047
4505	2047	5477	2047	6417	2047
4511	2047	5501	2047	6435	2047
4521	2047	5513	2047	6447	2047
4533	2047	5531	2047	6455	2047
4563	2047	5537	2047	6501	2047
4565	2047	5545	2047	6507	2047
4577	2047	5557	2047	6525	2047
4603	2047	5575	2047	6531	2047
4617	2047	5607	2047	6543	2047
4653	2047	5613	2047	6557	2047
4655	2047	5623	2047	6561	2047
4671	2047	5625	2047	6623	2047
4707	2047	5657	2047	6637	2047
4731	2047	5667	2047	6651	2047
4745	2047	5675	2047	6673	2047
4757	89	5711	2047	6675	2047
4767	2047	5733	2047	6711	2047
5001	2047	5735	2047	6727	2047
5007	2047	5747	2047	6733	2047
5023	2047	5755	2047	6741	2047

Table 5.2 (continued)

Degree (bold) and polynomial	Period	Degree (bold) and polynomial	Period	Degree (bold) and polynomial	Period
6747	2047	7175	2047	7553	2047
6765	2047	7201	2047	7555	2047
6777	89	7223	2047	7565	2047
7005	2047	7237	2047	7571	89
7035	2047	7243	2047	7603	2047
7041	2047	7273	2047	7621	2047
7047	2047	7311	89	7627	2047
7053	2047	7317	2047	7633	2047
7063	2047	7335	2047	7647	2047
7071	2047	7363	2047	7655	2047
7107	2047	7371	2047	7665	2047
7113	2047	7413	2047	7715	2047
7125	2047	7431	2047	7723	2047
7137	2047	7461	2047	7745	2047
7161	2047	7467	2047	7751	2047
7173	2047	7535	2047	7773	89

3. Divide each number in the list by all irreducible polynomial numbers of degree $\leqq r/2$ (Table 5.2). If it is an integral multiple of any of these, it is reducible, and can be thrown out.

4. All the remaining numbers represent irreducible polynomials of degree r; since $2^r - 1$ is prime, they all yield the maximum periods.

Golomb's more general method can be applied for any r, but it is too complicated to present here. It should be noted that $2^{19} - 1 = 524{,}287$. An r of 19 is the highest r that can be used with this computation method, given the fact that 11 is the highest r for which all irreducible polynomials are listed in Table 5.2. Thus, even if the shift clock frequency is as high as 100 kHz, the sequence will only repeat every 5.25 sec. If this is not a long enough period, Korn (1966) has compiled a list of some single-adder feedback configurations that can be used with shift registers of lengths up to $r = 33$. This is reproduced in Table 5.3.

Golomb proves that the output sequence $a_0, a_1, a_2, \ldots, a_n$ has certain properties that are surprisingly convenient, including

1. In every period, the numbers of zeros and ones differ only by one. Thus, for period $2^{19} - 1$, there are 2^{18} ones and $2^{18} - 1$ zeros, or 2^{18} zeros and $2^{18} - 1$ ones.

2. In every period, half the runs of successive ones have length 1, one fourth have length 2, one eighth have length 3, and so forth, as long as the number of ones so indicated exceed 1. Moreover for each of these run lengths there is the same

Table 5.3

Some maximum-length feedback configurations using a single modulo-2 adder. Feedback is from outputs r (last bit) and m, to serial input. (From Table 4-3, p. 4-9, in *Random Process Simulation and Measurement*, by A. G. Korn. Copyright 1966, by McGraw-Hill, Inc. Used with permission of McGraw-Hill Book Company.)

r	m	$2^r - 1$
3	1	7
4	1	15
5	2	31
6	1	63
7	1 or 3	127
9	4	511
10	3	1,023
11	2	2,047
15	1, 4, or 7	32,767
18	7	262,143
20	3	1,048,575
21	2	2,097,151
22	1	4,194,303
23	5 or 9	8,388,607
25	3 or 7	33,554,431
28	3, 9, or 13	268,435,455
31	3, 6, 7, or 13	2,147,483,647
33	13	8,589,934,591

number of runs of zeros as there are runs of ones, except there is one more run of length 1 of either zeros or ones, than of one or zero, respectively, because the period is of odd length.

3. The autocorrelation function is

$$C(t) = \begin{cases} \dfrac{p+1}{2} & \text{if} \quad t = 0 \\[2ex] \dfrac{p+1}{4} & \text{if} \quad 0 < t < p \text{ modulo } p, \text{ where } p = \text{the period.} \end{cases}$$

These properties, generated by a deterministic device, are surprising, because they describe a Bernoulli series (wherein the patterns of ones and zeros are random, analogous to heads and tails in a coin-flipping experiment), except for the periodicity. The binary output is useful in itself for generating pseudorandom intervals. Truly random intervals can be generated by discriminating an analog noise, such as a noise diode output or scintillation counter output.

The spectral output of the binary generator, assuming perfectly rectangular pulse shapes, is a line spectrum with peaks at $\frac{1}{N\Delta T}, \frac{2}{N\Delta T} \cdots \frac{1}{\Delta T}$, where ΔT is the clock interval and N is the period (number of clock cycles) of the shift register sequence. The height of these peaks is determined by a flat envelope (to within about 0.1 dB) out to about 8% of the clock frequency $1/\Delta T$. Of course, the clock frequency and its harmonics are also present. See Korn (1966) for a derivation of these spectral properties. We can use the digital output to generate a good approximation of white noise by using a bandpass filter. The bandpass limits should be at least the reciprocal of the period, $1/N\,\Delta T$ at the low limit, and one twentieth the clock frequency $1/\Delta T$ at the upper limit, with a sharp upper cutoff: say, 12–24 dB/octave. The same filter can be used, in fact, to select the desired bandpass; thus it is an element in the circuit that probably would have been used in any case. Because clock frequencies in excess of 1 MHz can be used, a bandpass of 50 kHz can be attained.

Figure 5.30 illustrates the configuration of the digital pseudo noise generator. It has options for external reset to a selected initial state and selection of characteristic polynomial. A clamping circuit is recommended to ensure uniform pulses into the filter; for most purposes, a common-emitter single-transistor inverting circuit is adequate if supply regulation is good.

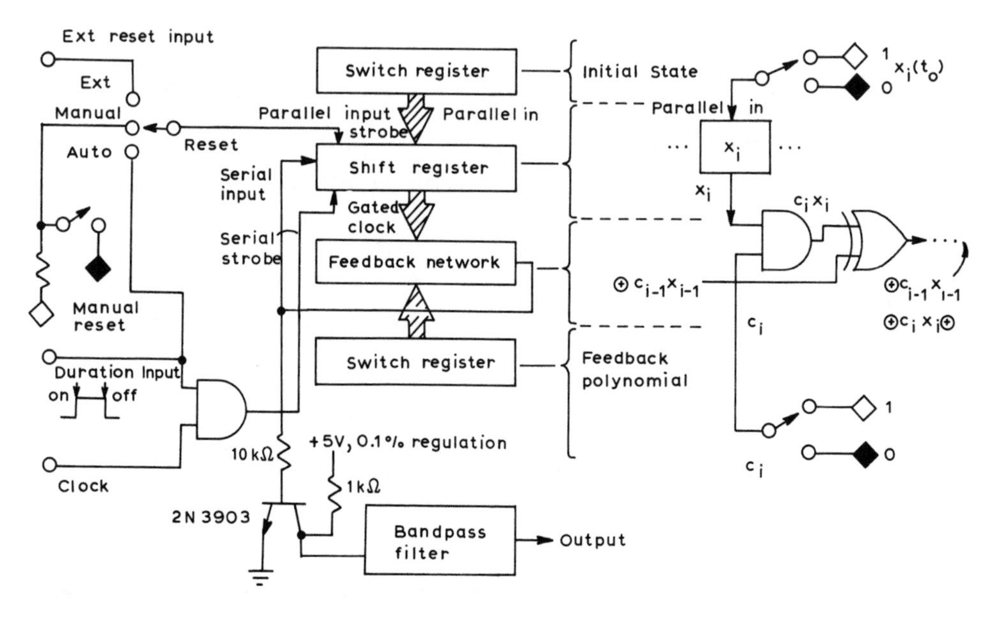

Figure 5.30
Digital pseudorandom white noise generator.

The digital pseudorandom noise generator and other digital wave-form generators presented here are elementary examples of digital wave-form processors. The field of digital wave-form processing is rapidly growing, with the advent of faster, smaller digital ICs. Thus, we should anticipate simple, inexpensive, and accurate digital wave-form generator modules, digital filters, and even digital FM and AM modules in the near future.

5.8 Active Filters

In Chapter 3, the discussion of integrators and differentiators introduced first-order active filters. These devices contained an op amp and a single resistor and capacitor for upper or lower frequency roll-off, or an RC pair for each, for band-pass filtering.

The order of an *RC* filter, n, can be defined as the number of *RC* pairs used to achieve the roll-off. The slope of the filter "skirt" (the portion of the filter spectral response describing the decreased response beyond the corner frequency) is 6 dB × (n/octave), for an nth-order filter.

Although there exist numerous designs for active filters, three types of filter are described in sufficient detail to allow the reader to design his own. These are (1) high-pass second-order Butterworth filter; (2) low-pass second-order Butterworth filter; and (3) twin-tee notch filter. Other designs can be found in the references at the end of the chapter.

All three filters described here depend on the use of a unity-gain op amp follower as the active element. Such an op amp must be selected for desired frequency response and input and output impedance. Examples of practical filters can be found in Chapter 9, in the design of a general-purpose amplifier.

The high-pass second-order Butterworth filter is illustrated in Figure 5.31. By using the following design equations, a filter can be designed for any desired cutoff (3 dB down) frequency, f_c:

$$C_1 = \frac{1}{2\pi f_c Z} \text{ farad,} \tag{5.13a}$$

$$C_2 = \frac{1}{2\pi f_c Z} \text{ farad,} \tag{5.13b}$$

$$R_1 = \frac{\sqrt{2}}{2} Z \text{ ohm,} \tag{5.13c}$$

$$R_2 = \sqrt{2}\, Z \text{ ohm,} \tag{5.13d}$$

where Z is the input impedance. If an input unity-gain follower is added to the

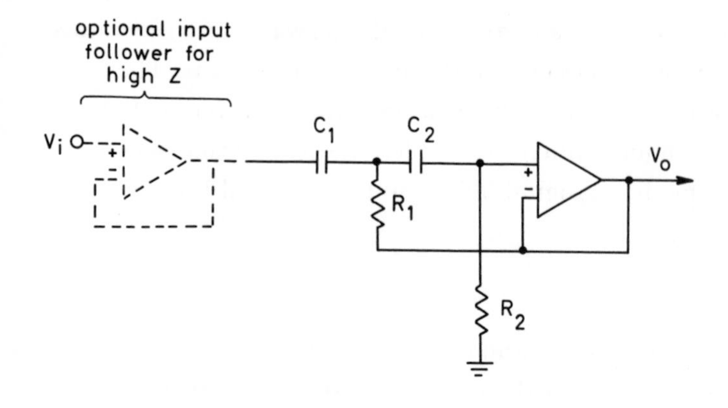

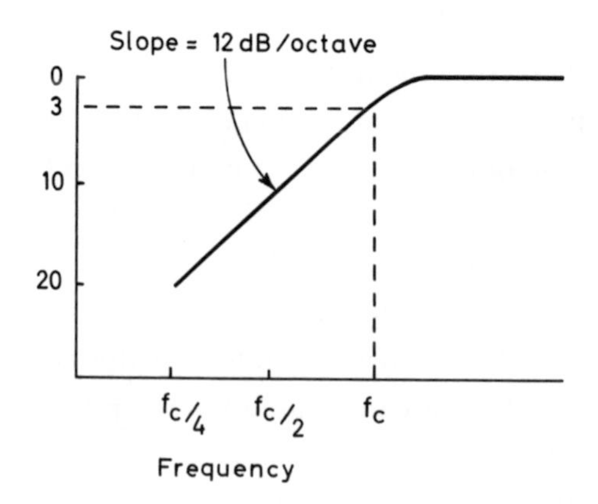

Figure 5.31
Second-order high-pass Butterworth filter.

circuit, Z may be varied over the range which the follower can tolerate as a load, with no change in the input impedance of the circuit as a whole. Most op amps, if a 50–100 Ω series output resistor is added, can drive loads of 1 kΩ or higher, with capacitances up to 0.2 μF. By using a high input-impedance op amp, Z may be as high as 10 MΩ, providing an effective range of allowable R from 1 kΩ to 10 MΩ, or four orders of magnitude. This is particularly useful if a switched band-pass filter is constructed, since a single value of C can be chosen and different R_1 and R_2 can be switched in for different low-frequency cutoffs.

A second-order Butterworth low-pass filter is illustrated in Figure 5.32. The design equations are

$$C_1 = \frac{5}{2\pi f_c Z} \text{ farad,} \tag{5.14a}$$

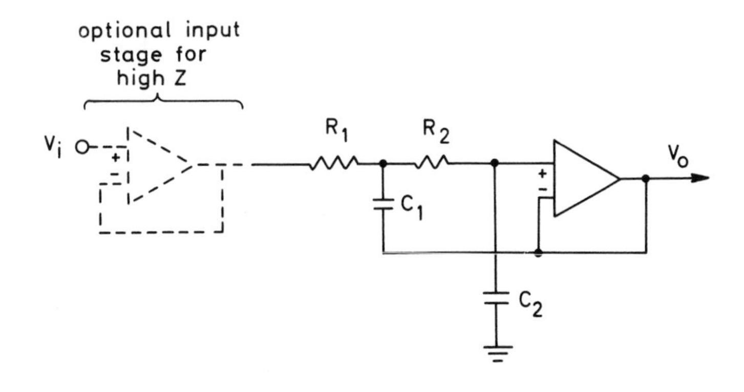

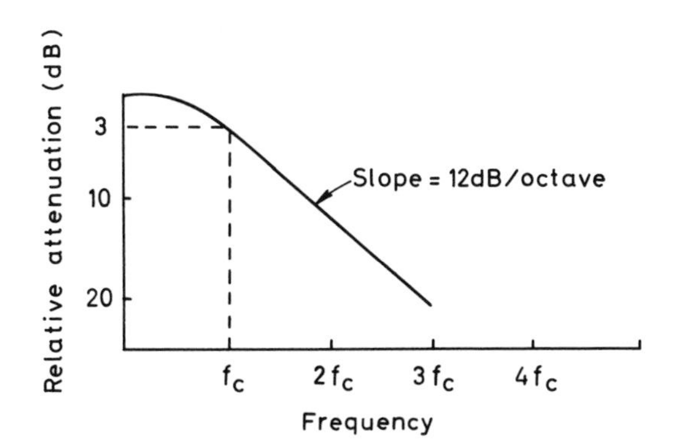

Figure 5.32
Low-pass second-order Butterworth filter.

$$C_2 = \frac{1}{2\pi f_c Z} \text{ farad,} \tag{5.14b}$$

$$R_1 = 1.25Z \text{ ohm,} \tag{5.14c}$$

$$R_2 = 0.16Z \text{ ohm.} \tag{5.14d}$$

These high-pass and low-pass filters may be cascaded for sharper cutoffs, or higher-order filters may be constructed (see references at the end of this chapter). Generally 12 dB/octave is adequate for filtering neurological signals. The Butterworth design has very flat spectral response out to the corner frequency, and very uniform roll-off.

The "twin-tee" filter of Figure 5.33 (Dobkin, 1969) is a very efficient method of achieving notch rejection of selected frequencies with a very deep notch (in excess of 30 dB), very sharp, narrow stop-band, and minimum distortion. The

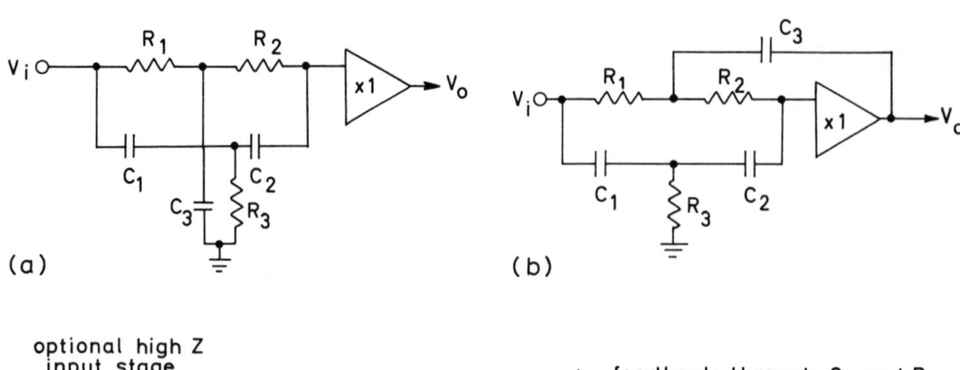

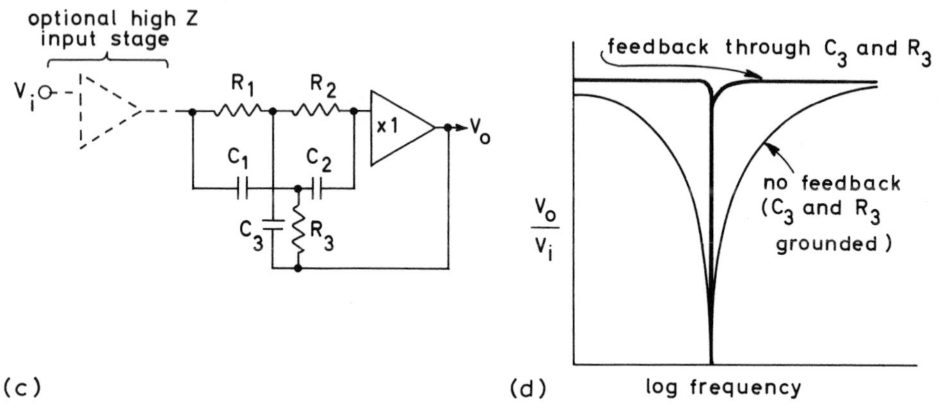

Figure 5.33
Twin-tee notch filters: (a) no feedback; (b) capacitor feedback; (c) feedback through R_3 and C_3; (d) response of notch filters with and without feedback.

design equations are

$$\frac{1}{2\pi f_c} = R_1 C_1 = R_2 C_2 \tag{5.15a}$$

$$R_2 = R_1 \tag{5.15b}$$

$$C_2 = C_1. \tag{5.15c}$$

Because of the very sharp tuning, use 1% resistors and 5% ceramic capacitors. Trim pots may be necessary for exact adjustment of notch frequency.

Selected References

Chabak, Eugene J. 1966. Resistance-capacitance active filters. Technical Report ECOM-2744, Clearing House for Federal Scientific and Technical Information.

Dobkin, Robert. 1969. High-Q active twin-T. *EEE 17*, 7: 46.

Eimbinder, J. 1969. *Designing with Linear Integrated Circuits.* New York: John Wiley & Sons.

Fairchild Semiconductor. 1970. *Semiconductor Integrated Circuit Data Catalog, 1970.* Mountain View, Calif.: Fairchild Camera and Instrument Corporation.

Federal Telephone and Radio Corporation. 1963. *Reference Data for Radio Engineers.* New York: American Book–Stratford Press.

Golomb, Solomon W. 1967. *Shift Register Sequences.* San Francisco: Holden-Day.

Hoeschle, David F., Jr. 1968. *Analog-to-Digital/Digital-to-Analog Conversion Techniques.* New York: John Wiley & Sons.

Holt, A. G. J., and R. Linggard. 1965. Active Chebyshev filters. *Electron. Lett. 1:* 130.

——— RC active synthesis procedure for polynomial filters. 1966. *Proc. Inst. Elect. Eng. 113:* 777.

Holt, A. G. J., and J. I. Sewell. 1965. Active RC filters employing a single operational amplifier to obtain biquadratic responses. *Proc. Inst. Elec. Eng. 112:* 2227.

Holt, A. G. J., and F. W. Stephenson. 1964. Design tables for active filters having 2nd and 4th order Chebyshev responses in pass and stop bands. *Proc. Inst. Elec. Eng. 111:* 1807.

Hove, R. G. 1964. An RC active network rejection filter. Dept. of Defense Documentation Center, Document #D2-90192-9.

Korn, Granino A. 1966. *Random Process Simulation and Measurement.* New York: McGraw-Hill Book Co.

Laning, J. Halcombe, Jr., and Richard H. Battin. 1965. *Random Processes in Automatic Control.* New York: McGraw-Hill Book Co.

Margolis, S. G. 1956. Design of active filters with Butterworth characteristics. *IRE Trans. Circuit Theory 3:* 202.

Philbrick/Nexus Research. 1968. *Application Manual for Operational Amplifiers.* Dedham, Mass.: Philbrick/Nexus.

Sallen, R. P., and E. L. Key. 1955. Practical method of designing RC active filters. *IRE Trans. Circuit Theory 2:* 74.

Signetics Corporation. 1969. *Application Memos.* Sunnyvale, Calif.: Signetics Corporation.

Strauss, G. G. 1971. An AF synthesizer for less than $200. *Elec. Design 19*, 17: 62.

Testronic Development Laboratory. 1971. *Some Comments and References on Pseudo-Random Sequences.* Las Cruces, N.M.: Testronic Development Laboratory.

6 CONSTRUCTION, TESTING, AND MAINTENANCE

Howard Moraff

A neurobiologist builds his own equipment in order to reduce costs or delivery time, or in order to fulfill special needs. Full realization of these advantages requires careful design, construction, and documentation.

When a construction project is completed, it must be tested to verify that it works. It is good practice to do as much testing as possible on the isolated unit before it is connected as part of a system of instrumentation or used in an actual laboratory experiment. The use of a test plan based on common sense and a few basic principles may prevent damage to other equipment and loss of valuable experiment time.

An electronic circuit or device is likely to need some form of maintenance service during its operating life. The devices presented in this book are composed mainly of integrated circuits, in which complex circuit functions are produced as a single chip of semiconductor material. This results in a substantial reduction in the number of discrete components and interconnections required. The reliability of these circuits is improved by a large factor over earlier technology that used discrete semiconductors and passive components wired together on printed circuit boards. Maintenance requirements are reduced, and in fact, drastically changed.

Manufacturers usually provide thorough documentation with their instrumentation products. This documentation is normally in the form of an operator's manual that describes the instrument, lists procedures for using it, explains the theory of operation, gives circuit schematics, and suggests maintenance procedures. The reader who builds his own circuits should spare no effort in producing this documentation for his own products, for this is the only way to ensure their continuing usefulness. In fact, the preparation of adequate documentation may require as much time and energy as the original design and construction tasks, but this must be regarded as an essential part of the total effort.

6.1 Construction Techniques

A circuit consists of electronic components wired together according to a schematic circuit diagram. The components or their sockets are fastened to a supporting substrate. Early circuits using vacuum tube technology were constructed by attaching the components to sockets, terminals, or standoffs fastened to a metal chassis. As component size decreased and circuit complexity increased, more advanced techniques were developed, which achieved higher packing density of components. A major advance was the development of the printed circuit board, composed of a nonconductive substrate with a pattern of metal strips for component interconnections. This reduced the labor required for circuit wiring and, ultimately, led to improved circuit reliability. Multipin connectors were developed for making electrical connections to these printed circuit boards. Printed circuit construction has essentially replaced discrete chassis wiring, except for very simple circuits, wiring of control panels and interconnections to large chassis-mounted components. Other types of circuit boards have been developed on which interconnections are made by means of discrete wiring. This approach is often used for construction of small numbers of circuits.

Printed circuit boards may be attached via their connectors to a main chassis that may be housed with other instruments in a cabinet. The chassis usually has a front panel to which are attached all of the controls that must be accessible during operation of the equipment.

An important benefit of circuit board construction over the older point-to-point chassis wiring is the resulting modularity. Modularity refers to the physical separability of circuit functions by the use of plug-in cables, connectors, and circuit assemblies. Modularity provides ease of servicing and alteration of an instrumentation setup. This is particularly important in a research environment in which the setup may be altered frequently. A major consideration in the design process is the matching of levels of functional complexity to levels of packaging modularity (Figure 6.1). It is often possible to design a single instrument that will perform all the functions needed for a given type of laboratory experiment.

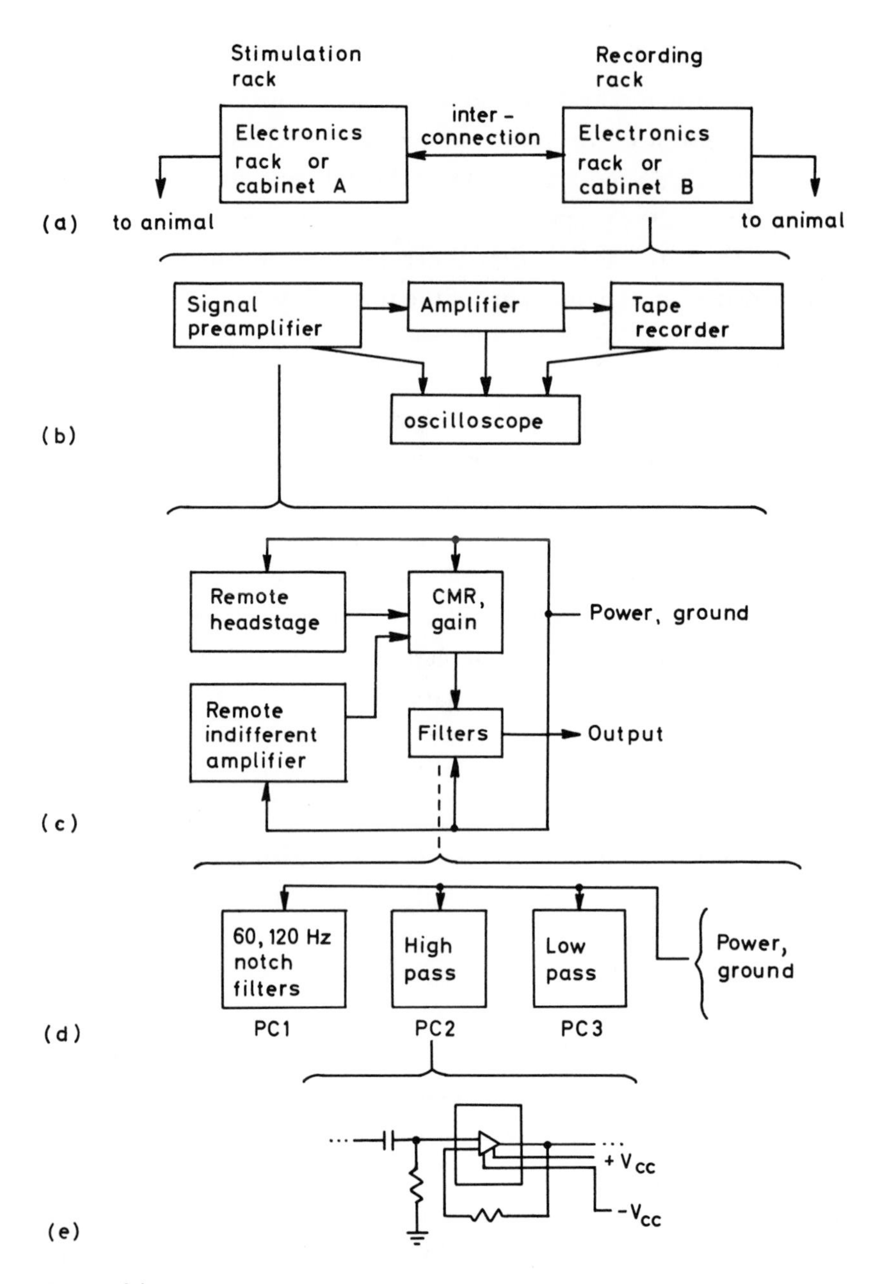

Figure 6.1
Levels of modularity. (a) Laboratory setup may contain several relay racks of equipment, which are interconnected. Each rack should be dedicated to some unified function. (b) Each rack will usually contain several instruments, grouped according to similarity and sequence of function. (c) Each instrument may consist of several subsections, arranged for minimum interconnections and unity of function. (d) Each subsection may consist of several PC cards. (e) Each card may have a variety of interconnected components.

Operation of such an instrument is relatively simple, and substantial packaging efficiency (small size, low power consumption and few interconnections) results. Alternatively, the same functions may be realized by temporarily interconnecting a set of modules. The modular approach permits relatively easy conversion of the apparatus for changing experimental requirements. Packaging efficiency is reduced, and operation of the equipment may be more complicated, but trouble-shooting and repair are facilitated. The degree of modularity of the instrumentation should be determined by the relative importance of packaging efficiency, ease of operation and maintenance, and functional flexibility in the laboratory environment.

6.1.1 Printed Circuit Boards

There are two basic types of printed circuit (PC) boards: the so-called universal PC board and the custom-designed board. A universal PC board has a regular pattern of printed wiring and holes designed to be usable in a wide range of circuit applications. Power and ground connections are made via the printed wiring pattern, and the circuit is completed with the use of wire jumpers. Universal PC boards are available from several manufacturers, with a variety of patterns. Some include such features as edge fingers for card connectors and printed lands for integrated circuit and discrete component mounting, and for mounting IC sockets (Figure 6.2).

Custom-designed PC boards, on the other hand, accommodate all or almost all of the circuit connections in printed wiring designed for a particular circuit. The choice between universal and custom PC boards may depend mainly on economics. It is cheaper and easier to design a custom board if multiple copies of the circuit are to be built, because the relatively high costs and effort of layout and artwork are distributed among the several copies. Universal boards may be a better choice for one-of-a-kind modules.

A printed circuit board consists of a sheet of insulating material plated with copper on one or both sides, from which copper has been removed selectively by an etching process, leaving a pattern of plated areas. Kits are available that provide all the necessary materials for good quality circuit board construction in the lab. The construction process consists of three main phases: layout, printing, and wiring.

In the *layout* phase, the spatial configuration of circuit components and wires is arranged so that a minimum number of wire crossings results. Where wire crossing cannot be avoided, insulated wire jumpers must be soldered to the finished board. If photographic masking is used during the printing phase (see below), then the pattern of circuit board conductors is expressed as artwork that can be

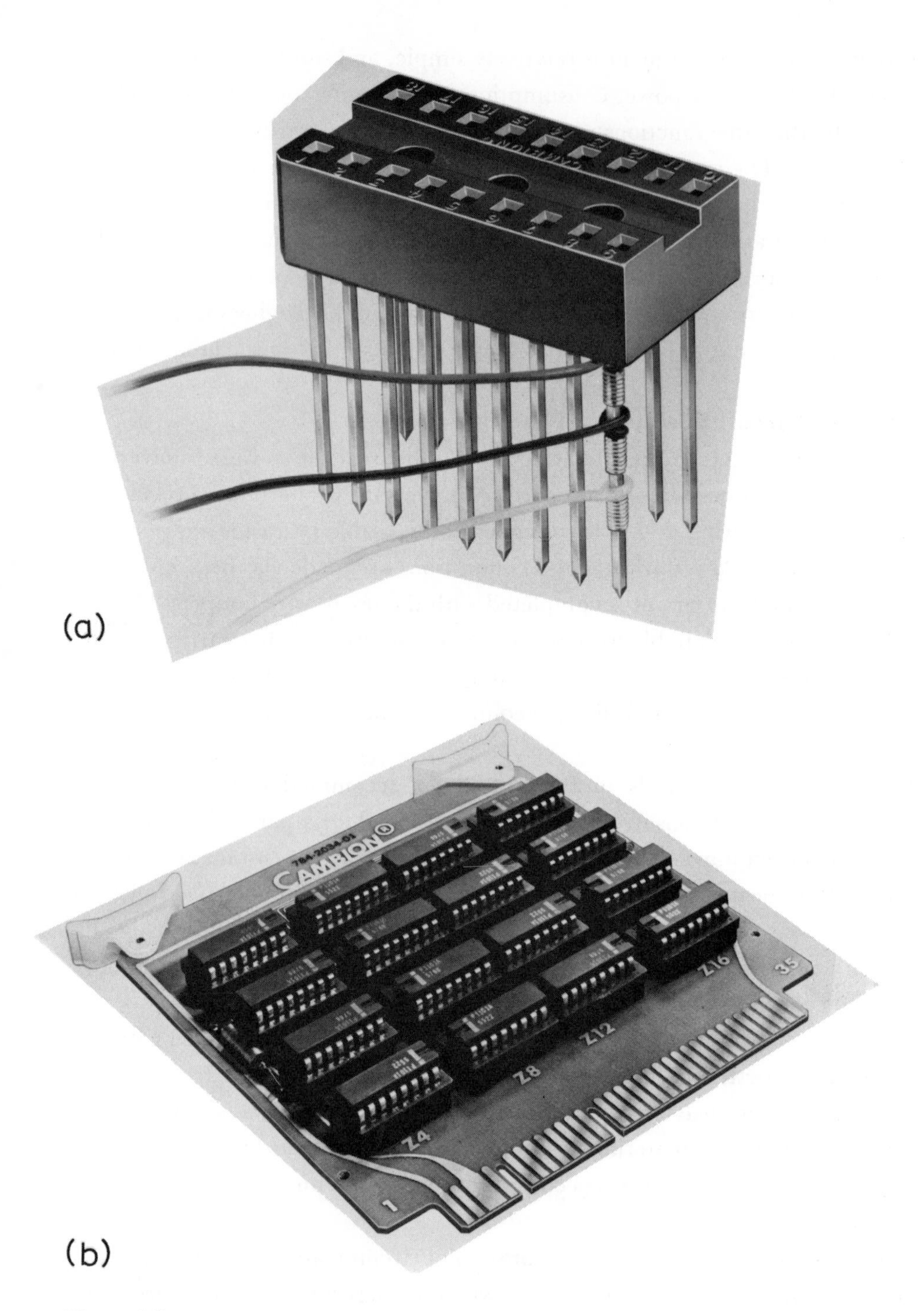

Figure 6.2

Modular assembly with universal printed circuits. (a) Integrated circuit wire-wrap socket. (b) Plug-in card with wire-wrap sockets. (c) Plug-in card with built-in, wire-wrap socket pins. (d) Rack-mount frame for plug-in cards. (Photographs courtesy Cambridge Thermionic Corporation.)

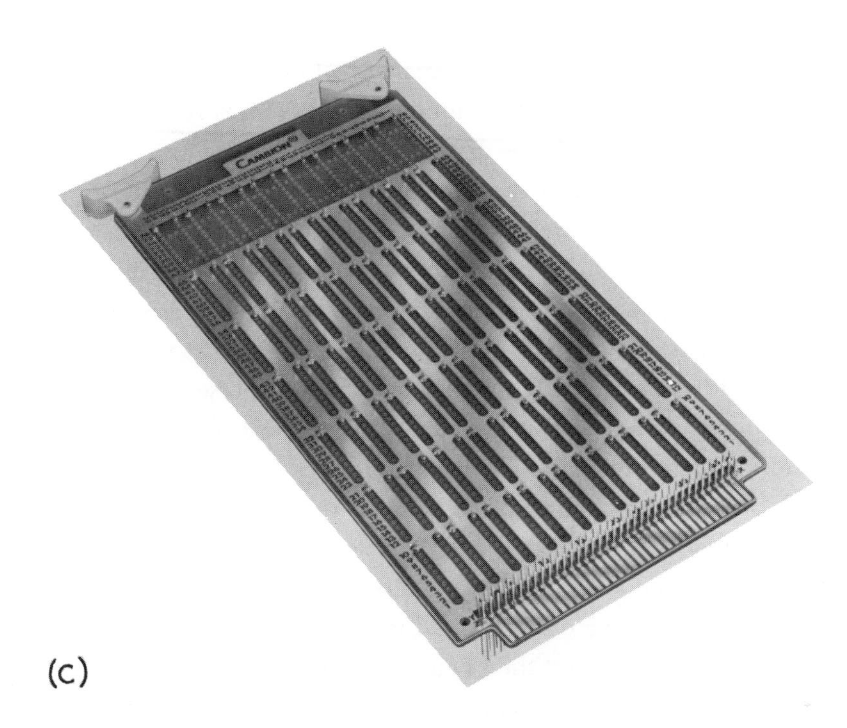

(c)

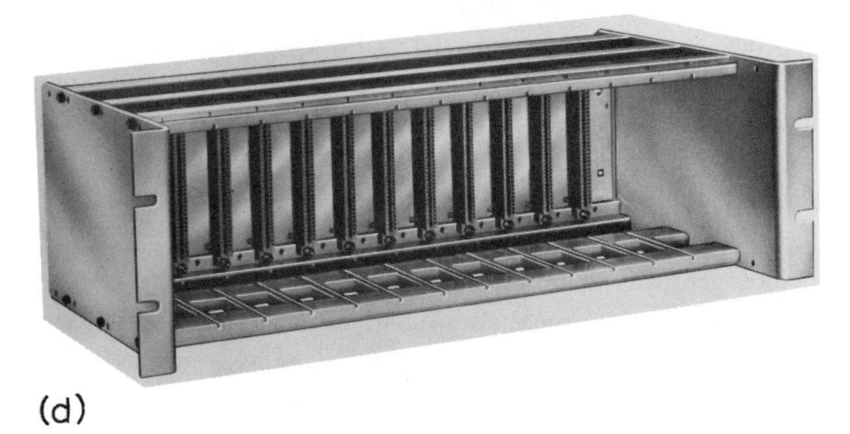

(d)

Figure 6.2 (continued)

reproduced as a photographic negative during the layout phase. The pattern of conductors is on the side of the board opposite the components. In order to facilitate the soldering of component leads, layout should thus be done with a bottom view of the circuit, including the components. In the case of photographic masking, artwork may be laid out as a top view, and the negative may be turned over during the printing process.

The first step in the printing phase is called *masking*, in which selected areas of the copper surface are protected from the etching solution. This is generally accomplished by one of two methods. Strips of an etch-resistant tape may be applied to the board where conductors or component lands are needed. Alternatively, boards can be obtained that are coated with a "resist," which upon exposure to light becomes insoluble in a "developer." The photographic negative of the circuit board artwork is placed on the resist-covered copper and used as a mask during exposure. When the board is developed, only the photographically exposed resist remains. With either process, the board is then immersed in a chemical etchant solution that removes the copper plate everywhere except under the tape or resist. The resist is then removed by immersion in a cleaning solution. If a tape resist is used, it is simply stripped off. The board is then ready for drilling of mounting holes for components.

The *wiring* phase consists of insertion of wire jumpers, component leads, and socket leads; soldering; and trimming of excess lead material. An air space should be provided between the component and the circuit board if much heat generation by that component is expected. The rosin flux accumulated during soldering is removed by washing the board with alcohol or another appropriate solvent. The finished board is then mounted and connected to the rest of the circuit.

Another type of circuit board (Figure 6.3) is often more convenient for production of small quantities of the same circuit. This is a perforated board, or *perf-board*, which is made of materials similar to that of PC boards but has no copper bonded to it. Instead, arrays of regularly spaced holes provide mechanical mounting of component leads, socket leads, or terminal posts. A board with spacing of 0.1 inch between holes is generally the most useful, since this corresponds to the spacing of DIP pins (0.1 inch and 0.3 inch). Leads and terminal posts are connected on the side of the board opposite the components, using American Wire Gauge (AWG) No. 26 or No. 30 insulated wire. Alternatively, stick-on conductors consisting of copper strips, printed socket lands, and assorted other printed conductors, bonded to transparent tape, may be used. These can be applied directly to the perf-board, to synthesize a *stick-on* printed circuit to which components are soldered. The components are mounted on the side opposite the stick-on conductors.

System modules that contain a large number of integrated circuit devices may be hard to build using printed circuit or discrete wiring techniques because of the very large number of interconnections required. Panels and plug-in cards are available which have a high-density array of integrated circuit sockets. The sockets have long terminal pins to which connections are made by wire wrapping (Figure 6.2a, b, c). This approach is expensive because of the sockets involved (sockets often cost more than the circuits they connect) but offers the advantage of compact construction and relatively easy modification.

Selection of wire types for solder joint and wire wrap construction is discussed in the sections on soldering and wire wrapping. Some general comments on wiring are made here. Where heating of insulation is anticipated during soldering or subsequent circuit operation, a high-temperature insulation such as Teflon or Kynar should be chosen. Solid wire must be used for wire wrapping and is convenient for other interconnection applications; but if the wire must flex or move about repeatedly during operation, solid wire would tend to break, and stranded wire should be used instead.

Traditionally, wire ends have been wrapped around terminal posts or socket pins before soldering. This is still advisable for commercial production of well-tested circuits or for leads that will be subjected to mechanical stresses. However, unless a bend around the terminal is required to hold a wire in place while other wires are added to the same terminal, the wire ends should not be wrapped around terminals where there will be no mechanical stresses, because the wrap makes replacement of components or circuit modification more difficult. If a wrapped conductor must be removed, it is often best to cut the conductor as close

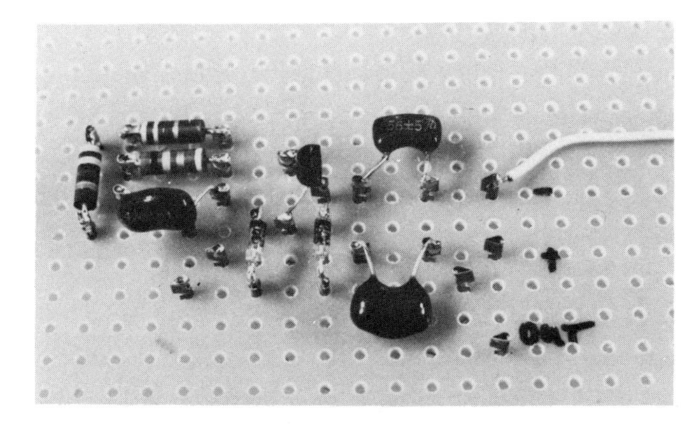

Figure 6.3
A breadboard and construction technique. Miniature pins (*flea clips*) are pushed into holes in perforated phenolic board. Components are soldered to clips on one side of board, and interconnecting wires are soldered to clips on the other side. If one clip is used for each lead, servicing is facilitated. Components may be laid out roughly according to the schematic layout for rapid location.

as possible to the terminal and solder on a new one, leaving the old wrapped conductor in place, in order to minimize exposure of other conductors and components to heat during the removal process.

Certain tricks may be used to facilitate wire tracing during servicing; the most common method is to use a number of wire colors during construction. The following color code is suggested:

Black = ground
Green = single-ended signal
Red = positive supply voltage
Yellow = negative supply voltage

Twisted pairs are usually used for differential signals, with two dissimilar colors of insulation. Twisted cables may be assembled rapidly by cutting all conductors to the proper length and tying them all at one end to a fixed object. All the conductors are then pulled tight at the other end and tied to a drill bit. The drill bit is inserted into an electric drill, lined up so the bit points down the length of the wires, and twisted until the wire has five to ten turns per foot.

If several wires run together from one point in a circuit to another, a cable should be fashioned and all the wires should be dressed along the side of the chassis for as much of the distance as possible; a different wire color should be used for each conductor. Ribbon conductors, consisting of several wires with different colors of insulation placed side by side and bonded together, provide a neat means of running a large number of conductors together. Since they run in parallel, their spatial arrangement at one end of the ribbon is the same as at the other end, facilitating assembly and wire tracing.

6.1.2 Handling of Components

Many electronic components are fragile and may be damaged by excessive mechanical stresses or heat. Care should be exercised in handling the leads and body of the component. The junction between the two is often a hermetic glass-to-metal seal that is easily fractured. The care required to prevent heat damage from soldering is discussed in Section 6.1.4.

Some MOS devices require additional precautions in handling. The silicon dioxide separating the gate from the source-drain circuit has such a high resistance that very high static voltages can accumulate across it. If the potential difference becomes great enough, the SiO_2 insulating layer may break down; if the charge is still present when the device is inserted into the circuit, the device, or other ones, may be damaged. These come with leads shorted together, and the leads should be kept shorted until after insertion in the circuit.

6.1.3 Tool and Component Inventory

An assembly bench should have a selection of tools including various sizes of regular and Phillips-head screwdrivers, Allen wrenches, adjustable wrenches, nut drivers, needle-nosed and square-nosed pliers, wire strippers, diagonal wire cutters (often referred to as *dikes*), vise-grip pliers, files, clamps or hemostats for lead heat-sinking during soldering, a wire terminal crimping tool, a bench vise, and a few soldering irons. Selection of soldering irons and solder are discussed in Section 6.1.4. Chassis punches and tapping and threading tools are also useful.

Component inventory should include resistors and capacitors. Passive components are inexpensive enough so that a good inventory may be kept on hand. Some form of records system is useful for guidance in reordering. Semiconductor components are somewhat more costly than passive components. A set of semiconductor components should be kept on hand to replace defective ones in existing circuits. One major advantage of working with ICs is the fact that the number of different active component types which should be stocked is greatly reduced: General purpose power transistors, power supply components, and diodes for digital and analog signal processing are all that are needed of discrete nonlinear components. Model 741 op amps and the most common SN7400N series TTL elements suffice for breadboard development of most new designs.

A selection of stranded and solid wire of various gauges is necessary, as well as a few selected types of cables and connectors. Structural components should include chasses or materials to make chasses, rack-mount panels, machine screws and nuts, self-tapping screws, flat washers, lock washers, heat sinks, power transistor mounting insulators, blank circuit cards, standoffs and brackets, and soldering lugs.

Machine tools are extremely useful in the fabrication of electronic instruments. Every electronics shop should have a drill press and a set of high-speed metal drills. Other equipment that might be included are listed here in the order of decreasing general utility, although some installations may have priorities other than those indicated: power hand drill; miniature high-speed hand tool with attachments for polishing and grinding; bandsaw; lathe; milling machine; power sanders and grindstones; and bending and shearing machines for shaping sheet metal. An electrically powered wire-wrap tool is recommended if wire wrapping is anticipated.

Several types of plug-in breadboards (Figure 6.4) are available for rapid assembly and testing of new designs; although these are expensive, they are invaluable for designers, because component leads may be quickly plugged in to assemble circuits for testing.

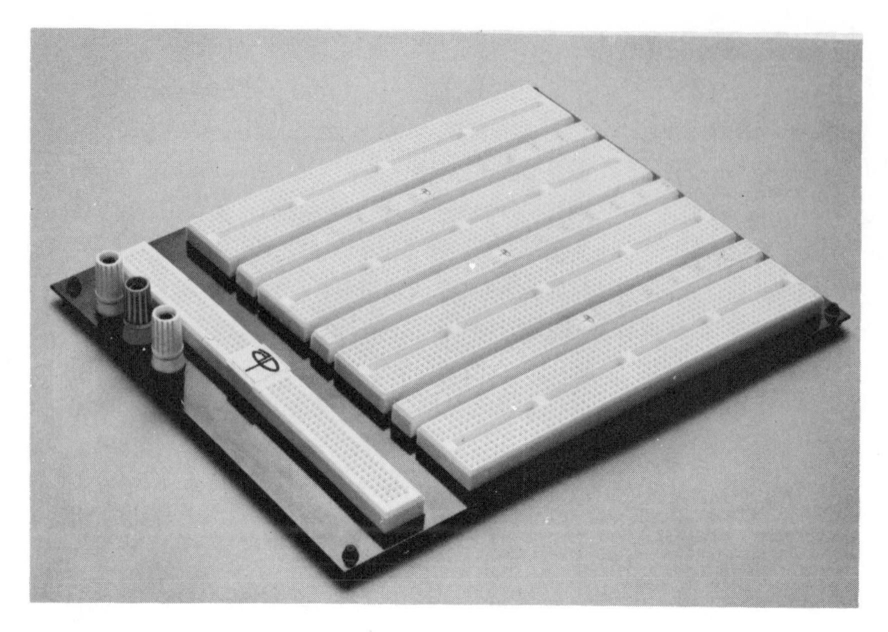

Figure 6.4
A breadboard assembly for testing integrated circuit configurations. Wires, component leads, and integrated circuit leads are pushed into socket holes. Columns of holes are connected together internally via metal strips to provide several parallel holes for each lead. No soldering or wire wrapping is necessary. (Photo courtesy of AP Inc.)

Electronic components are most easily obtained from a local distributor. If no local distributor carries the desired components, a mail order company is an alternative (for example, Allied-Radio Shack, Newark Electronics, Lafayette Radio Electronics). Listings of components and prices may be obtained from mail order catalogs or from the Radio Electronics Master (REM), a comprehensive volume obtainable from most distributors. A very useful listing of manufacturers' sources, local representatives, and distributors is contained in the Electronic Engineers Master (EEM), a companion volume to the REM. Both are listed in the references at the end of this chapter. The purchasing agent at your institution probably has the REM and EEM and should also have catalogs from several mail order suppliers. A direct request to the manufacturer will often yield data sheets, brochures, and catalogs of available components or equipment, including recommended sources. A valuable source of information and ideas is the wide variety of electronics trade journals available to qualified engineers and scientists and also found in the library. Some important ones are *Electronic Design*, *Electronic Products*, and *Computer Design*. These journals offer news and advertisements about products, information about circuit designs and principles of operation of new devices, and ideas in electronic design and development. Many other journals are also available, for more specialized applications. For example, the IEEE *Transactions on Biomedical Engineering* is a good source of useful circuits and ideas for neurobiologists.

6.1.4 Soldering

The process of soldering is the most critical in the construction effort. A poor soldering job can ruin a circuit. Soldering consists basically of the formation of a chemical bond between the solder and the metals to be joined. To ensure a good bond, the surfaces may require cleaning with the aid of a wire brush, knife blade, or metal file. Solder is an alloy of, typically, 60% lead and 40% tin, which has a low melting point. Solder intended for use with electronic components contains a core of rosin flux that, when heated, flows into the joint, further cleaning the metal surfaces. Acid flux should never be used for electronic construction. It is extremely corrosive. Silver solder is recommended for low-current, low-voltage circuits. Some metals, such as stainless steel, cannot be soldered with rosin-core solder: They require the use of special fluxes. These special fluxes should be used with fluxless solder.

A soldering iron or pencil having a power rating of from 40 to 60 W and a chisel-shaped tip with a width of about $\frac{1}{8}$ in. is recommended for most circuit construction. The soldering tip is normally of copper, for good heat conduction. Copper dissolves in solder, so that after some use, a copper tip will lose its shape and should be filed and tinned. Tinning is a process in which a clean surface is heated and solder is applied. The solder wets the surface and flows onto it, coating it completely. Tinning an iron improves its ability to transfer heat to the solder joint. Soldering tips are available that are clad in a metal such as nickel or iron. These tips are permanently tinned and will not dissolve in solder. They are relatively long lasting, and are worth their small extra cost in labor savings. Adjustable heat control is provided for some irons and increases the versatility of the iron for various soldering applications.

The most important consideration in soldering is the application of sufficient heat *to the connection* to allow the solder to flow into it, wetting the metal surfaces completely. The heat of the soldering iron is applied to the connection, not to the solder. The iron is held on the connection until solder flow is complete. This should take no longer than one second. Pre-tinning the members will facilitate quick soldering. Iron and solder are withdrawn, taking care to avoid jostling the connection while it is cooling. A good solder connection will be smooth and shiny. A coarse or grainy appearance indicates a *cold solder joint*, in which insufficient heat was applied or movement of the members occurred during cooling. Such a joint should be resoldered with application of additional heat, solder, and flux.

Solder provides a good electrical connection, but it is not mechanically very strong. If mechanical stress is expected on a soldered joint, the members should be twisted together or otherwise fastened to withstand the stress.

While heat is necessary to the soldering process, it is potentially damaging to the components (especially semiconductors), wires, and substrate. With an iron of sufficiently high power rating, it is possible to heat a joint sufficiently for soldering without inflicting heat damage on the components, wires, or board, since the duration of heat application is very short. Wire insulation having good heat resistance (such as Teflon or Kynar) is recommended for soldered connections, especially where the soldering is done in tight quarters. In situations where particularly delicate components must be soldered, the components may be protected by the use of temporary heat sinks. A pair of needlenose pliers or forceps may be clamped to component leads between the component body and the joint to be soldered. The tool should conduct away enough heat to protect the component. Hemostatic forceps are particularly useful since they leave both hands free to manipulate the solder and iron.

Insulation should be trimmed only far enough to expose enough wire for soldering (usually about $\frac{1}{8}$–$\frac{1}{4}$ inch). If a lead-to-lead connection must be insulated, a length of insulator tubing (called *spaghetti*) may be slid onto one lead, the joint

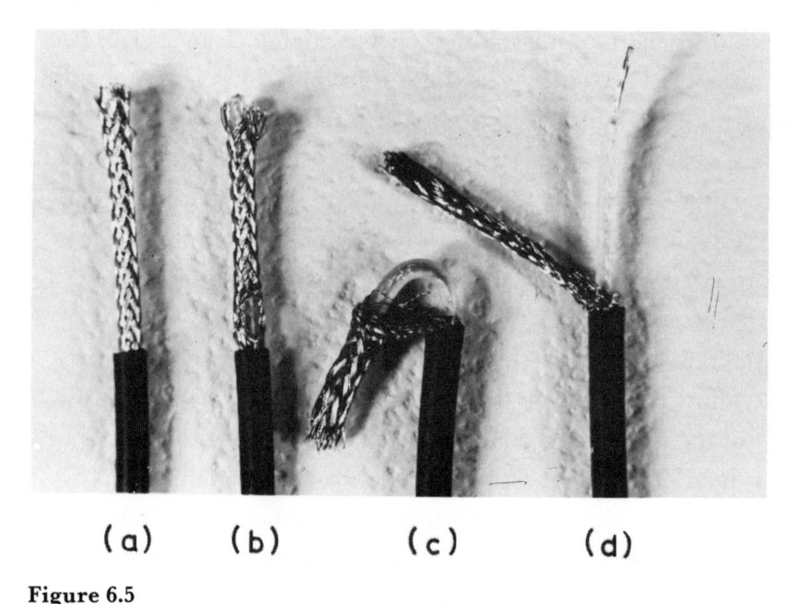

Figure 6.5
Soldering to coaxial cable (*coax*): (a) Remove outer insulation, taking care to avoid nicking shielding braid; (b) with a pointed instrument, poke a hole in the braid without breaking any strands; (c) bend cable sharply, pull insulated inner conductor through hole; (d) straighten braid. Tin the braid and inner conductor at their tips.

soldered, and the spaghetti slid over the connection. The spaghetti should fit tightly over the joint. Heat-shrinkable tubing may be used. Electrician's tape is useful for wrapping larger joints, for example, leads soldered to shielding braid or ac power-cord connections. The procedure for soldering to shielded coaxial cable leads is illustrated in Figure 6.5.

6.1.5 Mounting of Circuit Cards

A circuit card may be mounted by means of its edge connector, which is attached to a chassis, or by fastening it to chassis-mounted flanges, brackets, or standoff posts.

Edge-connector mounting is preferred when frequent insertion and removal of cards is expected, or when high packing density is desired. Card frames and files (Figure 6.2d) are available, in which the connectors are fastened in a row at the rear; edge guides aid in card insertion and provide supplementary support. Interconnecting wires are soldered to tabs on the connectors, on the back of the chassis. Card bins are sometimes used to achieve even higher packing density. The edge connectors are more closely spaced, and wire wrapping is used for interconnection.

Flange or standoff mounting may be used when only one or a few cards are mounted in a chasis. Interconnecting wires may go directly to eyelets in the PC board, or to an edge connector. The expense of the edge connector may be justified by facilitated maintenance.

6.1.6 Wire Wrapping

When systems are built that have a large number of interconnections, these connections are often made by wire wrapping instead of soldering. With a special tool, the bare wire end is wrapped tightly around a terminal post that has a rectangular cross section. The sharp corners of the post cut into the wire, assuring a highly reliable, low resistance connection. Solid wire of American Wire Gauge (AWG) No. 24 to No. 30 is recommended for wire wrapping. The wrap should start with one or two turns of insulated wire, continuing for four to eight more turns of bare wire depending on wire and terminal post size (more turns for thin posts and light wire). Teflon insulation should not be used for wire wrapping, because it tends to cut through or "cold-flow" and may eventually yield to pressure from terminal posts along the route of the wire, permitting the wire to make contact with a terminal. Kynar insulation has a much higher resistance to cut-through, and doesn't cold-flow. It is therefore preferred for wire wrapping. Wire wrap tools may be manual (operated by twisting a rod or pulling a trigger), electric, or air driven. A leading manufacturer of wire-wrap tools is the Gardner-Denver Company, Grand Haven, Michigan (Figure 6.6).

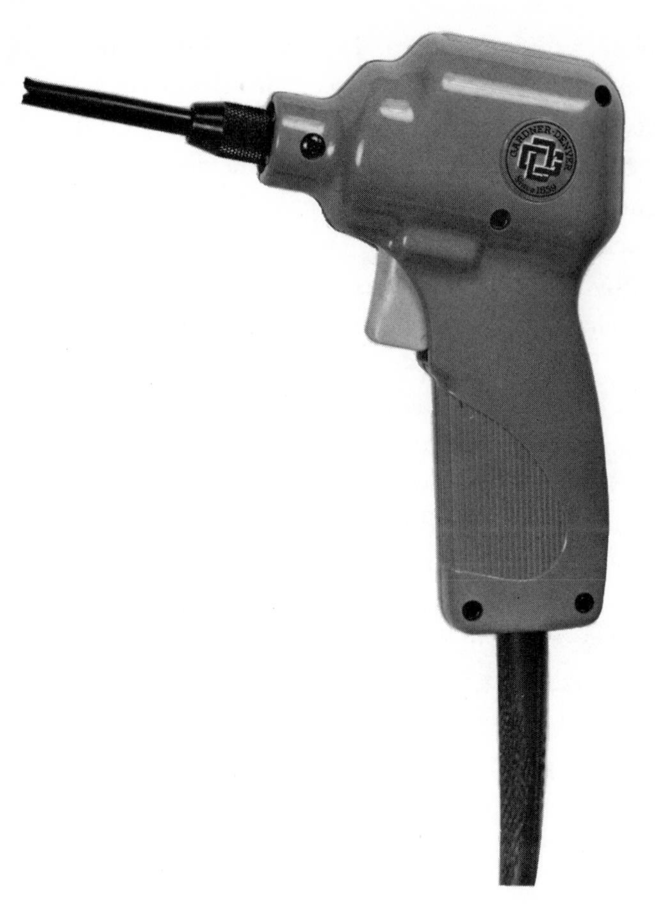

Figure 6.6
Electrical wire-wrap tool. (Photograph courtesy Gardner-Denver Company.)

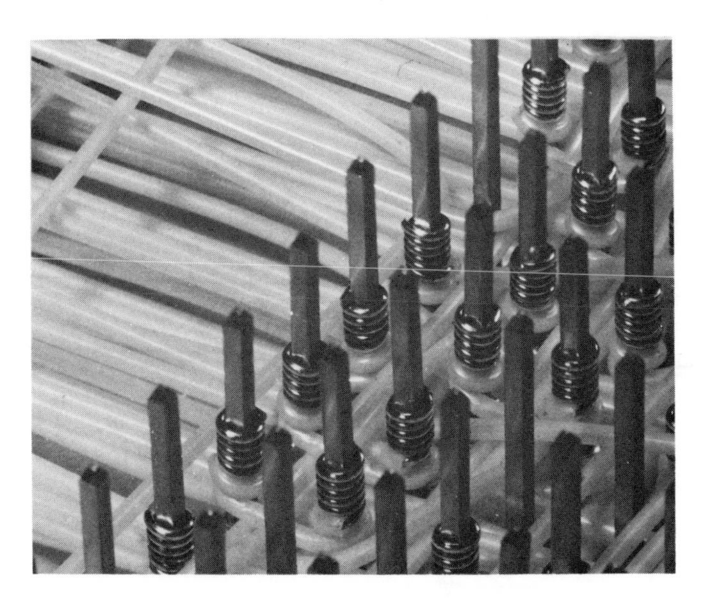

Figure 6.7
Close-up of portion of wire-wrap panel. (Photo courtesy Gardner-Denver Company.)

The use of an electric wire-wrapper is relatively simple. The straight-line distance between the two terminals is measured, enough length is added for the wire to be wrapped at each end, the wire is cut to length, and the insulation is stripped. Precision wire strippers are recommended; they prevent nicking of the fine wire. The wire is inserted as far as possible into the off-center hole in the wire-wrapping tool, and the tool is slid onto the terminal. The trigger is pressed to wrap the wire around the post, and the tool is withdrawn. Wires should be routed over paths that are as nearly straight as possible in order to minimize electrical pickup. A close-up of a portion of a wire-wrapped panel is presented in Figure 6.7.

6.1.7 Connectors and Cables

When a circuit is being built that contains a number of controls, these are best mounted on a panel for easy accessibility. Layout of this panel is quite important, because it will largely determine the ease of use of the circuit or instrument. Common sense is the important principle here. Controls should be spaced for easy handling and should be grouped according to function. All controls should be clearly labeled. A control that is rotated to change a variable such as frequency should normally be set to rotate clockwise for an increase in that variable. Switches that control on-off functions should have the *on* position up or to the right. Controls that are used sequentially should be arranged sequentially on the panel. A control that is used in conjunction with a visual indicator, such as a digital display or meter or panel lamp, should be placed close to that indicator.

Controls that are seldom used should be mounted on a rear panel or internal to the cabinet and may be adjusted by a screwdriver instead of a knob. Controls that require fine adjustment may be split into coarse and vernier sections or may make use of multiturn pots or screwdriver-adjusted trimmer pots. Connectors mounted on the control panel should be placed so that the cables or wires that connect to them do not interfere with operation of the controls. Connectors used infrequently, that is, for semipermanent wiring, should be mounted on the rear of the chassis.

A cable is composed of wire that ideally has zero impedance and thus conducts current from one place to another with no voltage drop and no distortion. Realistically, shielded cables have a nonzero impedance, the *characteristic impedance*, which varies with frequency. The impedance includes L, C, and R components. A cable is a form of transmission line. For more advanced considerations (for example, higher-frequency operations) see the reference on transmission lines at the end of this chapter. When a signal is applied to the end of a cable, it travels to the other end at almost the speed of light. Some of the signal is reflected back along the cable. The amount of reflection depends on the relation of the termination or load impedance to the characteristic impedance of the cable. The reflection may be made essentially zero by terminating the cable with a load equal to the characteristic impedance of the cable. Typically, this impedance is 50–100 Ω. Cable impedance is given in the manufacturer's specifications.

6.1.8 Grounding

A *ground* in electronics is a body that is at zero electric potential and can absorb an arbitrary amount of current from equipment without significantly changing potential. The earth itself is our primary ground.

In some nomenclatures, ground is just a reference point in the circuit; we will refer to such points as *common*. If the reference is connected to earth ground, we will simply refer to it as *ground*. In nomenclature where ground means common, zero potential is usually referred to as *earth*.

Secondary grounds include cold water pipes, special power line bus wires, and metal cabinets and chassis. Strips of metal plating and bus wires form local grounds on circuit boards; these are ultimately connected to earth through one or more of the secondary ground pathways. The connection from circuit to ground is called the *ground return*.

Equipment power cords have at least two wires, one the *hot line* that conducts current to the circuitry, and the other the ground return. If an ac outlet is remote from the earth ground, significant ac voltage may be induced in the return conductor. Therefore it should not be assumed that only one of the conductors has ac voltage on it.

Current leakage due to a defect or failure in the equipment can bring the housing or chassis to a dangerously high electrical potential. In most modern equipment, a three-wire power cord is provided for safety. The third, or ground wire, connects the chassis or housing directly to a special ground wire in the power line. This ground connection holds the equipment at ground potential, minimizing the shock hazard.

It is sometimes necessary to disable the third wire ground connection in laboratory instruments in order to minimize power line interference in recording of low-level signals. When this is done, the equipment should *always* be provided with an alternate ground return by connecting the chassis directly to an adequate ground in the laboratory. A long copper spike driven into the earth and connected to the laboratory by heavy braided cable is ideal for this alternate ground. The copper spike must be driven for at least part of its length into moist earth, for good conduction of ground return currents.

When several pieces of equipment or several circuits are connected to a common ground return path, it is important to consider the amount of current placed on the line by each unit. Units passing heavy current can produce transient or steady potentials on the ground wire that will affect everything connected to it. They should be connected to this wire at a point as close as possible to the primary ground to minimize this potential. A separate ground wire may be used for heavy current equipment. Ground wire size should be chosen such that its potential drop, with maximum current flowing, is suitably small. Ohm's law gives the magnitude of this voltage as equal to the resistance of the return line to ground, multiplied by the current. Thus, for 1 A of ac current, 1 mV of ac will be developed on a ground line that has a resistance of $10^{-3}\ \Omega$.

In designing a ground system, it is important to avoid creating ground loops. A *ground loop* is a closed circuit of ground conductors. It is vulnerable to induction of current by magnetic fields passing through it. Since the impedance of any real conductor is finite, the interference current will result in a voltage that could affect attached instruments. The tolerable size of this ground potential depends on the noise sensitivity of the equipment, but in no case should it exceed a few volts.

Within an instrument, the same grounding considerations apply. A ground bus scheme should be implemented with heavy wires connecting all circuits to a single instrument ground point. On a printed circuit card, unused areas may be left plated, and these plated areas may be connected together to form a *ground plane* that minimizes development of potential differences among individual circuit grounds. Even the addition of a ground conductor around the edges of a board, either in the form of a wire or plated copper, helps establish a useful ground plane.

6.1.9 Shielding

When a current is passed through a conductor, a magnetic field is produced in its vicinity. If another conductor is nearby, the magnetic field will induce a current flow in it. This induced current is a form of electrical interference called *cross-talk.* More specifically, this is inductive cross-talk or pickup. Capacitive pickup, in which electrostatic fields originating in one conductor produce voltages in another, is another source of interference. Typical sources of electrical interference include magnetic fields generated by transformers, motors, relays and coils, and electric fields produced by high voltages or sparks from switch or relay contacts. Electromagnetic fields contain both electrical and magnetic components, and constitute a third source of interference. These may originate in oscillators or radio or microwave transmissions. When circuitry is sensitive enough to be affected by interference, it is advisable to shield the circuit against the anticipated interference. Shielding against electric fields is best accomplished by surrounding the source of interference with a conductive shell. If this is not practical, the sensitive lines, circuits, or devices may be shielded by the conductive shell. Electric fields will not pass through a conductive shell that is grounded. Thus, any conductor or device contained within the shell will be unaffected by the field outside and conversely. In Chapter 9 on recording apparatus, *guard shields*, used to minimize capacitance between the "hot" conductor and ground, are discussed.

The shell used for shielding need not have a continuous surface. Wire screen is effective, provided that the largest hole in the screen is considerably smaller than the shortest wavelength present in the interference field. Shielded cables are used to protect long conductors from interference. They consist of one or more insulated conductors surrounded by a flexible metal braid or foil. Cables can be obtained with a wide variety of characteristics, such as number of conductors or twisted pairs in a common shield, individually shielded wires or pairs, or concentric coaxial shields.

For protection against magnetic fields, the shielding material must have a high magnetic permeability. Iron will often do, but for more demanding situations, special alloys such as mu-metal are available. Again, the most effective shielding is that which surrounds the *source* of interference, because the entire outside world is then protected with a single shield. A shield should not be used as a ground path for circuitry, because undesirable potentials may thereby be produced in the shield. When a wire or cable is shielded, one end of the shield conductor should be connected to ground, and the other end should be left unconnected to avoid ground-return currents and ground loops. The grounding should be done at the end of the shield nearer the signal source, if possible.

A twisted pair of wires is useful for reducing interference effects in transmitting signals. For single-ended signals, one of the wires carries the signal and the other is grounded. The grounded wire, because it is twisted around the other, may be regarded as a form of shield. In critical applications, interference effects may be further reduced by the use of differential rather than single-ended transmission. Any interference will tend to appear on both sides of the differential line, as a common-mode signal, and will therefore be rejected by a differential amplifier at the receiver.

6.1.10 Power Supply Decoupling

In electronic equipment, a number of circuits may share a common power supply. The wire, or *bus*, that connects the power supply to the circuits should be heavy enough to keep its voltage drop small under full current drain. Transient changes in loading of the supply bus by individual circuits will produce transient voltages on the bus which may affect sensitive circuits. The effect of such transients may be reduced by "decoupling" the power supply line at each circuit. Figure 6.8 illustrates the decoupling technique. The capacitor and resistor serve as a low pass filter that reduces the transient voltage change at each circuit. The resistor shown is normally the effective resistance of the power bus, rather than a discrete component. However, in circuits that process very low-level signals, R should be selected such that the maximum circuit current will produce a negligible voltage

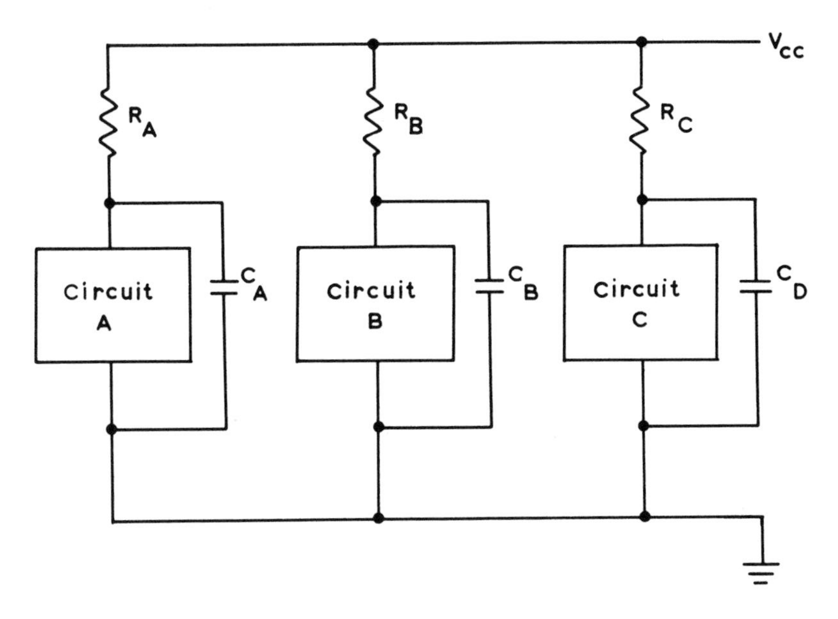

Figure 6.8
Power supply decoupling. See text.

drop across R (in order to preserve desired supply voltage), and C should be selected to reject the desired bandwidth of supply line noise. Thus, for a circuit drawing 100 mA of current and requiring ± 12 V $\pm$ 10%, each 12 V line should be decoupled with $R = 10\ \Omega$, 2 W. Since supply regulation can usually compensate for current fluctuations below 100 Hz with no difficulty, C can be 1000 μF or less. The electrolytic capacitor should be in parallel with a ceramic or mica capacitor, because electrolytics do not perform well as filters at radio frequencies. A fuse in series with R will protect the decoupling circuit and supply in the event that the instrumentation circuit is short-circuited. A rule of thumb for applications where supply ripple is regulated at 0.1% and signals are larger than 1 mV, is to decouple with $R = 0$, and $C = 0.01$ to 0.1 μF times the number of ICs, using a separate capacitor on each card. In critical applications, decoupling may be necessary at the power leads of a specific IC.

Fuses or circuit breakers prevent damage to both power supplies and circuits. The supply transformer primary and/or secondary should be fused at current levels between 1.5 and 2 times the anticipated maximum, and all components should be selected to tolerate at least double the fused value of current for the time required for the fuse or breaker to open. Either the regulator output should be fused to protect the regulator, or else overvoltage and short-circuit protection should be incorporated (see Chapter 11). Fuses may be added to individual circuits for further protection.

Isolation of power voltages from ground is possible to varying degrees both with batteries and transformer-driven power supplies. Batteries, if properly mounted, will have $>10^{12}\ \Omega$ and <1 pF to ground. Power lead length should be kept to a minimum, to minimize capacitive and inductive links to ground. Transformer-coupled supplies, using good isolation transformers, will have $>10^{11}\ \Omega$ and <10 pF to ground, but they are often bulkier than batteries, making long dc power leads (and hence, greater capacitive coupling to ground) necessary.

6.1.11 Construction for Easy Maintenance

If an instrument fails to operate properly during a laboratory experiment, it must be repaired or replaced as quickly as possible in order to minimize loss of experiment time. If economically feasible, pluggable spare circuits should be kept on hand for rapid replacement during the experiment, and for repair at more convenient times. Also, through careful design and layout, it is possible to construct a circuit which can be quickly repaired at the time of failure.

The most reliable of instruments may fail at some time. Therefore, maintainability and repairability should be maximized. In good designs the most common failures result from overloading input or output circuitry, and most failed components are semiconductors. It is generally advisable to use sockets for transistors and ICs. Both sides of PC boards should be accessible during testing. Pictorial and schematic diagrams are important elements in documentation, with appropriate codes for card function and location that match codes written on the cards themselves. Key components and test points should be labelled identically on the card and the schematic. Drawings should be included of anticipated wave forms at these test points, with detailed timing diagrams given for digital devices.

Component Reliability

It is important to consider component reliability during the design and construction phases. Precision instrument parameters such as gain and bandwidth are related directly to component tolerances. The incidence of equipment failure is related to component reliability. The added expense of high-reliability components in some cases is more than offset by minimization of lost experiment time and repair costs. This is especially true for components that may gradually drift out of tolerance, resulting in errors that may not be detected until several hours of artifact-ridden data have been collected. To achieve satisfactory reliability, components should be chosen that have appropriate temperature coefficients, tolerances, and heat dissipation capability. A component whose limits are exceeded in use may gradually change its properties until circuit tolerances are exceeded. Failure is much more likely for a component operated outside the safe range specified by the manufacturer.

Generally it is not necessary to compute failure rates of devices designed for use in the laboratory. Such computations require system engineering techniques and controlled manipulation of the environment in which the circuit is tested and are only practical in designing very high-reliability devices, as in life support systems for astronauts, or where reliability-cost trade-offs are computed for manufacture of large numbers of identical devices.

Component Tolerances

Component tolerances directly effect the performance of any circuit. Circuit designs should specify tolerances, if these are not obvious. We will assume 10% resistor tolerances and 20% capacitor tolerances in the circuits in this book, unless otherwise indicated. The effect of component tolerances on circuit performance specifications may be calculated by including the tolerance in the equations specifying those performance parameters. For example, 10% tolerances in feedback and gain resistors in a negative feedback inverting amplifier may produce a maximum gain error of 22%:

$$m_{\text{nominal}} = \frac{-R_{f\,\text{nominal}}}{R_{i\,\text{nominal}}} = -\frac{100\ \text{k}\Omega}{1\ \text{k}\Omega} = -100$$

$$m_{\text{max}} = \frac{-R_{f\,\text{max}}}{R_{i\,\text{min}}} = -\frac{110\ \text{k}\Omega}{900\ \Omega} = -122$$

$$m_{\text{min}} = \frac{-R_{f\,\text{min}}}{R_{i\,\text{max}}} = -\frac{90\ \text{k}\Omega}{1.1\ \text{k}\Omega} = -82$$

This is called a *worst-case calculation*, in which each component value is adjusted to the maximum or minimum within its tolerance range, such that every component value is at the extreme which produces the smallest result in the calculation, or all are adjusted to their opposite extreme to produce the largest calculated value. By shifting all component values in this way, the worst-case performance specifications are derived. More formally, any circuit performance parameter Y, which can be stated as a function of a component value X, will have a relative minimum within the tolerance range of the component value as well as a relative maximum. For linear circuits it is easy to determine the effect of variation of a component value, because dY/dX always has the same sign, although the magnitude may change. In some nonlinear circuits, however, even the sign of dY/dX may be partly a function of the values of other components or of applied voltages or currents.

Semiconductors, like other components, will have long lives in circuits if they have been properly selected for operating conditions. Failures occur most often when these limits are exceeded, even momentarily, or when the devices are not properly cooled. Heat sinks should be used wherever heat dissipation is required. These provide a path for conduction of heat away from the transistor or diode, through which heat is then dissipated into the air or the chassis. Since most power transistors have the collector tied to the case, and since the case is designed to be screwed down on the heat-sinking surface, an insulating mica cutout is provided with the transistor or can be obtained separately in order to prevent electrical contact with the heat sink or the chassis. It is often necessary to coat the transistor-insulator and insulator-heat sink interfaces with a specially prepared compound that has high heat conductivity and low electrical conductivity. These heat sink compounds are available from transistor distributors in the form of tubes or jars of greaselike material. The base and emitter leads of most power transistors emerge from the bottom of the case and are inserted through holes in the heat sink or the chassis. Stick-on masks are available for use as templates for drilling the lead and mounting holes. The leads must not touch the chassis or the heat sink, and metal filings and rough spots should be cleaned away before mounting. Each lead should be checked for isolation from the chassis or heat sink with an ohmmeter before soldering into the circuit. For low levels of heat dissipation ($<\frac{1}{2}$ W), the chassis itself may be the heat sink. The best heat sinks for dissipating large quantities of heat ($>\frac{1}{2}$ W) are extruded aluminum forms that have been painted dull black for maximum heat radiation. They have provision for mounting one or more power transistors, standoffs for mounting on the chassis and large-area fins for dissipation of heat into the air. Heat sinks should be aligned so that the fins are vertically oriented, for best air circulation. Heat sinks may also be used for high-power diodes, such as rectifiers and power zener diodes.

Sometimes small transistors or ICs in metal cans will generate relatively large amounts of heat that must be dissipated. Although there are heat sinks in which these can be embedded, which are then bolted to the chassis, slip-on miniature heat sinks with radiating fins may be adequate.

Power Supply Considerations

The effect of power supply ripple on circuit performance is often difficult to assess. However, for most of the circuits used in this book, a rule of thumb will suffice: Maintain supply ripple at a level at least one order of magnitude smaller than the minimum signal levels to be processed, and decouple individual cards. Generally, ripple of 0.1–1.0% is acceptable for neurophysiological apparatus. Further filtering and even regulation can be accomplished with the use of filters or IC regulators on those individual cards where less ripple can be tolerated. Supply current capability should be higher than the anticipated requirement to leave a margin for the addition of more equipment. Supply dc levels should generally be within 10–25% of nominal values. Common-mode ripple or dc error is cancelled out in many operational amplifiers.

Electrical Interference

RFI (radio frequency interference) and EMI (electromagnetic interference) may be eliminated by careful shielding. The amplitude of the interference is a function of conduction path impedance and length. Therefore the lengths of high-impedance paths and impedances of long conduction pathways should be minimized. The nature of possible sources of pickup in the environment should be determined in order to decide whether guard shielding, differential transmission, power boost stations, or transient protection is required.

Contaminants

Moisture, dust, and corrosive substances in the air can accumulate on circuit boards and switch contacts. If these effects are large enough to be deleterious to operation, the use of carefully sealed boxes or potting of circuitry in plastic or synthetic rubber may be necessary. If air cooling requirements preclude potting or the use of sealed housings, a fan with a built-in air filter should be used for forced air cooling, and the filter should be cleaned or replaced on a regular basis. The circuit cards themselves should be cleaned occasionally as well. The most susceptible areas are generally switch contacts and high impedance pathways.

Insulator or conductor breakdown may be prevented by choice of appropriate materials, with attention to environmental peculiarities, anticipated current levels, and heat generation.

Heat

If commercial-grade components are used rather than military-grade ones, the temperature range over which the circuit will operate is restricted; although if the ambient room temperature is within comfortable limits for humans and if the circulation of air through the equipment is adequate, most well-designed circuits will exhibit stable performance. Extremely temperature-sensitive devices should be kept within temperature-controlled enclosures. Air conditioning or fan ventilation may be required to maintain tolerable ambient temperature, especially in labs where a good deal of electronics is in operation. If ducted air conditioning is available, ducts and equipment should be arranged so that a large part of the cool air is blown down between a wall and the equipment, and pulled through the equipment with exhaust fans, if possible. This prevents cold and hot spots in the room that are not only annoying but also constitute a health hazard both for personnel and for experimental animals. Strategic location of the thermostat is essential. Air conditioning and heating should be controlled by means of individual thermostats in each laboratory.

Cabling

Exposed cables in the laboratory should be arranged for minimal stresses, by running them through areas where there is little walking traffic, such as behind racks of equipment, through false ceilings or floors, or in cable troughs. Stranded conductors should be used where any movement of the cable is anticipated. Connectors used to attach cables to each other or to chassis should be chosen as a compromise among requirements for structural strength, small size, low cost, ease of making and breaking connections, need for ground and guard shields, and number of conductors. Extra cable length should be allowed for possible future changes in cable route.

Modularization

Careful modularization of subassemblies facilitates servicing. Inter-connections between modules are minimized by intelligent choice of subassembly boundaries. The assembly should be divided into as few different module types as possible, in order to minimize the number of back-up modules required for temporary replacement, but the designer should try to minimize the total number of modules as well. In areas where PC cards are closely packed and access to either side of a board is restricted, an extender card may be constructed, with a female card connector at one end and a male at the other. This permits spacing the PC card away from the array of mounting connectors, for easy access to both sides for testing. Room must be allowed for the "spaced out" card within the chassis or in the chassis opening when the lid is removed, and standard card connectors should be used on all the PC boards so only one type of extender card is needed. The power should be turned off before unplugging or replacing a card, to prevent damage to components.

6.2 Testing and Maintenance

When a construction task is completed the device must be tested for proper operation. In general the testing should be done under conditions that simulate as closely as possible the range of conditions under which the instrument will be used. The device should be tested as thoroughly as possible before it is connected to the system in order to prevent damage to other instruments in the system by a defective circuit.

Access to and familiarity with test instruments is necessary for successful debugging of new designs and repair of older ones. The use of some of the more common test instruments is discussed in this section.

6.2.1 Testing of Components

For every type of electronics component, there exists either an instrument to test it or one may be devised. The more commonly used instruments include oscilloscopes; ohmmeters; voltmeters; ammeters; transistor testers; and resistance, inductance, and capacitance bridges. The functions of the ohmmeter, voltmeter, and ammeter are often combined in a single instrument called a *multimeter*.

Ohmmeters, ammeters, and voltmeters typically make use of a D'Arsonval meter movement, in which a coil of very fine wire is suspended by delicate pivot bearings and springs in the field of a permanent magnet. A current through the coil induces a magnetic field that interacts with the field of the magnet, producing rotation of the coil. The degree of rotation of the coil is proportional to the current through it. A pointer needle fastened to the coil indicates the rotation of the coil. This rotation is observed against a scale that indicates ohms, amperes, or volts. In the multimeter (Figure 6.9), panel switches select the function and range to be measured, by changing the configuration and component values of the circuit in which the basic meter movement is connected.

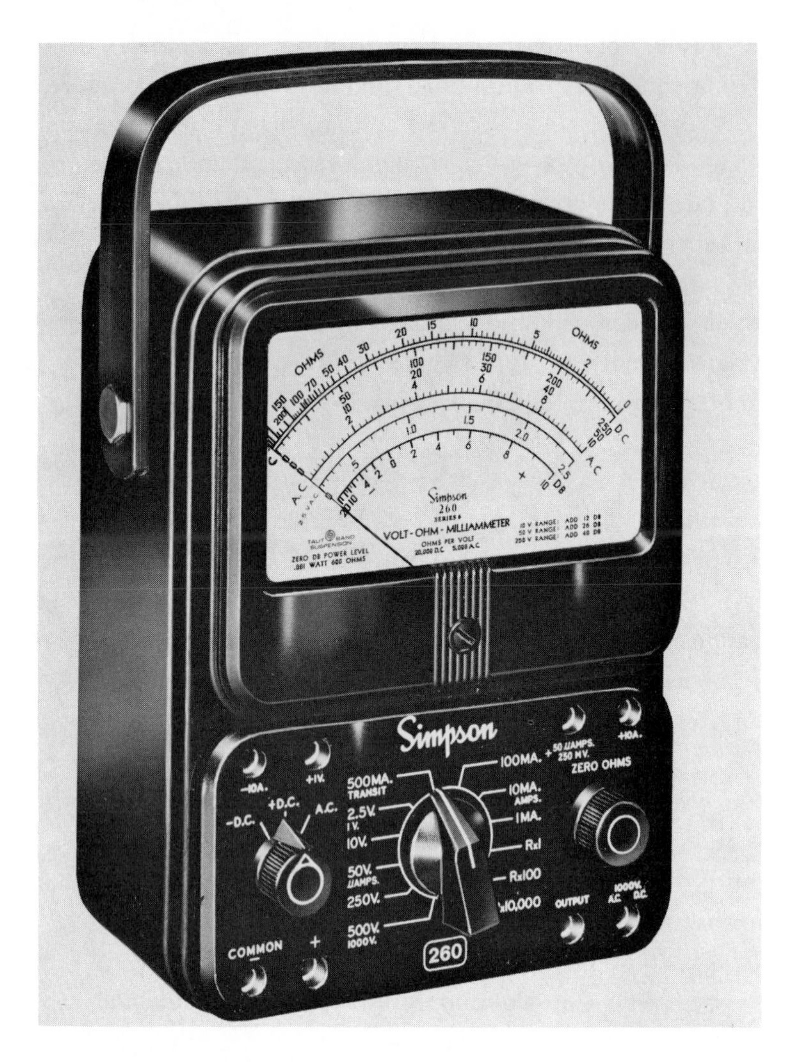

Figure 6.9
Volt-ohm-meter (VOM). Meter scales are labeled according to function and scale limit (for example, dc, 50) corresponding to selector switch settings (for example, ±dc, 50 V or 500 V). Normally, black meter lead (not shown) is plugged into COMMON (−), and red lead is plugged into +. When measuring dc, if red lead is positive with respect to black lead, use dc+; if red lead is negative, use dc−. The ac setting is used to measure rms level of a sinusoidal voltage. Current measurement requires placing meter in series with current source (red lead, dc+), and sink (black lead, dc−). Separate sockets are provided for red lead, for extended voltage and current ranges. Resistance measurement requires setting meter to zero ohms with leads shorted, using zero ohm adjustment. To avoid unnecessary battery drain, do not short leads unnecessarily in ohmmeter mode, and do not store with selector switch in ohmmeter position. If meter cannot be zeroed, batteries should be replaced. (Photo courtesy Simpson Electric Co.)

The leads of a meter may be connected between two points to measure the voltage across them, because the current flowing through the meter will be proportional to the unknown voltage. The sensitivity of the meter and hence the full-scale value is determined by the value of a switched series resistor in the voltmeter. Lead polarities are indicated on meters. The positive lead is usually red, and marked as +, *input*, or *test*; the negative lead is usually black, and labeled −, *common*, or *reference*.

Since full-scale value on a voltmeter is determined by a series resistor, the input resistance of a voltmeter is usually specified in ohms per volt (full scale). Thus, if the meter has a 20,000 ohm/volt input resistance and the full-scale setting is 20 V, the input impedance is 400 kΩ.

Whereas a voltmeter is used to measure voltage by connecting leads in parallel with the voltage drop to be measured, an ammeter is used to measure current by interposing it in the current path, with the current source tied to the positive lead and the sink tied to the negative lead. Ammeter sensitivity is regulated by switching various resistors in parallel with the meter coil. Voltages or currents that exceed the meter range by a great deal may exert considerable forces on the meter movement, damaging it. It is a good practice to start with a meter range that is higher than the anticipated input, and to switch to a higher sensitivity, if necessary.

An ohmmeter, or a multimeter operating in the resistance-measuring mode, is basically a voltmeter with a series-connected voltage source, often a battery. When the leads are connected across an unknown resistor, the current that flows through the meter is proportional to the resistance. Sensitivity is adjusted by changing resistances in the ohmmeter circuit. The meter should not be left in the ohmmeter mode when not in use as a means of preventing accidental battery drain in case the leads are shorted together. An ohmmeter's battery will change its properties with time; for this reason, most ohmmeters have a zero-adjust control. This should be set for a zero meter reading with the leads shorted.

A meter that measures only voltage or resistance is called a *volt-ohm meter* (VOM). In order to increase input impedance and/or sensitivity, some meters have preamplifiers built into them. If the meter amplifier uses vacuum-tubes, the device is referred to as a *vacuum tube voltmeter* (VTVM); a meter with a semiconductor amplifier is referred to as a *transistor voltmeter* (TVM).

The D'Arsonval movement of a dc meter can be damaged if it is used to measure ac voltages; however, many meters include rectifier bridges and filter circuits, and may be switched to operate in ac or dc modes. The ac reading is the *average* rectified dc voltage, which is proportional to ac power.

Ohmmeters have a variety of uses: They may be used to test continuity of wires, connectors, solder connections, and inductors. They are useful for tracing wiring connections. Semiconductor junctions are checked by measuring resistance in one direction and then the other. The dc meter will conduct much more current in one direction than the other if the semiconductor junction is functional. For example, base-to-collector and base-to-emitter resistances of a *pnp* transistor, when measured with the positive meter lead on the base, will have substantially higher values than if the leads are reversed, with the negative meter lead on the base. Forward semiconductor junction resistances are of the order of 10–100 Ω, and reverse resistances are typically 10^4–10^7 Ω. Low resistance in both directions indicates a shorted junction, and immeasurably high resistances in both directions suggest the junction is open. Collector-to-emitter resistances should be high in both directions, in junction transistors.

Transistor testers are variants on this type of testing, in which transistor sockets are mounted on the front panel, and panel controls allow selection of such parameters as collector-emitter voltage and base current. Qualitative measurement of transistor parameters such as current gain and leakage current are quickly performed with these instruments. More expensive models allow quantitative measurement of a variety of parameters. Although there are several varieties of integrated circuit testers, their cost is presently prohibitive for small laboratories engaged in building their own equipment.

RLC bridges are not generally of great use in a small electronics shop, because it is possible to have components selected at the factory for less than the cost of these devices. Qualitative testing is easily accomplished for most component values, by the use of an ohmmeter. Capacitors and inductors may be tested for serious shorts or open circuits, although not for small changes in values, with an ohmmeter. A capacitor may be charged by the ohmmeter current in series with a resistor chosen to provide an *RC* time constant of seconds. If the capacitor is initially discharged, the meter will initially register the resistance of the series resistor and the meter reading will increase exponentially to infinity. Larger capacitors (over 1 μF) can be tested without the series resistor. A shorted capacitor will have a zero resistance, and an open capacitor will have an infinite resistance, regardless of the presence of charging current in either direction.

Inductors generally may be tested for shorts or lack of continuity, although small shorts, such as between adjacent turns, may not be detected. If in doubt, compare the resistance reading with that for a new inductor that has never been used. This comparison-checking procedure may be used with confidence when testing semiconductors and capacitors as well.

Lower-valued capacitors (less than 0.01 μF) and inductors may usually be checked only with bridges or similar devices. Substitution of a new component in a circuit is often the simplest technique.

The cathode-ray oscilloscope (or simply, CRO, *oscilloscope* or *scope*), illustrated in Figure 6.10, is used in the neurobiology laboratory for monitoring of signals. It was invented by neurophysiologists specifically for this purpose. It is also useful for testing and maintenance of laboratory instrumentation. Therefore the principles of its operation are described and typical applications are given.

The heart of the oscilloscope is a *cathode-ray tube*, or CRT. It is similar to other vacuum tubes in that electrons are boiled off a hot cathode into the surrounding evacuated space (the process is called *thermionic emission*), and accelerated toward an anode. In contrast with most vacuum tubes, there are no control grids, and the anode is hollow. Therefore, the accelerated electrons pass through the anode. The cathode-anode assembly is called an *electron gun*. Vertically oriented metal plates are located on each side of the electron beam, and horizontally aligned plates are placed above and below the beam. By applying differential voltages to these two pairs of plates, the beam may be deflected horizontally or vertically, respectively. Focussing and astigmatism control are also achieved electrostatically by means of voltages applied to other electrodes in the CRT.

The electrons are thus focused into a very narrow beam, a fraction of a millimeter in diameter. The beam impinges on a flat glass face or screen at the end of the CRT, on which a phosphor coating has been deposited. If the intensity control is adjusted such that the beam electrons have derived sufficient energy due to acceleration by the cathode-anode potential difference, the phosphor will become excited and will glow, producing a bright spot on the CRT screen in the path of the beam. As the beam is moved by the deflection plates, the light spot moves about on the CRT screen, forming a *trace*. In modern laboratory oscilloscopes, the deflection amplifiers and CRTs are capable of displaying signals with a frequency range of dc to many megahertz.

Normally, the voltage applied to the horizontal deflection plates is a ramp, generated by a horizontal *sweep* generator inside the oscilloscope. The ramp slope may be varied for controllable sweep rate. The sweep rate is usually expressed in time/cm and it ranges from 0.1 μsec/cm to 1 sec/cm on a typical laboratory oscilloscope. Many oscilloscopes also provide connections for external horizontal input (X-input) for X–Y plotting. This is useful for graphing one signal as a function of another.

Both X and Y inputs generally have controls for adjustment of gain, and hence of *sensitivity*, expressed as volts/cm. Baseline position is adjusted by means of a

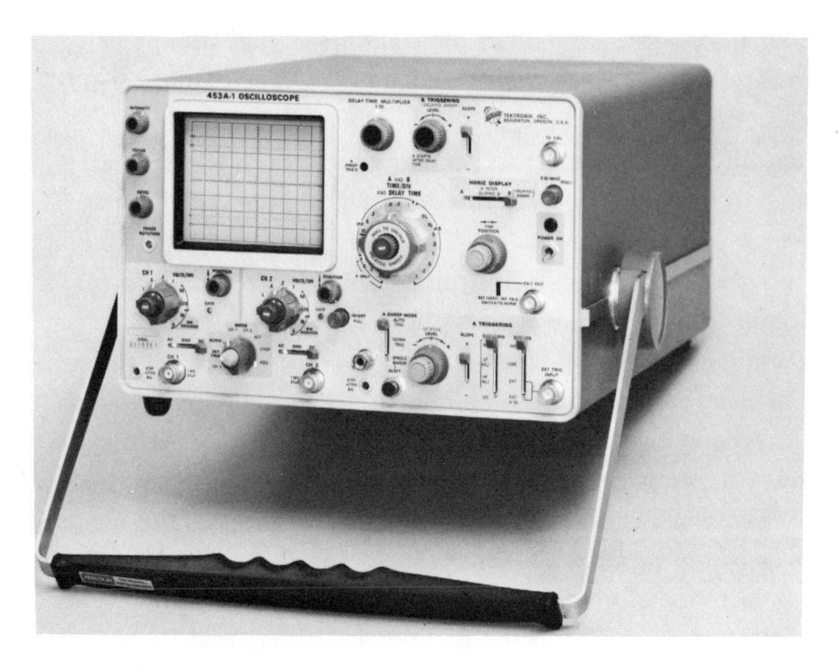

Figure 6.10
Tektronix 453A-1 portable oscilloscope. Beam intensity, focus, and astigmatism adjusted by controls at left of CRT. Below CRT are inputs for two vertical deflection signals, with gain and vertical position controls. Each vertical channel may be ac- or dc- coupled, or grounded (with input signal internally disconnected). Selector provides options for selecting either input alone, alternate sweeps, or chopped-trace display. Controls at lower right select trigger source (external, internal, or 60 Hz line frequency), trigger coupling, (ac, low-frequency reject, high-frequency reject, or dc), slope (rising or falling phase), threshold, and stability. Mode switch provides automatic or normal triggering or single sweep. Sweep controls permit adjustment of sweep speed from 0.1 μsec/cm to 0.5 sec/cm, delayed initiation and delayed triggerability of sweep, and intensification of a selected portion of the beam. (Photo Courtesy Tektronix, Inc.)

position control, which adds a dc differential offset to the horizontal or vertical deflection amplifiers. The vertical input sensitivity is usually adjustable from about 10 V/cm to 10 mV/cm, although some scopes have a maximum sensitivity of 100 μV/cm. For many purposes, neurophysiologists operate oscilloscopes at low sensitivity (for example, 1 V/cm) and achieve the necessary signal amplification with other electronics.

In order to observe several signals simultaneously, a multitrace oscilloscope may be used. Three methods are used to obtain multiple traces: multibeam guns, chopped trace, and alternate trace. The multibeam approach utilizes separate guns and deflection plates in a single CRT. Although the electronics for such a scope is slightly less expensive than that for chopped or alternate traces, the CRT is much more expensive. The major advantage of the multibeam approach is that the traces are completely independent, so that each may have its own time base as well as vertical position and sensitivity. The multibeam scope may also utilize the other methods for further multiplication of traces.

Chopping and alternation provide multiple traces with a single electron beam. Chopping consists of generating two separate deflection signals, derived from separate *Y*-inputs, each with its own sensitivity and position control, and then switching them to the vertical deflection plates in rapid alternation, typically at a rate of 10^5/sec. Each resulting trace appears to be a continuous representation of the associated input signal, except for sweep rates approaching the chopping rate, in which case the chopper wave becomes visible and the traces become discontinuous.

Trace alternation consists of a similar switching method, except that vertical inputs are each displayed as a continuous trace on alternate sweeps of the beam. The chopping artifact is eliminated, but if the signals vary from one sweep to the next, this method will not permit accurate comparison of simultaneous inputs. This mode is particularly useful for examining rapidly recurring, nonvarying signals, such as a sine wave at the input and output of an amplifier, or pulses generated by instrumentation.

The intensity of the beam may be controlled electronically by varying the cathode-anode potential difference. When using internal sweep-generation circuitry, the beam intensity is reduced to zero except during the sweep (a process called *blanking*). During the retrace of the beam, and between sweeps, it is blanked. It is then *unblanked* during the sweep. A connection to the cathode is usually provided for external unblanking.

The sweep sawtooth on most modern scopes may be initiated (*triggered*) by a Schmitt trigger. Input circuitry provides options for dc or ac coupling of the trigger signal, as well as a trigger threshold, hysteresis adjustment, and slope polarity selection. The trigger signal source may be one of the vertical deflection signals (*internal trigger*), an external signal, or the 60 Hz power line (*line trigger*). The sweep may also be restarted in a recurrent mode, wherein it begins again as soon as the retrace is completed, or in the automatic mode, in which the ac-coupled trigger signal causes a sweep trigger each time it crosses its mean value in the direction selected by the slope control. Manual control of triggering enables display of a single sweep by push-button operation, either immediately or upon the next electrical trigger after pressing the pushbutton. The trigger provides a means of synchronizing the display with an event that consistently occurs before the event to be displayed. This is essential in examining stimulus-response relationships, for example.

It is often desirable to generate a picture of a signal that can then be studied for some time. If the signal is repetitive, it may simply be displayed continuously on the screen. Nonrepetitive transients or signals that change over time may be permanently recorded by photographing the trace. There are cameras available, which attach to the face of the oscilloscope, and with which Polaroid or 35 mm photos may be taken. Polaroid film, while relatively expensive, has the advantage of an immediately available print.

Oscilloscopes are also available that have storage CRTs. The storage scope permits a single trace to be stored as a persisting glow on the screen. An image of reasonable quality may be retained for hours. Storage scopes also may be operated in the normal nonstore mode. In the store mode, the image may be erased quickly by operating an ERASE switch.

It is possible by using a storage scope or photographic methods to store successive traces of a signal, each deflected slightly further in vertical position either manually or by means of a simple staircase wave form generator, so that a *raster*, or many-trace picture of the signal, may be viewed. Long-term changes in latencies or time patterns of signals may be studied in this manner. Events marked by occurrence of impulses, such as neuron spike trains, may be represented in such a raster by using the impulse to unblank the beam that is normally held blanked by adjustment of the intensity control. The time pattern of event occurrence will then appear as a raster of dots on the screen. This type of display, and others, will be discussed in Chapter 10. While the storage scope offers economy compared with film, the results are of course not permanent, and there are disadvantages: The storage scope has relatively poor resolution and contrast, relatively limited life, a more expensive CRT, and a need for considerable periodic adjustment of the internal circuitry.

Many oscilloscopes offer the flexibility of removable units for horizontal and vertical input channels, including deflection amplifiers with a variety of characteristics, for example, sweep generators with special features such as expansion of a selected segment of the main sweep.

6.2.2 The Systems Approach to Troubleshooting

When a piece of electronics apparatus breaks down, the symptoms should be examined in such a way as to "focus in" on the defect by a logical process of successive elimination. The first thing to determine is whether the inputs to the system are correct—this includes the power supply voltages. If turning the power switch on and off seems to have no effect, an unplugged power cord, blown fuses, or disconnected power supply leads may be responsible. Inadvertently disconnected ground leads sometimes have the same effect as absent power voltages. If these tests do not reveal the trouble, the power supply output voltages should be checked, with the load still connected. Use of an alternate power supply will provide a definitive check on whether the device or the supply is defective. If the power supply fuses are blown (line fuses and circuit breakers or fuses in a malfunctioning circuit may be blown as well), the problem may not be solved simply by replacing the fuse, because it presumably blew in the first place due to an overload. All devices powered by the supply should be disconnected one at a time, turning the supply off each time a connection is changed to prevent damage to the instrumentation. If no single device blows the fuse, some device is marginal or too many devices are being powered by the same supply. If one single device is the source of the trouble, high-current pathways should be checked for faulty components, and portions of the circuit should be isolated from the supply line, until the portion of the circuit that is responsible has been found. Checking component resistances with an ohmmeter is usually adequate for locating the defective component at this point. A search may be made for charred components or boards, and for peeling paint or blistered insulation. A burnt smell is often the giveaway sign. Characteristic odors are produced by various overheated components.

Panel controls or indicators that seem to malfunction may simply be connected to malfunctioning subassemblies. If a complex assembly fails, the first step should be to determine which board or other subassembly is faulty. Following the input signal through the circuit, a procedure called *signal tracing*, is often a rapid means of localizing the site of the failure. Signal tracing between instruments (for example, finding the point at which the signal is lost, from microelectrode through preamplifier, through discriminator, cable transmitter, and computer interface) is accomplished at their respective inputs and outputs. Within a single instrument constructed from several cards, the signal should be traced on the back-panel wiring or at the card connectors. Once the point has been found where the signal no longer is correct, the fault will almost always be found in the card preceding that point or in a card to which that signal is connected; the latter can cause disappearance or distortion of the signal if the signal is overloaded. Disconnecting the load will quickly determine whether the loss of signal is due to an overload. If overloading occurs, it can be the fault of the *transmitter* card if the current capability has been diminished by failure of some component in the output circuit, or of the *receiver* card if a failure of some component or a mechanical short has caused a decrease in the input impedance of the receiver circuit.

If a signal cannot be traced from one card to another, but both cards seem to work properly, it is possible that the fault lies in a bad solder joint or a broken wire: Continuity should be checked between the two points with an ohmmeter, with the power off. The resistance will be large if a discontinuity has occurred. Alternatively, the signal may have shorted to ground or to another signal wire by defective insulation.

The failure may be due to a defective source, an increased load, or a broken or shorted connection. The occurrence of a decreased load resistance due to one component failure can cause another component to fail in the signal source. An overvoltage at the input of one stage may propagate through to the next, damaging both. Daisy-chain effects such as this can damage several stages in a signal-processing instrument, unless each stage is short-circuit and overvoltage protected.

A signal generator is useful for signal injection during the signal-tracing process. Choice of wave form depends on the circuit to be tested, but generally a source of recurrent TTL pulses of variable frequency and duration is sufficient for testing of digital logic, and a source of sine waves of variable frequency and amplitude is sufficient for testing of analog devices. Circuits described in Chapter 5 should be adequate for most signal-generation applications.

Signal tracing is most easily accomplished with an oscilloscope. The scope should be selected for appropriate input impedance, sensitivity, number of beams, and frequency response. It should have a triggered sweep in order to synchronize the sweep with the injected test signal. An audio monitor with input overvoltage protection is useful for tracing ac signals.

Once the defective circuit stage has been located and the defect has been localized as well as possible by signal tracing, the circuit schematic should be examined for those components whose failure (usually but not always an open or short circuit) could produce the observed change in the signal. Except in more complicated circuits, there is usually a limited variety of component failures that can give rise to the observed alteration of the signal. Components may be checked in place with an ohmmeter, if care is taken to calculate the effect of the rest of the circuit on the resistance measured across the component.

Note that supply voltages must not be applied during checks with an ohmmeter. In addition, some circuits may contain capacitors that discharge slowly when the power is turned off and that may give spurious (even negative!) resistance readings, even at distant points in the circuit. Large capacitors ($>10\ \mu F$) should not be discharged by simply shorting them; a small resistance should be used instead, with a wattage determined by R, C, and suspected Q. Thus, a 1000 μF electrolytic originally charged to $+100$ V may have as much as 10^{-1} coulombs of charge on it. If a 100 mA discharging current is tolerated by the electrolytic, a shorting resistor of 1 kΩ can be used, with a power rating of at least 10 W. Discharge to 10% of the original charge will take about 4 RC sec, or 4 sec, after which a 100 Ω, 1 W resistor can be used to remove the remaining charge.

If an open circuit component is suspected, the component may be paralleled with a similar one in order to see if proper circuit performance is restored. Shorted components will be indicated by an unreasonably low or even zero resistance and may be tested by cutting or unsoldering one lead at the solder junction and paralleling with a new component. If the component is found not to be at fault, it may be resoldered.

Locating the defective component in a complicated digital or analog feedback network is generally more difficult. The alternative methods for finding the bad component consist of (a) simplifying the problem by opening the loop and simulating the proper feedback response if necessary (especially useful in digital networks); (b) paralleling suspected passive components (especially in analog circuits) with new ones of the same value to see if the circuit performance is altered in the manner predicted by theory; or (c) swapping of suspected active components with spares. In cases of suspected multiple failure, *all* active components should be replaced and each new one should be replaced, one at a time, with the original one, discarding and permanently replacing any of the originals that do not work. Power should be turned off before connecting or disconnecting active components.

Besides acting as a simple short, improper loading of a signal can also result in distortion or reduction of signal amplitude, or oscillation due to excess capacitive loading of an op amp output. Improper frequency compensation can have similar effects, as can improper power supply decoupling. These effects may be due to design error or defective components. Bad layout can cause pickup and parasitic oscillations. Cold solder joints have been known to cause unusual effects, especially at high frequencies. Wire insulation may melt during soldering, resulting in short circuits between wires or between a wire and a component lead, terminal post, chassis, or housing. Some components have metal cases that are electrically connected to a component lead. For instance, some junction transistors have the collector internally connected to the case. These cases should be isolated or insulated from wires, leads, and chassis.

Open connections from one point in a circuit to another may be the result of an open component, a missing or misplaced connection, or a broken wire. Wires that have been repeatedly flexed may have breaks underneath the insulation, especially solid wires. Nicks and gouges incurred during wire stripping will sometimes result in breaking of the wire after several hours of use, due to stresses caused by temperature changes, movement, or vibration. Stresses on component leads should be minimized, because some components have fragile mechanical connections of the leads to the component body.

Whenever troubleshooting is performed on a design for the first time, the faults may be caused by incorrectly wired connections, rather than bad components—indeed, the former may be a direct cause of the latter. Incorrect design calculations or even typographical errors in the schematic may cause improper assembly; the design should be checked for possible explanations of the malfunction.

6.2.3 Preventive Maintenance

A regular schedule should be followed for testing and calibrating of equipment. Batteries should be checked on a schedule determined by expected battery life. A dead battery may leak, depositing corrosive substances in the housing. Recalibration and adjustment of offset, common mode rejection, and gain may be scheduled largely on an empirical basis: A record of weekly values of these operating variables should be kept, without performing any readjustments, in order to determine the length of time that elapses before these adjustments drift out of the acceptable range. Many variables are a function only of passive components, whose properties vary little with time. This is an advantage of operational amplifier feedback circuits in general. Any equipment in which components or batteries are changed should be completely recalibrated.

Air filters on devices cooled by forced-air circulation should be replaced on a regular basis. If there are no instructions with the device, the frequency with which such changes should be carried out may be determined empirically: Dust will gradually clog a filter, and the air flow through the filter will be impeded as dust accumulates.

The most important aspect of preventive maintenance is the equipment check-out before each experiment. This is particularly important in a laboratory where the same equipment is used in different configurations for different experiments. It is essential to duplicate all the conditions of the experiment, with the subject or biological preparation replaced by an appropriate electronic analogue.

A particularly useful procedure in the detection of marginal components, or for forcing intermittent failures to become consistent, consists of varying supply voltages to determine the margin of supply voltage error that the device can tolerate. Such a *margin test* generally consists of slowly decreasing the supply voltage until the device fails. Bipolar supply voltages should be decreased together. Design of supplies that permit simultaneous variation of the positive and negative supply voltages is simple; the voltage adjustment potentiometers are combined, using a ganged dual pot. A separate series trimmer pot is inserted into the adjustment circuit of each supply. The trimmer pots are used to match the two circuits, and the ganged pots are used to vary the two voltages in parallel. Operating an instrument on a marginal supply voltage may help detect a faulty component. Troubleshooting should then be carried out at the marginal supply voltage until the faulty component is located.

6.2.4 Selection of Test Instruments

Equipment that is designed and built in-house will also be tested and maintained in-house. It may also be desirable to have local facilities for at least minor service work on some commercial equipment, because full service maintenance, when provided by the equipment manufacturer, is typically expensive and may involve undesirable delays. An inventory of equipment must be kept on hand for such repairs, and it is a good rule to maintain replacements for all components, because serious delays can be encountered in ordering replacement parts after a component fails.

With respect to the types of repair equipment that should be kept on hand, the following are suggested: It is often wise to invest in a separate oscilloscope designated specifically for the electronics bench. A good multimeter can be obtained for very little expense, and with these two instruments most defects can be tracked down quickly. Signal generators are so inexpensive to build that no laboratory should be without some. A collection of appropriate power supplies, including, if possible, current-limited and metered varieties, is helpful not only for powering devices being tested on the bench but also for providing test dc signal levels. Additional useful devices for the laboratory include RMS meters, counters, and special-purpose devices such as dB meters, spectrum analyzers, stroboscopes, and specially designed signal generators for special applications. Some of the latter may actually be built into the devices to be tested, for ease of maintenance.

Selected References

Catalogs

Allied-Radio Shack Corp., *Industrial Electronics Catalog*, Allied-Radio Shack Corp., 100 N. Western Ave., Chicago, Ill. 60680.

Cramer Electronics, Inc., *Catalog*, Cramer Electronics, Inc., 85 Wells Ave., Newton, Mass. 02159.

Electronics Buyer's Guide (annual). McGraw-Hill Book Co., 330 W. 42 St., New York, N.Y. 10036.

Newark Electronics Corp., *Catalog*, Newark Electronics Corp., 500 N. Pulaski Rd., Chicago, Ill. 60624.

United Technical Publications, *Radio Electronic Master* and *Electronic Engineers Master*, United Technical Publications, 645 Stewart Ave., Garden City, N.Y. 11530.

Trade Journals

Computer Design, Computer Design Publishing Co., Winchester, Mass. 01890.

Electronic Design, Hayden Publishing Co., Inc., 50 Essex St., Rochelle Park, N.Y. 07662.

Electronic Products, 645 Stewart Ave., Garden City, N.Y. 11530.

Manufacturers' Literature

Application notes on instrumentation and measurements are available (with index) from Hewlett-Packard Co., 1501 Page Mill Road, Palo Alto, Calif. 04304.

Several semiconductor manufacturers (for example, Texas Instruments, Motorola, National Semiconductor, Fairchild) offer application notes on their discrete and integrated circuit products.

Literature on wire wrap techniques is available from the Gardner-Denver Co., Wire Wrap Div., Grand Haven, Mich. 49417.

Books

Simpson Electric Co., 1965. *1001 Uses for the 260 Volt-Ohm-Milliammeter*. 5200 West Kinzie St., Chicago, Ill. 60644.

Strong, Peter. 1970. *Biophysical Measurements*. Beaverton, Ore.: Tektronix, Inc.

7 FLUIDICS

Paul B. Brown

The term *fluidics* refers to the use of fluid pressures and flows for control, communication, and other processes, in a manner that is analogous to the use of electromotive forces and electron flow in electronics. Most of the current development has been applied to the use of pressurized gases rather than liquids. The latter, frequently distinguished by the term *hydraulics* (which unfortunately has other connotations as well), has not been developed to as advanced a level and will not be discussed here.

In some applications it is convenient to directly control the flow of gas across a pressure differential, using properties of gaseous flow to achieve the control. This avoids the necessity of electrical wave form generation and electrical-to-gaseous interfacing with solenoid-driven valves. One powerful application of such an approach is in the implementation of a compressed air positive-pressure respirator like the Bird Mark II, that can operate in the absence of electrical power. Another application, which we shall discuss in the chapter on stimulation methods, is control of sapid solutions in gustatory physiology, using fluidic rather than electronic control, to avoid the troublesome magnetic fields, audible switching noise, and mechanical vibrations generated by solenoid-driven valves and stopcocks. An additional application that we shall propose is the fluidic control of olfactory stimulation.

7.1 Passive Fluidics Components

From Equation 1.83, it is known that a series *LRC* circuit will obey the equation

$$L\frac{d^2q}{dt^2} + R\frac{dq}{dt} + \frac{q}{C} = V. \tag{7.1}$$

The same expression applies to gaseous flow, substituting pounds of gas for charge and pressure differential for emf. Frictional effects are referred to as resistance. From Equation 7.1, if $L = 0$ and $C = 0$,

$$\frac{\Delta q}{\Delta t} = W = \frac{\Delta P}{R}, \tag{7.2}$$

in which q is quantity of air in pounds; ΔP is the pressure differential (*pressure drop*) in pounds per square inch (psi, #/in.^{2}); W is gas flow in pounds per second (#/sec); and R is resistance in sec/in.^{2}. Perhaps the more convenient cgs, or

P_1 W P_2 R

$P_2 < P_1$

$W = \frac{\Delta P}{R} = \frac{P_1 - P_2}{R}$

(a)

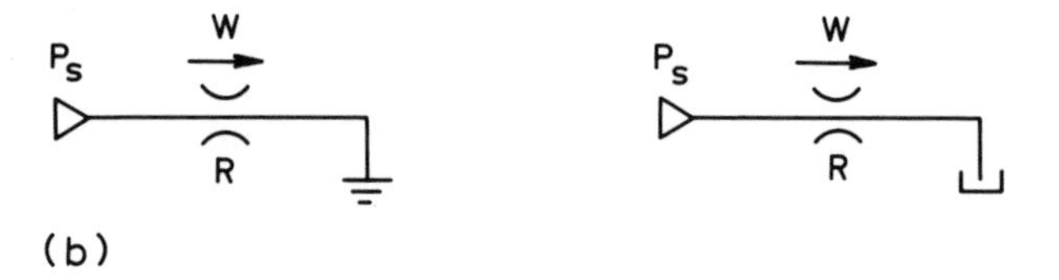

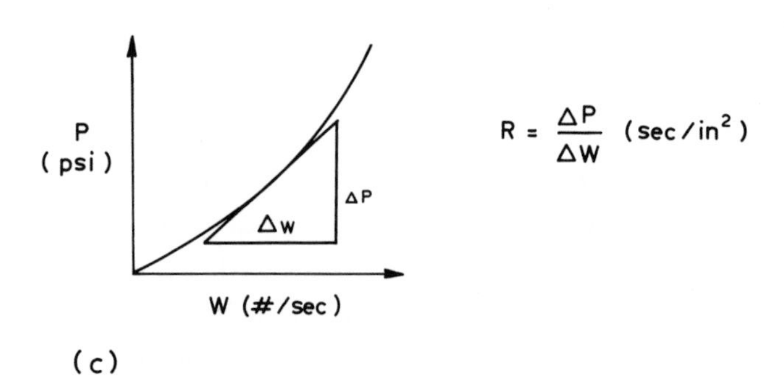

Figure 7.1
Fluidics Restrictors: (a) flow through a fluidics restrictor; (b) flow from pressure supply to ground; (c) pressure-flow relation for a fluidics resistor.

metric, terminology will be substituted in the future, but at present American industries still adhere to this system.

We can schematize flow through a fluidics resistor as shown in Figure 7.1a. If we take ambient air pressure as *ground*, *reference*, or *common* pressure, we can refer to ΔP as $P_{\text{source}} - P_{\text{ambient}} = P$, as illustrated in Figure 7.1b.

The practical limit for most fluidic resistor applications is about 10^6 sec/in.^{2}. Unfortunately most restrictors (fluidic resistors) are nonlinear in their flow-impedance characteristics (Figure 7.1c).

Within the limitations imposed by nonideal resistors (restrictor technology is improving, however), all the rules for resistive circuit analysis apply to the analogous fluidics resistive flow.

Referring again to Equation 7.1, we can derive the voltage-charge relationship for fluidic capacitors, if $R = 0$, and $L = 0$:

$$q = CP \tag{7.3}$$

where capacitance is expressed as in.^{2}. Differentiating, we have

$$i = \frac{dq}{dt} = C\frac{dP}{dt}. \tag{7.4}$$

The fluidic equivalent of capacitance is the ability of a fixed volume of compressible gas to store and release additional gas (to "charge" and "discharge") when subjected to external pressure variations. The capacity of air at room temperature is approximately 2.1×10^6 in.^{2} per in.^{3} of volume. Figure 7.2a illustrates the symbol for a fluidics capacitor.

The rules for *RC* network analysis in fluidics are analogous to those in electronics. Common values of C range from 10^{-7} to 2×10^{-5} in.^{2}.

Once again, Equation 7.1 can be used to derive the properties of a passive component type, this time for inductors, setting $C = 0$ and $R = 0$:

$$L\frac{di}{dt} = P. \tag{7.5}$$

Figure 7.2b illustrates the symbol for a fluidics inductor. Physically, inductance is the inertial property of a fluid that resists flow changes caused by pressure changes.

Figure 7.2
Schematic symbols for fluidic (a) capacitance, (b) inductance.

Inductances can range from 0.1 to 50 $sec^2/in.^2$. Inductive reactance in fluidics circuits is generally insignificant below 100 Hz; larger values of inductance, as in electronics, are associated with a resistive component. The L/R time constants are generally less than 0.5 msec.

7.2 Digital Fluidics

Most nonlinear fluidics devices rely on two physical principles for their operation: the wall-attachment effect, sometimes called the Coanda effect (after the discoverer), and the principle of momentum transfer. The Coanda effect is illustrated in Figure 7.3a. A jet of air tends to attach to a solid wall and will tend to flow along the wall. This tendency can only be overcome by the application of a force directed away from the wall surface.

The second effect, transfer of momentum, is illustrated in Figure 7.3b. A jet of air is deflected by transfer of momentum from a jet applied normal to the direction of flow. Essentially the momentum of the deflected jet is the sum of the momenta of the two input jets. For example, if the supply jet has only a Y-component, and

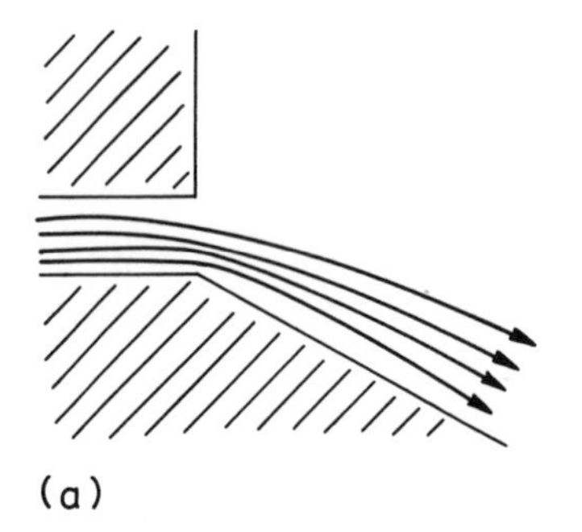

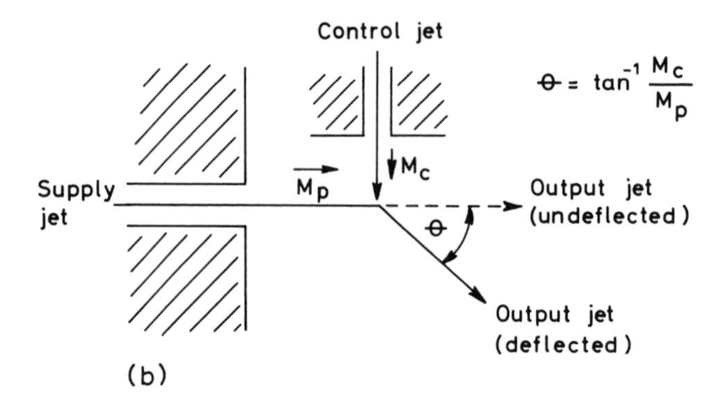

Figure 7.3
Hydrodynamic principles used in fluidics: (a) wall-attachment (Coanda) effect; (b) transfer of momentum.

the control jet has only an X-component, the single output jet will have a momentum vector whose Y-component is that of the supply jet and whose X-component is that of the control jet.

The design for fluidics devices that will probably become the most popular is a laminar form, wherein a thin metal, glass, ceramic, or even plastic, *silhouette* is sandwiched between two plates through which holes are bored for supply pressure, *vent* (ground), and *control* (input) and output *ports*.

The silhouette is a punched or etched channel connecting the various ports in such a way as to use the Coanda and momentum-transfer effects to realize logical functions or, as described later, analog functions. Some metal-plate silhouette devices can be taken apart and cleaned periodically to remove contaminants; some plastic silhouettes are so inexpensive they can be discarded and replaced when contaminated; and the fused-glass (ceramic) devices described later and some fused-metal devices can be cleaned with detergents or by ultrasonic washing.

For binary fluidics devices, we use the convention that at any pressure above a certain threshold, the *switch pressure*, the signal is considered to be "on," and at pressures below a lower level, called the *return pressure*, the signal is "off." We will discuss the Corning line of FICM (Fluidics Industrial Control Modules) fused-glass (ceramic) fluidics logic elements, although several other manufacturers provide extensive lines of modules as well. Material from Corning's manuals is reprinted here by their kind permission. In the FICM series, switch pressure is 10 to 30% of supply pressure (P_s), and return pressure is 0 to 2% P_s. Supply pressure may be anything between 3 psi and 10 psi. These devices have a fanout of 4 when mounted on Corning's interconnected assembly manifolds (Figure 7.4). When connected with plastic tubing, they have a fanout of 3. Unfortunately, there is no industry-wide convention relating to standard switching and return pressures, or even supply pressures. However, standard symbols exist for fluidics logic elements, which we will use.

Consider the operation of a wall-attachment fluidics flipflop (Figure 7.5). Once a state has been established, say, O_1 is one, O_1 will stay on (Figure 7.5a) until pressure is applied to C_2 (Figure 7.5b), at which time O_1 goes off and O_2 goes on. Then O_2 stays on (Figure 7.5c) until C_1 goes on. This effect depends upon the fact that in the absence of input, the stream can go through O_1 or O_2 with equal facility, but once it is diverted to go through one channel exclusively, the wall-attachment effect is adequate to maintain exclusive flow down that channel in the absence of any further input. When a control input goes on, the resulting transfer of momentum is adequate to force the stream into the channel opposite the control input, overriding the wall-attachment effect. Obviously, if both C_1 and C_2 go on, the

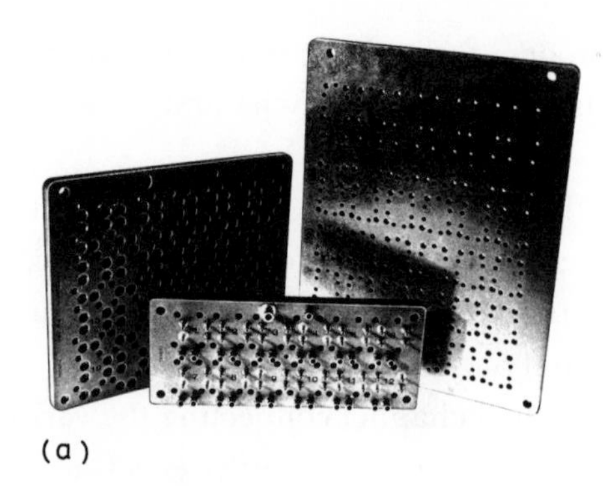

(a)

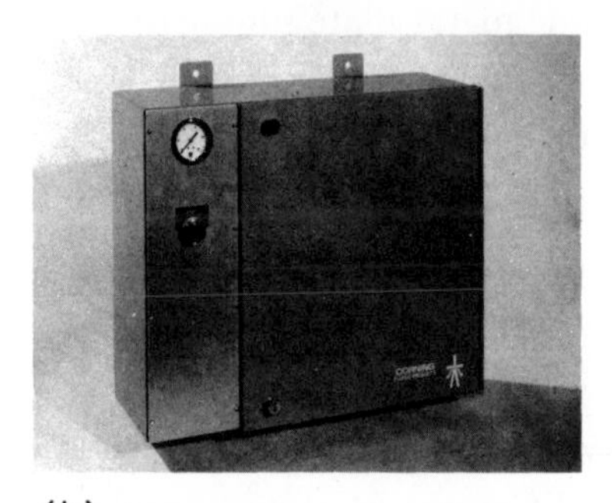

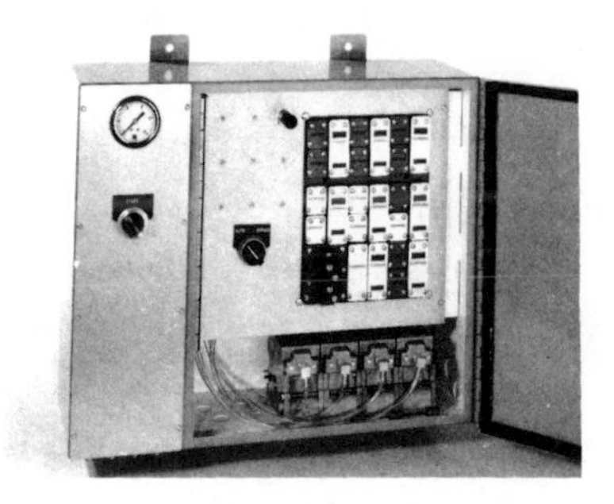

(b)

Figure 7.4
Fluidics assembly manifolds: (a) manifolds; (b) fluidic system consisting of modules mounted on manifold, air pressure regulator and filter, and fluidics interface valves, enclosed in a 19 × 16 × 6 in. enclosure. (From *Fluidic Industrial Control Modules: Logic Components*, 1970, by Corning Glass Works. Used with permission of Corning Glass Works.)

stream could go either way, or it could be split between O_1 and O_2, depending on the relative pressures of C_1 and C_2. We will consider this property in our discussion of proportional amplifiers. The additional vents on the two output legs, below the control jet intersections, are for venting back pressures when the output is off.

The logic symbol for a fluidics flipflop is shown in Figure 7.5d. The O_1 goes on if C_1 OR C_3 is on; it will stay on until C_2 OR C_4 goes on, at which time the output signal goes to O_2 and stays there until the beam is once again deflected by C_1 or C_3. Output is indeterminate if opposing inputs are on, and when power P_s is first applied.

An OR/NOR gate is diagrammed in Figure 7.6. Note that in the absence of any control input, the O_2 output is on, because the air jet tends to be straight as long as no sideward deflection is present. Actually, the symbol is largely schematic; the O_2 output is drawn to symbolize the one stable output when all control inputs

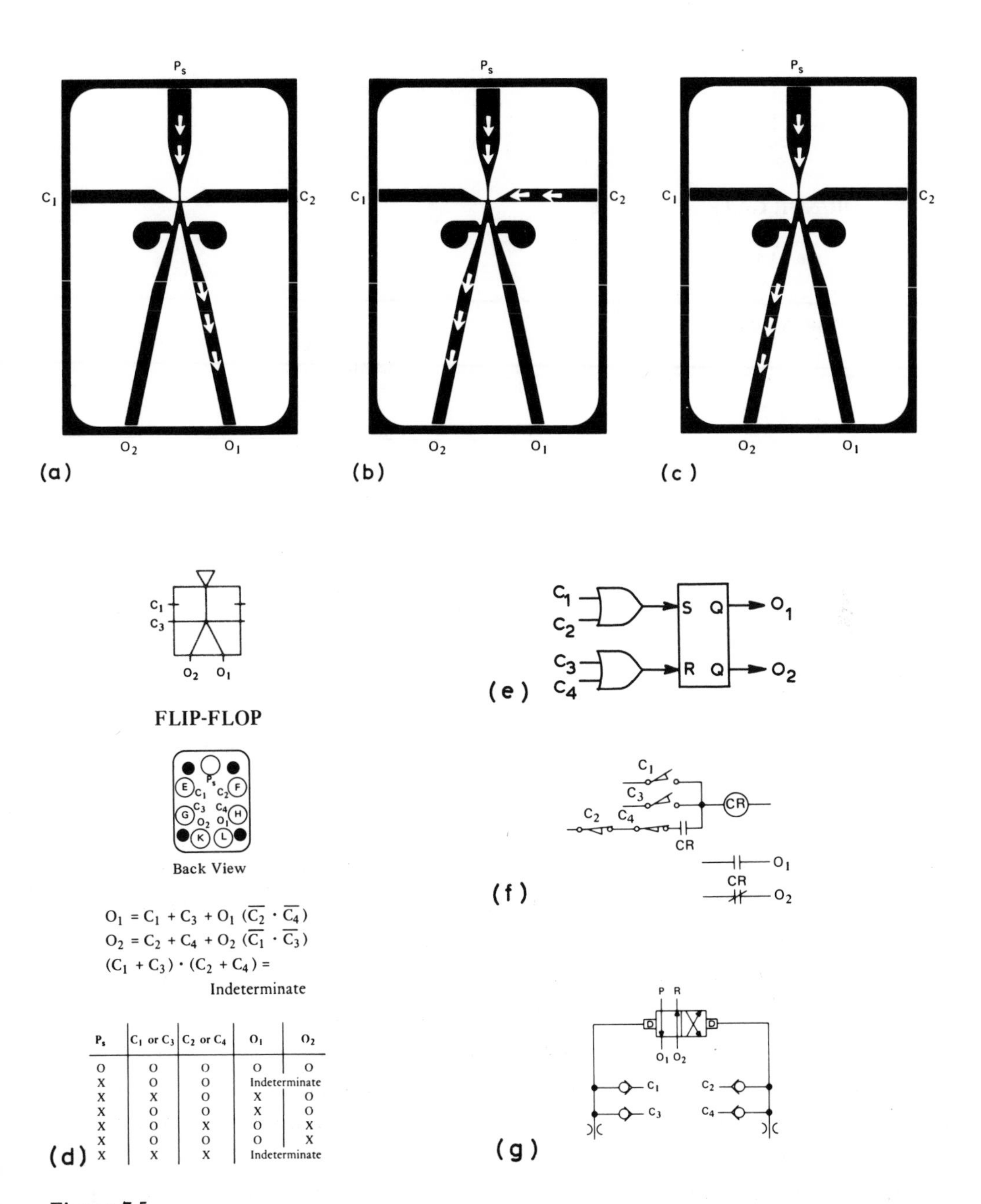

P_s	C_1 or C_3	C_2 or C_4	O_1	O_2
O	O	O	O	O
X	O	O	Indeterminate	
X	X	O	X	O
X	O	O	X	O
X	O	X	O	X
X	O	O	O	X
X	X	X	Indeterminate	

Figure 7.5
Fluidics flipflop: (a) initial state; (b) C_2 input pressure applied; (c) output O_2 maintained after C_2 goes off; (d) Corning FICM series flipflop and fluidics logic symbol; (e) digital logic equivalent; (f) hydraulic equivalent; (g) pneumatic equivalent. Letters shown in port openings indicate manifold port designations. (From *Fluidic Industrial Control Modules: Logic Components*, 1970, by Corning Glass Works. Used with permission of Corning Glass Works.)

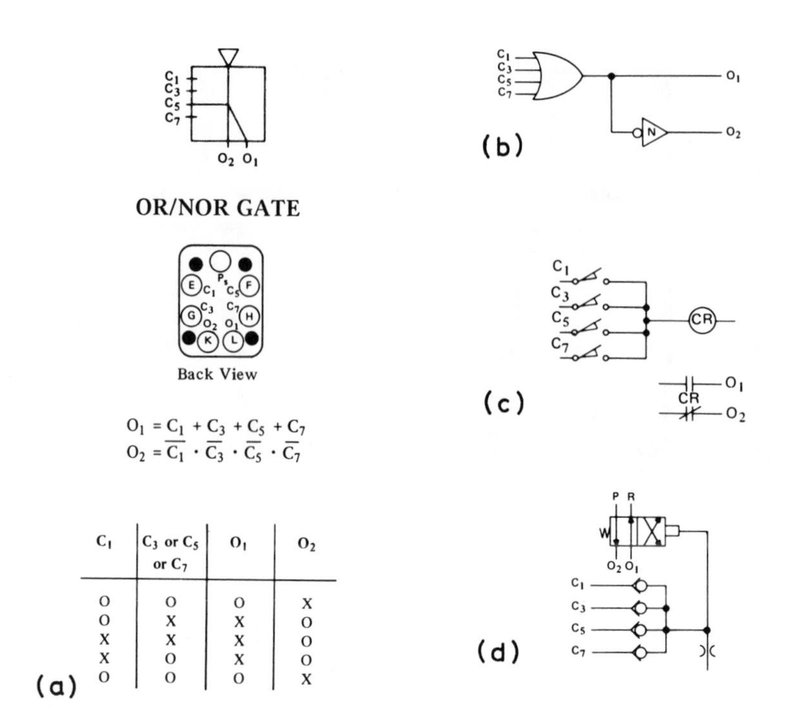

C_1	C_3 or C_5 or C_7	O_1	O_2
O	O	O	X
O	X	X	O
X	X	X	O
X	O	X	O
O	O	O	X

Figure 7.6
Fluidics OR-NOR gate: (a) fluidic logic element; (b) logic equivalent; (c) electrical equivalent; (d) pneumatic equivalent. (From *Fluidic Industrial Control Modules: Logic Components*, 1970, by Corning Glass Works. Used with permission of Corning Glass Works.)

are off; the deflected line O_1 represents the only stable output direction when any of the control inputs is on. The symbols for fluidics devices do reflect the basic principles of their operation, however; in this respect they have a considerable advantage over corresponding symbols for complex electronics devices. When any control jet goes on, it is deflected to O_1. Thus, $O_1(1)$ occurs whenever $C_1 \vee C_3 \vee C_5 \vee C_7 = 1$, and $O_2(1)$ occurs when $C_1 \wedge C_3 \wedge C_5 \wedge C_7 = 0$. In this device, the wall-attachment effect is not adequate to hold the stream in the O_1 channel, in the face of a pathway that is more direct (O_2), and in the absence of any deflecting air jet.

The AND/NAND gate (Figure 7.7) is similar to the OR/NOR gate, except that if C_1 or C_3 is off, any pressure from the other input is vented into the input that is off, instead of traveling down the common control channel to deflect the output jet. This means that, unless C_1 and C_3 are both on, no deflecting jet will drive the signal jet to O_1. Therefore $O_1 = C_1 \wedge C_3$ and $O_2 = C_1 \overline{\wedge} C_3$.

The inhibited OR gate (Figure 7.8) consists of a pair of ORed control inputs C_1 and C_3, opposed by an inhibit input C_2, which is sufficiently powerful to prevent

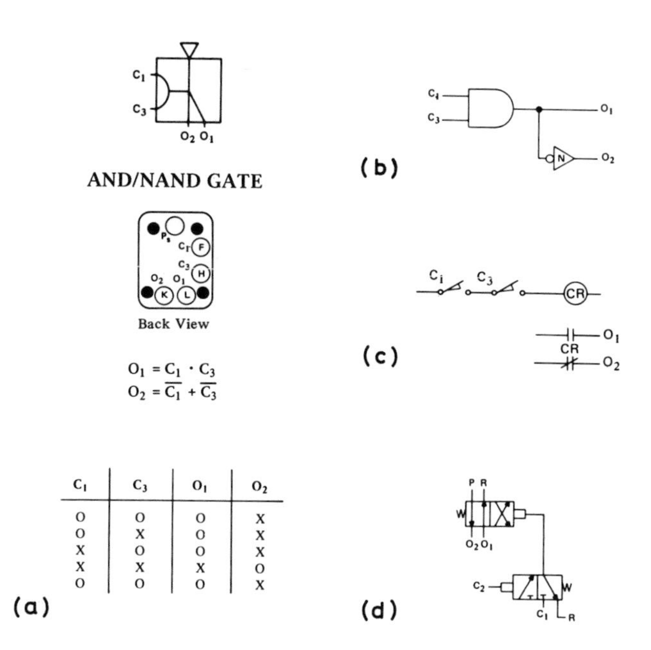

C_1	C_3	O_1	O_2
O	O	O	X
O	X	O	X
X	O	O	X
X	X	X	O
O	O	O	X

Figure 7.7
Fluidics AND/NAND gate: (a) fluidics module; (b) logic equivalent; (c) electrical equivalent; (d) pneumatic equivalent. (From *Fluidic Industrial Control Modules: Logic Components*, 1970, by Corning Glass Works. Used with permission of Corning Glass Works.)

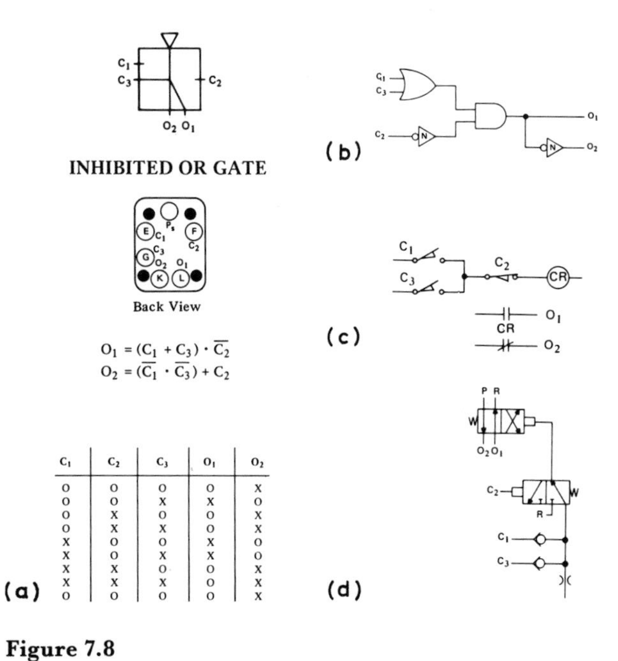

C_1	C_2	C_3	O_1	O_2
O	O	O	O	X
O	O	X	X	O
O	X	O	O	X
O	X	X	O	X
X	O	O	X	O
X	O	X	X	O
X	X	O	O	X
X	X	X	O	X
O	O	O	O	X

Figure 7.8
Fluidics Inhibited OR gate: (a) fluidics module; (b) logical equivalent; (c) electrical equivalent; (d) pneumatic equivalent. (From *Fluidic Industrial Control Modules: Logic Components*, 1970, by Corning Glass Works. Used with permission of Corning Glass Works.)

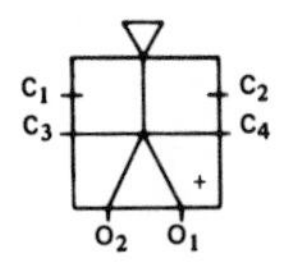

PREFERENCED FLIP-FLOP

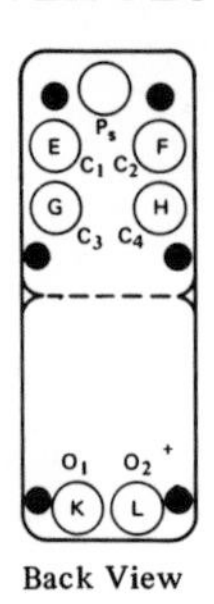

$O_1 = C_1 + C_3 + O_1 (\overline{C_2} \cdot \overline{C_4})$

$O_2 = C_2 + C_4 + O_2 (\overline{C_1} \cdot \overline{C_3})$

$(C_1 + C_3) \cdot (C_2 + C_4) =$ Indeterminate

P_s	C_1 or C_3	C_2 or C_4	O_1	O_2
O	O	O	O	O
X	O	O	X	O
X	O	X	O	X
X	O	O	O	X
X	X	O	X	O
X	O	O	X	O
X	X	X	Indeterminate	

Figure 7.9
Fluidics preferenced flipflop. (From *Fluidic Industrial Control Modules: Logic Components*, 1970, by Corning Glass Works. Used with permission of Corning Glass Works.)

either or both C_1 and C_3 from deflecting the signal jet into O_1. Therefore, $O_1 = (C_1 \vee C_3) \wedge \overline{C_2}$.

Figures 7.9 and 7.10 illustrate the preferenced flipflop and binary counter, operating on the same principles as the devices already discussed.

The preferenced flipflop is the same as a regular flipflop, in that O_1 goes on if C_1 or C_3 goes on and stays on until C_2 or C_4 goes on, and so forth. It differs from a regular flipflop in that when P_s is turned on, output O_1 goes on in the absence of any control signals. This ensures proper initialization when pressure is first turned on. Output is indeterminate if opposing inputs are on at the same time.

The binary counter consists of more complicated fluidics circuitry, but it is essentially a fluidics flipflop with *toggling*. It requires differential inputs C_3 and C_4. Toggling occurs once per input cycle; a C_4 positive level enables the C_3 input,

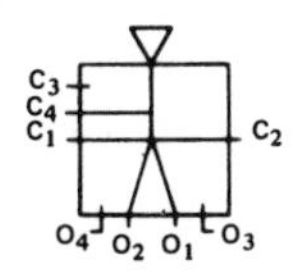

BINARY COUNTER

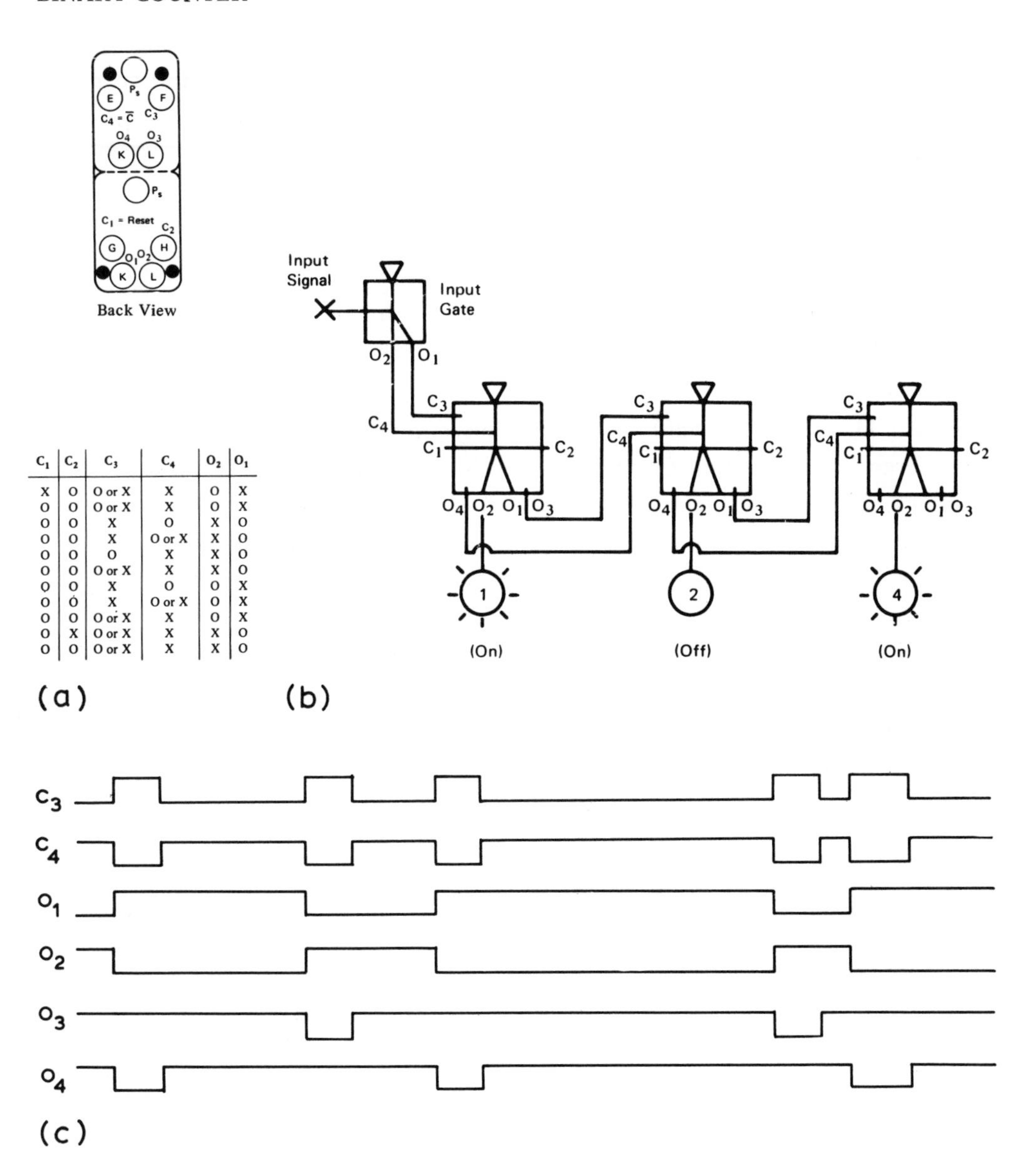

C_1	C_2	C_3	C_4	O_2	O_1
X	O	O or X	X	O	X
O	O	O or X	X	O	X
O	O	X	O	X	O
O	O	X	O or X	X	O
O	O	O	X	X	O
O	O	O or X	X	X	O
O	O	X	O	O	X
O	O	X	O or X	O	X
O	O	O or X	X	O	X
O	X	O or X	X	X	O
O	O	O or X	X	X	O

Figure 7.10
Fluidics binary counter: (a) fluidics module; (b) ripple-counter; (c) wave forms at outputs of units counter. (From *Fluidic Industrial Control Modules: Logic Components*, 1970, by Corning Glass Works. Used with permission of Corning Glass Works.)

such that when C_3 goes on, the flipflop toggles. At the C_3 on-transition, then, O_1 and O_2 reverse states. Also, C_1 and C_2 are available for *preset* and *clear* functions.

In multibit operation, O_3 and O_4 are used for driving other counters. Whereas O_1 and O_2 remain in their new states until the next toggle, O_3 and O_4 produce *pulses*. Output O_3 goes off for the duration of the C_3 on-state only when O_1 goes off, that is, on every other cycle. Output O_4 goes off for the duration of the C_3 on-state, only when O_2 goes off, that is, on alternate cycles. Thus, O_3 and O_4 go off alternately, and they cannot both be off at once. Their states may be expressed as follows:

$$O_3 = C_3 \overline{\wedge} O_2$$

$$O_4 = C_3 \overline{\wedge} O_1.$$

These provide very useful signals to drive successive binary counters, as illustrated in Figure 7.9a. Wave forms at inputs and outputs of the first counter are illustrated in Figure 7.9b.

Figure 7.11 illustrates a Schmitt trigger, consisting of an OR gate set up for a fixed reference pressure C at C_1 or C_2 and an input signal of variable pressure at the other input. The output switches when the control (input signal) pressure equals the reference pressure: $O_1(1)$ when $C_1 > C_2$; $O_2(1)$ when $C_2 > C_1$.

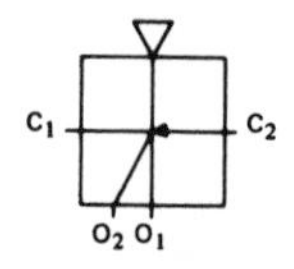

SCHMITT TRIGGER

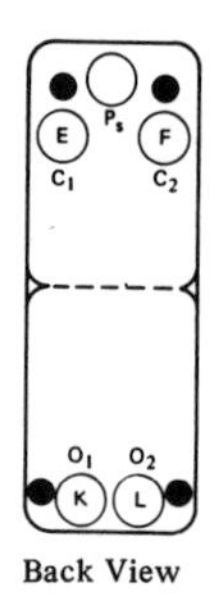

Back View

$O_1 = C_1 > C_2$
$O_2 = C_1 < C_2$

Figure 7.11
Fluidics Schmitt trigger. (From *Fluidic Industrial Control Modules: Logic Components*, 1970, by Corning Glass Works. Used with permission of Corning Glass Works.)

Corning's back-pressure switch (Figure 7.12) is similar in concept, except there is an internal connection between supply and control ports; thus, when the control port is blocked (that is, when the supply pressure is divided across the internal and external restrictors, and the external restrictor exceeds a certain value), the O_1 goes on. This can be a mechanism for providing manual control; if a button is used to block the air vented through S_1, the O_1 goes on for as long as the button is depressed.

The device, or variants of it, can be used as level detectors on liquid reservoirs, as can the Schmitt trigger. If the biasing port is tied to a tube venting into the bottom of the liquid reservoir, the back pressure will be a function of the height

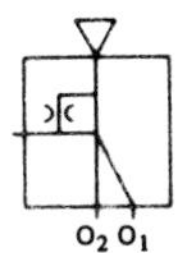

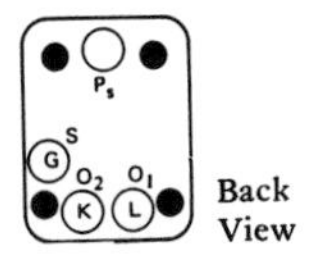

Figure 7.12
Fluidics back-pressure switch. (From *Fluidic Industrial Control Modules: Logic Components*, 1970, by Corning Glass Works. Used with permission of Corning Glass Works.)

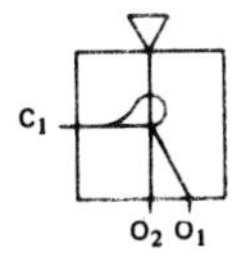

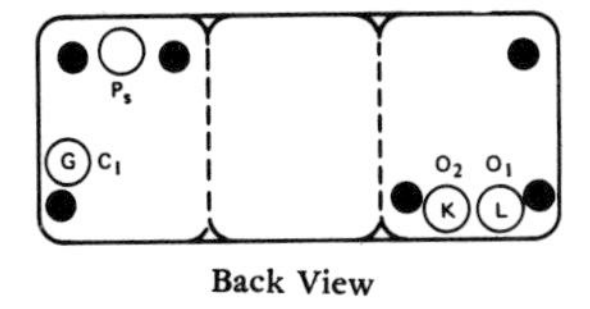

Figure 7.13
Fluidics one shot. (From *Fluidic Industrial Control Modules: Logic Components*, 1970, by Corning Glass Works. Used with permission of Corning Glass Works.)

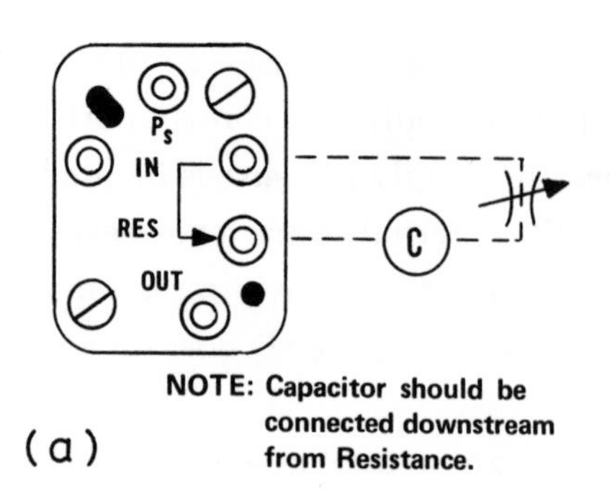

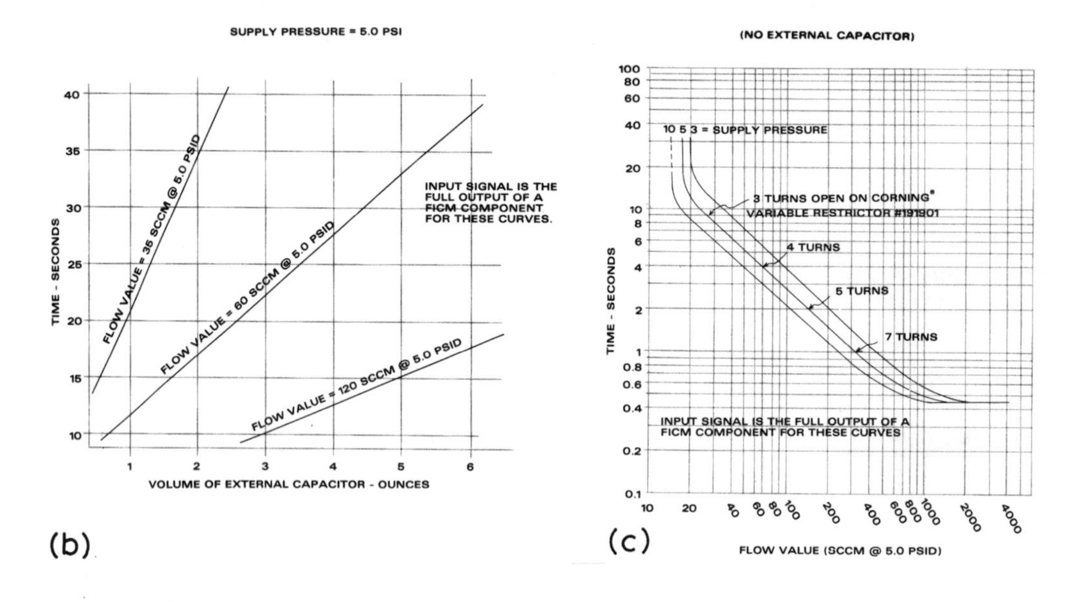

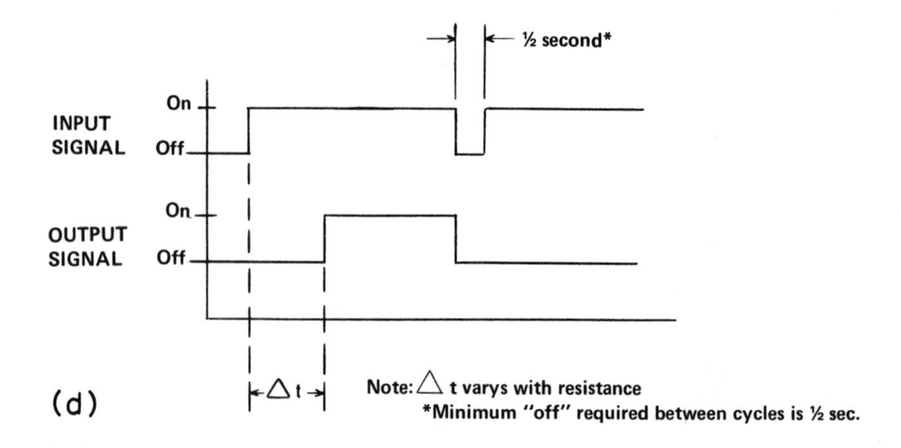

Figure 7.14
Fluidics time-delay relay: (a) fluidics module; (b) delay duration as a function of capacitance; (c) time delay as a function of flow; (d) input and output waveforms. (From *Fluidic Industrial Control Module Time Delay Relay*. (Advance Fluidics Product Data FAD-465), 1969, by Corning Glass Works. Used with permission of Corning Glass Works.)

of the liquid; such devices can be used, with variable reference pressures, as fairly sensitive regulators of liquid height.

A one shot is illustrated in Figure 7.13. The device is the familiar flipflop, except both control jets are derived from a single port, with the right jet traveling a longer distance than the left one. If a pressure pulse is applied suddenly to the C_1 input, a deflecting jet at the left appears before an equal pressure can reach the right deflector input. The O_1 output therefore goes on until the compensating pressure reaches the right control jet; at that time, the O_1 output goes off again, because there is no net lateral pressure differential. The delay is about 10 msec. If the C_1 pulse is shorter than 10 msec, the output will last for the duration of the C_1 pulse. If C_1 is longer than 10 msec, the output will last for the first 10 msec of the input pulse. A related device, the time delay relay, is illustrated in Figure 7.14. The output goes on some fixed or adjustable time after the input and goes off at the same time the input goes off.

Since the fanout of these devices is small, digital amplifiers with a fanout of 5 to 8 have been developed (Figure 7.15). For noninverting amplification, tie O_1 of the driver device to C_1, and tie O_2 to C_2.

The most convenient method of mounting these devices is on standardized mounting manifolds. This is not only a convenient and compact method, but it increases the fanout of most Corning modules.

The proper operation of fluidics devices requires reasonably well regulated supply pressure and very clean air. Compressed air is dehydrated with $CaCl_2$ and filtered through a millipore filter. Supply pressure regulation is introduced

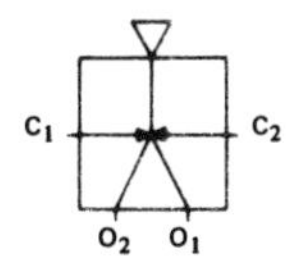

DIGITAL AMPLIFIER

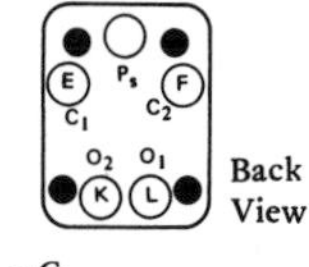

$O_1 = C_1$
$O_2 = C_2$
$(C_1 \cdot C_2) + (\overline{C_1} \cdot \overline{C_2}) =$ Indeterminate

Figure 7.15
Fluidics digital amplifier. (From *Fluidic Industrial Control Modules: Logic Components*, 1970, by Corning Glass Works. Used with permission of Corning Glass Works.)

after filtering. The degree of purity required, the supply pressure, and regulation depend on the devices used and the manufacturer. Corning and other manufacturers supply contamination indicators, which are useful for the detection of eventual collection of contaminants in the modules.

For complex circuits that are to be produced on a large scale, integrated circuit technology is available. These devices, consisting of stacked laminar modules or custom-designed modules, are expensive in small lots, however, and are not economical for the research laboratory except for widely used integrated circuits sold by some manufacturers.

7.3 Analog Fluidics

To date, there has been little application of analog fluidics. The major drawbacks in fluidics analog applications are the low gain of proportional amplifiers, limited frequency range and dynamic pressure range, cross-coupling effects among analog devices, and the limited range of values of fluidics resistors, capacitors, and inductances. Since consumer and military applications do exist and since these promote the greatest incentive to industry, we can expect improvements in analog fluidics. Certainly we may expect analog and digital fluidics control to appear in appropriate consumer devices, ranging from automobiles to washing machines. Fluidics circuits are already used in weapons of war. A major impetus in the development of fluidics has been, regrettably, the need for backup control systems in guided missiles that would be reliable in the presence of mechanical vibration or attempts to "jam" the control system with RF interference. On a saner note, fluidics is being used to control anaesthesia and respirator units, with resulting portability and independence from a less and less reliable power source, electricity. Undoubtedly, these will become popular in hospitals in the large cities within blackout and brownout zones in the next few years.

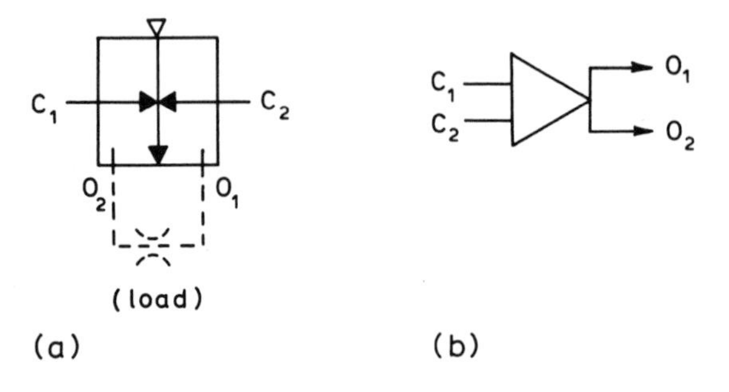

Figure 7.16
Fluidics analog amplifiers: (a) proportional amplifier symbol; (b) operational amplifier symbol.

A fluidics analog amplifier is built in much the same fashion as a fluidics flip-flop, with the difference that the Coanda effect is minimized, and the momentum-transfer effect is enhanced. The symbol, Figure 7.16a, emphasizes the difference from a digital amplifier or flipflop. The jet is split between O_2 and O_1, in a proportion that is linearly related to the ratio of pressures of C_2 and C_1. High-gain amplifiers, designed for use as operational amplifiers, are symbolized by the usual differential op amp symbol, as in Figure 7.16b. These devices are usually built by cascading several proportional amplifiers in an integrated circuit. Within the limitations of low gain, poor frequency response, interaction among components connected to the same supply, and audio "crosstalk" caused by vibrations, these devices can be used in much the same manner as electronic op amps.

7.4 Fluidics Sensors and Interfaces

A large variety of sensors and interfaces is available. Fluidics-operated electronic switches provide electrical output, and relay-operated fluidics switches provide the inverse function. Fluidics pushbutton switches, selector switches, and visual indicators find use in circuits such as the ones to be described in Chapter 8 on stimulation techniques. Proximity sensors, using back pressure in a jet of air, find most use in industrial applications but may also prove useful in neurophysiological work. As a rule, interface and sensor devices can be found or devised that parallel most electronic devices in this category.

We will discuss only those interface devices that will be used in fluidics circuits in later chapters. These include the Schmitt trigger, already discussed, manual pushbuttons, toggle switches and rotary selector switches, on-off indicators, and fluidics interface valves.

A variety of fluidics switches is illustrated in Figure 7.17. These devices are entirely analogous to electric switches, except for higher resistances and capacitances in their on-states, due to the properties of fluidics passive components in general, a subject discussed earlier. The devices are simple valves enabling or disabling air-flow.

Fluidics indicators, such as those illustrated in Figure 7.18a, are used to provide visual or electrical indication of "on" or "off" pressure states of fluidics devices. The visual indicators consist of light-weight colored disks that are pushed against gravity or some other source of passive back resistance, into a viewing window when the monitored signal is a logical 1. The electrical fluidics-operated switches (Figure 7.18b) are usually simple low-force switches driven by diaphragms, in normally-on or normally-off configuration, using a back-force derived from the diaphragm's elasticity to hold the quiescent on or off position in the absence of a fluidics pressure.

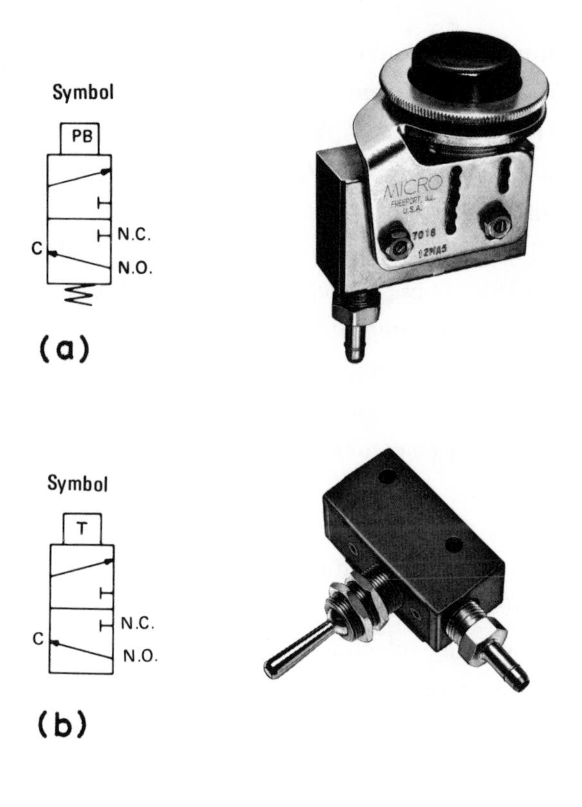

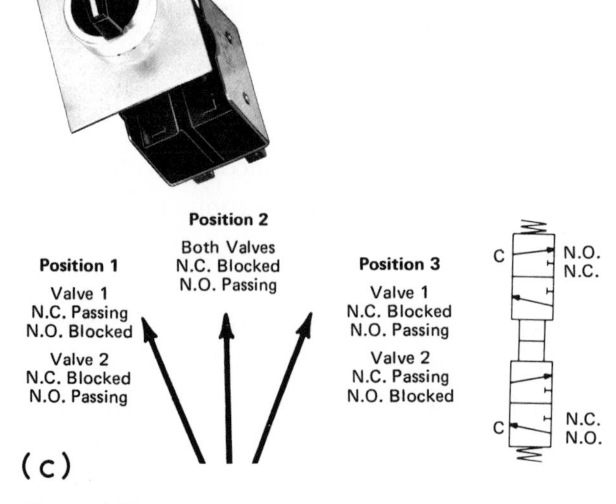

Figure 7.17
Fluidic switches: (a) pushbutton (manufacturer: Micro Switch); (b) toggle (manufacturer: Mead Fluid Dynamics); (c) 3-position selector (manufacturer: Micro Switch). (From *Fluidic Industrial Control Modules: Sensors and Interfaces*, 1971, by Corning Glass Works. Used with permission of Corning Glass Works.)

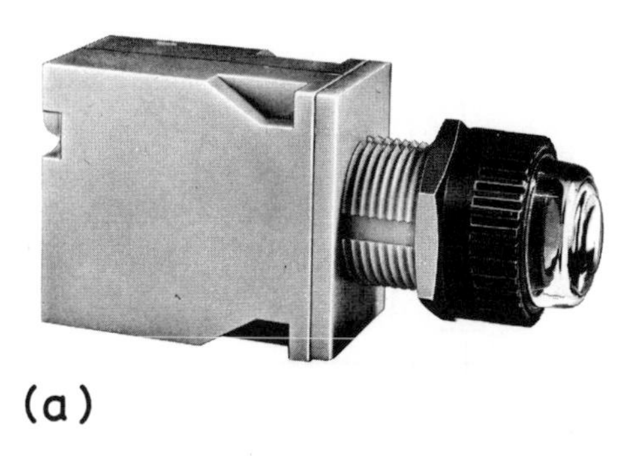

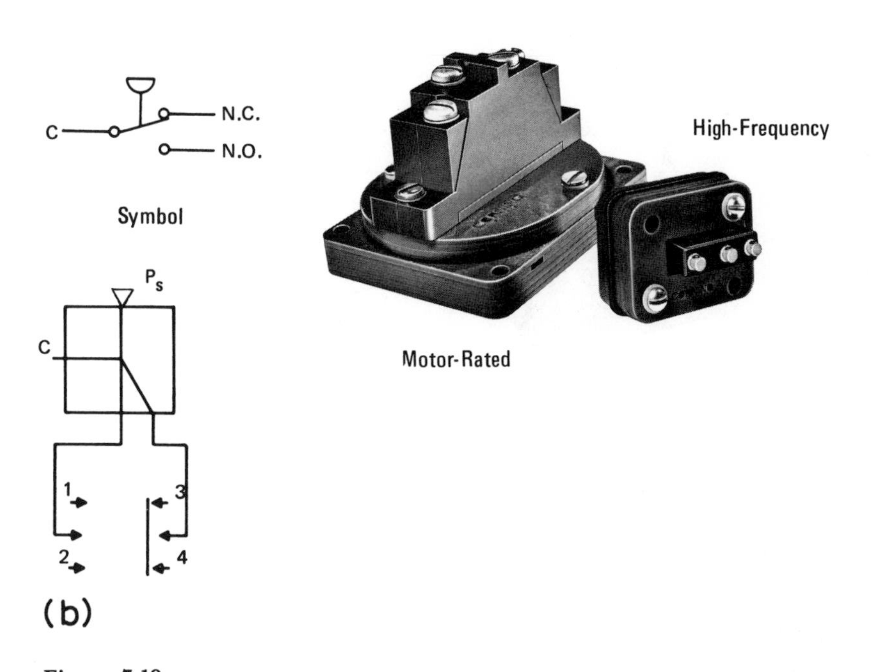

Figure 7.18
Fluidics (a) logic level indicator (manufacturer: Micro Switch); (b) pressure-to-electric switch interface (manufacturer: Corning Glass Works). (From *Fluidic Industrial Control Modules: Sensors and Interfaces*, 1971, by Corning Glass Works. Used with permission of Corning Glass Works.)

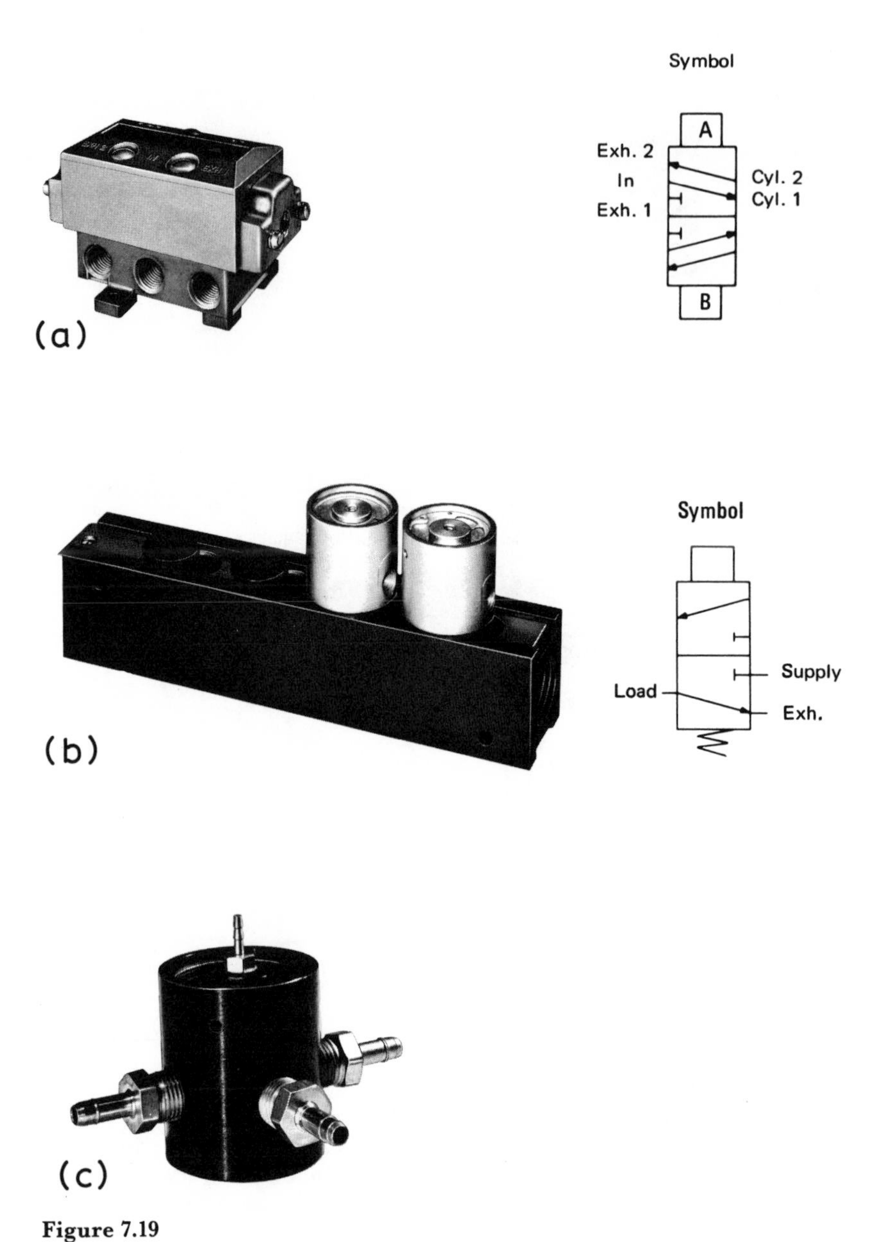

Figure 7.19
Fluidic interface valves: (a) Allcon Products interface valve; (b) Fluidamp® interface valve (manufacturer: Northeast Fluidics); (c) Corning interface valve. (From Fluidic *Industrial Control Modules: Sensors and Interfaces*, 1971, by Corning Glass Works. Used with permission of Corning Glass Works.)

Fluidic interface valves are illustrated in Figure 7.19. These devices use the relatively small pressures at output ports of fluidics logic modules to control valve position, using diaphragms to provide quiescent condition, mechanical coupling to the valve, and isolation from the valved pressure and flow. These devices are particularly useful when using fluidics logic to switch the flow of gases other than the compressed air or nitrogen used to power the fluidics logic, or to control gases at pressures outside the range of permissible fluidics supply or signal pressures. They must be driven with one digital amplifier per interface valve.

Interfaces also exist for pneumatic and hydraulic applications. Undoubtedly, pneumatic logic devices will be devised that will allow direct control of large pressures and flows of less highly purified gases, and hydraulic control devices will also be evolved, permitting direct control of liquid flows. We will examine the use of fluidics in the sections on gustatory and olfactory stimulation, in Chapter 8.

Selected References

Conway, Arthur (ed). 1971. *A Guide to Fluidics.* N.Y.: Elsevier.

Corning Glass Works. 1969. *Corning Fluidics Industrial Control Module Time Delay Relay.* (Advance Fluidics Product Data FAD-465). Corning, N.Y.: Corning Glass Works.

Corning Glass Works. 1970. *Fluidic Industrial Control Modules: Logic Components.* Corning, N.Y.: Corning Glass Works.

Corning Glass Works. 1971. *Fluidic Industrial Control Modules: Sensors and Interfaces.* Corning, N.Y.: Corning Glass Works.

Doherty, Martin C. 1968. "Applying fluidic operational amplifiers." 23rd Annual ISA Conference. G.E. Fluidics reprint 6165.

Imperial-Eastman Corporation. 1966. *Fluidics Systems Design Guide.* Chicago, Ill.: Fluidonics Division, Imperial-Eastman Corporation.

Shinners, Stanley M. 1967. *Techniques of System Engineering.* N.Y.: McGraw-Hill Book Co.

Woodson, C. W. 1968. "AC fluidics." Western Electronic Show and Convention, August, 1968. Schenectady, N.Y.: General Electric Specialty Fluidics Operation.

8 STIMULATION TECHNIQUES

Paul B. Brown,
Leonard Smithline, and
Bruce Halpern

In order to study the transducing or integrating function of some part of the peripheral or central nervous system, it is usually necessary to perturb that portion of the system with an appropriate stimulus. Such input may be in the form of adequate stimulation of a receptor or electrical or chemical stimulation of some portion of the nervous system. We will consider some of the techniques in use today and propose a few that, at least theoretically, should constitute an improvement in the controllability of stimulation over the present state of the art. Emphasis will be on electronic control and quantitation of stimuli, using the simplest means available. Although the physical principles behind the operation of the various transducers will not be examined, the behavior of these devices will be described in sufficient detail to allow the reader to modify intelligently the specific designs presented.

8.1 Electrical Stimulation

Electrical stimulation methods may be divided, according to the structures stimulated, into two main classes: intracellular and extracellular methods. The former have the advantage of enabling the experimenter to activate selected single elements in the central nervous system, but the technical difficulties inherent in intracellular stimulation severely limit the utility of the method. Extracellular techniques generally suffer from the disadvantage of activating poorly identified elements except in a few specific preparations. On the other hand, extracellular electric stimulation is much simpler to accomplish. The technical problems involved in controlling such stimuli are all related to the quantification of the stimulus, for purposes of calculation of the physical parameters involved in the generation of the membrane response as well as for purposes of reliably repeating the same stimulus under varying conditions. Stimulus parameters that must be controlled for pulsatile stimulation consist of pulse timing, duration, and amplitude. Multipulse control requires the programming of numerous additional parameters all at one time.

The amplitude of an electrical stimulus is perhaps best monitored by recording the depolarization of the stimulated electrical membrane. However in most situations, this is not possible and some other measure of the stimulus must be selected, to provide quantitation. When stimulating via an intracellular electrode (Figure 8.1a), all the current applied passes through the electrode and the cell, but only a fraction of the applied voltage is dropped across the cell. This fraction is variable, depending on electrode and cell resistance. It is not surprising, then, that the best stimulus quantification is obtained when a so-called *constant-current stimulator* is used. This device, consisting of a voltage-to-current converter, produces a current that is proportional to the voltage applied at its input, regardless of the load, within its operating limits. Thus, regardless of electrode resistance, the current applied to the cell is a fixed multiple of the control voltage. Current control is limited by output voltage range: A device with ± 10 V output limits cannot deliver more than $\pm 1\ \mu$A through a 10 MΩ microelectrode. For this reason, selection of an appropriate constant-current device should include specification of required current, anticipated electrode and cell resistances, and calculation of required output voltage range; using Ohm's law, we have

$$\pm V_{\text{max}} = \pm I_{\text{max}} \times (R_{\text{electrode}} + R_{\text{cell}})_{\text{max}}.$$

Generally, a ± 100 V limit is adequate, except for some intracellular muscle stimulation where high currents are required to depolarize the large areas of membrane involved.

There is another application for constant-current devices: passing current through a microelectrode to deposit dye from a micropipette or metal ions from a metal microelectrode. Current is obviously the parameter that should be controlled, because

$$\text{number of ions} = \frac{Q}{\text{valence}} = \frac{\int i\,dt}{\text{valence}},$$

and the amount of dye or metal ion is thus roughly proportional (the presence of

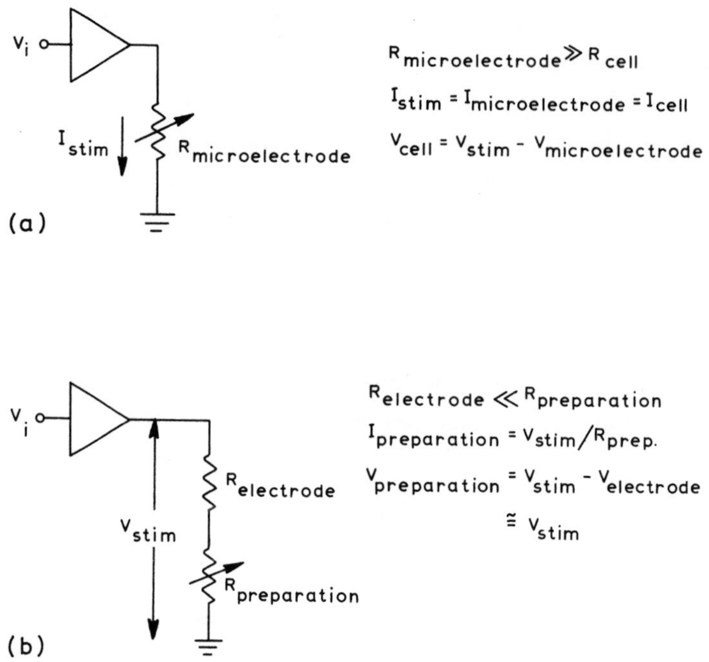

(a)

$$R_{microelectrode} \gg R_{cell}$$

$$I_{stim} = I_{microelectrode} = I_{cell}$$

$$V_{cell} = V_{stim} - V_{microelectrode}$$

(b)

$$R_{electrode} \ll R_{preparation}$$

$$I_{preparation} = V_{stim}/R_{prep.}$$

$$V_{preparation} = V_{stim} - V_{electrode} \cong V_{stim}$$

Figure 8.1
Electrical stimulation through microelectrode and gross electrode. (a) Microelectrode stimulation requires current-source stimulus for reproducible stimulus with variable microelectrode resistance. (b) Gross electrode stimulation requires voltage-source stimulation for reproducibility with variable preparation resistance.

other ions and electrode reactions may prevent perfect linearity) to current times duration. Variations of electrode resistance will not affect these parameters, within the operating range of the current source, a factor that is important during passage of marking current, because electrode resistance may change considerably during the marking process. Generally, dyes are anions and metal ions are always cations; therefore, the electrode should be cathode or anode, respectively, for proper marking of electrode location. Note that, for most of the devices in this book, the input stage can only tolerate $\pm V_{CC}$, or ± 10–15 V. For higher voltages, reed switches can be inserted in the headstage to switch in the marking current circuit and switch out the headstage input during current application.

When stimulating through electrodes whose impedance relative to the tissue impedance is negligible, it is generally more appropriate to control the stimulus voltage, as can be seen from the equivalent circuit of Figure 8.1b. The variable impedance of the preparation (for example, a peripheral nerve) results in a variable current through each element (for example, each nerve fiber) if a constant current is applied. However if a constant voltage is applied, that does not vary as a function of tissue impedance, then the voltage across, and current through, each element will be less subject to variation. Thus, the appropriate stimulator for such an application is a device whose output voltage does not vary over the anticipated range of resistive loads. Since these loads can vary from perhaps 500 Ω to several megohms, the voltage source should have a current capacity of ±30 mA if output limits of ±15 V are specified. Once again, output voltage limits and current limits should be calculated using Ohm's law:

$$\pm I_{max} = \frac{IV_{max}}{(R_{preparation})_{min}}.$$

Notice that the *minimum* preparation resistance is used to determine the maximum current requirement, since it appears in the denominator.

A voltage source can also be used for electrophoresis of dyes through axons, a technique that has recently been developed and that should become very popular with time. The applied voltage is the appropriate parameter for such electrophoresis, because the ion migration rate is a direct function of voltage gradient rather than applied current.

In general, when recording is accomplished with high-gain techniques, it is necessary to ensure that the artifact due to stimulation does not swamp the recording. Differential amplification is usually employed, but this is only half the solution; an electrically isolated stimulus is also usually required. Figure 8.2 compares the equivalent circuits using isolated electrical stimulation and a common-indifferent arrangement.

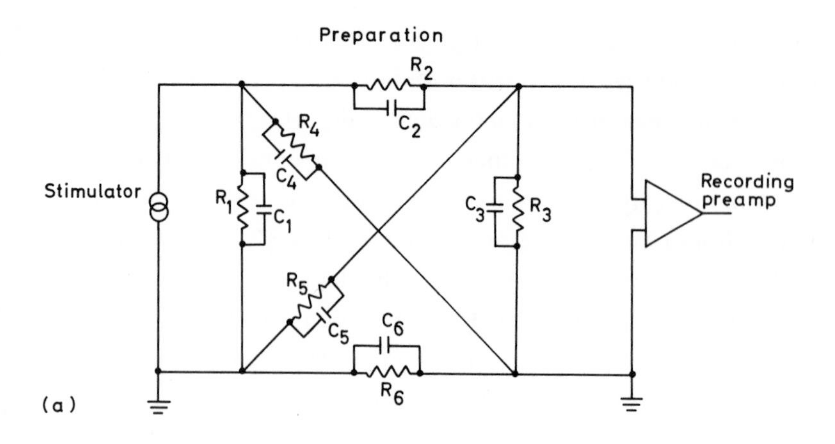

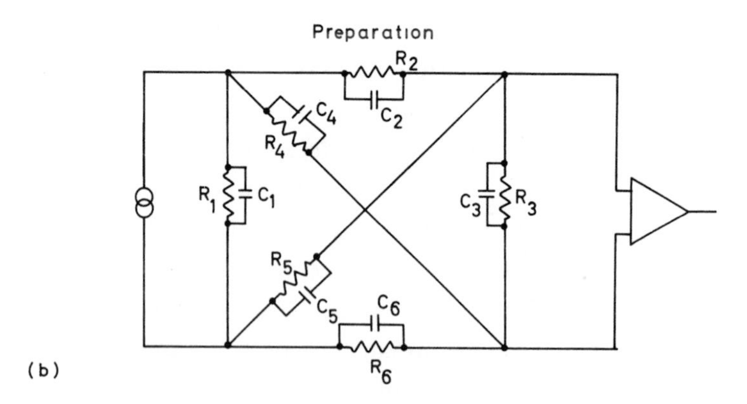

Figure 8.2
Comparison of isolated and ground-referenced stimulator in ground-referenced recording system. (a) Common-indifferent (ground): R_6 and C_6 are shorted, unbalancing "bridge." (b) Floating stimulator and recording input: R_6 and C_6 are not shorted, "bridge" is more easily balanced.

The equivalent circuits through the preparation are indicated in an over-simplified fashion by the resistor-capacitor network. The network can be recognized as a distributed *bridge* circuit, which is balanced as long as

$$R_1 = R_3, \quad R_2 = R_4, \quad R_5 = R_6,$$

$$C_1 = C_3, \quad C_2 = C_4, \quad C_5 = C_6.$$

The recording device will see no differential input due to the stimulus as long as the bridge is balanced (Figure 8.2a). However, if the indifferent leads of the stimulator and recorder are connected together, either as a common ground or even as a common floating indifferent, the bridge is clearly unbalanced, and a large differential voltage can appear at the input to the recorder (Figure 8.1b), due to the shorting of R_6 and C_6. This can result not only in a large artifact but also in a recovery time from the overload at the input that outlasts the stimulus by several orders of magnitude, as the distributed capacitances in the preparation, recording leads, and the recording amplifier itself discharge.

The circuits of Figure 8.2 are actually gross oversimplifications, because there is in reality a much greater complexity of current paths, and there are distributed inductances as well. Balancing the bridge is difficult under the best of situations; often it is necessary to try different electrode arrangements to determine the optimum geometry. Generally, it is best to have the recording leads as close together as possible, and as far from the stimulating leads as possible. Keep the stimulating leads close together as well. Placing preparation ground between stimulating and recording sites is often helpful.

It is necessary to devise a means of isolating the two circuits. Both devices could be run by batteries, but this is an expensive solution. Generally the entire recording apparatus is powered by a transformer-driven, ground-referenced power supply. A similar technique can be used for powering an electrical stimulator, without referencing to ground; batteries can be used if anticipated current requirements are not too great. The resistance between the signal and ground should be at least two orders of magnitude greater than the resistance from the stimulating electrode through the preparation to ground. This is easily accomplished by any of a number of different methods. The capacitance to ground must also be very low, say 10 pF or less. This means that the isolation should be accomplished as close as possible to the stimulation site; power must be derived from batteries if the capacitive links to ground via an ac supply's transformer and power leads are to be avoided. As a rule of thumb, a floating ac supply is adequate for stimulation when differential low-gain recording is used, such as in intracellular microelectrode mode, but batteries are still the best power source for a stimulus isolator when high-gain recording is used.

Stimulus isolation is not particularly helpful when stimulating through a recording microelectrode, except in instances where the recording circuit (including the preparation) is isolated from ground for some reason and hence the stimulator must be isolated as well, or when the stimulus source must be attached in series between electrode and amplifier.

Ground-referenced devices are usually used to generate the desired stimulation wave form, and this wave form is then transmitted to the floating output stage of the electrical stimulator. Radio frequency coupling has been employed by using the stimulus wave form to amplitude modulate the carrier at the ground-referenced transmitter and by demodulating at the receiver, transmitting across a small air

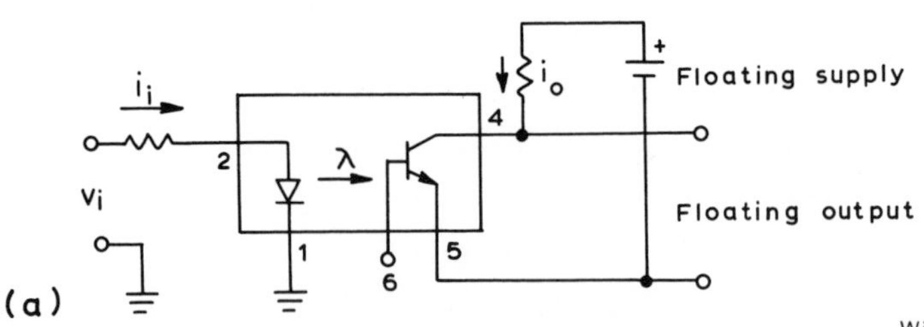

With an I_F of 20 mA, the opto-isolator has a minimum current transfer ratio (CTR) of 20% with a V_{CE} of 10 volts.

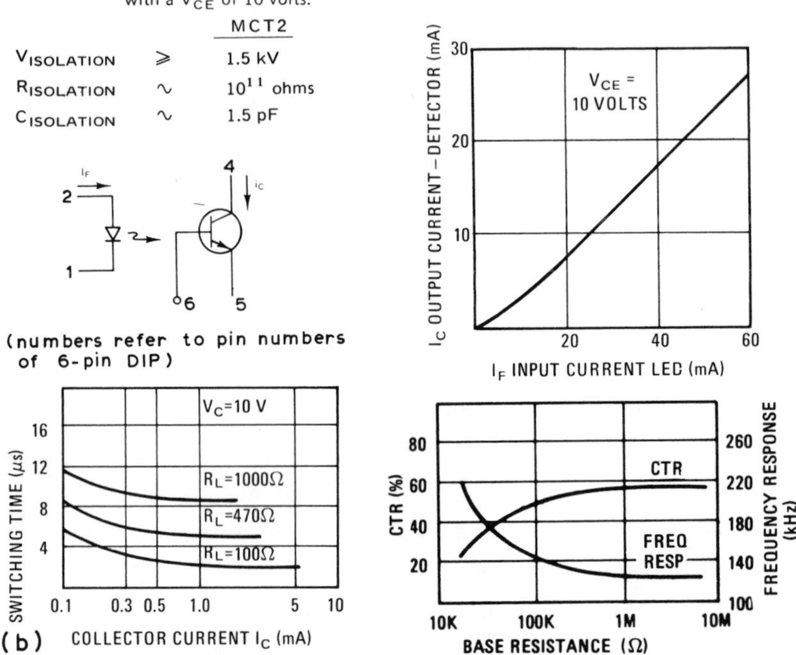

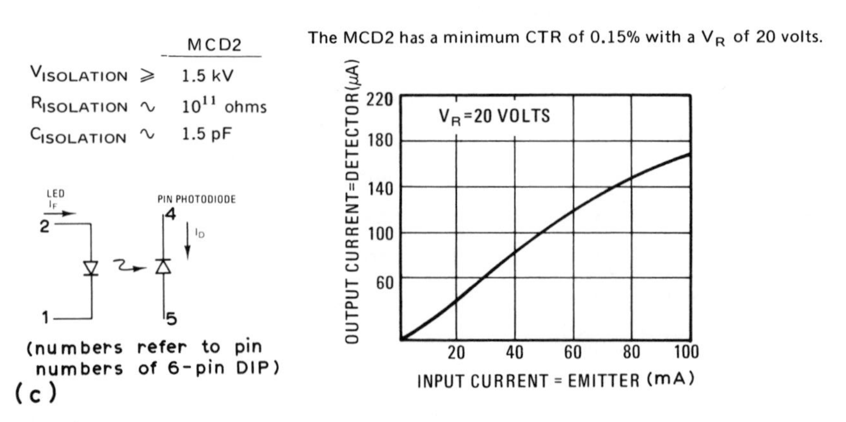

Figure 8.3
Opto-isolators. (a) Simple proportional-output optical coupler. (b) Characteristics of Monsanto MCT-2 opto-isolator. (c) Electrical characteristics of MCD-2 opto-isolator. (Sections b, c, from *GaAslite Tips*, 1970, by Monsanto Electronic Special Products. Used with permission of Monsanto Electronic Special Products.)

gap. The entire circuit must be well shielded. Optical coupling has also been used. MOSFETS can provide the same degree of isolation as optical couplers, $>10^{11}$ Ω and <10 pF relative to ground, but they are less easily applied, usually require at least two separate supply voltages, and generally do not allow as large a voltage differential between input (gate) and output (source-drain) circuits.

Figure 8.3a illustrates the use of a photon coupler in driving a floating stimulator. The positive pulse at the input generates a current through the light-emitting diode (LED), which emits light. The light causes the phototransistor (PT) to conduct, decreasing the output voltage. Commercially available optical isolators include the LED and the PT in a light-tight can the size of an integrated circuit. The electrical characteristics of the Monsanto MCT-2 opto-isolator are illustrated in Figure 8.3b.

Figure 8.3c illustrates the details of an opto-isolator using a photodiode (PD) as the receiver, the MCD-2 (Monsanto). When compared with the PT receiver, the PD has the disadvantage of lower current transfer ratio (I_o/I_i = CTR) and the advantage of higher frequency response.

The output current, which is the relevant parameter in intracellular stimulation and iontophoretic injection and for deposition of metal ions from stainless steel electrodes, is dependent on the output voltage and the load impedance, including the electrode impedance. Since the electrode impedance is often highly variable and may even change during the stimulus, an output stage is usually added to regulate the current. There are several techniques for achieving this, but they are all means of increasing the effective output impedance of the device to well above the load impedance (Figure 8.4).

If a genuine high impedance is used for R_o, V_o must be very large. This is one possible approach. Generally a 10^8 to 10^9 ohm resistor is used for microelectrode work. Instead we will use a feedback technique to control the output current directly and to simulate a high output impedance.

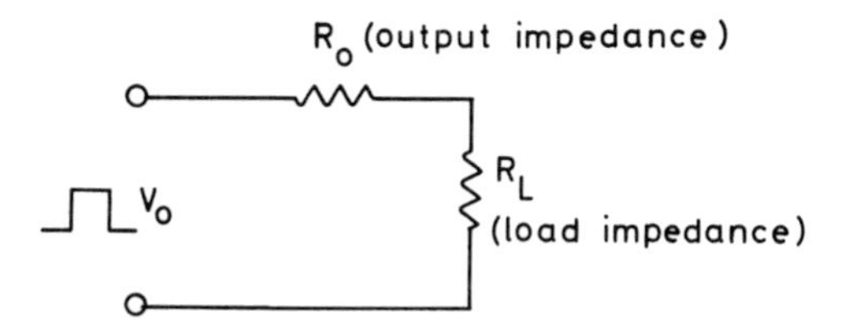

Figure 8.4
Current source output impedance.

$$I_o = \frac{V_o}{(R_o + R_L)} = \frac{V_o}{R_o}, \qquad \text{if } R_o \gg R_L.$$

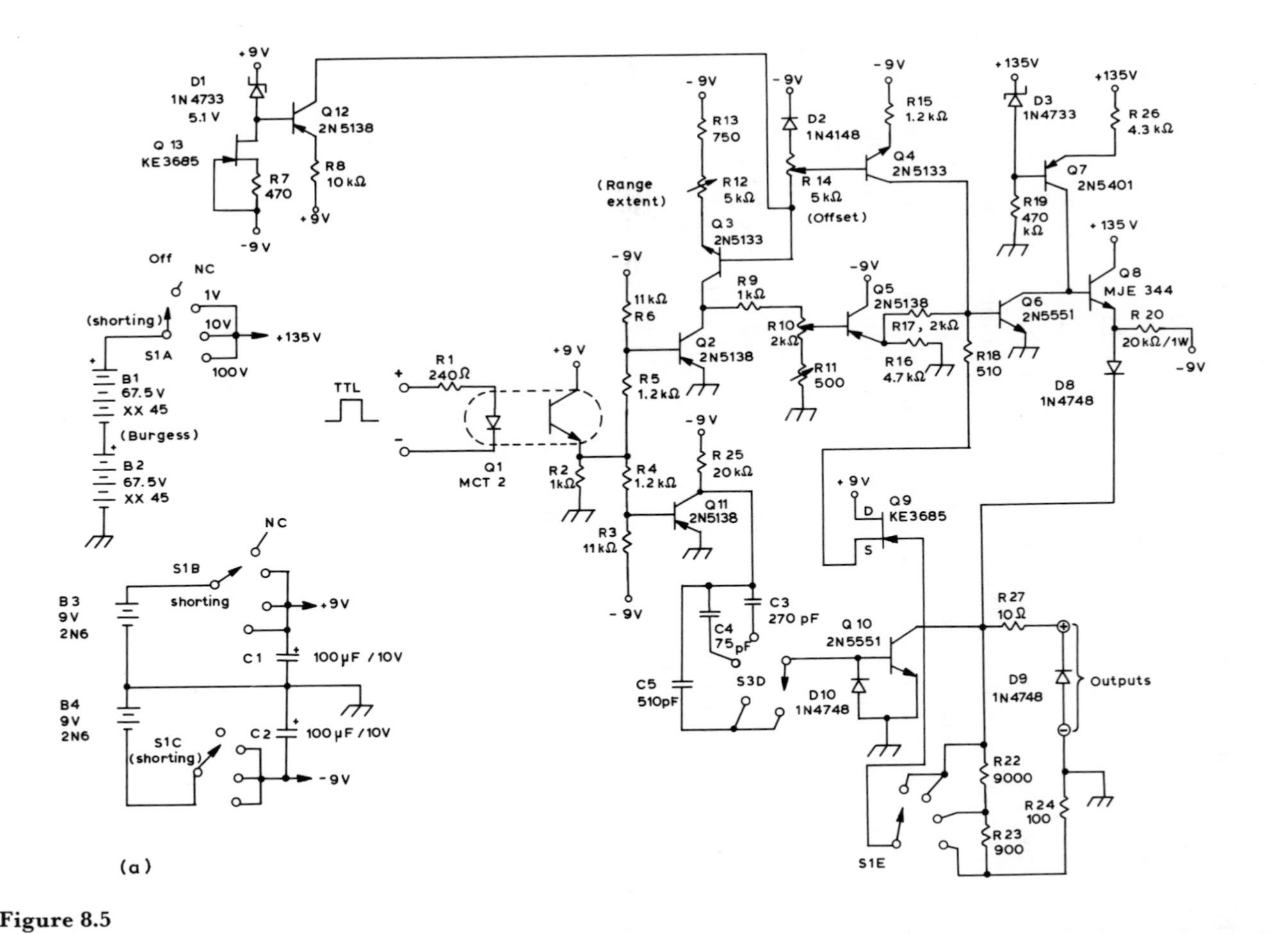

Figure 8.5
Stimulus isolation units. (a) Digital version produces pulse of preselected voltage, whose time-course matches that of input TTL pulse. (b) Analog isolator produces output wave form, either bipolar (±50 V range) or monopolar (0–100 V range), which is proportional to input wave form. Current-source and voltage-source modes can be selected and battery output test circuits indicate failure to produce desired stimulus due to overdriven input or output, or weak batteries.

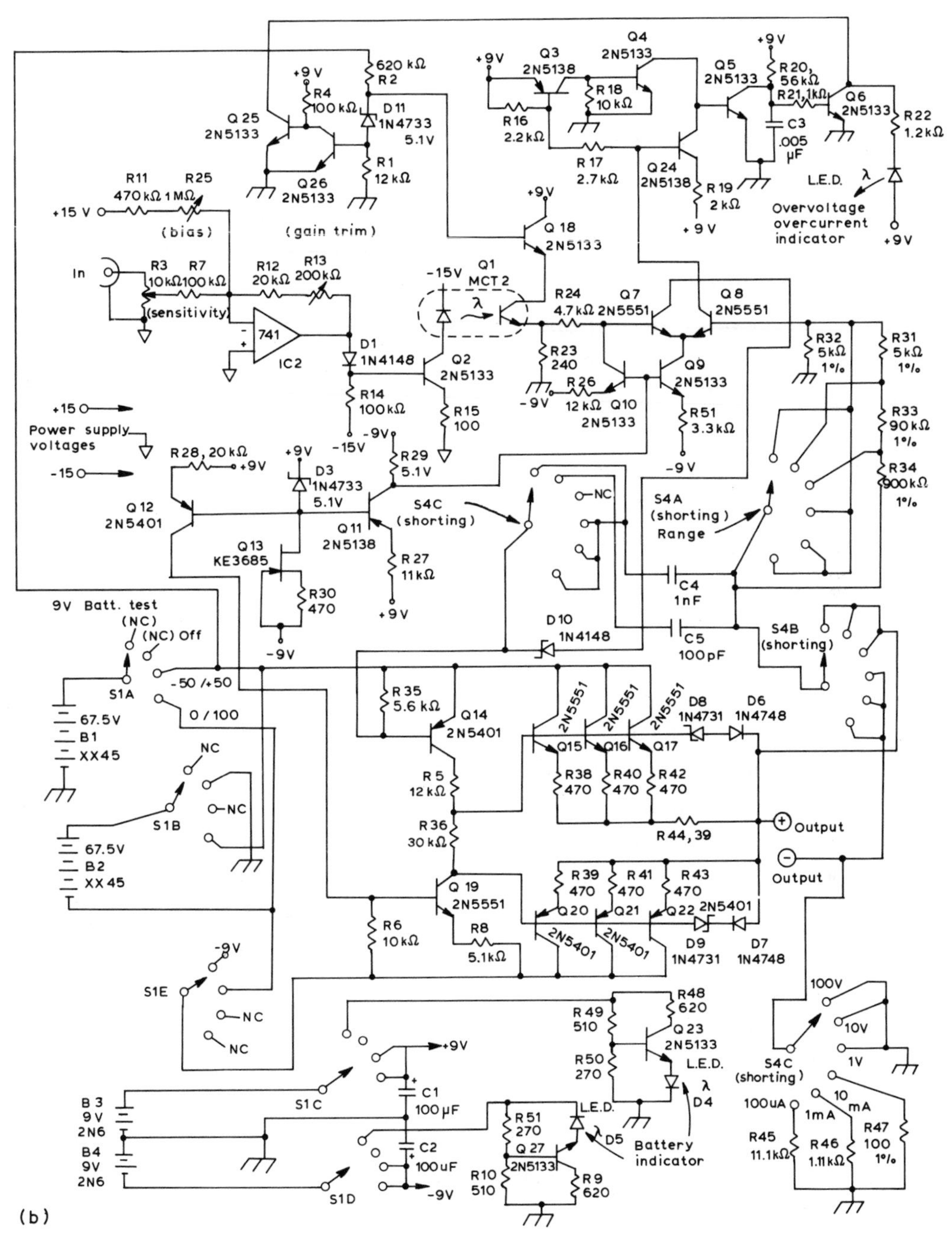

Figure 8.5 (continued)

There are presently no IC designs for constant-current stimulus isolation units available. Lansing Research Corporation has kindly granted us permission to reproduce the schematics of discrete-component digital and analog isolation units, in Figure 8.5a and b, respectively. Frederic Haer, Grass, and ORTEC also make similar devices.

The output of the digital isolator can take on only two possible values, zero and an adjustable monopolar voltage: the stimulus level. The analog isolator will reproduce an input wave form. Both isolators have attendant advantages:

1. The digital isolator is simpler and less expensive.
2. It requires less quiescent current, and therefore batteries will last longer.
3. It can produce pulses with shorter rise and fall times than can the analog isolator.
4. The analog isolator can produce a much wider variety of wave forms and has controlled-current output mode as well as a voltage output mode.
5. The wave forms out of the analog and digital isolators are controlled, as much as possible, in the ground-referenced portion of the isolators, thus reducing experimenter-preparation interactions.

First, consider the digital isolator (Figure 8.5a). A positive voltage at the input causes a current to flow in the LED (emitter portion) of an opto-isolator. This is optically coupled to a phototransistor and current flows in the collector-emitter circuit. Note that no current flows when the input voltage is zero (*idling*). This is an important consideration, for batteries have a much shorter life and higher cost than comparable ac supplies.

The output from Q_1 is amplified by a *squaring amplifier* Q_2, used to gate a controlled current from Q_3. An emitter follower, Q_5, serves as an input buffer for the voltage amplifier, composed of Q_{6-9}. Selection of the feedback circuit R_{22-24} controls the gain of the high voltage amplifier. The amplifier can only provide unidirectional current flow. This is sufficient for resistive loads. When energy is stored in the load (for example, capacitors), it is necessary to provide a reverse current path for negative-going voltage transitions (even though the voltage level itself never goes negative). This is the function of the transient return path Q_{10} and Q_{11}.

One underlying goal of the circuit design is low current drain for long battery life and insensitivity to supply voltage changes so that even as the batteries wear out it is not necessary to consider them useless until they are quite thoroughly derated. To this end circuits have been designed that draw very little idle current. The periods of heavy current drain occur only when the input goes high. Also regulator circuits have been added to decrease the sensitivity to supply voltage changes. This is primarily the function of Q_8, D_1 and D_3. The 9 V batteries can derate to approximately 5 V before the circuits fail. At the current levels typical for this circuit (2–4 mA) a reasonably small 9 V battery will last approximately

400 hr with continuous use. The XX45 67 V batteries will permit full 100 V output for about 200 hr but will permit operations at lower voltages for considerably longer periods.

The analog isolator (Figure 8.5b) has a design that is similar to the digital one. Signals are interfaced to the LED using an op amp. Now the operating point is crucial. The amplifier now consists of a differential amplifier Q_7, Q_8, and Q_9, driving a complementary class B amplifier, Q_{17-22}. Again this is a technique for efficient operation. This amplifier can provide bipolar outputs. Once again, the supplies are regulated via Q_{10-13}, and D_3 and D_{11}.

This particular circuit has three additional features:

1. It can provide current source outputs.
2. It has built-in current limiting. The output current is not allowed to exceed 13 mA.
3. There are built-in facilities for checking the batteries. The 9 V batteries are checked manually. The high voltage XX45 batteries are checked continually while in operation. Only when they are not strong enough for the specific task at hand is a failure indicated by LED D_2 lighting and signaling failure.

Monitoring stimulus current through a microelectrode can raise difficulties whenever very high voltages are used, and the monitor must not interfere with recording. Figure 8.6 illustrates two techniques. The simple circuit of Figure 8.6a is adequate for situations in which stray capacitance does not constitute a significant return path, bypassing the series monitor resistor. Note the usefulness of an isolated stimulator in this circuit. To directly monitor the current in the path to the microelectrode, it is possible to use an opto-isolator to overcome the disadvantage of the large differential between the current-path voltage and the recording reference, as well as to maintain a high degree of isolation from ground. However, this technique only works for relatively large currents. By using a FET-input op amp with low leakage and bias current (say, less than 50 pA) a resolution of less than 0.1 μA should be possible. Keep in mind the fact that the stimulator voltage must not exceed the input limit of the recording amplifier. Although high-voltage FET-input op amps are available, they are usually expensive and large in size. A phototransistor opto-isolator will provide a higher current transfer ratio and enhanced sensitivity at the cost of increased rise time. Presently, new opto-isolators with much higher CTR are appearing on the market.

8.2 Mechanical Stimulation

There are two types of transducers, each with its unique advantages and disadvantages, generally used for mechanical stimulation: *piezoelectric* and *dynamic elements*. The former are characterized by high-frequency capability, small size,

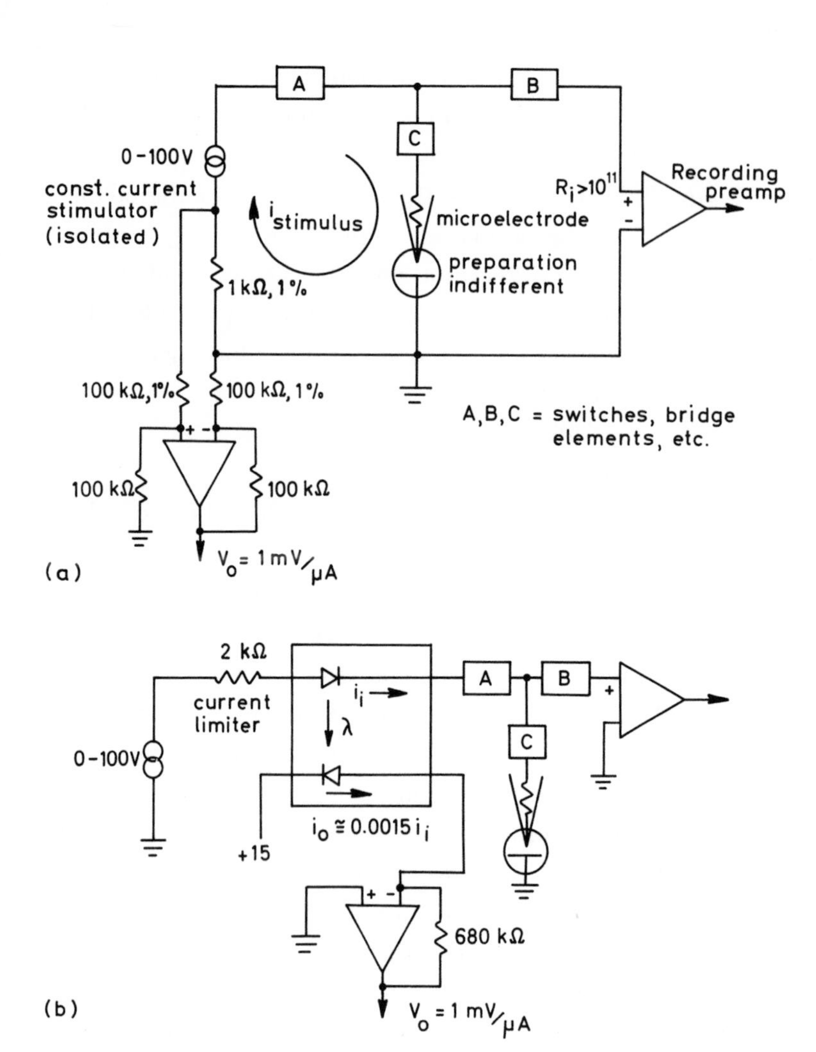

Figure 8.6
Current monitors for high-voltage stimulation via recording electrode. (a) Monitor in return path. (b) Monitor in electrode circuit.

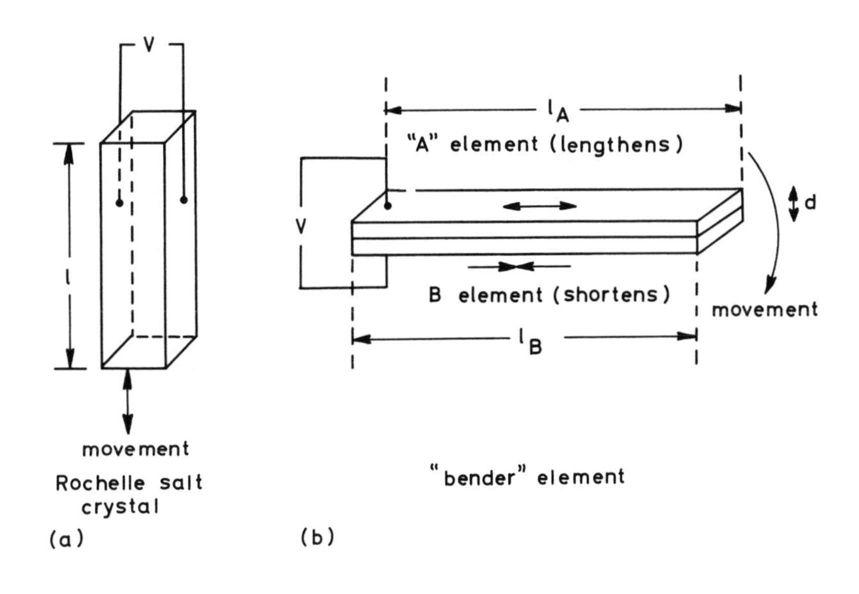

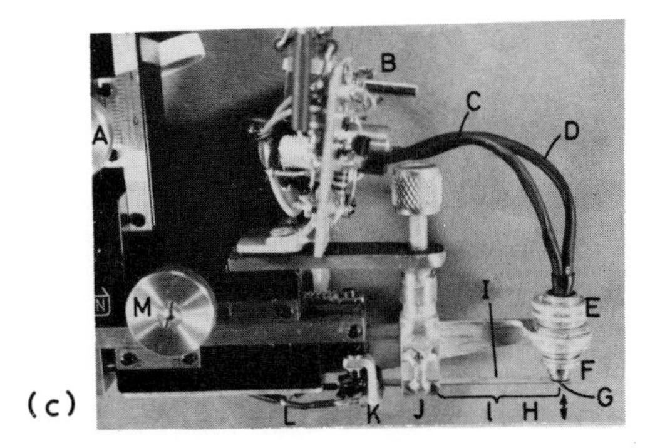

Figure 8.7
Piezoelectric devices used for mechanical stimulation. (a) Rochelle salt crystal. (b) Bender element. For bender, $l_A = f(V)$, $l_B = -f(V)$. Therefore, $\theta = K_1 f(V)$ for small θ, and $d = K_2 f(V)$ for small θ. (c) Photograph of ceramic bimorph resonance stimulator:

A. Manipulator (vertical position adjust).
B. Illuminator lamp and phototransistor monitor circuit.
C. Pickup fiber optics bundle.
D. Illuminator fiber optics bundle.
E. Vertical position adjustment for fiber optics.
F. Mixed fiber optics bundle.
G. Reflective foil.
H. Direction of movement.
I. Crystal.
J. Moveable clamp.
K. Fixed clamp.
L. Electrical lead to crystal.
l. Length of crystal free to move.
M. Manipulator (crystal length adjustment).

The *fixed* clamp (rigidly attached to the crystal), the crystal itself, and the fiber optics are all moved relative to the *movable* clamp (which is rigidly attached to the fixed portion of the manipulator), thus varying the length l of free crystal, and hence the resonant frequency. The stimulator probe, consisting of a small silver wire with a ball at the tip, is not attached to the tip of the crystal in this photograph.

high mechanical impedance, and high electrical impedance. The latter have lower frequency capability, larger size, and lower mechanical and electrical impedance.

The piezoelectric transducers utilize the property of piezoelectric materials, whereby they change their length when a voltage applied to an appropriate axis is varied. The change of length can be used directly, as with Rochelle salt crystals, to move a stimulator probe (Figure 8.7a) or in *bender elements*, in which two crystals change length in opposite directions, causing bending of the element (Figure 8.7b).

The photograph of Figure 8.7c illustrates a bender-element stimulator that uses a ceramic bimorph (Brush-Clevite) as the transducer. The device was designed and built in the laboratory of Dr. D. N. Tapper, at Cornell University. When used as a vibrator, it provides adequate displacement for stimulating low-threshold cutaneous receptors at frequencies from 100 Hz to 600 Hz and higher. These transducers have a frequency response similar to that graphed in Figure 8.8a.

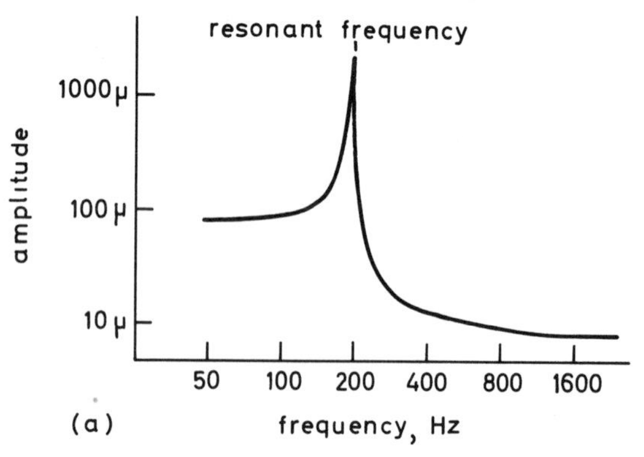

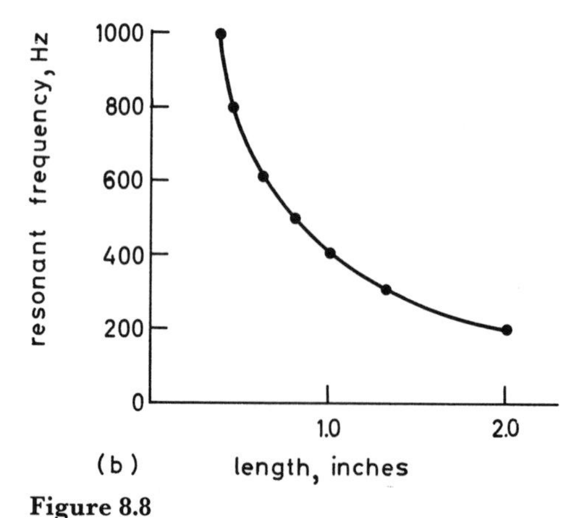

Figure 8.8
Characteristics of ceramic bimorph. (a) Resonance of a mechanical vibrator with high Q. (b) Crystal length versus resonant frequency. Resonant frequency $\cong K/\text{length}$.

Note that at frequencies below resonance, the device can only produce displacement of 100 μ or less, and at frequencies above resonance, the displacement is much less. However, at the resonant frequency, sinusoidal oscillations of several hundred microns can be maintained. The stimulator of Figure 8.8 is designed to vary the resonant frequency by varying the length of bender element which is free to vibrate, by means of a sliding clamp. The relation of crystal length to resonant frequency for this particular bender element is graphed in Figure 8.8b.

The monitor for the device consists of a *Y*-bundle of randomly mixed fiber optics, coupled to a light source and a phototransistor on the two branches of the *Y*-bundle. The main bundle is brought to within approximately 1 mm of the surface of the bimorph tip, to which is glued a piece of metal foil in order to increase reflectance. The circular foil has the same diameter as the fiber optics, about $\frac{1}{8}$ in. The amount of light reflected back to the pickup fibers is a function of the light intensity transmitted by the illuminator fibers and the distance between the *Y*-bundle tip and the surface of the bimorph. If variations of the distance are small relative to the resting distance (say, one-tenth the distance), the amount of light picked up will vary more or less proportionally with the distance from the resting position. The relation of the output voltage to the distance from a large (2×2 cm) reflecting surface is plotted in the graph of Figure 8.9. Using a smaller reflector, like the one on the stimulator, the peak is closer to zero, and the 1 mm resting position is on the relatively linear portion of the falling slope. Calibration is accomplished by plotting monitor output *vs.* amplitude of oscillation as observed with stroboscopic illumination, through a microscope with a calibrated ocular scale.

Fairchild has recently introduced an integrated-circuit reflectance monitor, the FPLA 850, which may be ideally suited to measuring displacements. This device is small enough ($0.25 \times 0.185 \times 0.092$ in.) to replace directly the fiber-optic bundle in most applications and has a distance *vs.* output current curve that is similar to that used here. This approach should be much more inexpensive and convenient than bulky and expensive fiber optics methods. The light source (an LED) and the detector (a phototransistor) are mounted in the same device on the same face. Thus, the only light from the emitter reaching the detector is that which is reflected back.

Figure 8.10 illustrates a simple amplifier configuration for the phototransistor monitor. There are a few integrated-circuit devices in which op amps are built into the same can as the phototransistor, but these are presently prohibitive in cost. The amplifiers of Figure 8.10 should be placed as close as possible to the phototransistor in order to minimize stray electrical pickup. Be sure to shield the

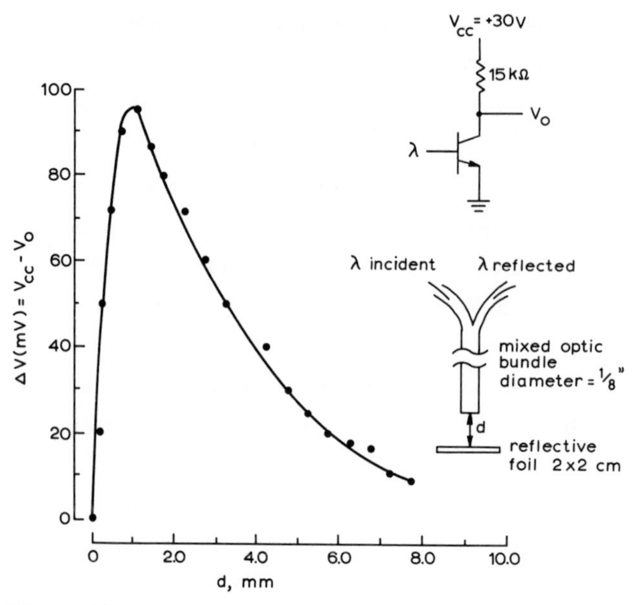

Figure 8.9
Characteristics of optical monitor used in ceramic bimorph resonant stimulator.

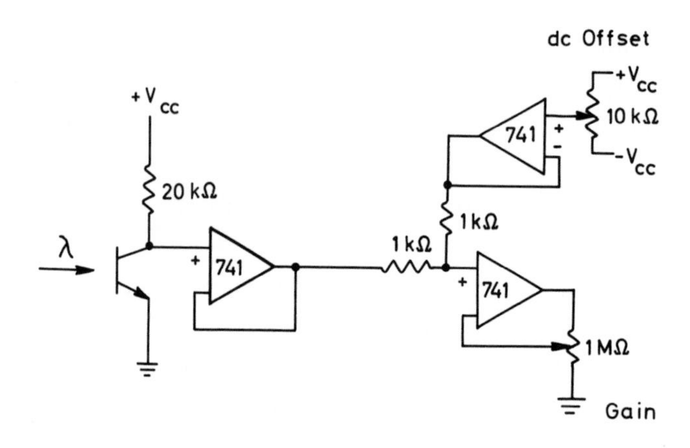

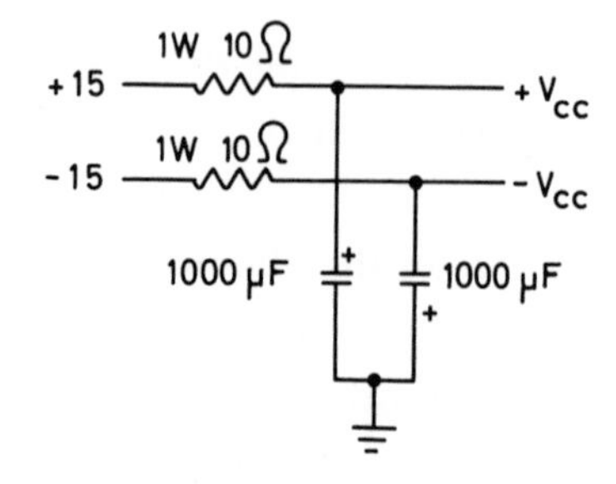

Figure 8.10
Amplifier for phototransistor monitor.

monitor-bimorph tip area from ambient room light. The vertical position of the *Y*-bundle should be adjustable, because the tip of the bimorph has a tendency to move up or down slightly when the clamp is moved, in the process of tuning the stimulator to the desired resonant frequency. The dc level at the monitor output can be used for this purpose. When monitoring the actual movement of the bimorph tip, use ac-coupled or bias-compensated methods to monitor the relatively small voltage variations riding on the large dc component. The latter method allows adjustment of resting position and monitoring of movement without changing sensitivity or coupling at the oscilloscope, if the vertical movement of the bender tip relative to the *Y*-bundle with different clamp positions is not too large.

The circuit of Figure 8.11 was found useful in generating sine wave "pips," when used in conjunction with the digital counter/pulse generators of Figure 5.16.

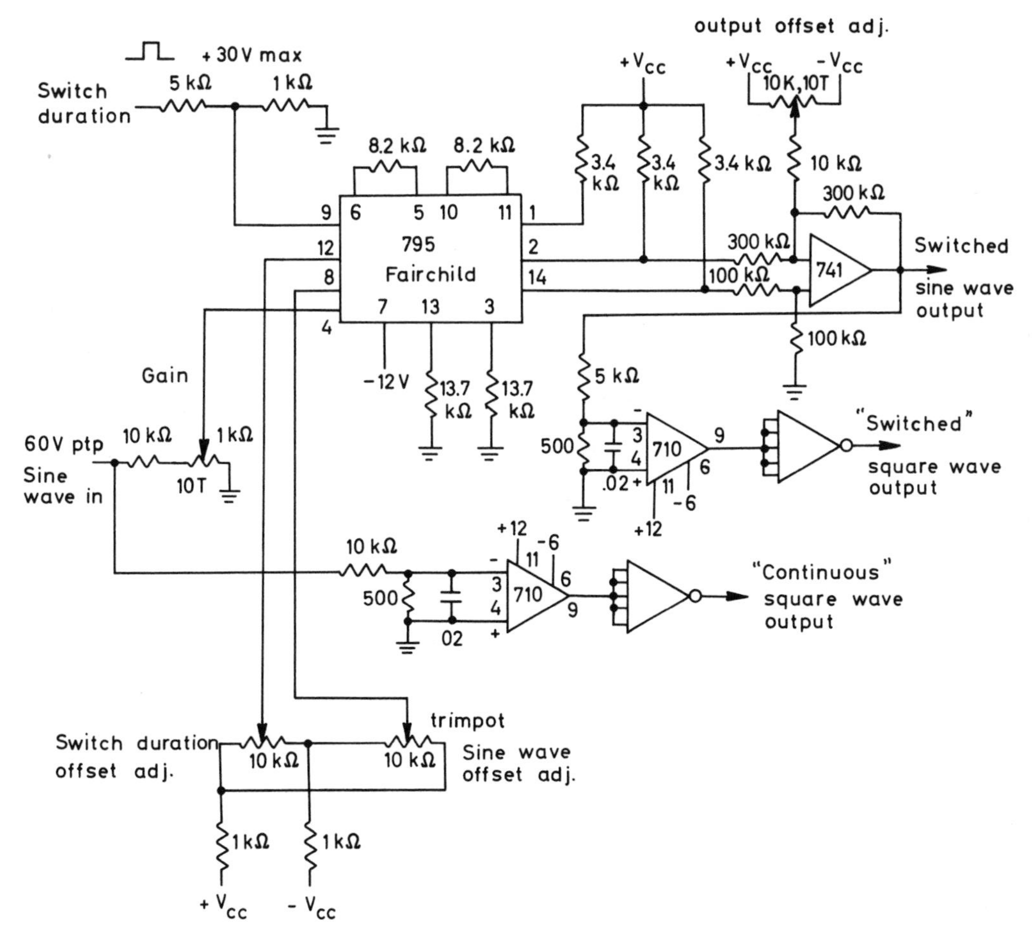

Figure 8.11
Tone pip generator. Vary envelope by varying input to *switch duration*.

The multiplier serves as an analog switch to turn the sine wave on and off; the discriminators provide square waves derived from the input and output sine waves—these are useful for triggering the control logic in order to turn the vibration on and off with consistent phase relations (in this case, on positive-going zero crossings) and in order to count number of oscillations for control of duration or delay relative to another stimulator. Control logic can be assembled from digital modules in a configuration similar to that of Figure 5.23a. By varying the amplitude of the *duration* pulse, the amplitude of the pip is directly controlled. If gain is to be separately controlled as is advisable for output voltages of less than 100 mV (due to thresholds of the comparators), switching can be accomplished by an analog switch, with a gain-control amplifier at the output. This way, the maximum output from the analog switch can be used to drive the comparator, regardless of the voltage actually used to drive the stimulator. An additional advantage of such an alternative is the higher voltage limit that can be obtained by using a high-voltage operational amplifier to drive the crystal. Some types of crystal will tolerate driving voltages in excess of 100 V.

Figure 8.12 illustrates a ±30 V pulse amplifier design based on a circuit communicated by Dr. D. Domizi of the University of Chicago. The variable output

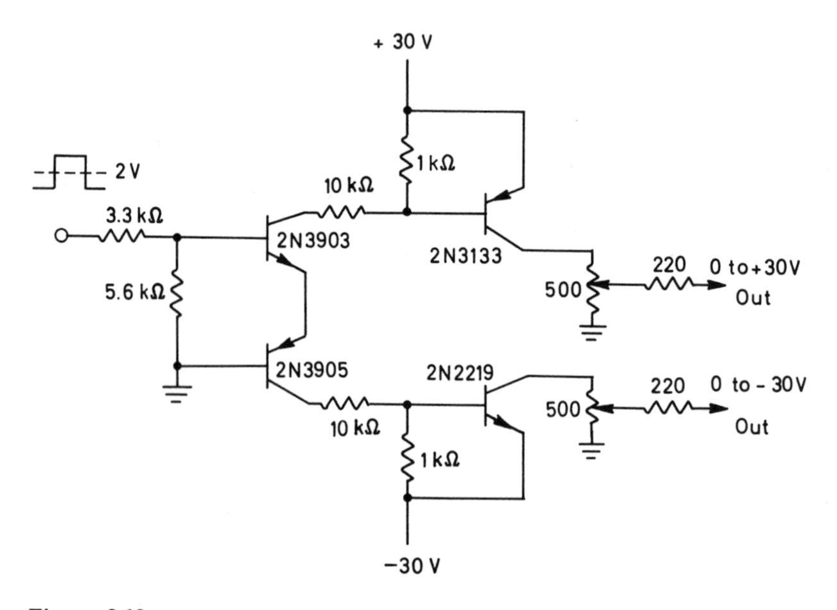

Figure 8.12
Pulse amplifier, ±30 V. All transistors have $BV_{CEO} > 30$ V. Use power transistors if lower output impedance is required. Output transistors, $P_D = 600$ mV. Adjust (*) resistors so all switching transitions occur when input crosses +2 V. The values shown are adequate for most purposes. (Schematic courtesy of Dr. D. D. Domizi.)

voltage can be used to drive the SWITCH DURATION input of the analog multiplier.

Another transducer that is commonly used to deliver mechanical stimuli is the dynamic loudspeaker. Expensive dynamic vibrators produced commercially are not recommended, except in a few rare applications where large displacements are required at high frequencies. They have no advantage other than their greater power output and extended frequency range. Figure 8.13a illustrates the configuration of a stimulator used in the laboratory of Dr. D. N. Tapper at Cornell University. The loudspeaker, a 3-in. tweeter-type dynamic device, has built onto its frame an armature that supports a lever assembly. One end of the lever is tied to a rod glued to the center of the speaker cone, and the other end carries a small glass, metal, or plastic probe, used to deliver the stimulus. The fulcrum is a precision bearing from a clock, with little resistance to movement and little lateral movement.

The monitor for this device is a photocell that detects the amount of light passing a flag glued to the rod connecting the lever to the cone. A long-life bulb provides illumination, and the flag cuts off a variable amount of the light as a function of the cone displacement. With appropriate changes in the optics, the photocell can be replaced by a phototransistor with a consequent gain in frequency response. The frequency responses of some photocells are poor; roll-off may be as low as 25–100 Hz. A phototransistor will always handle much higher frequencies, far higher in fact than any produced by the loudspeaker. In this configuration, the upper useful frequency limit for mechanical vibration is around 200 Hz. If, alternatively, the configuration of Figure 8.13c is used, frequencies up to 400 Hz can be obtained without much difficulty. Calibration of the monitor is accomplished by displacing the stimulator probe by known amounts, either with a micrometer or with an electrical bias applied to the speaker; in the latter case, it is necessary to monitor the actual displacement with a microscope and calibrated ocular. A static displacement, instead of a dynamic one, can be used only when it is certain that the frequency response of the monitor is adequate to reproduce the fastest movements of the stimulator. Thus, it can be used for calibration of phototransistor or photodiode responses, including the response of the ceramic bimorph stimulator, but it is only adequate for calibrating a photocell response if photocells are chosen with frequency responses that are flat within the frequency range which will be used. Otherwise, frequency response curves must be obtained, using different vibratory frequencies and observing movement with stroboscopic illumination.

The monitor may be used to generate a feedback signal, compensating for nonlinearities of loudspeaker response (Figure 8.14). A monitor circuit is illustrated in Figure 8.15a.

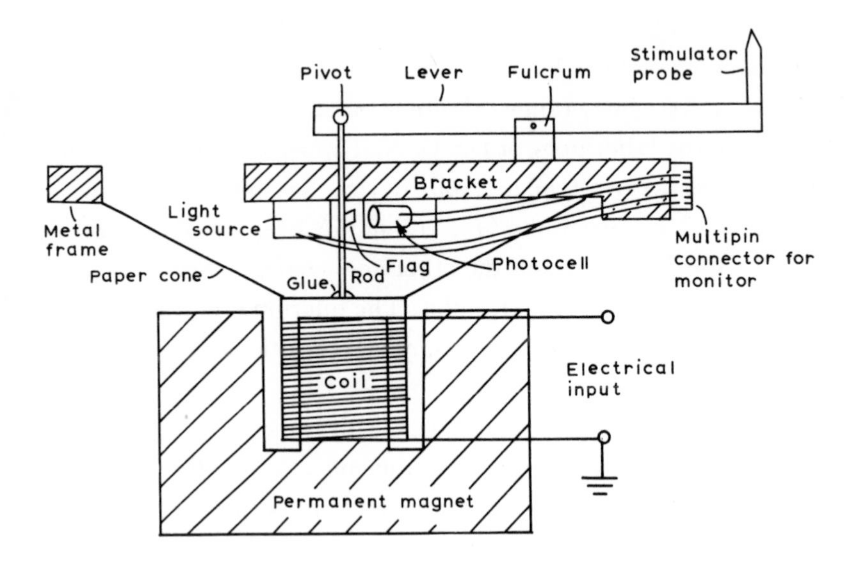

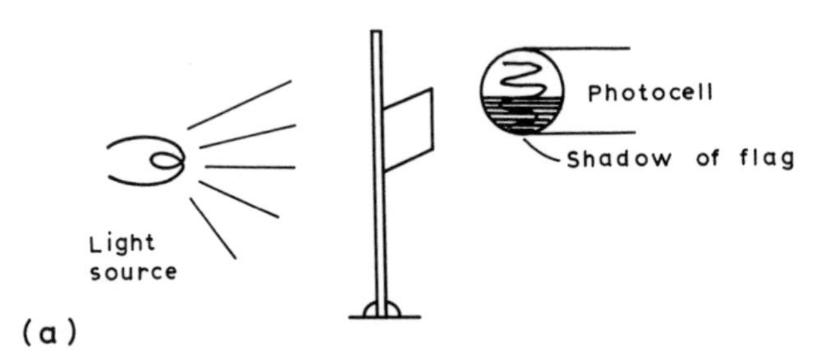

Figure 8.13
Dynamic vibrators. (a) Dynamic loudspeaker mechanical stimulator (after a device designed by Dr. D. N. Tapper), and illustration of flag-photocell displacement monitor. (b) Photograph of lever-type stimulator (courtesy of Dr. D. N. Tapper): A, Loudspeaker; B, Connector for driver and monitor signals; C, Manipulator; D, Coupling of rod to lever; E, Fulcrum; F, Lever; and G, Stimulator probe. (c) Direct coupling with diaphragm for lateral alignment.

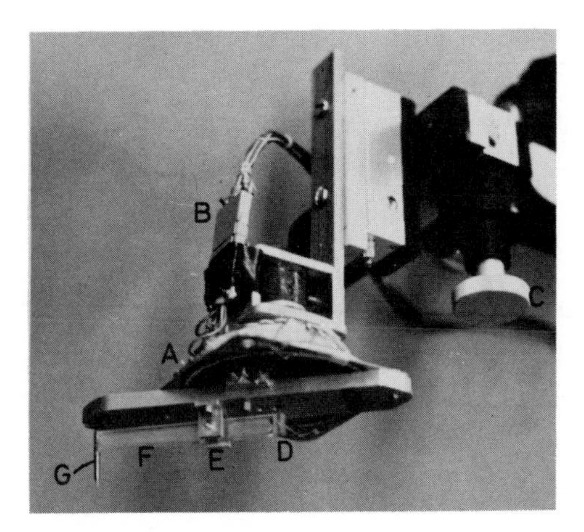

(b)

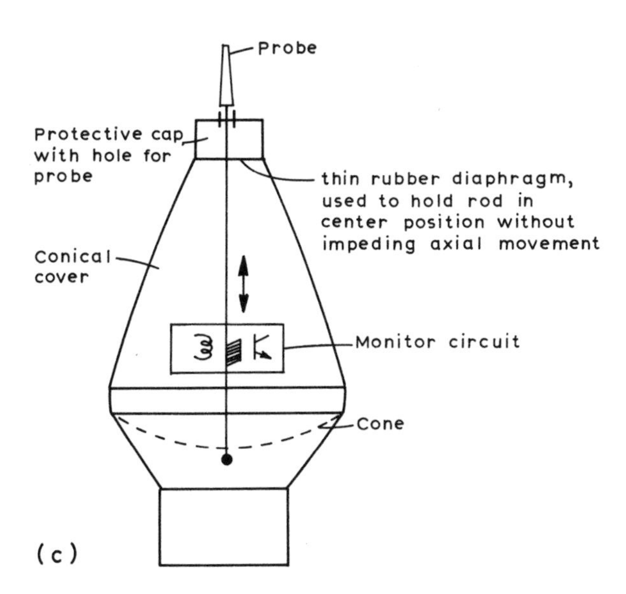

(c)

Figure 8.13 (continued)

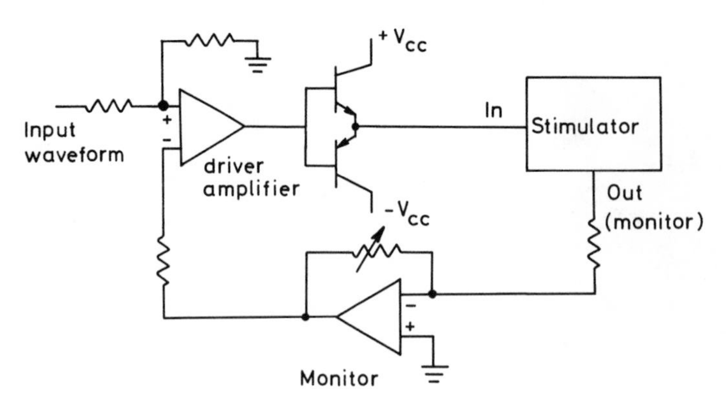

Figure 8.14
Negative feedback compensation of loudspeaker response.

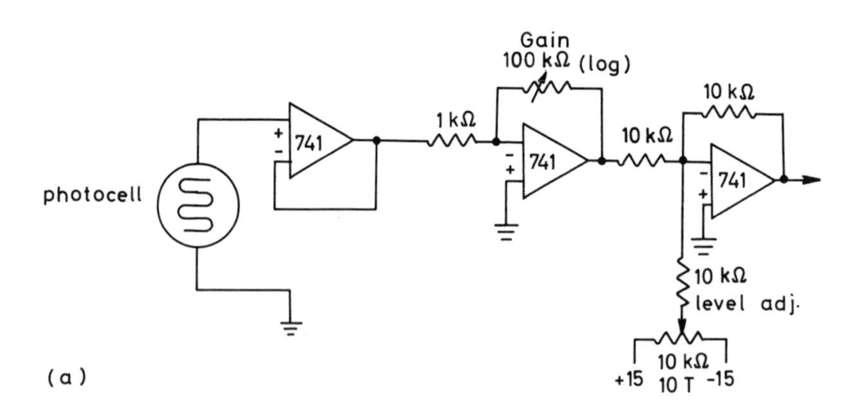

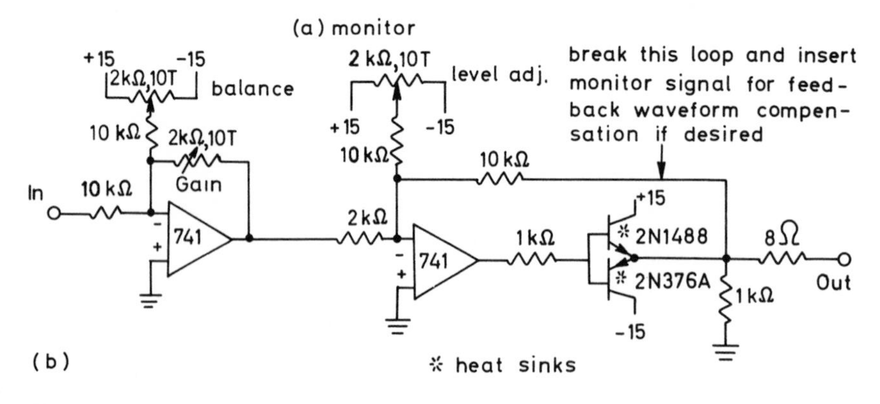

Figure 8.15
Monitor (a) and driver (b) circuits for dynamic stimulator.

Wave form generation is accomplished either by directly synthesizing the desired wave form or, as in Figure 5.22, by combinations of triggerable generators. The latter is recommended for greater flexibility. Since the dynamic stimulator has a low impedance, use a power-boost output stage to drive the device. Voltage range need not exceed the usual ± 10 V op amp range. A suggested output driver is diagrammed in Figure 8.15b.

It is frequently necessary to determine the time at which the action potential is generated at the receptor, in order to synchronize an averaging sweep or a pulse interval timer when monitoring the cutaneous nerve response (see Chapter 12 for a description of these techniques). It is generally adequate to indicate when the probe touches the skin or the accessory structure being stimulated; this time can vary considerably, even using fast (5 msec) pulses, because the skin tends to move slightly with respiration and changes in blood pressure. This slight movement, when superimposed on the small stimuli used to activate single cutaneous receptors (2–20 μ, for tactile pads), is often enough to cause variations of as much as 1 msec in contact time.

Contact detection can be accomplished with varying degrees of success by several methods; we will describe the one that we consider to be the most potentially fruitful, although the technique is still in the experimental stages. This consists of an optical method similar to that used for the displacement monitor of the bimorph stimulator, except we will make use of the portion of the distance *vs.* reflected light curve which has a positive slope, that is, that portion from zero distance to some small distance (of the order of 100 μ). As would be expected, there is a minimum of reflected light when the fiber optics *Y*-bundle of Figure 8.16 is actually in contact with the receptor (in this case, a tactile pad), because both the illuminator and pickup fibers are blocked. The *Y*-bundle, which is the stimulator probe, is placed at a distance from the receptor within the operating range of the monitor, and contact is detected when the light current drops to a minimum during the stimulus. A standard discriminator circuit could be used to detect this drop, once the output of the phototransistor is amplified.

The optical contact detector has another potential use: Since the device would provide a signal with a monotonic relation (for small distances) to the distance from the skin surface, a negative feedback signal could be derived to compensate for the relation between the skin and the probe, allowing the device to *track* the skin as it moves, thus minimizing jitter in contact time from one stimulus to the next.

Unfortunately, other techniques do not work well for small stimuli and contact areas. Other methods include the grounding of a small offset voltage connected

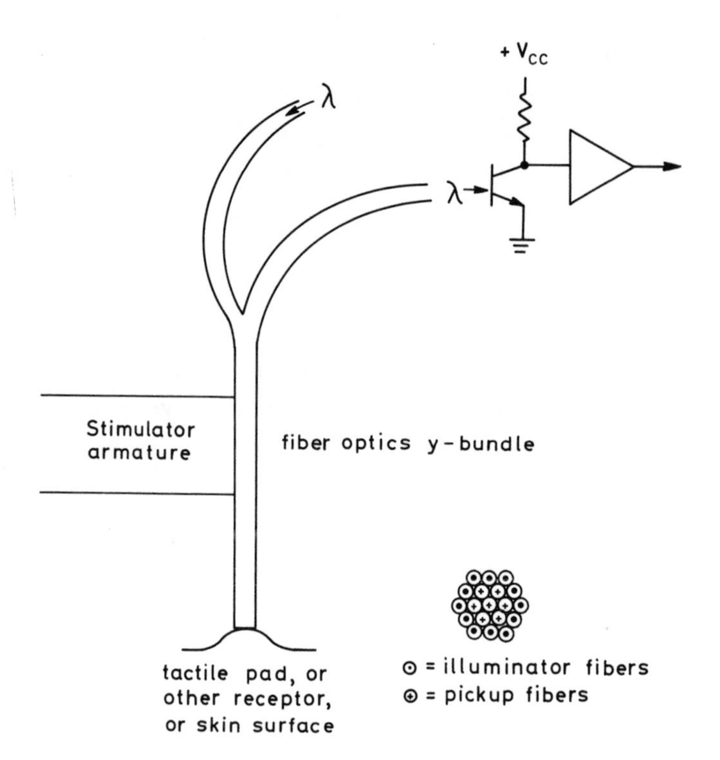

Figure 8.16
Optical contact detector.

through a large (10^9 Ω) resistor to a high-impedance amplifier, when a conductive stimulator probe touches the animal's skin; or taking advantage of the variable capacitance of the probe relative to ground, with the preparation serving as ground, by using a capacitance-meter coupled to a conductive stimulator probe. For larger amplitudes (over 100 μ) and contact areas (over $100^2\ \mu^2$) these methods are usually adequate.

Only one other currently available technique is capable of resolving contact time, although it is not recommended for precisely that application. If a small bimorph bender crystal is mounted in series between the stimulator probe and the armature of the mechanical stimulator, the bending of the crystal caused by the force exerted against the receptor can be used to indicate the time of contact. Unfortunately, the force used to drive the inertial mass of the probe and the crystal is generally greater than that delivered to the receptor, and the resulting signal caused by pressure on the receptor is small relative to the voltage caused by bending of the crystal when the stimulus is delivered in air. Thus computational methods are necessary to subtract the *in air* signal from the *on receptor* signal. Although this is a useful technique for measuring the minute forces exerted to drive a cutaneous

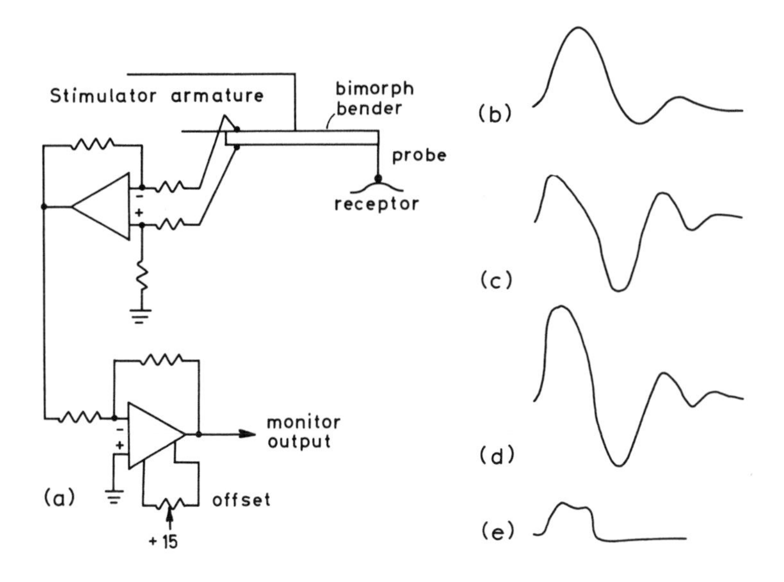

Figure 8.17
Force monitor for mechanical stimulation. (a) Schematic. (b) Probe movement monitor. (c) "In air" response of bender element. (d) "On skin" response. (e) Difference signal = (*d*) − (*c*) = force delivered to skin.

receptor to threshold, it is not a practical method for signaling time of contact on a trial-by-trial basis. This force-monitor technique is diagrammed in Figure 8.17.

8.3 Vestibular Stimulation

Depending on the receptors or the central nervous elements under study, vestibular stimulation will generally consist of either linear or angular acceleration of the animal, or for short distances, of the animal's head relative to his body. We will concentrate on angular acceleration of the whole animal.

For analysis of input-output relations of a system, it is customary to use wave forms whose analytic functions are simple, such as angular velocity sinusoids, ramps, or fixed velocities. It is impractical in vestibular studies to use impulses or steps as stimuli, because the devices used for spinning the animal are generally too massive to give a good approximation of a unit impulse: Their frequency limits are generally under 50 Hz, and their maximum accelerations are much less than the physiological maximum.

Wave form generation can be accomplished using the circuits of Chapter 5. The electrical wave form is generally translated into angular velocity (rather than, say, position or acceleration). Thus a voltage trapezoid produces a constant acceleration up to a constant velocity, which is maintained for the duration of the voltage plateau, followed by a constant deceleration to the original baseline velocity.

Spinning tables are manufactured by a relatively small number of manufacturers. The device used by Drs. Goldberg and Fernandez of the University of Chicago is a spinning table with slip rings that provide electrical pathways for power and signal voltages to and from the recording amplifier mounted on the table with the animal. The animal is mounted on a rigid frame built onto the table top, centered, and positioned by rotating around two axes to place the desired canal in the horizontal plane (the plane of rotation), with the curvature of the canal centered at the center of the table (the axis of rotation). The electrode is positioned with the usual microdrive, and manual spinning of the table is used as an intermittent probe stimulus.

The Inland Controls Model 712 Rate Table System has a servomechanism built in, in order to follow electrical inputs, producing accelerations up to $\pm 100°/\text{sec}^2$ with a maximum angular velocity of 1500°/sec. Frequency response is DC-25 Hz. A monitor (tachometer) signal is available directly from the device. The machine should be securely bolted to the floor, and all joints, pivots, and so forth, should be tightly locked before spinning is commenced. Remove all loose objects from the table top before spinning: It is wise to build a sturdy safety barrier surrounding the device in case any of these precautions are inadvertently omitted.

Linear accelerations are more difficult to control; we are not familiar with any simple, inexpensive method of varying linear acceleration as a function of some input voltage, over anything approximating the entire physiological range.

8.4 Auditory Stimulation

Generally, free-field auditory stimulation with a loudspeaker is extremely unreliable in terms of controlling both absolute and relative intensity of sound delivered to the two ears, diffraction and interference patterns, reflections, and time of arrival of the stimulus at the eardrum. Although there are situations in which such stimuli are adequate or even necessary (for example, when studying echolocation in bats), considerations are restricted here to stimuli delivered from earphones through tubes directly to the tympanum.

A typical configuration used for delivering auditory stimuli is diagrammed in Figure 8.18. The time for sound conduction to the eardrum is simply the entire length of the air column (use tubing lengths that are equal for both ears when using binaural stimuli) divided by the speed of sound in air (331.7 m/sec).

The 1 cc cavities in the earphone holder and at the ear probe are used to achieve approximate acoustic impedance matching. Isolation between the two ears is determined primarily by bone conduction if a good seal with the auditory canal

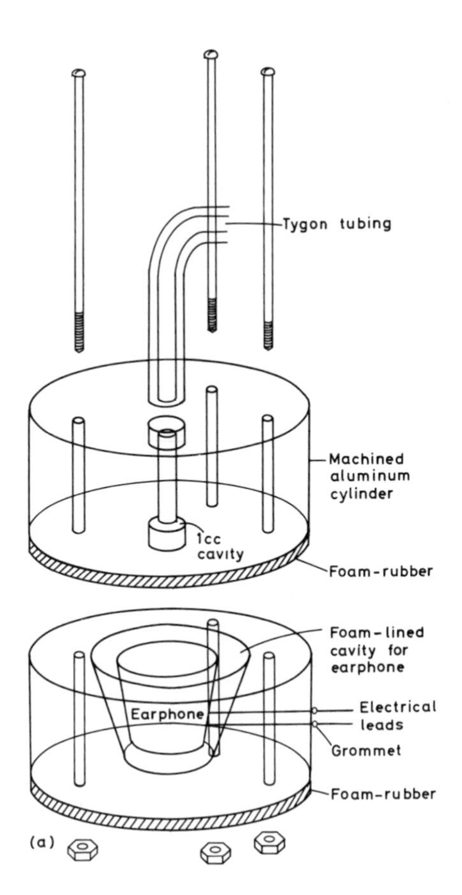

Figure 8.18
Coupling of auditory stimulus. (a) Chamber for ear phone. (b) Ear probe assembly. (c) Phase delay control for 125 Hz, using a 0–2 msec. delay line:

Left°	Right°	Delay° (Right–Left)
0 to 90	0 to 90	−90 to +90
0 to 90	0	−90 to 0
0 to 90	180	90 to 180
0 to 90	180 to 270	90 to 270
0	0 to 90	0 to 90
0	0	0
0	180	180
0	180 to 270	180 to 270
180	0 to 90	−180 to −90
180	0	−180
180	180	0
180	180 to 270	0 to 90
180 to 270	0 to 90	−270 to −90
180 to 270	0	−270 to −180
180 to 270	180	−90 to 0
180 to 270	180 to 270	−90 to +90

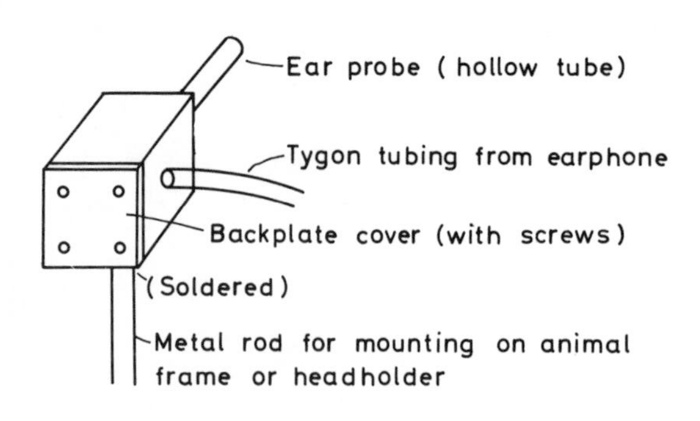

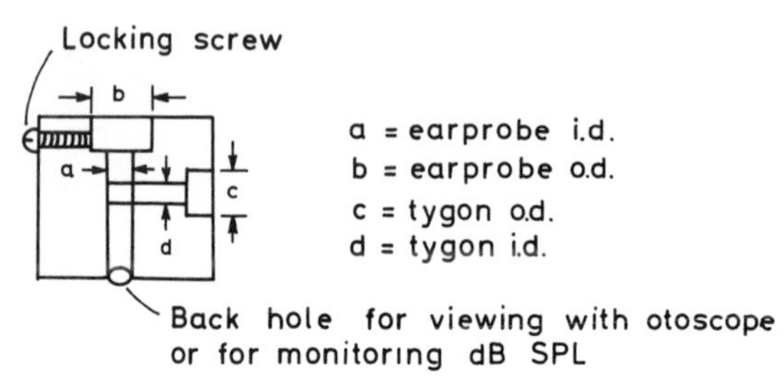

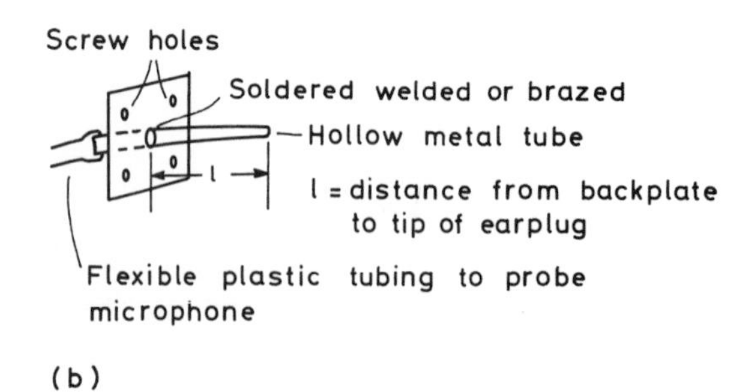

Figure 8.18 (continued)

is maintained. Mites, wax, bubbles, or films of fluid can attenuate sound by at least 10 dB and often more than 30 dB. For accurate monitoring of the sound levels at the ear, it is useful to insert a probe through the back of the earpiece and lead the sound to a calibrated probe microphone for measurement of intensity. Rather than monitor continuously, it is sometimes adequate to precalibrate on one animal and rely on calibration curves. These are probably not more than ± 10 dB accurate over the full audible spectrum and from one preparation to the next, but such accuracy is usually adequate for most studies, as long as it remains constant throughout an experiment.

Earphones may be dynamic, or condenser microphones may be used as earphones. The latter have a better frequency range, but they should always be monitored directly due to loading effects. For ultrasonic stimulation use a crystal transducer rated for the desired frequency range. Calibration and monitoring

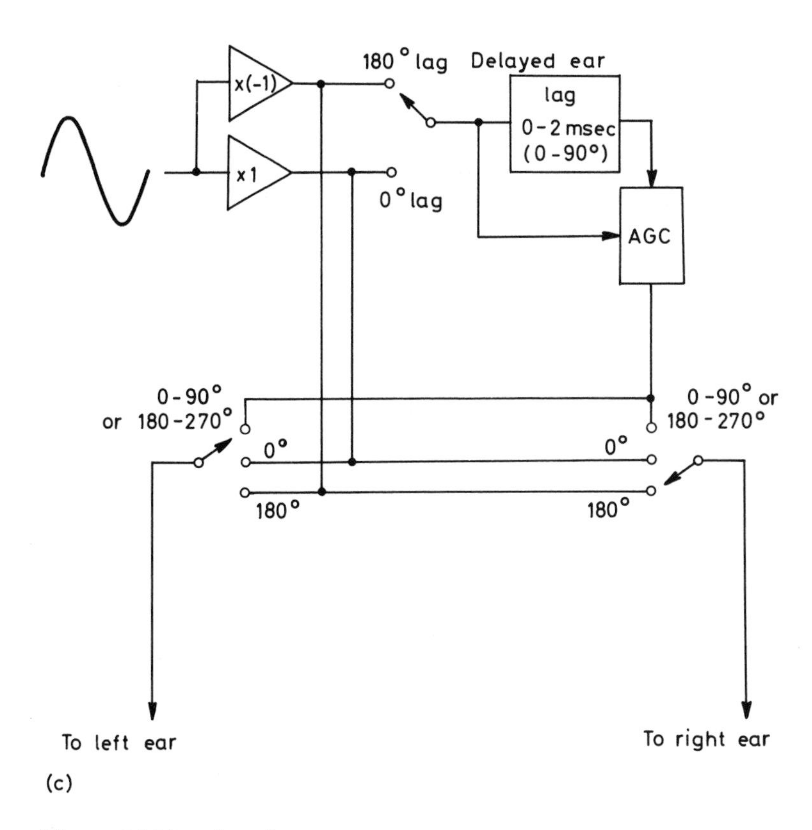

Figure 8.18 (continued)

equipment is generally too difficult and expensive to build and it is simpler to use a good calibrated probe monitor such as those made by Breuel and Kjaer or Hewlett-Packard. All calibration equipment should be traceable to the National Bureau of Standards, if intensities of tones are to be specified in dB SPL (that is, *re* 0.002 dynes/cm^2).

Stimuli generally consist of clicks, tone pips, tones that are amplitude or frequency modulated, or noise bursts. Low-noise amplifiers must be used in the stimulus-generating circuits, and the sine waves must be harmonically pure. If home-made generators are used, include an AGC in the tone-generator and delay circuits and perform harmonic analysis to verify low harmonic distortion of tones, because an auditory neuron may respond to harmonics of the fundamental tone. One percent harmonic distortion implies that all harmonics have a total power that is 40 dB down *re* the fundamental; this should be adequate for most purposes. When checking harmonic distortion with a wave-form analyzer, measure successive harmonics and keep a running total of their power until the total is changed by 1% or less by each new harmonic; the lower harmonics usually contain most of the energy produced by distortion in analog generators. When checking digital generators, check the nth harmonic and integral multiples of it, where n is the number of clock cycles per sine wave period; also check low-order harmonics of the sine wave and the clock. Noise must be filtered to the desired bandwidth, and uniform spectral density should be verified. Additional filtering to compensate for earphone properties may be necessary; condenser microphones have the flattest spectral responses. Logarithmic attenuators are available, calibrated in dB, for amplitude control. Analog switches or multipliers may be used for turning tones and noise bursts on and off.

For amplitude modulation the Motorola 1596 modulator or any of a number of other IC balanced modulators may be used. Balanced modulation (an AM signal with the carrier suppressed) will usually require direct coupling of carrier and modulator inputs with careful bias compensation to prevent dc components on any input. The dc drift or temperature changes may vary the carrier suppression, which should be checked before and, if necessary, during each experiment. Multipliers may also be used for suppressed-carrier AM if dc offsets are carefully trimmed to zero. To gain some notion of the dc offset precision required, consider the hypothetical requirement of carrier suppression of -60 dB *re* a total output of ± 10 V. If the two input angular frequencies are ω_A and ω_B and their corresponding dc offsets are K_A and K_B, the output is

$$\begin{aligned}(K_A + A\cos\omega_A t) \times (K_B + B\cos\omega_B t) = {} & \{K_A K_B + K_A B\cos\omega_B t + K_B A\cos\omega_A t\} \\ & + \{\tfrac{1}{2}AB[\cos(\omega_A + \omega_B)t \\ & + \cos(\omega_A - \omega_B)t]\},\end{aligned}$$

where the last two frequency components are those desired from true suppressed-carrier AM, and the first three components are contaminating frequencies due to input dc offsets. The $K_A K_B$ term could be eliminated by ac-coupling the output, but the $\cos\omega_B t$ and $\cos\omega_A t$ terms must be eliminated by bias-compensating K_A and K_B.

For the sake of simplicity, assume that we wish to determine the dc voltage K below which K_A and K_B must both be trimmed for the desired suppression of input frequencies. For the sake of further simplicity, assume that A and B are equal and adjusted to $\sqrt{10}$, so the output peak-to-peak amplitude is ± 10 V and effects of differential offsets are minimized and equal for both inputs. Setting $K_A = K_B = K$, and $A = B = \sqrt{10}$, we have

$$20 \times \log_{10}\left(\frac{K\sqrt{10}\cos\omega_B t + K\sqrt{10}\cos\omega_A t}{5[\cos(\omega_A + \omega_B)t + \cos(\omega_A - \omega_B)]}\right) = -60,$$

or

$$K\sqrt{10}\,(\cos \omega_B t + \cos \omega_A t) = 0.005[\cos(\omega_A + \omega_B)t + \cos(\omega_A - \omega_B)t].$$

If we further assume that the load on the output signal is constant for all anticipated output frequencies, which is a reasonable assumption in a well-designed system, then the frequency terms may be neglected:

$$K\sqrt{10} = 0.005,$$

$$K \cong 1.6 \text{ mV}.$$

Input offsets for most op amps are of the order of 10–100 mV, and must therefore be compensated. Offset drift is usually of the order of 75–200 μV/°C, and therefore if initially $|K| < 100\ \mu$V, a temperature range of, say, ± 7°C can be tolerated. If the multiplier is operated under low-current conditions in a well-ventilated space, ambient air temperature fluctuation will generally not seriously degrade carrier suppression.

Narrow bands of noise with very sharp frequency cutoffs can be obtained by amplitude modulating a sine wave of frequency CF (center frequency) with a dc to X Hz noise where X equals the desired half-bandwidth. The result of this modulation consists of a flat spectrum from (CF $-$ X) to (CF $+$ X) with a large peak at CF. The roll-off is usually 6–12 dB/octave with respect to the *original* noise bandwidth, depending on type of bandpass filter. Thus, if a 50 Hz noise bandwidth with a 6 dB/octave roll-off is used to modulate a 1 kHz tone, a band of noise from 950–1050 Hz is obtained, with a 5 dB/50 Hz roll-off. The spectral peak at the carrier frequency is usually eliminated by using a balanced modulator and by rejecting dc in the narrow-band noise, in which case a notch occurs at CF. If carrier rejection is poor, a peak may still occur at CF. Suppression should be checked with a harmonic analyzer.

Commercial analog delay lines are available that can provide delays of as much as 10 msec for auditory stimuli. An AGC is needed to compensate for the variable attenuation introduced by the delay line at various delays. These devices can be used to obtain the full range of relative phase relations of tones delivered to the two ears for frequencies as low as 125 Hz if the technique of Figure 8.18c is used. A 2 msec delay range is more than adequate for reproducing the physiological range, up to head widths of about 65 cm.

A setup for auditory stimulation that is capable of delivering a variety of stimuli to the two ears is shown in Figure 8.19. Of course, if digital methods are used to synthesize the sine waves, the analog oscillator and delay circuitry can be omitted.

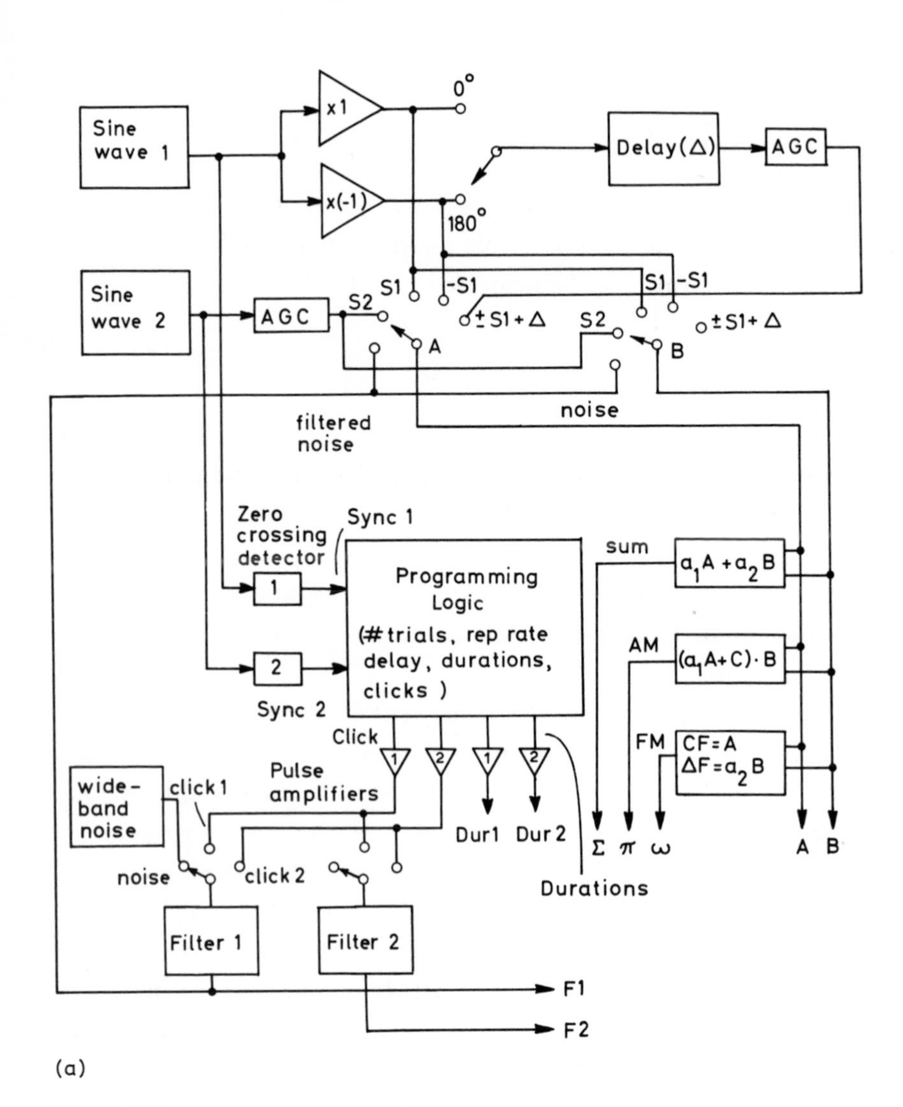

Figure 8.19
Stimulus programming for dichotic stimulation. A, B = sine waves 1 (with various delays) or 2, or filtered noise (from filter 1). R, L = $\{[A, B, \text{sum, AM, FM, or filtered noise}] \times [\text{DUR1 or DUR2}] \vee [\text{filter 1}] \vee [\text{filter 2}]\} \times$ attenuator R, L. All leads must be shielded, with output buffer resistors on op amps. Carefully avoid ground loops, and use low-noise, low-distortion circuits.

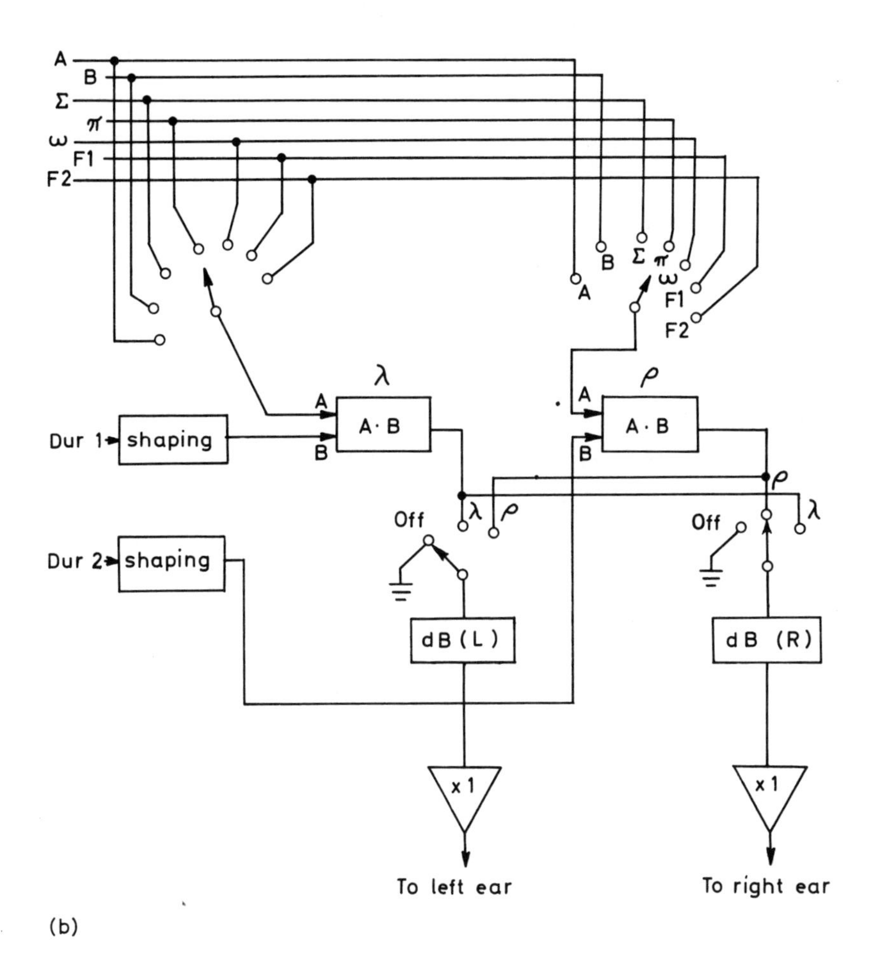

Figure 8.19 (continued)

8.5 Visual Stimulation

We will consider here both the generation of visual patterns and monitoring of the muscular activity of the eye.

8.5.1 Simple Pattern Generation

There are more variables involved in visual stimulation than in any other sensory system. Wavelength, intensity, and spatiotemporal patterns might be considered "primary qualities," and "secondary qualities" derived from these might include contrast (both color and intensity) relative positions, shapes, and sizes of different stimuli, movement, orientation, and temporal modulations of intensity, color (hue), saturation, and other parameters.

Corresponding to this bewildering array of visual parameters are a host of technical difficulties involved in their control. The techniques and principles involved in visual stimulation are reviewed here with an emphasis on mechanisms for controlling these parameters electronically. Examples are chosen that illustrate the principles of quantitative control. Some of the techniques described have not been used for the purposes suggested, but they will be based on practical methods derived from other fields.

The wavelength of colored light can be varied by several techniques; if truly monochromatic light is desired, the only method of obtaining it at high intensities is with a laser. These devices are becoming less expensive, but only a few wavelengths are available in the lower price range. Tunable lasers have recently been introduced, but their cost is presently prohibitive for most physiologists and psychologists. A disadvantage of purely monochromatic coherent light is the grainy quality of images caused by interference patterns developed in the eye itself.

Traditionally, optical filters have been used for bandpass filtering of white light. For narrow bands a prism or diffraction grating is generally used in conjunction with a narrow slit which passes a narrow spectral band. *Diffraction filters* are available that pass selected narrow spectral bands. The light source must be chosen to provide the desired spectral band, of course; xenon arc lamps are commonly used. One advantage of using prism or grating devices is the fact that the wavelength is "tunable"; a colorimeter or spectrophotometer can be used to great advantage for this purpose. Electronic control of wavelength is then obtained by using a servomotor or stepping motor to rotate the prism or grating under electronic control. The speed with which tuning is accomplished can be quite high and controlled; interesting color modulation techniques could easily be developed. Alternatively, the technique described later for pivoting a mirror with a loudspeaker could also be used to obtain changes of tuning over more limited ranges. However, the intensity of different spectral bands may vary widely. If intensity variations must be minimized, some form of AGC must be used to hold intensity constant. Several manufacturers produce inexpensive and reliable rotary position controllers that can be used to open and close an f-stop.

The intensity of a patterned or unpatterned light stimulus can be varied by controlling the amount of light generated at the source (Figure 8.20). Although the amount of energy applied to the light-emitting source such as the current through a bulb filament can be varied, this is generally inefficient, and the emitted spectrum may vary with the filament current. If polarized light is acceptable, a fixed polarizer can be placed in front of the source with a rotating analyzer in front of it. A rotary position control is used for electronic control. The output light intensity is determined by the following equation:

$$I_o = I_i \quad [B + (A \cos \theta)], \tag{8.1}$$

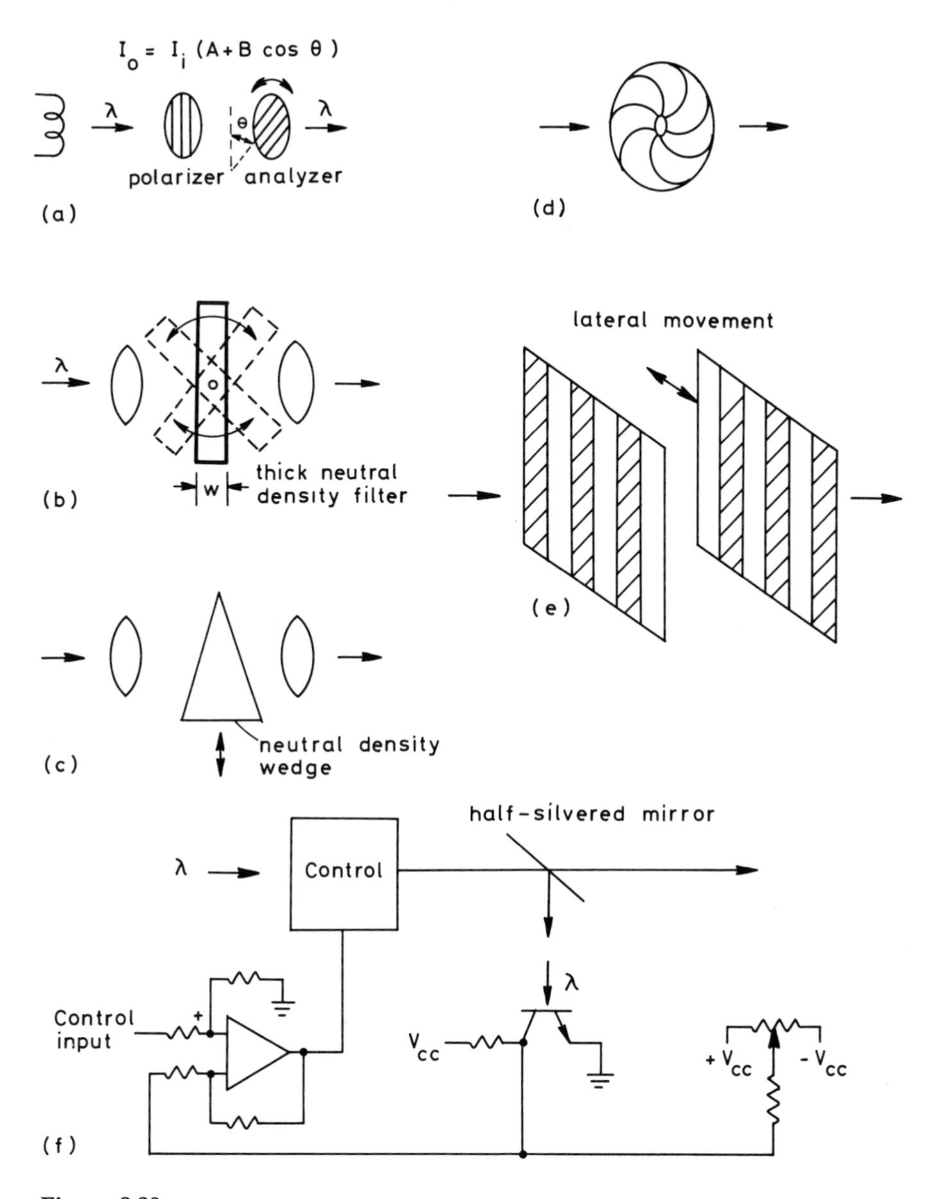

Figure 8.20
Control of illuminator intensity. (a) Crossed polarizers. (b) Tilted neutral density filter. (c) Moveable neutral density wedge. (d) Variable aperture. (e) Moving slats. (f) Feedback control.

where

I_o = output intensity,
I_i = intensity of light transmitted by polarizer,
θ = angle between polarizing axes of polarizer and analyzer,
A = correction for attenuation at all angles due to polarizer and analyzer optical densities,
B = correction for leakage when the axes of the polarizing elements are exactly crossed.

If polarized light is not acceptable (some organisms are sensitive to the polarization of light), the intensity of the illuminating light can be varied by interposing neutral density filters or variable apertures. The former method is simple and cheap; neutral density filters of calibrated optical density are available, as are neutral density wedges whose optical density is a function of linear position and circular filters whose optical density is a function of angular position. Electronic control of density is often accomplished by sliding or rotating neutral density wedges or disks; alternatively, an electronically controlled aperture can be placed in the illumination path prior to collimation. Modulating techniques that can be used up to audio frequencies include using a pattern of fixed slats with the slat width equal to the gap width in conjunction with a similar series of slats placed in front of this and moved normally to the slat orientation by a loudspeaker with a large displacement capability. The total light passed is proportional to the displacement if the resting position is one in which the slats of one shutter completely block the light passed by the other shutter.

Liquid crystals can be used to vary light intensity, but they are presently too expensive.

A fraction of the illuminating light can be used to activate a phototransistor in order to monitor the light intensity. This monitor voltage, of correct polarity and gain, can even be fed back as an error signal to the controlling device in order to compensate for nonlinearities and to serve as an AGC.

The generation of images, depending largely on their complexity, is a process which can be achieved in any of several different ways. Simple light rectangles of varying width, length, and location, can be generated with electronic control of each variable using the system of Figure 8.21. A pair of slats is moved by a pair of loudspeakers to control length and width of a rectangular "window," and another pair of loudspeakers is used to tilt mirrors over very small angles in orthogonal planes; using a long projection path, the small angles are translated into relatively large deflections of the rectangular light pattern projected on a screen.

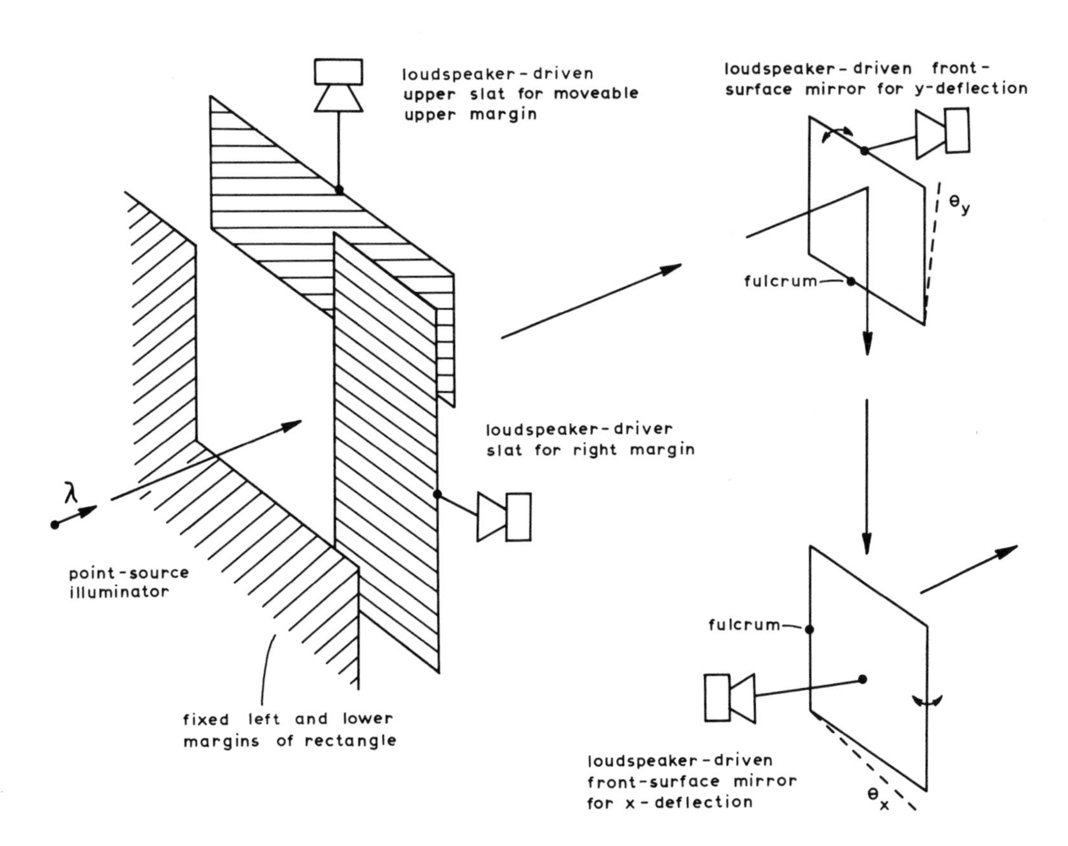

Figure 8.21
Light rectangles of varying width, length, and position.

For small angles such as these, that is, limited to a degree or two, the screen position is a nearly linear function of the speaker deflection. Actual monitoring of position for feedback compensation of speaker properties can be achieved either by photoelectric monitoring of the loudspeaker cone position using a monitor similar to that of Figure 8.13, or by detecting the position of the light beam directly with a system similar to that of Figure 8.22. Signals that are directly proportional to displacement along each of the two axes and that can be used both as monitors and for feedback compensation are thus obtained.

A good alternative method of deflecting light beams consists of using a mirror mounted on a polygraph pen driver. The polygraph electronics can be used to control static position and gain of the system.

The inverse of the light-on-dark pattern, that is, a shadow cast on a bright ground, is obtained by a different technique, illustrated in Figure 8.23. A shadow is cast by an opaque, thin target illuminated by a point source of light. The target is glued onto a glass plate, which can be moved in three dimensions by a servomotor such as those used in X-Y plotters or by dynamic loudspeakers.

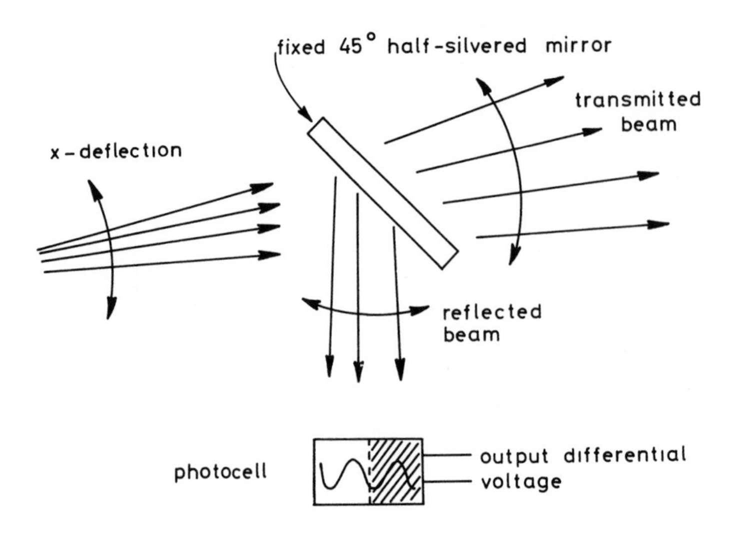

Figure 8.22
Position monitor for deflected light beam. Variable area illuminated by reflected beam is proportional to deflection angle θ_x. If beam is of variable intensity or size, use a dummy beam whose image is blocked before reaching projection screen.

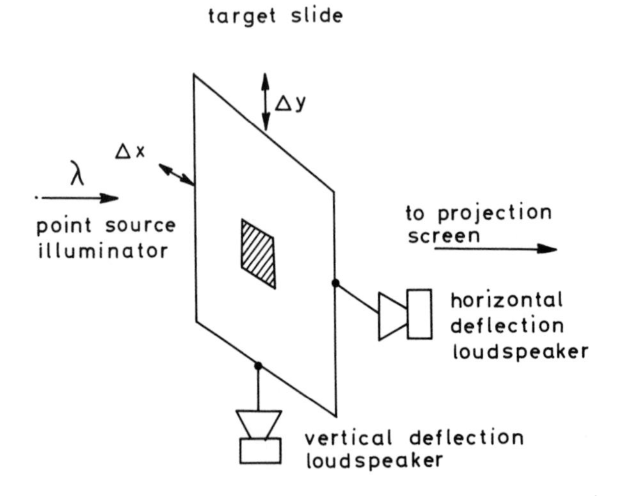

Figure 8.23
Generation of dark rectangles.

Such simple stimulus patterns can be very useful in the study of visual coding; the controls described thus far are adequate for determination of most receptive field properties of retinal cells with the added advantage that quantitative variations of stimulus parameters is possible, with consequent potential for quantitative studies of visual processing by these and other neurons.

Simple geometrical figures can be generated with appropriate slides or by rapid "scanning" of a light or dark dot through the locus of a geometrical figure, using appropriate wave forms to drive light-deflecting loudspeakers at high speeds. This technique suffers from being limited to audio frequencies, which may or may not modulate the responses of some photoreceptors, confusing the experimental results. For some studies, this should not be a serious limitation, because it is an easy matter to exceed flicker fusion frequencies with these methods.

Prepared films or videotapes of naturally occurring scenes or animated drawings, or even filmed, videotaped, or directly displayed computer-generated graphics, allow a greater variety of patterns, although the limitations of film videotape and computer displays, such as flicker rate, limited dynamic range, limited resolution, and the like, must be taken into account. Whenever using color film, keep in mind the fact that the actual spectral composition does not match that of the original source.

We will now consider means of monitoring the properties of the eye, such as orientation, pupil size, and accommodation. In order to study the latter, a technique for controlling blur is also discussed.

8.5.2 Oculomotor and Accommodative Systems

It is the function of the oculomotor and accommodative systems to correct for movements of the object of regard. In order to stimulate these systems optically, it is necessary to move a test target along the visual axis to stimulate accommodation and/or, in a plane perpendicular to the visual axis, to stimulate eye movements. The simplest approach to producing these stimuli is of course to move the target, using servomechanic techniques. Two orthogonal rectilinear transports are provided by X-Y plotters, which can be modified for transporting visual test targets.

Mechanical transports are slow and usually noisy. To produce movement suitable for stimulating the oculomotor system, the dot formed by the beam of an oscilloscope may be used. If the persistence of the CRT phosphor is short there will be no apparent tail as the target moves around. Use of this oscilloscopic technique is restricted to producing target movements perpendicular to the visual axis. It also has the disadvantage of greatly restricting the target characteristics of color, size, shape, intensity, and so forth.

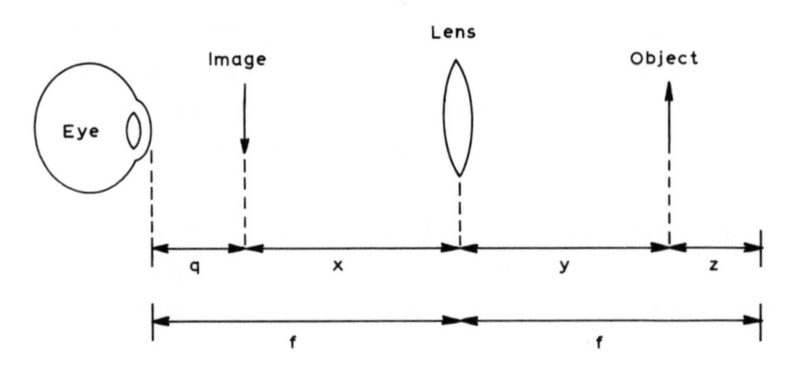

Figure 8.24
Maxwellian view.

Use of mechanical transports to produce sufficient axial movement is limited, because the range of interest extends from points as close as 10 cm from the eye to points as far as 10 m (optical ∞). Using a simple optical trick called *Maxwellian view*, the range of necessary distances to the target may be compressed. Maxwellian view has the property that effective reciprocal distance in diopters (1 D = 1 diopter = 1 m^{-1}) is directly proportional to target movement.

Maxwellian view is schematized in Figure 8.24. It is achieved by placing a lens a distance from the eye equal to its focal length f. An object (test object) is placed distance y behind the lens. The eye now sees its image located a distance x in front of the lens. The lens formula can be used to relate x and y:

$$\frac{1}{x} + \frac{1}{y} = \frac{1}{f}. \tag{8.2}$$

The distance of the image from the eye is q and the amount of *accommodative stimulus* Q is given by

$$Q = 1/q. \tag{8.3}$$

Observe that

$$q = f - x. \tag{8.4}$$

Then by the lens formula,

$$f^2 = (f - y)q. \tag{8.5}$$

Set $z = f = y$. Then,

$$q = f^2/z$$

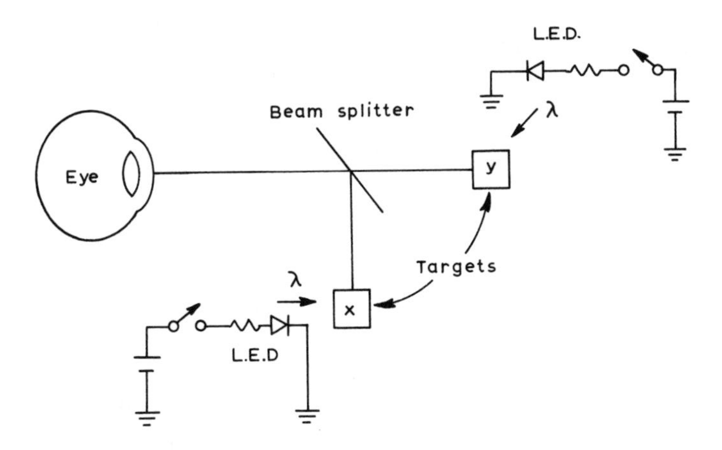

Figure 8.25
Source gating technique.

or

$$Q = z/f^2. \quad (8.6)$$

Let us state two other properties of Maxwellian view without proof:

1. The angular size of the image at the eye does not vary with Q.
2. The apparent brightness of the image does not vary with Q.

The techniques discussed are all designed to be capable of providing analog control of target parameters. In many instances step functions or pulses of stimuli are adequate. If we can sacrifice the facility of analog control, then we can take advantage of the tremendous flexibility of the *source gating* technique (Figure 8.25). Separate sources of illumination of two or more targets are used (for example, LEDs): LED_x and LED_y illuminate targets X and Y. Positions of X and Y are optically superimposed with a beamsplitter. Targets are selected to have the desired properties (for example, position, color, size, and contrast gradient). If a target is not illuminated, it is invisible. By gating the associated light sources in a mutually exclusive way, the effective target state will be changed. Gated light sources may be purchased that use mechanical or liquid crystal shutters, LEDs, gas bulb, or lasers. This technique offers the advantages of speed, quantitative control capability, and versatility.

8.5.3 Monitoring of the Muscular Adjustments of the Eye

Some of the light that hits the retina is diffusely reflected. It therefore acts as a secondary source. As it travels back out of the eye, it undergoes an optical variation that recapitulates in a reverse order the exact variation which it suffered when it originally entered the eye (*principle of optical reversal*). If we monitor the characteristics of this return light, we obtain a direct indicator of the optical significance of the anatomical alterations in question. Hence, this is termed a *primary measurement.*

For all primary measurements we shall use an IR test source. Infrared light behaves much like visible light with respect to the optics of the eye, yet the eye is insensitive to infrared light. Therefore the system will not be appreciably disturbed (uv light is not advised; it irreversibly breaks down the photopigments of the retina).

One may also monitor the anatomical changes directly and then deduce the optical significance of them; this is termed a *secondary measurement.* There is no restriction to the measurement method. Mechanical and electrical techniques have been tried (see Alpern, 1969, for a survey). We shall restrict our treatment to optical techniques, because they tend to disturb the system the least. Again IR light will be used since the receptors are insensitive to it.

Both types of measurements have advantages. The primary measurements require no assumptions about the relationship between the anatomy and the optics. These relationships are, in general, complex and highly variable both within and among species. Also, primary measurements have signal-to-noise ratios that are much lower than corresponding secondary measurements.

8.5.4 Measurement of Eye Movements

The principle of reversibility tells us that an image of the retina will be formed in the outside world by the eye's lens system. It will give an exact indication of the optical correspondence between points on the retina and points in the outside world. By picking at least two landmarks (two are necessary to eliminate possible ambiguity that might arise from torsional eye movement around a single point), we may deduce the orientation of the entire retina. The position of the eye may be deduced from the retina position. This technique has not been used extensively; a discussion can be found in Comsweet (1958).

Secondary measurements, on the other hand, have been employed successfully. Various devices have been mounted on contact lenses to help indicate the position of the eye.

It is possible to determine the position of the globe with no attachments. One such method has been described by O'Neill and Stark (1968). The corneoschleral region is flooded with IR light (Figure 8.26). Two photocells are then positioned near the eye to pick up the light reflected from the eye in the region of the corneoschleral junction. Because of the difference in reflectances in the two regions, the output of the photocells will vary as the eye rotates in their plane. If the difference of outputs of the two photocells is generated electrically, this signal provides an

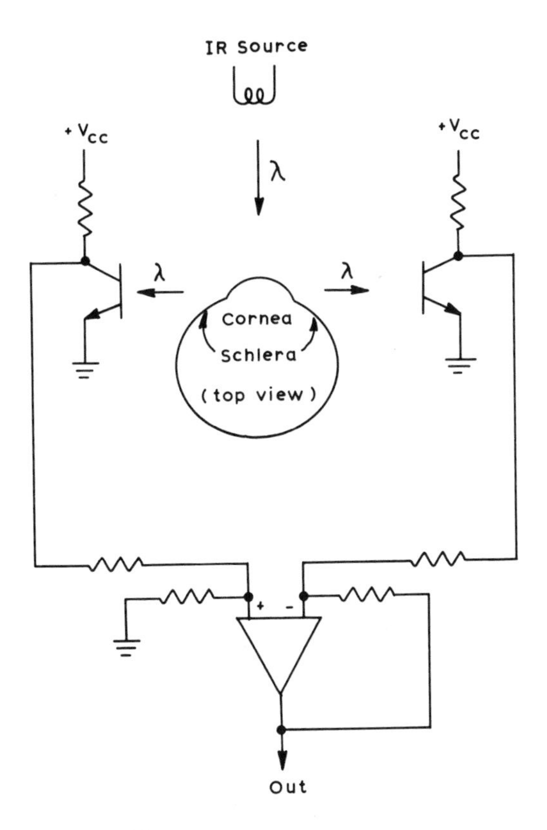

Figure 8.26
Monitoring lateral eye movements.

indication of the position of the globe. If the photocells are positioned just below the visual axis, the vision of the eye will not be impaired.

The method described here is simple to set up and requires no ocular attachments. However, if vertical or torsional eye movements are to be detected, contact lens techniques become necessary. Contact lens techniques as a rule provide a larger range of measurement.

8.5.5 Monitoring Refractory State of the Eye

The ocular state of refraction that we shall call Q is the reciprocal of the distance for which the eye is focused q. By the principle of reversibility, we know that if the eye is focused for a distance q then any light originating at a point on the retina will come to a focus at a distance q from the eye. Let us assume we have a source of light on the retina of no vertical width: a line source. If we put a double slit aperture in front of the eye, we permit only two peripheral sheets of light to return from the retina (Figure 8.27a). If we now put a screen a distance S from the eye, we will form two slit images on it, and the spacing between the slits e will be directly

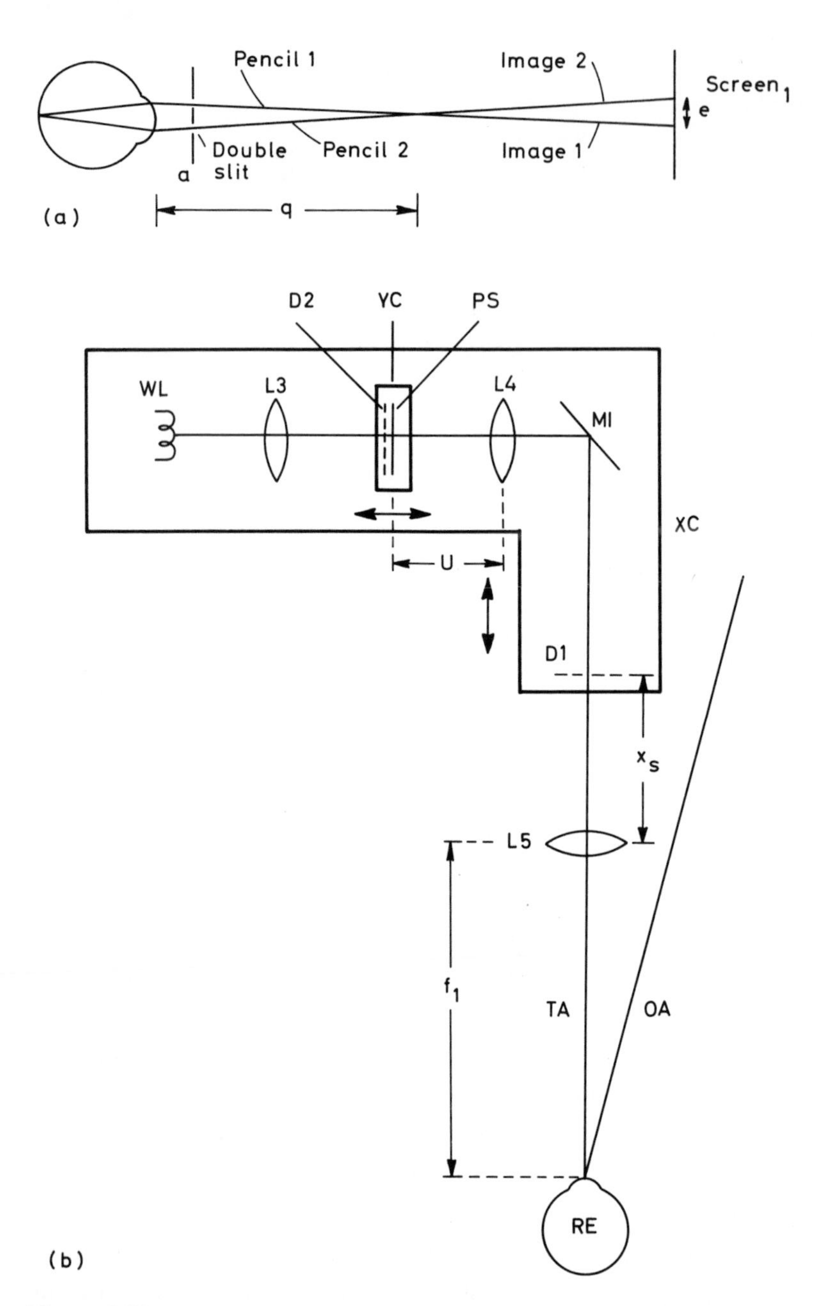

Figure 8.27
Monitoring accommodative state. (a) Image of a line source on retina of an eye accommodated for a distance q, projected on screen with double slit arrangement. (b) Stimulus apparatus consists of tungsten filament lamp (WL), condenser lens (L3), and diffusing filter (F2), providing diffuse light to illuminate photographic slide (PS) from the rear. Image of PS is projected onto fine-grain diffusing screen (D1) via lens L4 and front-surface mirror M1. This image is the test target, and may be replaced by a direct-viewed target if only reversible blur is used. Movement of plotter carriage *XC* is used to vary X_S. $Q = X_S/f_5^2$, where f_5 is focal distance of lens L5. Thus movement of carriage of *XC* produces reversible blur. Irreversible blur can be produced by movement of Y_C (pen holder of X-Y plotter).

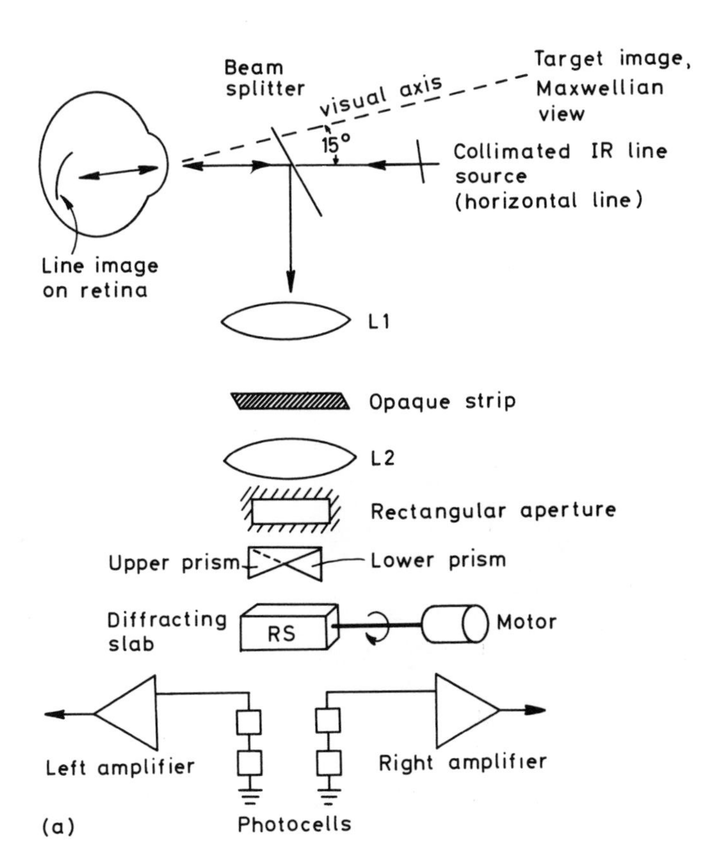

Figure 8.28

Dynamic monitor for accommodative responses to reversible or irreversible blur stimuli. (a) Scanning method for monitoring image derived from retinal line source. See text for complete description. (b) Effect of rotating slab (RS) on the image position Y. (c) An optometer. All optical shields removed. Labels on photograph:

A. Blur target.
B. Target slide.
C. Target projection lens (L4).
D. Mirror.
E. Target screen.
F. Photocells and preamplifiers.
G. Rotating slab (RS).
H. Opaque strip, L2, aperture, prisms.
I. Motor for rotating RS.
J. Mirror.
K. "Gunsight" for axial eye alignment.
L. L1.
M. Bite bar.
N. Optics for Maxwellian view (L5).
O. X-Y plotter.

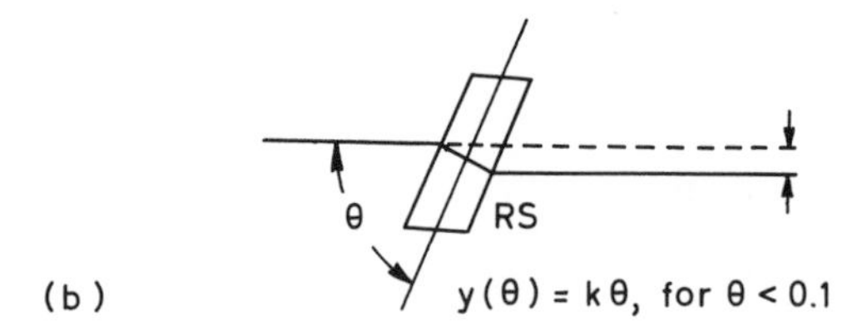

(b)

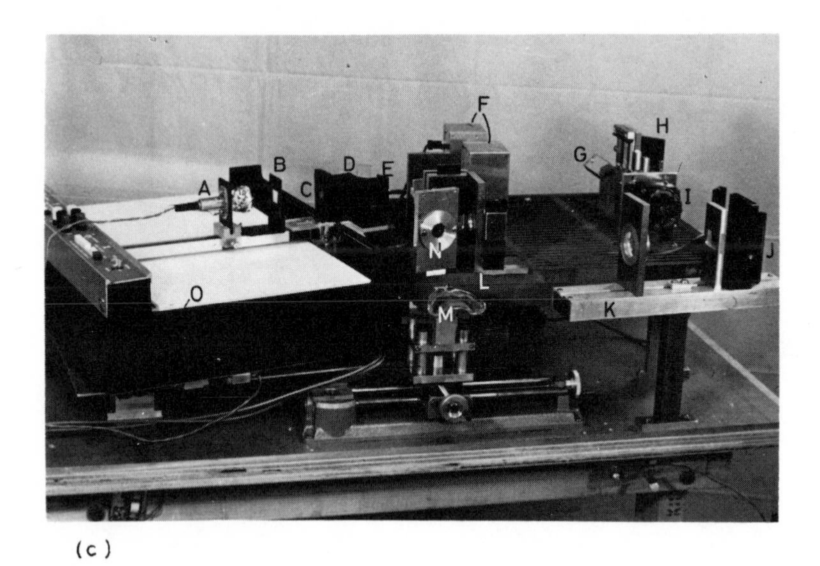

(c)

Figure 8.28 (continued)

proportional to $Q = 1/q$. Figure 8.28a illustrates the implementation of this technique. A beam splitter is used to enable the injection of high intensity IR light into the eye. The return light is reflected off the beam splitter to the detector optics starting with lens L1. Lens L1 is arranged so that the iris of the eye is optically conjugate with a horizontal opaque strip. The purpose of L1 is to reconstruct an optical equivalent of the situation diagrammed in Figure 8.27a; now the vision of the eye is not occluded. The old double-slit aperture has been implemented using two separate components: a rectangular aperture and an opaque strip. If the image of the pupil in its most constricted state completely bounds the rectangular aperture, pupil size will have no effect on the measurement. The opaque strip also serves to eliminate a strong corneal reflection, which is brought to a focus on the opaque strip and therefore blocked.

The addition of lens L2 converges the return light on the photocells.

The problem that remains is to determine the vertical separation in the slit images. This is accomplished using the prisms, a rotating refractory slab, and photodetectors. The upper prism is placed in the path of the upper slit. The lower prism is placed in the path of the lower slit. They are arranged apexes to bases. They thus effect left and right horizontal displacements of the upper and lower slit images, respectively. The refractory slab displaces the images vertically by an amount y, which is a function of the orientation of the refractory slab. For small θ ($\theta < 0.1$ rad), $y(\theta) = K\theta$.

The possibility of obtaining perfect slit images is precluded by imperfect retinal line sources, a nonideal double slit aperture, and the effects of diffraction. In actuality, the slit images are blurs whose intensities are shown qualitatively in Figure 8.29a.

Two photodetectors are arranged one above the other and are wired back-to-back to form the difference voltage (Figure 8.29b). As the blur is swept across them, the output voltage V is as shown in Figure 8.29c. The center of the blur (maximum intensity), which corresponds to the ideal location of a perfect slit image, is detected when the blur pattern symmetrically straddles the photodetector pair ($y = y_0$), resulting in $V = 0$. This is essentially a spatial differentiation, and we search for a negative-going zero derivative V.

With a photodetector (PHD) pair for each slit image (four PHDs in all), the relative positions may be discerned by noting the required change in θ between conditions of $V_1(y) = 0$ and $V_2(y) = 0$. The outputs of the PHD pairs are V_1 and V_2.

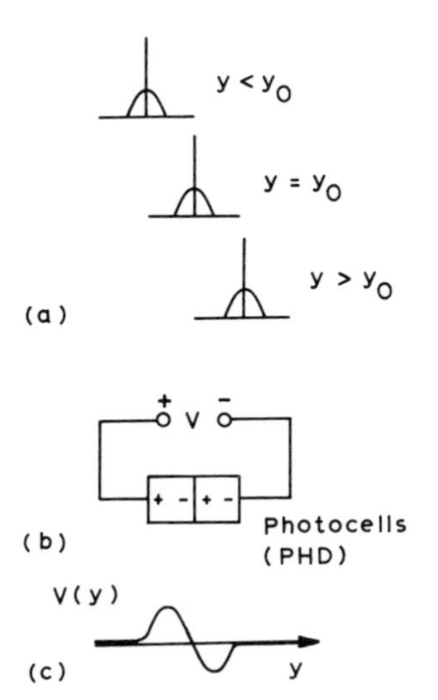

Figure 8.29
Effect of RS position on photocell output. (a) Qualitative sketches of intensity of illumination of blurred slit image. Three different displacements due to effect of RS are shown. (b) Differentiating arrangement of photodetectors. (c) Photodetector pair output as a function of location of blur pattern.

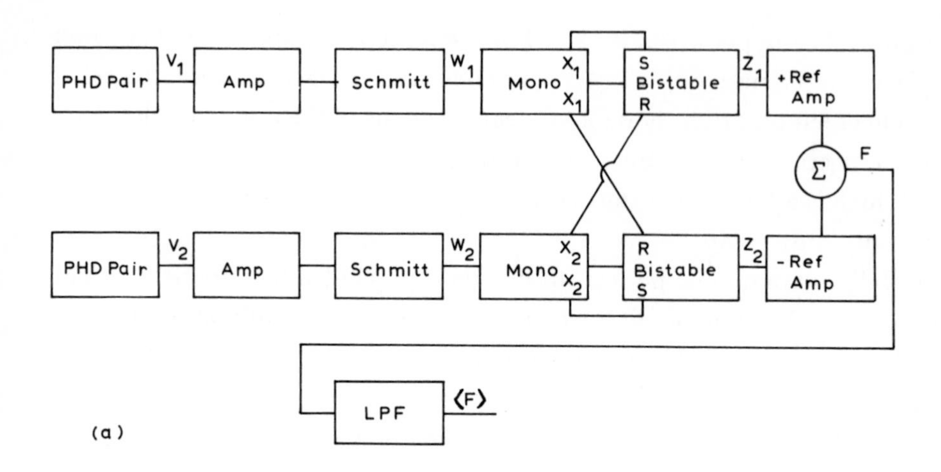

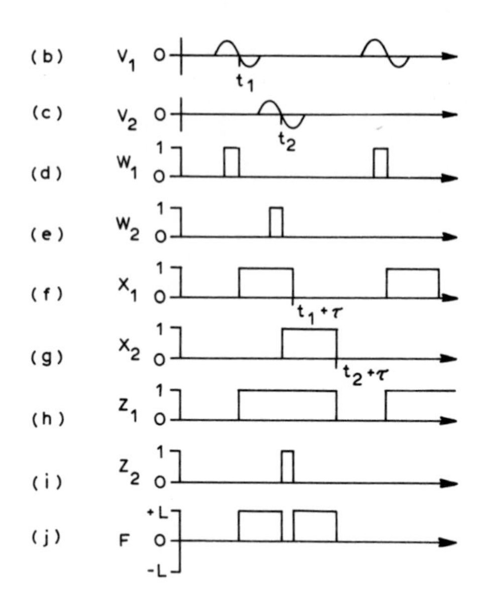

Figure 8.30
Phase detector. (a) Block diagram; (b–j) typical waveforms at indicated points in block diagram.

Spinning RS at radian frequency ω (that is, $\theta = \omega t$), we have, from Figure 8.29,

$$y = \omega t K \tag{8.7}$$

for small θ where K is a constant. (For large θ the images, $Y1$ and $Y2$, are not passing over the PHDs; therefore, the functional dependence is not important.) The periodic waveforms shown in Figures 8.30b and 8.30c result. From symmetry arguments the negative-going zero crossings correspond to the conditions of $y = e/2$ for $Y1$ and $y = -e/2$ for $Y2$, where e is the spacing between the two blurred slit images. Letting t_1 and t_2 be the times of occurrence of negative-going zero crossings of V_1 and V_2, respectively, we obtain from Equation 8.7

$$e = (t_2 - t_1)\omega t K. \tag{8.8}$$

The electronic scheme used to detect $t_2 - t_1$ is diagrammed in Figure 8.30. Signals V_1 and V_2 are amplified and used to switch associated Schmitt triggers. The Schmitts are adjusted to set on a rising portion of V and reset on the negative-going zero crossing. This results in Schmitt trigger outputs W_1 and W_2 (Figures 8.30d and 8.30e). Monostables are triggered on the reset transitions of their associated Schmitt triggers; they are adjusted to have equal quasistable periods τ. The logical equivalent outputs of the monostables X_1 and X_2 are shown in Figures 8.30f and 8.30g. Bistable #1 is set by X_1 and reset by $\bar{X}_2$; its output (Z_1, Figure 8.30h) gates the $+L$ reference amplifier. Bistable #2 is set by X_2 and reset by X_1; its output (Z_2, Figure 8.30i) gates the $-L$ reference amplifier. The outputs of the gated reference amplifiers are summed to produce

$$F = \begin{cases} +L & \text{if } Z_1\bar{Z}_2 = 1 \\ -L & \text{if } \bar{Z}_1 Z_2 = 1 \\ 0 & \text{if otherwise} \end{cases}$$

(Figure 8.30j). The average value of F is obtained by putting it through a low pass filter (LPF):

$$\langle F \rangle = L\omega(t_2 - t_1)/\tau. \tag{8.9}$$

Thus,

$$\langle F \rangle \cong kR, \tag{8.10}$$

where k = constant.

As an alternative to the primary measurement that we have examined, it is possible to monitor anatomical properties of the eye in order to obtain a secondary measurement of accommodation. In human accommodation mechanics, the

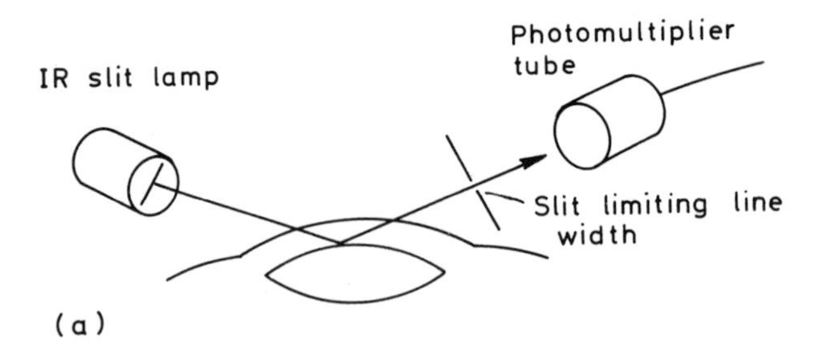

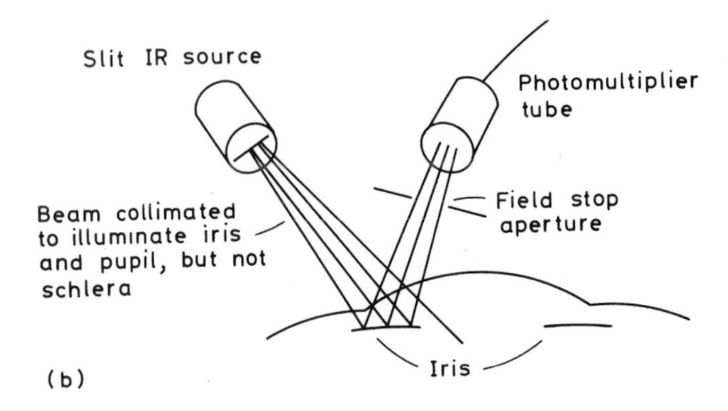

Figure 8.31
Secondary measurements of (a) accommodation, and (b) pupil diameter.

primary anatomical change is in the position of the anterior surface of the lens. The reflection of this surface may be monitored to provide a secondary measurement of refractive state (Figure 8.31a). The lens is illuminated from the side and the light is reflected off the anterior surface. A photomultiplier is positioned to receive this reflected light. A field-limiting stop permits different amounts of light to reach the photomultiplier tube depending on the position of the anterior surface of the lens. Then the refractive state is deduced.

8.5.6 Measurement of Pupil Size

For the discussion of pupil size measurements, we recall two previous methods. We may obtain pupil size information by noting the magnitude of $V(y)$ (Figure 8.29), using a light source that illuminates the entire pupil. The only quantity that will affect this amplitude is the strength of the retinal source. This is determined by the strength of the collimator source, the pupil of the eye. If the source is such that light flux enters the eye through the entire pupil area, the retinal source (and the amplitude of $V(y)$) will depend directly on the pupil area. If light flux is bundled in a slit geometry, the dependence will be on pupil diameter.

The secondary measurement of pupil size (Figure 8.31b) is carried out using a technique similar to the one described for position measurement. The width of the iris is monitored in this way, providing a difference indication that reflects pupil size. The iris and lens are illuminated by an IR slit lamp. Variations in the diffuse reflection received by a photocell located as in Figure 8.31b arise from variations in the diameter of the pupil.

8.6 Gustatory Stimulation

The chemical senses, which can detect very small quantities of some substances, require precisely controlled stimuli for investigation of their mechanisms. Temporal control of the type, concentration, and location on the tongue of sapid solutions often must be attained at least at the level where thresholds can be accurately determined and stimuli can be reliably repeated. This means, given prepared taste solutions, that delivery of the stimulus to the tongue must be precisely controlled. Preferably, physiological ranges should be attainable. This means that the duration of a taste stimulus should be controllable down to 20–100 msec, the duration of a lick for some species, up to several seconds.

A fluidics stimulus control system used in the laboratory of Dr. Bruce Halpern, of Cornell University, is illustrated in Figures 8.32 to 8.34. Fluidics logic is used to control air-driven valves, for automatic control of taste solution flow through the tongue chamber.

The fluidic sequence control (programming controller) was designed by application engineers at Corning Glass Works and was custom-built from Corning FICM components. The device presents a specified volume of sapid solution for a predetermined length of time at a predetermined constant flow rate with rapid onset and cessation of flow. The minimum stimulus duration is about 50 msec if a special Corning time delay relay (TDR) is used. Flushing can be automatically performed after each stimulus, from the HOLDING CONTAINER to the four-way valve (Chromatronix CAV-4060, with PA-875 pneumatic activators) leading to the taste chamber. If desired, the final connections to the tongue can be blown dry with the prepure nitrogen used to drive the liquid. For brief stimuli, with rapid onset and cessation, a low vacuum (1.5–2 psi) is connected to the four-way valve.

An alternative program can be selected through a fluidic selector switch. The alternate program (AUTO WASH) follows the stimulus with a series of tongue water washes with duration and flow parameters identical to those of the stimulus. These rinses are repeated until the AUTO WASH program is discontinued.

The device consists of five major components. These are (1) the fluidic Sequence Control, (2) the Selector Switches and Pressure Controls, (3) the Stimulus Liquids

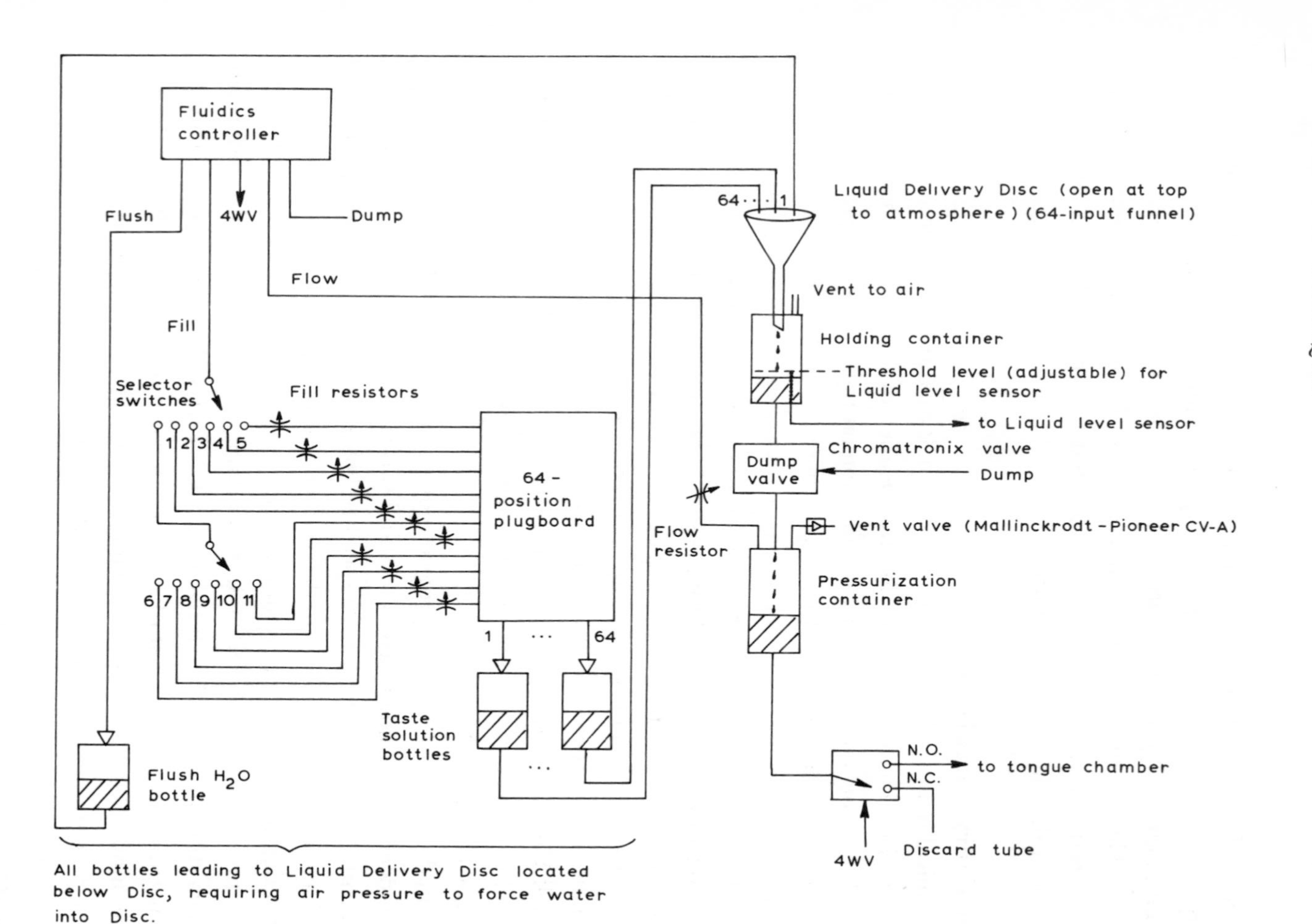

Figure 8.32
Gustatory stimulator, block diagram.

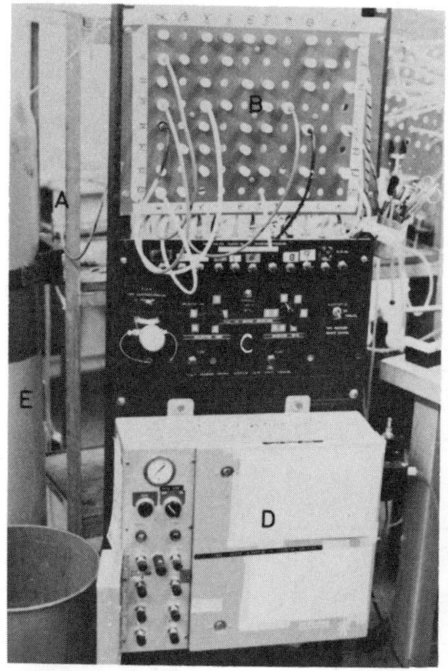

(a)

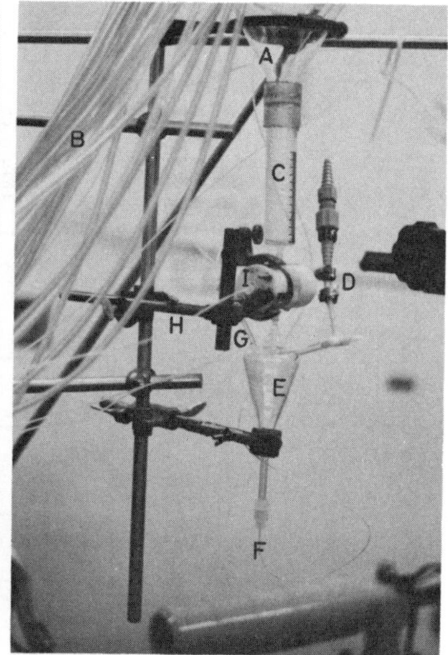

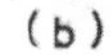

(b)

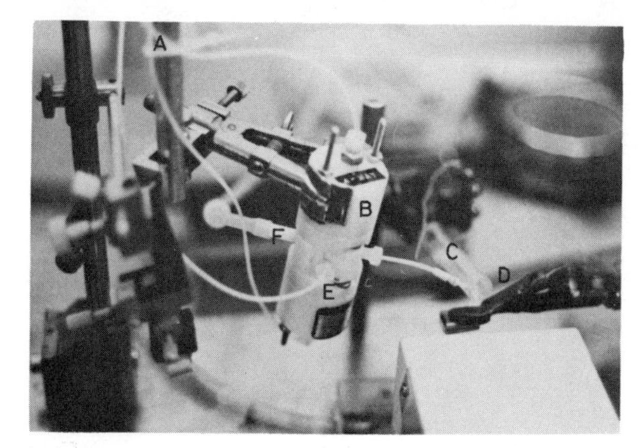

(c)

Figure 8.33
Gustatory stimulator.

(a) Fluidics controller:
A. Solution bottles.
B. Plugboard.
C. Variable resistors, switches, indicators.
D. Fluidics logic manifolds.
E. Prepure nitrogen cylinder.

(b) Liquid delivery system:
A. Liquid delivery disc.
B. Tubes from taste solution bottles.
C. Holding container.
D. Vent valve.
E. Pressurization container.
F. To 4-way valve.
G. FLOW, from fluidics interface valves in fluidics.
H. Dump logic manifold chassis.
I. Dump valve.

(c) 4-Way valve:
A. From 4 WV interface valve in fluidics logic manifold chassis.
B. 4-Way valve.
C. Drain.
D. Tongue chamber.
E. From pressurization container.
F. Drain.

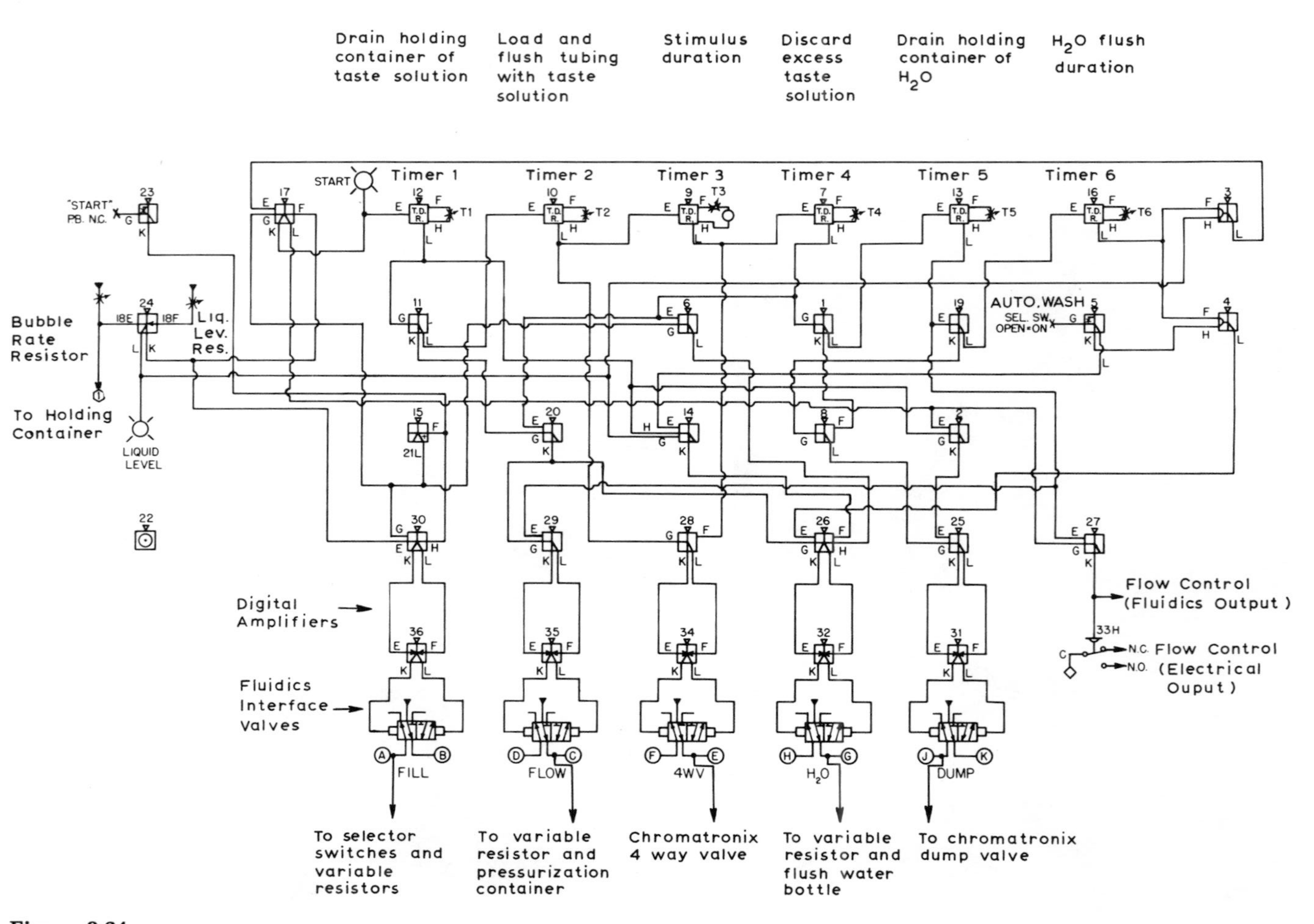

Figure 8.34
Fluidics controller.

Storage Bottles and their pressure input and liquid output connections, (4) Liquid Delivery Disc and the HOLDING and PRESSURIZATION containers, and (5) the two pneumatically operated valves: the DUMP VALVE (Chromatronix CAB-2060 with PA-875 pneumatic activators) and the 4-WAY VALVE. These are illustrated in the photographs of Figure 8.33.

8.6.1 Fluidic Sequence Control (modified Corning SK-70-144-1)

The Fluidic Sequence Control (Figure 8.34) carries out a series of timed logical operations that control (a) the position of the fluidic interface valves; (b) the presence or absence of a fluidic output signal (FLOW CONTROL), which may be used to run logic elements added at a future time, and a switch closure (fluidic-to-electric); and (c) the positions of the visual indicators. The fluidic time delay relays (TDR) are remotely controlled by six high-flow variable resistors. As the resistor is closed (R increases), the duration of the timer that it controls increases. The theoretical maximum timer duration at a 5 psi air supply pressure is 30 sec. This can be extended, however, by providing external capacitance between the variable resistor and the timer. Timer 3 is a special TDR and has an external capacitor. Therefore durations longer than 30 sec are possible. When a special short-duration TDR is used for timer 3, maximum duration is 10 sec and minimum duration is 50 msec. The variable resistor for timer 3 is a nonrising stem valve with a digital control knob.

Two additional variable resistors control the fluidic sensor. This sensor is a back-pressure sensing system which is used for determining correct initial liquid volume (Liquid Level).

8.6.2 Selector Switches and Interface Valve Output-Pressure Controls

Selector Switches

Two six-position rotary fluidics selector switches (Chromatronix R60) determine where the FILL N_2 pressure from position A of the FILL interface valve is directed. (Position B is not used.) Since the two rotary switches are interconnected, there are 11 active output positions.

Pressure Controls

FILL Resistor. For each of the 11 output positions of the rotary switches, there is a graduated, resettable, variable resistor (Hoke 1325 M4B) to determine output pressure from that switch position. The output from each of these eleven variable resistors is brought to a male quick-disconnect through color-coded Tygon tubing.

FLOW Resistor and Regulator. A variable resistor and a gauge-equipped regulator (Mead Fluid Dynamics miniature regulator, 5–50 psi, with 0–60 psi gauge) control output pressure from position C of the FLOW interface valve. Position D is not used. Position *C* provides nitrogen pressure into the PRESSURIZATION CONTAINER (see Multiplexing of Outputs below), which moves liquids from the PRESSURIZATION CONTAINER through the rest of the system.

FLUSH Resistor. A variable resistor controls pressure from position *G* of the H_2O-FLUSH valve. (Position *H* is not used.) Position *G* provides N_2 pressure for the FLUSH cycle, and for the water delivered in the AUTO WASH program. As needed, other variable resistors may be added to control the output pressure of other interface valve output positions.

Multiplexing of Outputs

The output of any of the interface valves can be divided into two or more streams and used to control pneumatic devices or to move liquids other than those presently controlled (in addition, visual indicators may be added to the rotary switch and pressure control panel at some time, in order that the program state can be directly determined). The same gas N_2 is supplied to, and delivered by, all interface valves. This gas is supplied from a tank of *prepure* nitrogen through two stages of regulation.

8.6.3 Stimulus Liquids Storage Bottles and Delivery Tubes

The stimulus liquids are stored in 32 oz polyethylene aspirator bottles. At the top of each bottle is a female quick-disconnect that brings to that bottle nitrogen pressure from the FILL interface valve. The FILL pressure, as noted earlier, passes through the rotary selector switches and a variable resistor. Between the 11 variable resistors and the stimulus liquid bottles is a 64-position plug board. The front plug-board connectors are female quick-disconnects. The outputs of the 11 variable resistors can be connected to any position in the plug board. Each stimulus liquid bottle is connected to one of the positions in the plug board through a rear connector. The output of each stimulus liquid bottle is through the aspirator connection at the bottom of the bottle. When a stimulus bottle receives nitrogen pressure from the plug board, the liquid contents are forced out through Tygon tubing. The outputs of all the stimulus liquid bottles are brought to the LIQUID DELIVERY DISC located above the HOLDING CONTAINER.

The temperature of the stimulus liquid is normally controlled by setting the ambient temperature as desired. If this is impractical (that is, very high or low temperatures are required), stimulus bottles can be put in a water bath at temperatures above or below ambient temperature. In that case, however, the final delivery temperature will be different from the water bath temperature because of temperature changes between the bottle and the tongue. Consequently, measurement of temperature at the tongue will be necessary. This is not the case when the ambient temperature is used as the stimulus liquid temperature.

8.6.4 Containers

The stimulus liquid from the FILL-pressurized stimulus liquid bottle is delivered into the HOLDING CONTAINER through a Tygon tube placed in the LIQUID DELIVERY DISC. The HOLDING CONTAINER has, at its bottom, the sensing tube of the LIQUID LEVEL sensor. Stimulus liquid accumulates in the HOLDING CONTAINER until the volume determined by the LIQUID LEVEL variable resistor is obtained. When LIQUID LEVEL is reached, the liquid in the HOLDING CONTAINER transfers to the PRESSURIZATION CONTAINER. The PRESSURIZATION CONTAINER is vented by a one-way valve (Mallinckrodt-Pioneer CV-A) to permit rapid transfer of liquid into it.

8.6.5 Pneumatically Operated Valves

DUMP Valve

The DUMP valve is a two-way pneumatically operated valve which, when open, allows the transfer of liquid from the HOLDING to the PRESSURIZATION CONTAINER. When closed, it permits an accumulation of liquid in the HOLDING CONTAINER, and a build-up of nitrogen pressure in the PRESSURIZATION CONTAINER. The DUMP valve is closed when the DUMP interface valve is in the *K* position, and open when the DUMP interface valve is in the *J* Position.

4-WAY VALVE

The 4-WAY VALVE controls stimulus liquid access to the tongue. When the 4-WAY interface valve is in position *F* (normal rest position), the input connection to the 4-WAY VALVE from the PRESSURIZATION CONTAINER is connected to the discard tube, and a low vacuum is connected to the tongue chamber input. When the 4-WAY interface valve is in position *E* (duration of timer 3), the PRESSURIZATION CONTAINER output is directed towards the tongue.

8.6.6 Basic Operational Sequence

We will discuss the operation of the device without going into detail on its actual internal workings. A summary is presented in Table 8.1.

Single Stimulus Presentation Program (Selector Switch in OFF position)

Pressing the START button initiates a stimulus presentation cycle. The first event in the cycle is the beginning of FILL pressure (through position *A* of the FILL interface valve, the rotary switches, and a FILL pressure fluidic variable resistor). FILL pressure continues until the accumulation of liquid in the HOLDING CONTAINER produces enough back pressure to trigger the LIQUID LEVEL sensor. When the LIQUID LEVEL sensor is triggered, FILL pressure stops (the FILL interface valve returns to position *B*). The LIQUID LEVEL and START indicators become green, the flow control fluidic and electrical output go on, and the

Table 8.1
Operating sequence of fluidics gustatory stimulator.

5.0 psig Air												FLUIDIC SEQUENCE CONTROL	
55 psig Main N_2 (to Interface Valves)										40 psig LL N_2 (Stimulus bottles)			
		INPUTS			INDICATORS		OUTPUTS						
Setting (+30 mm)	STEPS	LIQUID LEVEL	START push button	AUTO. WASH switch	LIQUID LEVEL	START	FLOW CONTROL	DUMP	H_2O FLUSH	4-WAY VALVE	FLOW	FILL	Fluidic-to electric switch
		LL	PB	SS	LL		6	5	4	3	2	1	Jack
	0	O	O	O	O	O	O	O	O	O	O	O	O
	1	O	P	O	O	O	O	O	O	O	O	X	O
3.9		5–30 ml (set via BR)											
	2	X	O	O	X	X	X	X	O	O	O	O	X
2.8		1–85 sec later (set via T-1)											
	3	X	O	O	X	X	X	O	X	O	X	O	X
4.6		1–15 sec later (set via T-2)											
	4	O	O	O	O	X	X	O	X	X	X	O	X
Digital		0.05–10 sec later (set via T-3)											
	5	O	O	O	O	X	X	O	X	O	X	O	X
3.7		1–6 sec later (set via T-4)											
	6	O	O	O	O	X	X	X	O	O	O	O	X
3.5		1–150 sec later (set via T-5)											
	7	O	O	O	O	X	O	O	O	O	X	O	O
3.3		1–30 sec later (set via T-6)											
	8	O	O	O	O	O	O	O	O	O	O	O	O

	0	O	O	O	O	O	O	O	O	O	O	O	O	
	1	O	P	X	O	O	O	O	O	O	O	X	O	
3.9		5–30 ml (set via BR)												
	2	X	O	X	X	X	X	X	O	O	O	O	X	
		1–85 sec later (T-1)												Auto .
	3	X	O	X	X	X	X	O	X	O	X	O	X	Wash
4.6		1–15 sec later (T-2)												Sequence
	4	O	O	X	O	X	X	O	X	X	X	O	X	
Digital		0.05–10 sec later (T-3)												
	5	O	O	X	O	X	X	O	X	O	X	O	X	
3.7		1–6 sec later (T-4)			(X)									
	6	O	O	X	O	X	X	X	O	O	O	O	X	
3.5		1–150 sec later (T-5)												
	7	O	O	X	O	X	O	O	O	O	X	O	O	
3.3		1–30 sec later (T-6)												
	8	O	O	X	O	O	O	O	X	O	O	O	O	
		Do not change SSw between steps 8 & 9												
	9	X	O	X	X	X	X	X	O	O	O	O	X	
	10	X	O	O	X	X	X	X	O	O	O	O	X	

Note: Timer 1 is running.

Symbols: SSw = selector switch
PB = push button
X = "ON"
O = "OFF"
P = "PULSE"
T = "TIMER"
BR = bubble rate variable resistor
LL = liquid level

pneumatically controlled Chromatronix DUMP valve is switched from closed to open (DUMP interface valve goes to position *J*), allowing transfer of the liquid in the HOLDING CONTAINER into the PRESSURIZATION CONTAINER. A plastic one-way (Mallinckrodt-Pioneer CV-A) valve vents the PRESSURIZATION CONTAINER at this time, permitting rapid liquid transfer, using gravity feed. The LIQUID LEVEL indicator will become red when sufficient liquid drains out.

When Timer 1 runs out (maximum duration of about 85 sec), the Chromatronix DUMP valve closes (DUMP interface valve goes to position *K*), thus sealing the input to the PRESSURIZATION CHAMBER and closing the bottom outlet of the HOLDING CONTAINER. The FLOW INTERFACE VALVE moves to position *C*. Flow pressure is supplied through the FLOW variable fluidic resistor and pressure regulator into the PRESSURIZATION CONTAINER. FLOW pressure will continue for the duration of Timers 2, 3, and 4. Simultaneously, the H_2O-FLUSH interface valve moves to position *G*, and H_2O-FLUSH pressure passes through the FLUSH fluidic variable resistor to the H_2O-FLUSH distilled water bottle. This produces movement of distilled water toward and into the HOLDING CONTAINER. The H_2O-FLUSH pressure will continue through Timers 2, 3, and 4. When sufficient water accumulates, the LIQUID LEVEL indicator will become green, but the back-pressure sensor will *not* operate.

Timer 2 begins running as soon as Timer 1 times out and goes on. No change in operation can be seen during the running of Timer 2. When Timer 2 times out, the 4-WAY VALVE interface valve moves to position *E*, and N_2 pressure is led directly to and changes the position of the 4-WAY VALVE through which stimulus liquids pass to the tongue. The 4-WAY VALVE continues in this "timed input" position (with the 4-WAY VALVE in this position, the liquid in the PRESSURIZATION CONTAINER is delivered to the tongue) for the duration of Timer 3 (50 msec to 45 sec). Timer 3 is controlled by a Matheson N.R.S. valve, with a numerical counter.

When Timer 3 times out, the 4-WAY interface valve returns to position *F*, thus moving the 4-WAY VALVE to its "rest" position (liquid in the PRESSURIZATION CONTAINER is delivered to the discard tube). The 4-WAY VALVE is in this position throughout the cycle *except* during the operation of Timer 3. The low vacuum immediately empties the input to the tongue chamber and dries it. A normally closed manual fluidic switch is in series with the output from position *F* of the 4-WAY INTERFACE VALVE. If this switch is opened before Timer 3 starts, the 4-WAY VALVE will remain in its input position, and liquid will be delivered to the tongue chamber until Timer 4 times out.

When Timer 4 times out, FLOW and H_2O-FLUSH pressure stop, but pressure continues at position *F* of the 4-WAY VALVE interface valve, thus keeping the Chromatronix 4-WAY VALVE switched such that the PRESSURIZATION CONTAINER is connected to the discard tube and the vacuum is connected to the tongue chamber input. The DUMP interface valve goes to position *J*, and therefore N_2 pressure is led to and opens the Chromatronix DUMP valve. This causes a flushing of the HOLDING CONTAINER by the flush water which accumulated during the cycles of Timers 2, 3, and 4. The flush water now transfers to the PRESSURIZATION CONTAINER, which is vented through its one-way valve. As the water drains out, the LIQUID LEVEL indicator becomes red.

When Timer 5 times out, the Chromatronix DUMP valve closes (DUMP interface valve to *K*), thus sealing the liquid input to the PRESSURIZATION CONTAINER. At the same time, the FLOW interface valve moves to position *C*, causing onset of FLOW pressure, thus moving the FLUSH WATER out of the PRESSURIZATION CONTAINER. The FLOW pressure remains on for the duration of Timer 6. If the manual switch in series with output *F* were opened before Timer 3 started, and is still open at this time, the FLUSH water will pass into the tongue chamber.

When Timer 6 times out, the START indicator changes from green to black, and the stimulus cycle is completed. No further events will occur until a new cycle is initiated (it should be noted that after one cycle has run, if liquid is placed in the HOLDING CONTAINER from any source, a full presentation cycle will be initiated, if liquid level is reached).

Stimulus Presentation with AUTO WASH PROGRAM

If the Selector Switch is placed in the ON position, and a stimulus cycle is initiated by pressing the START PUSH BUTTON, a stimulus liquid will be presented exactly as described above. However, when Timer 6 times out, the H_2O-FLUSH INTERFACE VALVE will move to position *G*, thus bringing water into the HOLDING CONTAINER. Flow of water into the holding container will continue until LIQUID LEVEL is reached. At this time, the LIQUID LEVEL indicator will become green, the back-pressure sensor will trigger, and the START indicator will become green. The system now proceeds as described above. Once again, however, when Timer 6 times out, the H_2O-FLUSH interface valve will move to position *G*. This automatic initiation of another wash cycle will continue indefinitely until the Selector Switch is returned to the OFF position. It should be noted that the Selector Switch must *not* be moved from ON to OFF between the time that Timer 6 times out and the time that LIQUID LEVEL is reached.

8.6.7 Operation

The timers must be set to provide the stimulus cycle necessary for a particular experiment. Timer 1 must be set long enough so that the liquid in the holding container will completely drain into the pressurization container. Timer 1 should be set no longer than necessary, since this will needlessly prolong the stimulus or H_2O-WASH cycle.

The LIQUID LEVEL and the FILL fluidic variable resistors should be set such that the desired volume of liquid enters the HOLDING CONTAINER.

Timer 3 is set with the numerical counter variable resistor to give the desired stimulus duration.

Timer 4 removes the remaining contents of the PRESSURIZATION CONTAINER from the system.

Timer 5 should be set long enough to permit the FLUSH-H_2O to drain from the HOLDING CONTAINER to the PRESSURIZATION CONTAINER.

Timer 2 should be set long enough so that the FLOW pressure will move liquid from the PRESSURIZATION CONTAINER to the Chromatronix 4-WAY VALVE, through the valve, and into the discard tube before Timer 2 runs out. This provides a flush of most of the system with the liquid that will be presented to the tongue during the duration of Timer 3 (see below). Also, Timer 2 duration must be long enough for flow pressure to reach a constant value (measured on the FLOW regulator gauge). Timer 6 controls duration of the FLOW pressure following Timer 5. If Timer 6 has sufficient duration, all liquid will be blown from the system, except the connection to the tongue from the Chromatronix 4-WAY VALVE.

The fluidic-to-electric switch, which can be used to automatically operate a tape recorder or other electronics, will turn off when Timer 6 starts.

8.6.8 Common Problems

1. *The LIQUID LEVEL and the START indicators alternate between their two color states. The fluidics sequence control will not operate:*
Check the air pressure supply. About 60 psi must be supplied to the system filter and regulator to provide 5 psi fluidics working pressure.

2. *Liquid continues to accumulate in the HOLDING CONTAINER after the START button is pressed, and reaches an excessive volume.*
(a) Check the setting of the LIQUID LEVEL variable fluidic resistor. (b) Check to see that the LIQUID LEVEL sensor tube is appropriately placed in the HOLDING CONTAINER. (c) Reduce the FILL pressure. (d) Check BUBBLE RATE variable resistor.

3. *The Fluidic Sequence Control program advances to some step, and will not move beyond that point:*

Check the setting of the timer variable resistor that controls the duration of that step of the program. It probably has been increased such that the step now has an infinite length.

4. *After the DUMP valve opens, liquid will not drain from the HOLDING CONTAINER to the PRESSURIZATION CONTAINER or drains very slowly.*
(a) Check the one-way valve on the PRESSURIZATION CONTAINER to see if it is operating correctly. (b) Check the stopcock on the PRESSURIZATION CONTAINER to see if it is in the correct position, that is, the PRESSURIZATION CONTAINER is connected to the one-way valve. (c) Check the position of the one-way valve. The one-way valve should be placed such that its arrow points toward the PRESSURIZATION CONTAINER.

5. *After liquid enters the PRESSURIZATION CONTAINER, the liquid does not move out during Timers 2, 3, 4:*
(a) Check the one-way valve; it may not be closing. (b) Check the position of the stopcock connected to the one-way valve; it may be continuously venting the CONTAINER. (c) Check for mechanical blockage of the output tubing.

6. *No liquid enters the tongue chamber during the operation of Timer 3:*
(a) Check the duration of Timer 3; it may be excessively short for the flow pressure that you are using (for brief stimuli a 16 psi flow pressure is used). (b) Check the 4-WAY VALVE; its connects may be blocked or it may not be operating.

8.6.9 System Maintenance

1. *Air supply.* The air supply to the Fluidic Sequence Control unit must be dry and thoroughly filtered. There should be an initial filter and an initial regulator on the output from the main air supply. The second filter (Corning) should be placed after the main air supply filter. The filter should be changed once every six months and more often if any sign of liquid appears. The output of the filter is led to a second regulator (Corning) connected to the air input to the Fluidic Sequence Control unit. This air is used only to operate the fluidics, and does not reach the stimulus liquids.

2. *Contamination Gauge.* The Fluidic Sequence Control contains a contamination gauge. This is a device with a glass window. The window clouds if the air supply is contaminated. The gauge should be checked monthly. *If* the gauge shows contamination, the fluidic logic elements may require cleaning by high pressure, clean air. Washing or ultrasonic cleaning may be necessary. Also, the gauge window should be replaced.

3. *Nitrogen Supply.* Two tanks of *prepure* (that is, very dry) nitrogen are required for system operation. They are used to drive the stimulus liquids, not for powering the fluidics. One tank is connected through a two-stage regulator to the input

for the interface valves. The second tank is connected through a two-stage regulator to the pressure input for the Liquid Level fluidics element.

4. *Liquid Supply Tubes.* Salts may crystallize in the tubes that carry liquids from the stimulus liquid bottles to the HOLDING CONTAINER. Such tubes should be flushed with water. Tubes which carry sugars, amino acids, and so on, should be flushed before every experiment.

5. *Stimulus Liquids.* The conductivity, refractive index, and/or pH of all stimulus liquids, including the FLUSH water, should be checked before each experiment.

6. *Delivery System Cleanness.* Unless precluded by the experimental design, each stimulus should be presented through a system and to a tongue chamber which contain no traces of previous stimuli. The number and volumes of washes necessary to accomplish this is determined by either using the animal's response as a criterion, or by measuring the conductivity or some other index of solute strength, after washing.

The electrical conductivity of the stimulus solution is of importance when using a *lickometer*, a conductance-measuring trigger used to detect contact of the tongue with the stimulus solution. Such a device may consist of a high-impedance ($10^{12}\ \Omega$) high-gain (10,000) amplifier biased with a very small voltage (say, 0.1 mV) through a large resistance ($10^{9}\ \Omega$). The stimulus solution is grounded, and shunts the bias voltage where it touches the tongue, to which the amplifier ground is attached. This results in a voltage change, which can be discriminated. However, lickometers can cause electrical artifacts during neurophysiological recording, unless special precautions such as the use of an isolated voltage supply for the input bias and careful head placement are used.

Alternatively, a light and phototransistor can be used to detect the advancing fluid optically by reflected light. This method is more difficult but does not run the risk of electrical stimulation of the tongue and eliminates artifacts. Capacitance changes can be detected when liquid enters the tongue chamber. Either of these devices can be calibrated with a lickometer before and after an experiment.

8.7 Olfactory Stimulation

The primary concern in olfactory stimulation over recent years has been control of the stimulus quality: Some odorants are effective at very low concentrations, and when present as contaminants they may confound interpretation of olfactory responses. For this reason, some workers, such as Dr. Maxwell Mozell of the State University of New York in Syracuse, have turned to gas chromatographic methods for assaying the purity of their odorants and even for preparation of chromatographically pure stimulus substances. Most of the material presented here is based on discussions with Dr. Mozell.

Concentration of an odorant in the delivery system is generally expressed as partial pressure of the material in the air delivered to the mucosa. At the very low concentrations that are used, several precautions must be taken, which we will briefly mention here. Deodorized air is sometimes prepared by passing it through columns of activated charcoal and silica gel after drying with $CaCl_2$. The air is tested for olfactory neutrality using the lack of response of the experimental preparation as a criterion.

The deodorized air is remoisturized, to prevent drying of the mucosa, and used to produce a mixture of air and odorant by one of two methods: serial dilution or flow dilution. These are diagrammed in Figure 8.35. In both techniques, a mixture of odorant in air at a known partial pressure is generated first, generally by saturating the air at a carefully controlled temperature.

In the serial dilution method, the saturated air is mixed in a known volume with a known volume of remoisturized deodorized air, thus diluting it by a known ratio. This is continued serially until the desired dilution is attained. Precautions must be taken, however, to ensure that the odorant is not adsorbed on the walls of the mixing chamber(s), or the concentration may be much less than that expected from the serial dilutions. This can be a troublesome effect, especially if several successive dilutions are performed in separate containers. Careful, thorough mixing is essential, as in any serial dilution. Also, at the low final concentrations required to work at physiological levels for some substances, such as pheromones, the concentration cannot always be monitored directly, and extrapolation techniques must be relied on.

The flow dilution technique avoids some of the problems involved in serial dilution by mixing flows of saturated and deodorized air in a mixing vessel; the dilution ratio is equal to the ratio of flow rates of odorant-saturated remoisturized air and deodorized air. The major difficulty with the technique lies in ensuring good mixing, because the saturated air flow may be several orders of magnitude less than the deodorized air flow. Much of the substance is lost in the technique, because the material is constantly vented through the mixing chamber exhaust.

Delivery systems consist of pumps or other means of generating pressure differentials, causing the mixed air to flow over the mucosa; the system of Figure 8.36, used by Dr. Mozell, generates artificial "sniffs" of about 20 cc per minute, by applying gentle suction via the nasopharynx, pulling the stimulus air in through the cannulated nares. Most animals must be artificially respired through a tracheal cannula in order to bypass the nose. The frog is an exception in that it can respire through its skin if the skin is kept moist.

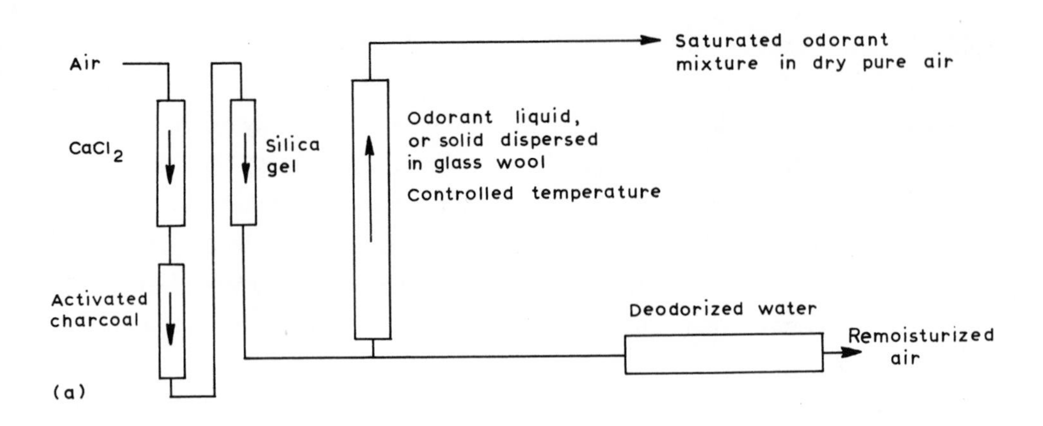

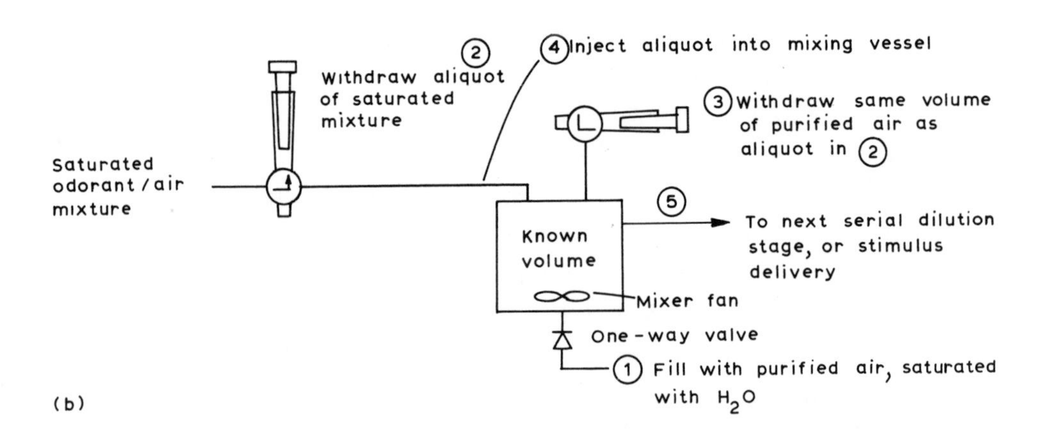

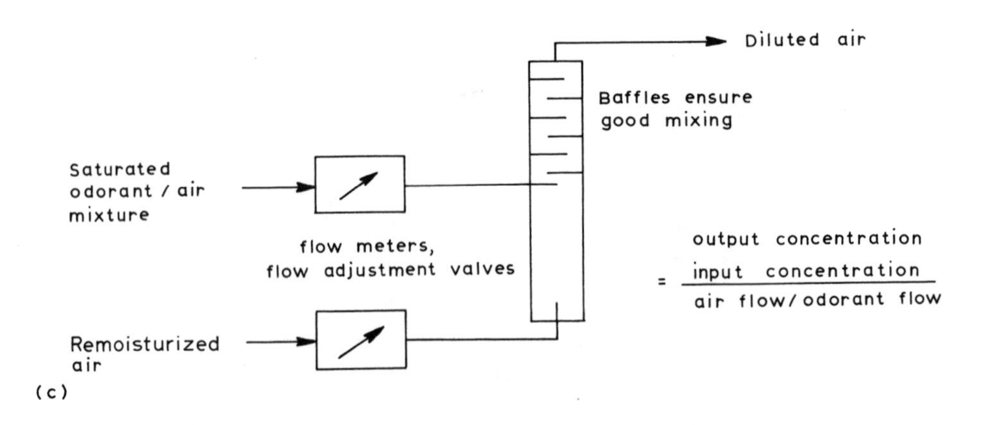

Figure 8.35
Methods for controlled dilution of odorants. (a) Purification of air, saturated odorant mixture. (b) Serial dilution technique. (c) Flow dilution technique.

Vent
Odorant evaporator
Dilution chamber
nares
nasopharynx
Pure air
negative pressure pump
Remoisturized air
Entire section within dotted lines is changed whenever odorant is changed

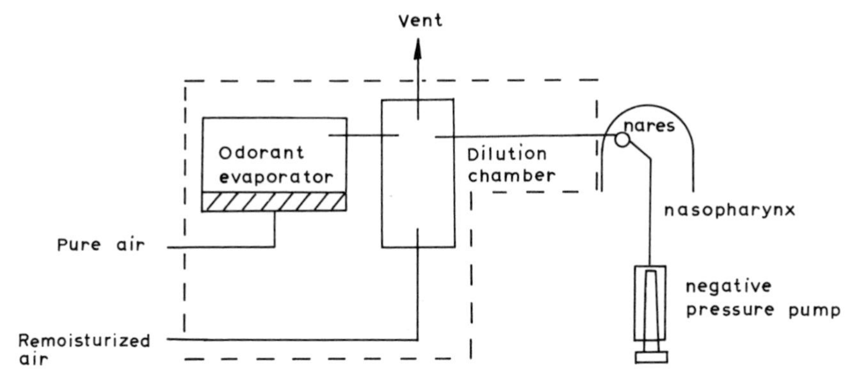

Figure 8.36
Delivery system for odorants.

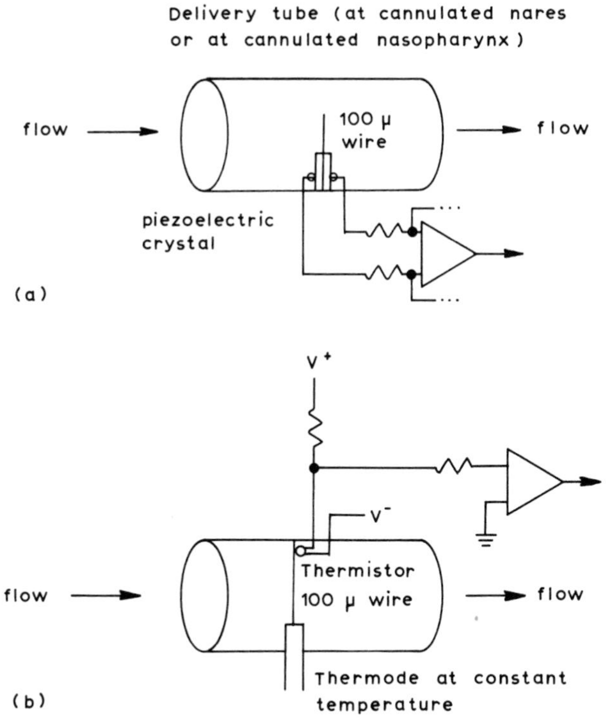

Delivery tube (at cannulated nares or at cannulated nasopharynx)
flow
100 μ wire
flow
piezoelectric crystal
(a)
V+
V-
flow
Thermistor
100 μ wire
flow
Thermode at constant temperature
(b)

Figure 8.37
Suggested methods for monitoring air flow.

There is no developed system for either precisely controlling the wave form of linear flow versus time, or for monitoring flow, in present olfactory stimulation systems. Monitoring of air flow can presumably be accomplished by one of the methods of Figure 8.37, although none of these has been tested in the laboratory.

The first method consists of detecting small forces exerted on a fine wire inserted into the air stream. The wire diameter should be sufficiently small relative to the delivery tube diameter to prevent undesirable turbulence.

Another monitoring technique might consist of measuring the temperature of a heated surface in the delivery tube. If the thermode temperature is very stable, the temperature of the surface in contact with the flowing air should be a function of the rate of flow. Small temperature differentials should be used, with a small transfer surface, in order to prevent fluctuations in the temperature of the stimulus

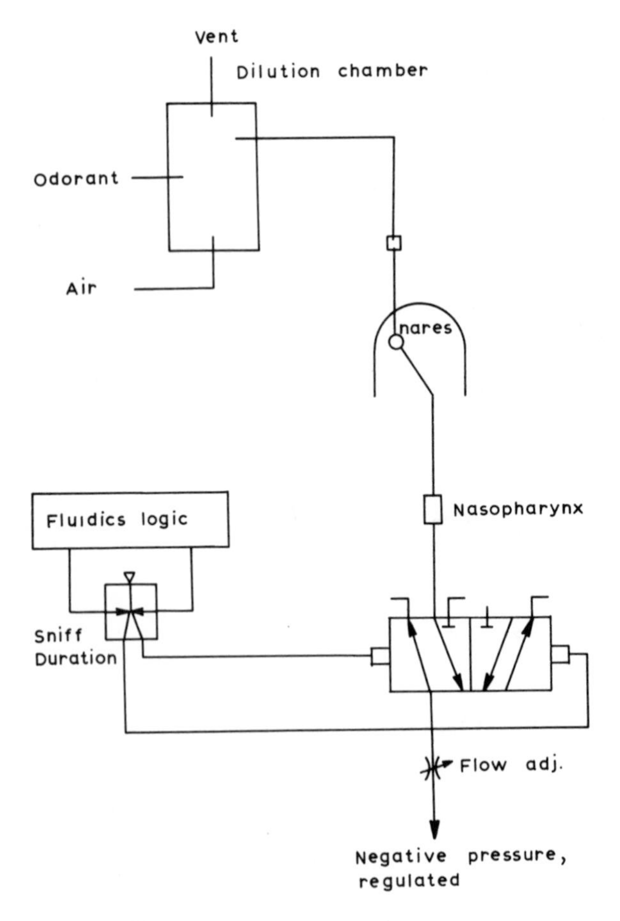

Figure 8.38
Proposed fluidics sniff generator.

air at the mucosa. Also, the incoming stimulus air must be carefully temperature controlled. This is a precaution that is generally advisable in any case.

Control of air flow could presumably be accomplished by fluidic logic. The device depicted in Figure 8.38 is proposed as a first step in the synthesis of such a system. In order to more accurately reproduce the natural sniff, switching of valves is performed at the nasopharynx end rather than the nares end of the air passage. When the exhaust valve is open, the pressure differential should be similar to that during a sniff; when it is closed, the flow should stop with the same time course as a sniff. By monitoring flow during natural sniffs a close approximation should be possible.

8.8 Thermal Stimulation

Formally, thermal stimulation consists of the control of heat flow into or out of the tissue stimulated in order to obtain some degree of control of the tissue temperature as a function of time. This is generally accomplished by apposing a heat source or sink whose temperature is controllable and monitoring the tissue temperature, either at the point of contact or at a relevant point nearby, with a thermistor.

Until recently, the best sources and sinks of heat were thermodes constructed from good heat conductors, such as silver or copper, through which were circulated heated or cooled liquids. Today, a better method exists; the use of the Peltier effect, whereby a semiconductor acts as a variable heat source or sink, depending on the magnitude and direction of electrical current across the junction of two dissimilar metals. The use of electrical current of course provides opportunity for temperature wave form generation by direct transduction of an electrical wave form. Since thermistors provide rapid, accurate transduction of temperature into voltage, feedback control is easily attained.

Figure 8.39a schematizes the heat pump principle used in the Peltier effect. As current is passed across the junction, the device acts as a heat pump, conducting heat from one side of the junction to the other. Depending on the heat source and sink reservoir capacities, a temperature gradient of variable size can be built up across the device. Figure 8.39b schematizes the equivalent circuit for a *heat circuit*, representing the heat pump, internal resistance (inverse of thermal conductivity) and capacitance, and the equivalent resistance and capacitance of the two reservoirs. If one reservoir is assumed to have infinite capacity and infinitesimal resistance, it can be used as a reference temperature; in practice, circulating air or water can be used to hold one end of the heat pump at a constant temperature.

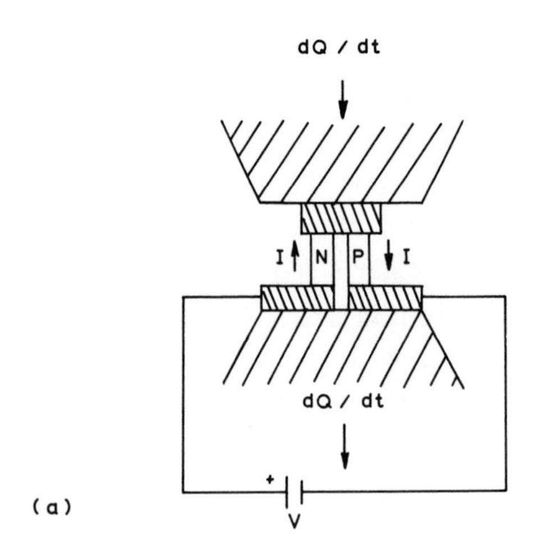

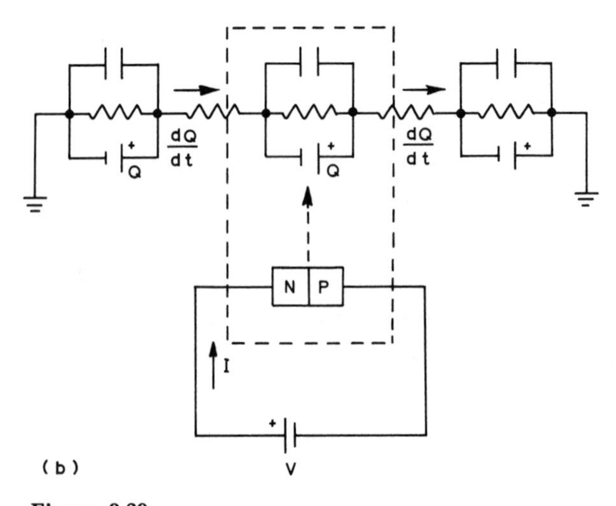

Figure 8.39
Heat pumping using Peltier effect: (a) Block diagram of heat flows and current flows in Peltier effect; (b) thermal equivalent circuit.

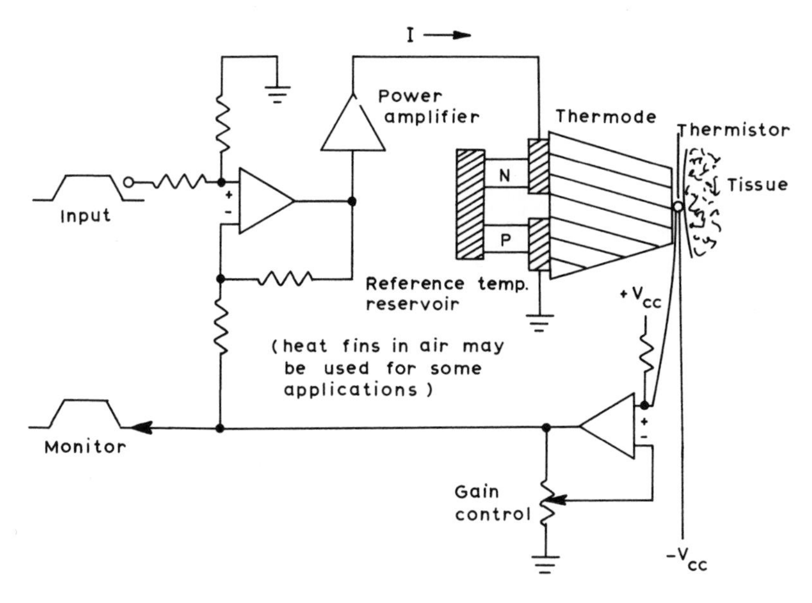

Figure 8.40
Basic driver-monitor circuit for temperature control.

Figure 8.40 schematizes a possible setup for electrical control of temperature. Temperature may be controlled absolutely, or relative to the temperature of some portion of the animal—for example, if stimulating skin, the thermode temperature can be referred to nearby skin temperature.

Choice of Peltier device is dependent on two parameters: (1) the desired temperature range of the device, which should exceed the desired stimulus range, because negative feedback control is optimal if large heat spikes can be used to drive the thermal load of the thermode during rapid temperature changes; and (2) the desired heat-pumping capability, also primarily dependent on the thermode. A large variety of Peltier-effect devices is available. Low-voltage, high-current sources for the Peltier devices are also available, which can be modified to be driven by external electrical wave forms.

Most heat pumps are limited by the maximum temperature drop that can be tolerated by a single junction; often these gradients are not as large as might be desired. In order to increase the gradient across a heat pumping device, several heat pumps can be stacked, as in Figure 8.41a, such that their thermal dipoles are connected in series; this results in a summation of their temperature drops, raising the magnitude of maximum acceptable temperature drop across the whole device. If the diodes are electrically connected in parallel, using a substance with high thermal and low electrical conductivity to separate cells in the heat battery,

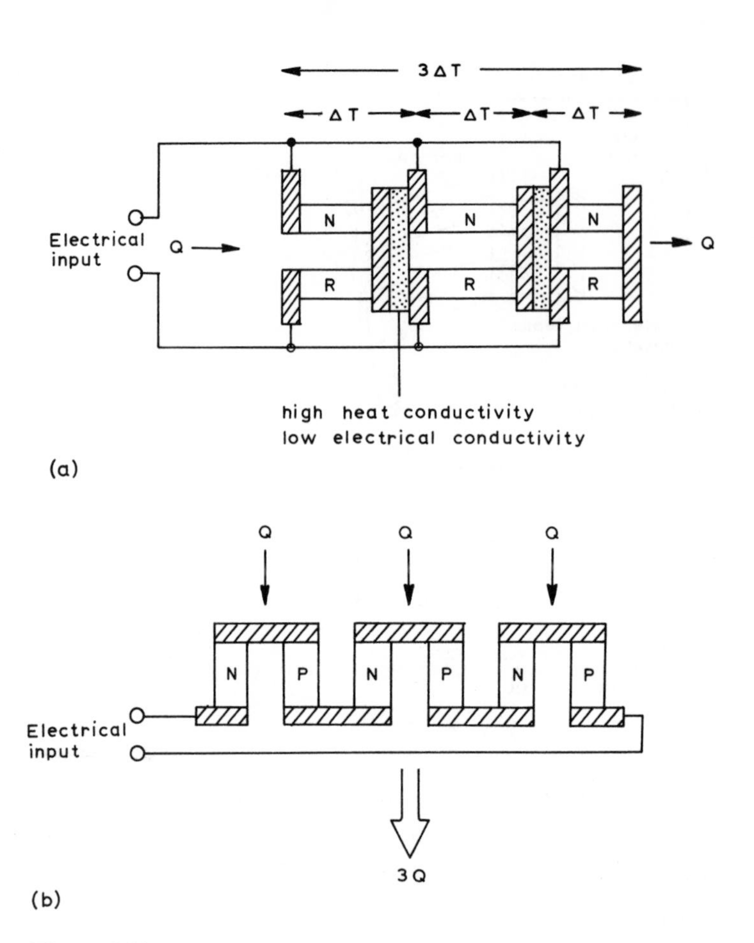

Figure 8.41
Stacking Peltier devices for (a) increased thermal gradient or (b) increased heat flow capability.

all the diodes can be driven by a single low-voltage, high-current driver. Such stacked assemblies are commercially available in several configurations.

Arrays of couples whose thermal dipoles are in parallel are also available for increased heat-pumping capacity (Figure 8.41b). Performance data are tabulated for different configurations in Bird and Yamamura's useful *Cambion Thermoelectric Handbook* (1971).

Choice of thermode geometry is of course a function of the application. For rapid temperature changes, use as small a thermode as possible, constructed from a good heat-conducting metal with low heat capacity. The monitoring thermistor should be on the surface, which is in contact with the tissue being stimulated, or embedded in the tissue.

Selected References

Araki, T., and T. Otani. 1955. Response of single motoneurons to direct stimulation in toad's spinal cord. *J. Neurophysiol. 18:* 472.

Bird, Gordon, Jr., and Akira Yamamura. 1971. *The Cambion Thermoelectric Handbook.* Cambridge, Mass.: Cambridge Thermionic Corporation.

Bureš, Jan, Mojmir Petráň, and Josef Zachar. 1967. (P. Hahn, translator). *Electrophysiological Methods in Biological Research.* New York: Academic Press.

Comsweet, T. N. 1958. A new technique for measurement of small eye movements. *J. Opt. Soc. Am. 48:* 808.

Fein, H. 1966. Passing current through recording glass micropipette electrodes. *IEEE Trans. Bio-Med. Engr. BME-13:* 211.

Rubio, R., and G. Zubieta. 1961. The variation of the electric resistance of micro-electrodes during the flow of current. *Acta. Physiol. Latino-amer. 11:* 91.

Ito, M. 1957. The electrical activity of spinal ganglion cells investigated with intracellular micro-electrodes. *Jap. J. Physiol. 7:* 297.

Monsanto. 1970. *GaAslite Tips, Vol. 1 and 2.* Cupertino, Calif.: Monsanto Electronic Special Products.

Morrison, Ralph. 1967. *Grounding and Shielding Techniques in Instrumentation.* New York: John Wiley & Sons.

Nastuk, William L. 1964. *Physical Techniques in Biological Research,* Vol. V: *Electrophysiological Methods, Part A,* and Vol. VI: *Electrophysiological Methods, Part B.* New York: Academic Press.

O'Neil, William, and Lawrence Stark. 1968. Triple-function ocular monitor. *J. Opt. Soc. Am. 58:* 570.

Roth, Niles. 1965. Automatic optometer for use with the undrugged human eye. *Rev. Sci. Instr. 36:* 1636.

Vaughan, W., and S. Locke. 1971. A circuit for stimulating and recording through a single-capillary micropipette. *IEEE Trans. Bio-Med. Engr. BME-18:* 71.

9 RECORDING APPARATUS

Paul B. Brown

In this chapter we will consider some of the various devices that must be interposed between the source of a bioelectric signal and the display or recording device. We will also very briefly consider some methods for monitoring physiological parameters, as well as various amplifiers that are useful in the laboratory for signal transmission.

9.1 Electrode Amplifiers

By electrode amplifiers we mean amplifiers used to amplify electrical signals generated by organisms, as recorded via various types of electrodes. The approach here will be to develop the rationale for a general-purpose electrode preamplifier that can be used under a wide range of operating conditions. The reader should be able from the discussions to devise variants that are cheaper and of more specific utility for particular applications. A method is given for passing current through a recording microelectrode while recording evoked membrane potential changes.

Before developing amplifier circuits, however, we will briefly review some rules for minimizing pickup of unwanted electrical signals, or *noise*. Such noise includes local radio broadcasts, radar signals, 60-cycle harmonics from transformers, fluorescent and incandescent lights, brush noise and ignition noise from electric motors and automobile engines, switching noises, and even unwanted biological signals such as the EKG, which can contaminate EEG and other recordings.

Electrostatic pickup is best eliminated by shielding all low-voltage or high-impedance conduction paths. In fact, it is a good rule to shield all signal lines. Shielded cables, braided wire on unshielded wires or cables, and Faraday cages (special mesh or foil cages surrounding the recording setup) are often essential. The shielding should be grounded securely to a stake driven into the ground, if possible, using a heavy busbar, braided wire, or copper tubing to conduct the stray currents to ground. If a stake is not available, use a plumbing drain; do not use gas lines. When running shielded cables carrying low-level signals from one device to another and when both devices have a common ground, ground the shield at only one end of the cable in order to prevent *ground loops*. A useful convention is always to ground the shield at the source end of a transmission line and not at the receiver.

If a coaxial cable is used to transmit signals between two devices that are grounded via different ground paths (that is, devices in separate rooms or buildings), a ground should be carried through between the two machines. In this case, each coaxial shield usually should be carried through at both ends; furthermore, for good rejection of common-mode noise, differential transmission and pickup usually should be used (see the description of video cable transmitter and receiver later in this chapter).

Sources of interference should be shielded. Sometimes these sources can be located by attaching an antenna consisting of a 1 ft piece of wire to a sensitive amplifier and searching for the source by moving the antenna around on the end of a length of shielded cable. The pickup is maximum when the antenna is pointed along a line that goes through the source and increases as the source is approached. If a suspected source can be disconnected from its power, this is a simple means of determining whether unwanted signals are emanating from it. Once it has been located, it can be removed, turned off, or shielded to prevent electrostatic radiation. The shielding should be grounded, preferably via a separate ground circuit from that used for shielding of recording pathways.

Magnetic pickup is more difficult to prevent. Shielding is difficult except with large amounts of soft iron or with expensive alloys such as mu-metal. Distance between source and pickup is an important factor, as is alignment of magnetic field and pickup circuit. Magnetic radiation can be expected from transformer and solenoid circuits and from conductors carrying large currents.

A mention of Faraday cages should be made at this point. These are double-walled enclosed volumes, in which the walls are made of conductive material, each of which is grounded at only one point. These enclosures may consist of whole rooms covered with grounded sheets of copper or aluminum, or smaller cages consisting of a supporting framework over which are applied the sheets of metal. Instead of metal sheets, which are expensive, wire mesh may be used. Generally galvanized steel chicken wire with $\frac{1}{4}$ in. grid spacing is adequate, except in environments where RFI is intense. It is very important that the resistance between different parts of the screen be minimized, with good solder joints between the various sheets of metal or screen, or ground loops will develop.

Grounded shielding of signal paths essentially reduces pickup by surrounding a signal path with a potential surface that is unchanging and, although it acts as a capacitative load, does not allow the introduction of any spurious signals. An alternative method is called *guard shielding*, in which the signal is led through a conductance path that is surrounded by another conductor whose potential exactly matches that of the signal. If the surrounding conductor has a high conductivity and is driven by a low-impedance source (for example, the output of a unity-gain follower), pickup on the higher-impedance input signal circuit will be less, because the major component of the electrostatic field in which it is immersed is at the same potential as it is. This method is useful in shielding high-impedance (low-current) circuits and will be used in the microelectrode amplifier described later in this chapter. The technique also has the advantage of minimizing the effective capacitive load on the input signal, an important consideration in some applications.

It is not uncommon, in the measurement of small signals originating from high-impedance sources, to guard the input circuit and to shield the guard shield with a grounded shield.

Each device used in the same laboratory should be grounded through a single secure connection to avoid ground loops. These are current "loops" through which ground currents can circulate, generating considerable interference. To this end it is often good strategy to isolate the third pin of a grounded power cable with a three-pin to two-pin adapter or to disconnect the ground pin (the third pin) on the outlet. Then when the ground lug on the chassis of the device is tied to the ground circuit, a ground loop will not result. If the ground pin on the power plug has been disconnected, it is *imperative* that the device be grounded securely to the laboratory ground stake, to prevent electrical shock hazards. *UNGROUNDED EQUIPMENT HAS RESULTED IN MANY DEATHS BY ELECTROCUTION*. Never operate an ungrounded device; in fact, never plug one in. Power supplies should have their ground returns tied to a grounding system separate from that used for recording, because the large currents in the power circuits are likely to generate unwanted pickup in the sensitive recording amplifiers. This is accounted for quite simply. Imagine a ground line that is 0.01 Ω off ground. If ± 10 A of 60 Hz ac current is passed through it, an ac voltage of ± 0.1 V will be developed. If this line is used as the reference for recording, the ± 100 mV will appear on the recording device. Both lines must be tied to a common ground at some point; this point should be as close to the ground stake as possible.

Microelectrode recording poses a set of special problems, which can be met using some of the ICs that have recently become available. Although extracellular and intracellular recording present somewhat different obstacles, they can profitably be discussed together.

Since microelectrodes generally have impedances ranging between 1 and 100 MΩ, it is necessary to place the first stage of amplification, even if it is only a unity-gain impedance reduction stage, as close as possible to the recording electrode. ICs are ideally suited to this purpose, and the design we will present allows connection of the electrode directly to the input lead of the op amp. This minimizes pickup and shunt capacitance. Further reduction of shunt capacitance is accomplished by using a guard shield, as will be described later.

FET-input op amps have an appropriate input resistance, input current, and band width for microelectrode recording, and except in instances where very little noise can be tolerated, their noise levels are low enough for both intracellular and extracellular recording.

Noise requirements vary, but a few useful facts about noise should be mentioned here. For high-impedance electrodes, the noise level of the AD503JH, the FET-input op amp we will use, is less than 10% of the theoretical minimum thermal noise calculated for a pure resistance.

The rms noise level of a 20 MΩ microelectrode, at 25°C, over a bandwidth of 100 kHZ, is thus (Equation 3.50):

$$V_{20\,\mathrm{M}\Omega} \cong 7.4 \times 10^{-12} \times \sqrt{20 \times 10^{6} \times 10^{5} \times 298} \cong 160\ \mu\mathrm{V\ rms}.$$

The noise level of any device can be predicted rather simply, using the manufacturer's specifications. These specifications are based on recordings of the output noise level of an op amp with the input shorted to ground. Generally the noise is determined primarily by the input stage, because gain of that stage maximizes the percent contribution at the input. That is, if the input stage has 60 dB of gain, subsequent stages with equal amounts of noise will contribute only 0.001 as much noise to the final output level. Thus, if the first stage had 10 μV rms noise, the second stage could inject 100 μV of noise and still contribute only 1% as much to the output noise level. For most applications it is therefore adequate to refer the output noise level back to the input by dividing by the gain of the device, regardless of the nature of the device. If the gain or bandwidth of the device is varied, the output noise level varies as though it were almost entirely generated right at the input.

We will take advantage of this fact wherever possible, by achieving as much voltage gain as possible in the first stage of any high-gain device. In this way, the contribution of subsequent stages is minimized. The actual amount of gain that can be achieved at the input stage without distortion is a function of the application, however, and the decision concerning amount of gain in the first stage must be based on anticipated signal levels at the input.

Noise can be reduced by appropriate use of common-mode rejection to remove pickup and by filtering out all frequencies outside the desired bandpass. Notch filters and differential amplification will suffice to remove 60 Hz harmonics to the point where Faraday cages can often be dispensed with even for high-gain ac recording in the presence of fluorescent lights and other sources of 60 Hz. The location of notch and band-limiting filters in the chain of signal processors is determined largely by the relative sizes of different signal and noise components. Although thermal noise of op amps is reduced best by placing gain stages near the input, sometimes 60 Hz or rf noise must be filtered out before much gain can be achieved. Perhaps the optimal method would consist of a modular setup, in which the stages can be arranged in any order, although to the author's knowledge this approach has never been tried. Generally the designer can anticipate the magnitudes of different noise components and optimize the arrangement of signal conditioning stages accordingly.

The importance of differential recording should be emphasized here. If the inputs of a differential amplifier are tied to electrodes located very close together, the pickup on both electrodes should be nearly identical. If, further, one electrode is much closer to a small signal generator, such as a neuron, than the other, then the neuron's signal will be recorded with much less attenuation at that electrode than at the other. Therefore the output of the amplifier should be:

$$\underbrace{(V_{\text{cell}} + V_{\text{interference}})}_{\text{active electrode}} - \underbrace{(V_{\text{interference}})}_{\text{indifferent electrode}}.$$

Thus, theoretically, all the interference is canceled.

Although many differential devices are specified to have better than 60 dB common mode rejection ratio (CMRR), actual common mode rejection will usually not be better than 60 dB because of asymmetries external to the point of common mode rejection, unless the CMRR is adjusted carefully under each recording situation.

Decoupling capacitors should be used in all circuits. This prevents current surges in one device from showing up as voltage spikes on the power inputs to another device powered by the same supply.

A microelectrode preamplifier, to be used for differential or single-ended recording of extracellular or intracellular potentials, using a variety of electrodes, should have the following characteristics:

1. At least 50 dB common mode rejection at high frequencies, 70 dB common mode rejection at dc-100 Hz.
2. High input impedance. Since electrode impedances can be as high as 100 MΩ, at least 10^{10} Ω is required, single-ended and differential.
3. Low noise, preferably less than 10 μV rms, because some signals may be as small as a few microvolts.
4. dc-50 kHz unity gain bandpass, or dc-50 kHz bandpass at desired gain of input stage.
5. Low input current, in order to prevent iontophoresis at the electrode tip and interaction with excitable tissue. Input current should be less than 100 pA. For some applications it must be less than 10 pA, but this is rarely necessary.
6. Low drift, offset adjustable to less than 0.5 mV.

The Analog Devices AD503JH, which we will use in our electrode amplifier, has the following characteristics:

Unity gain bandpass: dc-1 MHz
Input impedance: 10^{11} Ω
Input offset current: 0.5–15 pA
Input offset voltage: 20–50 mV (can be compensated to zero)
Input bias current: 5–25 pA
Gain: 20,000 to 50,000
Noise: 7 μV rms
Input capacitance: 2.0 pF to ground.

The device is packaged in a TO-99 can with a diameter of 0.370 in. and a depth of less than 0.25 in.

If the only function of a microelectrode preamplifier were to present a high input impedance to the microelectrode and provide low impedance output for subsequent stages, the circuit of Figure 9.1 would be adequate. This primitive design has the advantage of small size, low cost, and elegant simplicity. The input current, bandwidth, and noise level are all appropriate to the task. The simple modification of Figure 9.2 would provide a means of differential amplification of microelectrode and indifferent inputs by taking the difference of the outputs of two AD503s.

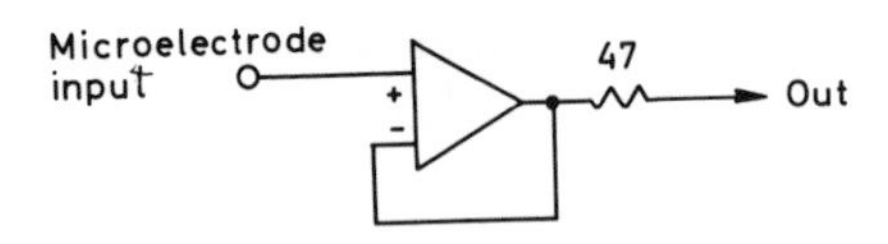

Figure 9.1
Primitive design for microelectrode preamplifier.

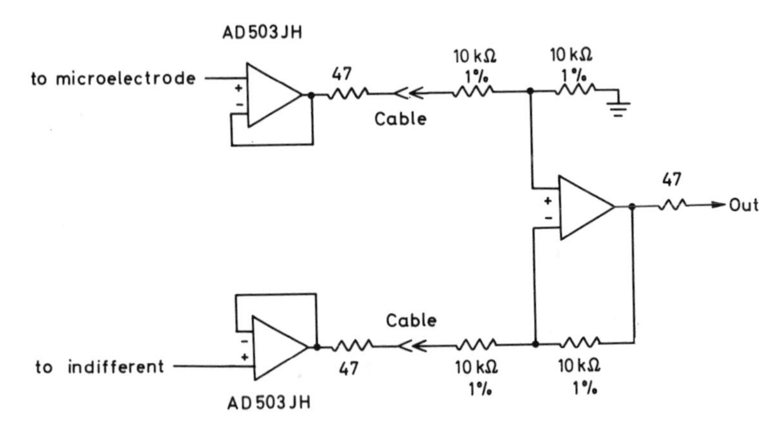

Figure 9.2
Primitive differential amplifier for microelectrode recording.

Unfortunately, the input time constants of such configurations are generally too high due to input capacitance of the amplifier and shunt capacitance of the microelectrode. Figure 9.3a presents the equivalent circuit for the input network, somewhat simplified for the purposes of this discussion. The microelectrode and amplifier capacitances are lumped into one capacitor C_e.

Typically,

$10^6\ \Omega \leqq R_e \leqq 10^8\ \Omega$

$10^{-2}\ \text{F} \leqq C_e \leqq 10^{-10}\ \text{F};$

therefore, 10^{-6} sec $\leqq \tau_e \leqq 10^{-2}$ sec,

usually in excess of 1 msec.

In order to compensate for this low-pass filter effect, a method called *negative capacity feedback* is used. The input signal is amplified and fed back through a small capacitance (<25 pF) to the input. This positive feedback boosts the high frequencies that were attenuated by the input capacitance and has no effect on lower frequencies if the gain of the feedback is properly adjusted. Since this feed-

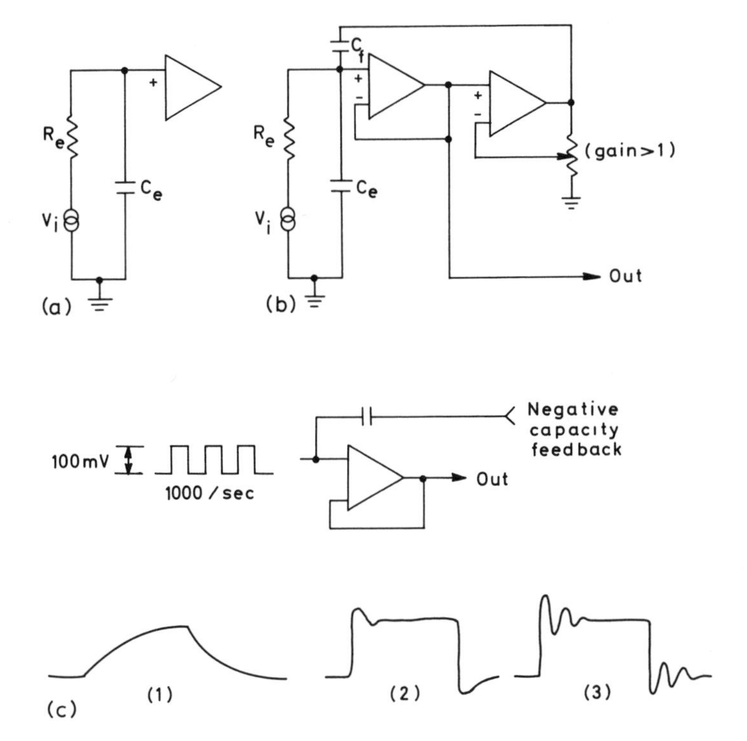

Figure 9.3
Compensation for input capacitance. (a) Equivalent circuit for microelectrode input. (b) Negative capacity feedback. (c) Adjustment of feedback: (1) undercompensated (feedback gain too low); (2) properly compensated (overshoots exaggerated for purposes of illustration); (3) overcompensated (feedback gain too high).

back boosts *all* high frequencies, the high-frequency noise components are increased as well.

Finally, in order to reduce input capacitance of any shielding used to protect the input or electronics from pickup, a guard shield is generally used. This is a shield that is connected to a low-impedance source of voltage equal to the input voltage. Minor dc offsets are tolerable, because the purpose is to reduce the effect of capacitance, and dc performance is not affected by capacitance. That is, the input capacitance acts as a shunt only for ac signals; therefore, dc offsets are of no great consequence as long as the signal on the shield always has the same time derivative as the input signal.

The circuit of Figure 9.4 is recommended, therefore, for a dc or ac microelectrode preamplifier. The microelectrode headstage is shielded by a 125 Ω guard signal, which is in turn shielded by a grounded shield. The grounded shield can usually be dispensed with, but it is included here as the best procedure. The indifferent headstage uses an AD503JH primarily for good matching of bandwidth

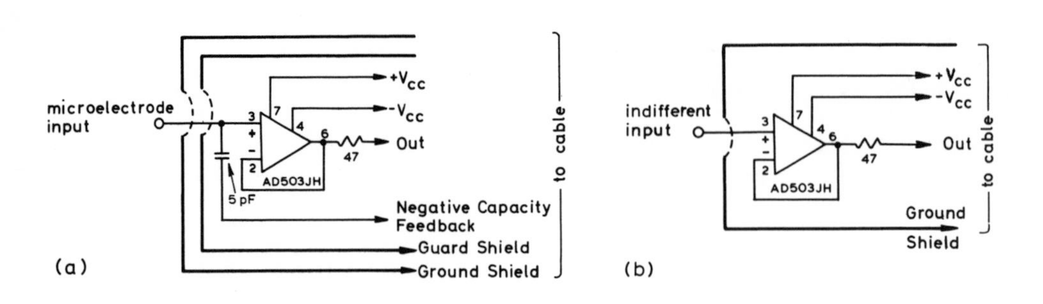

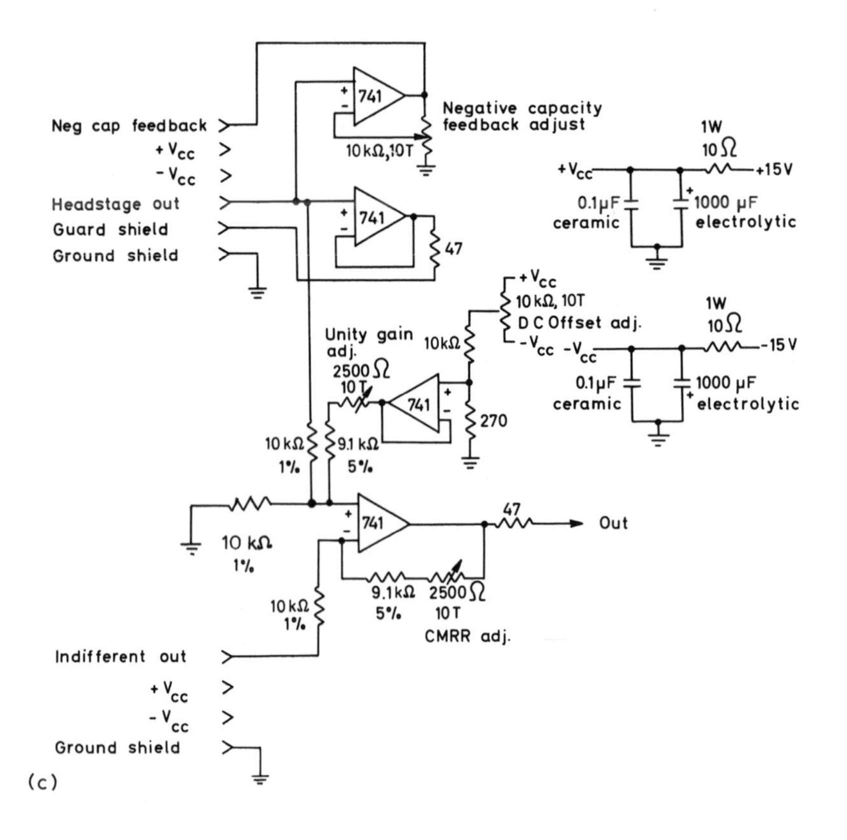

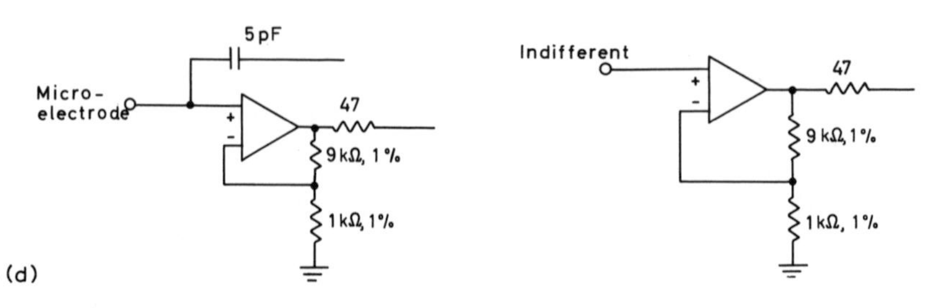

Figure 9.4
General-purpose headstage. (a) Remote microelectrode buffer amplifier. (b) Remote indifferent buffer amplifier. (c) Differential amplifier section. (d) × 10 Input gain stages.

properties. No negative capacity feedback or guard shield is necessary in most instances because the indifferent input is generally attached to a low source impedance, such as an Ag-AgCl plate embedded under a skin flap or an alligator clip clamped to muscle near the microelectrode. The headstage amplifier includes a 5 pF capacitor (ceramic) tied to the input, for negative capacity feedback. Both headstages use a 47 Ω output resistor to decouple the output from the capacitive load of the cables in order to prevent instability.

The remote amplifiers should have some gain if this is at all feasible. Generally a × 10 gain can be tolerated for most applications. Use potentiometric feedback, as illustrated in Figure 9.4d, in order to maintain high input impedance. The × 10 gain will help minimize the effect of pickup in the cable leads, and noise contributions by subsequent stages will be of no consequence. Note, however, that dc offsets (differential) of more than 1 V will result in clipping at the output, unless ac coupling is used at the input or dc is rejected at the differential amplifier.

The main chassis of the preamplifier, Figure 9.4c, contains electronics for generating guard signal (attenuate the input to the guard amplifier by a factor of 10 if a × 10 input gain is used), negative capacity feedback (attenuate this signal also if × 10 input gain is used), and single-ended output. Common-mode rejection is achieved by use of an adder-subtracter configuration, with injection of a variable dc bias compensation. The dc offsets of the AD503JHs can be of the order of 50 mV, therefore the offset null of the 741 cannot be used. Minor dc offsets due to electrode potentials can also be balanced. If a × 10 input is used, it may be necessary to use a larger range of dc balance, which is achieved by increasing the 270 Ω resistor on the voltage divider. By buffering the dc balance voltage with an op amp, we ensure that the adder resistance arm is of constant resistance in order to prevent interaction of dc balance with gain or CMRR. The gain and CMRR may be adjusted with back-panel or internal trimpots, because they will need readjustment only once per year or so, unless op amps are switched.

Although considerable decoupling of $\pm V_{CC}$ is provided in this design, use a supply with 0.1% ripple and 1% regulation, or better. One-ampere current capability will provide adequate power for subsequent signal conditioning apparatus as well.

Note that the negative capacity feedback has no series resistor. This is intended to maximize rise-time capability of the circuit, and rise times of less than 50 μsec are easily obtained even with 50 MΩ microelectrodes. However, if the cable has too high a capacitance to the shield, instability may result. The guard amplifier may be tied to the output of the negative capacity feedback amplifier in this case in order to guard the feedback signal. The input will still be guarded appropriately with some negative capacity feedback via the guard shield itself.

Note: The AD503JH TO-99 can is internally connected to $-V_{CC}$. It is therefore necessary to insulate it carefully. Also, the device is unusually sensitive to heat; if soldering directly to the leads, clamp the leads between the point of heat application and the case, to heat sink them. Analog Devices has recently released a new op amp, the AD523, which is similar to AD503 but has the case floating with respect to the circuit. A separate pin is tied to the case, for a guard signal or ground.

Stimulation through microelectrodes has been accomplished by a number of methods. The technique used by Mentor in their dc amplifier, similar to the method of Fein (1966), is the one illustrated in Figure 9.5, although different operational amplifiers are used.

In this circuit, the microelectrode and indifferent amplifiers (A1, A2) and the negative capacity feedback circuit (A3) are similar to ones already described. However, an additional feedback circuit is added to the microelectrode section.

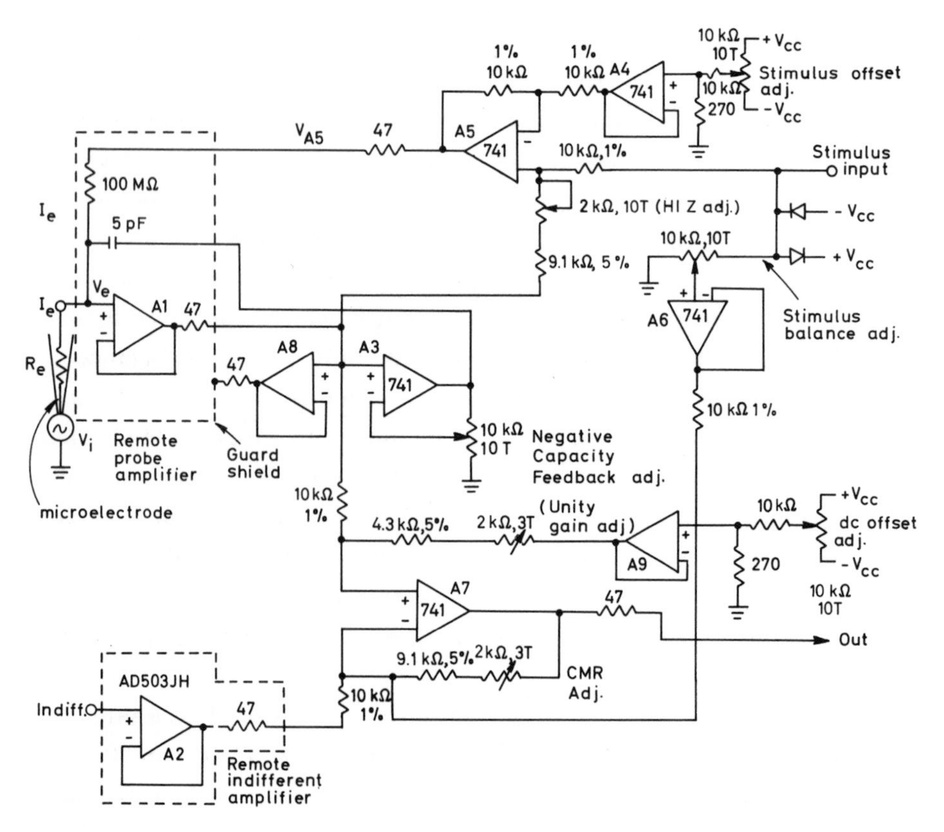

Figure 9.5
Circuit for passing current through recording microelectrode.

The output of the microelectrode amplifier is summed with a stimulus voltage and fed back to the microelectrode input through a 100 MΩ resistor. Assume perfect unity-gain summation of V_e, the electrode voltage, and V_{STIM}, the stimulus input voltage, by amplifier A5, whose output voltage V_{A5} must be

$$V_{A5} = V_e + V_{STIM}. \tag{9.1}$$

Given an input impedance of A1 of 10^{12} Ω, all the current through the 100 MΩ resistor must pass through the microelectrode resistance, for all microelectrode resistances within practical resistance limits. We can solve for the current I_e through the microelectrode R_e, by using the known IR drop across the 100 MΩ resistor:

$$I_e = \frac{V_{A5} - V_e}{100\ \text{M}\Omega},$$

which, substituting for V_{A5} using Equation 9.1, gives

$$I_e = \frac{V_e + V_{STIM} - V_e}{100\ \text{M}\Omega} = \frac{V_{STIM}}{100\ \text{M}\Omega}. \tag{9.2}$$

Thus, I_e is related to V_{STIM} by a constant 100 MΩ proportionality factor, regardless of V_i, V_e, or R_e, within the operating limits of the device. If $V_{STIM} = 0$, $V_{A5} = V_e$, and $I_e = 0$, because there is no voltage drop across the 100 MΩ resistor. This means that the feedback presents an infinite shunt resistance in the absence of a stimulus voltage.

In the absence of any I_e, $V_e = V_i$. However, when stimulus current is applied,

$$V_e = I_e R_e + V_i.$$

If $V_i = 0$ and V_{STIM} is some known signal, V_e can be measured and used to determine electrode resistance:

$$R_e = \frac{V_e}{I_e} = \frac{V_e \cdot 100\ \text{M}\Omega}{V_{STIM}}. \tag{9.3}$$

The current-passing limit of the amplifier is reached when $V_{A5} = \pm V_{max}$. Therefore, since

$$I_e = \frac{V_{A5} - V_i}{R_e + 100\ \text{M}\Omega},$$

$$I_{e(max)} = \frac{\pm V_{max} - V_{A5}}{R_e + 100\ \text{M}\Omega}. \tag{9.4}$$

Therefore, assuming maximum $\pm V_{A5}$ of ± 10 V, and $V_i \cong 0$, we find that

$\pm I_e(\max) = \pm 9.9 \times 10^{-8}$ A, if $R_e = 10$ MΩ, or $\sim \pm 10^{-7}$ A for $R_e \leqq 10$ MΩ;
$\pm I_e(\max) = \pm 6.67 \times 10^{-8}$ A, if $R_e = 50$ MΩ;
$\pm I_e(\max) = 5 \times 10^{-8}$ A, if $R_e = 100$ MΩ, and so forth.

Higher current limits can be realized with lower resistances in place of the 100 MΩ resistor, although quiescent input currents will be higher for a given offset of A5.

The quiescent input current through the microelectrode, if we neglect input current through the AD503, is

$I_e = V_{A5}/100$ MΩ.

Therefore, V_{A5} must have a very precise gain of 1 for the sum $V_e + V_{STIM}$ and a very low dc offset. Specifically, for 10^{-12} A, $V_{A5} - V_e \leqq 100$ μV. The offset and gain of A5 may be adjusted with a differential amplifier, such as the one described in the next section, which has been adjusted for CMRR of at least 60 dB, preferably 80 dB. The stimulus input should be grounded for all these adjustment procedures. Apply a 1–10 V square wave to the microelectrode input and the indifferent input of the resulting recording system and adjust CMRR, such that there is a minimum output signal and no dc error. Next, interpose a 10–100 MΩ resistor in the path to the microelectrode input, and adjust the negative capacity feedback for best square wave at the output of A1. Now, any signal fraction or dc error at the output of the differential amplifier, other than the negligible imbalance of CMRR or dc offset, which have been adjusted to be negligibly small, will be due entirely to dc offset and gain error of A5. Adjust these until the signal is minimum and the dc error is minimum. If, for example, the total error has been adjusted to less than 1 mV, and the input resistor to the microelectrode input is 100 MΩ, the error current must be less than 1 mV/100 MΩ $= 10^{-11}$ A.

The microelectrode input may be protected against overvoltages with low-leakage diodes tied to the supply voltages, such that they are reverse-biased for acceptable voltages and forward-biased for overvoltages. This cannot be done with the record-only amplifier, because there is no dc current feedback available for compensating the still appreciable leakage of the diodes.

The output stage is modified to provide means for cancelling the stimulus voltage, by subtracting a fraction of the stimulus from the difference between microelectrode and indifferent amplifier outputs. We know that the appropriate fraction for cancellation of the stimulus is less than unity, from Equations 9.1 to

9.3, if $R_e < 100\ \mathrm{M\Omega}$:

$$V_e = V_i + I_e R_e$$
$$(V_e - V_i) = R_e V_{\mathrm{STIM}}/100\ \mathrm{M\Omega}.$$

If lower resistances are substituted for the 100 MΩ resistor and if R_e is greater than the new resistance, the stimulus fraction will have to be greater than unity for cancellation.

The fraction of V_{STIM}, $R_e/100\ \mathrm{M\Omega}$, which must be subtracted from V_e to obtain V_i, is a linear function of the potentiometer setting. If a 10-turn vernier dial calibrated in tenths of a turn is used, the dial can be read as 10 MΩ/turn, or 1 MΩ per $\frac{1}{10}$ turn. Verniers calibrated in hundredths of turns will give readings accurate to the nearest 0.1 MΩ if the potentiometer is sufficiently linear. This provides a convenient method not only for determining electrode impedance and for balancing out stimulus voltage while recording but also for determining changes in the impedance of the V_i source, which we have lumped into R_e. Actually,

$$R_e = R_{\mathrm{microelectrode}} + R_{V_i},$$

where R_{V_i} is the source impedance of V_i. Thus, a high-frequency sine wave (say, 20 kHz) could be used to measure changes of membrane impedance during membrane events such as action potentials or local excitatory processes. Direction of change in membrane impedance would be signaled by polarity of the recorded sine wave. Note, however, that, when recording from muscle fibers, movement of the fiber during a twitch can result in bending the microelectrode, causing a change of the *microelectrode* resistance. Also, microelectrodes with very small apertures not uncommonly change their resistances when large currents are passed through them.

Since the rise time of the recording amplifier is about 1–20 μsec, depending on R_e and C_e, spikes will remain at the beginning and end of the stimulus that can only be canceled by wave shaping the stimulus-cancellation signal out of the balance potentiometer. Although this is possible, judicious filtering with a reasonably sharp cutoff at about 50 kHz is generally adequate for elimination of these spikes.

9.2 Amplification and Signal Conditioning

Requirements for high-gain amplifiers vary according to their application, but generally gain of more than $\times 10$ is reserved for ac recording. The exception to this rule is dc recording in which a well-calibrated dc bucking voltage is used to null the input, providing high-resolution measurement of membrane potential.

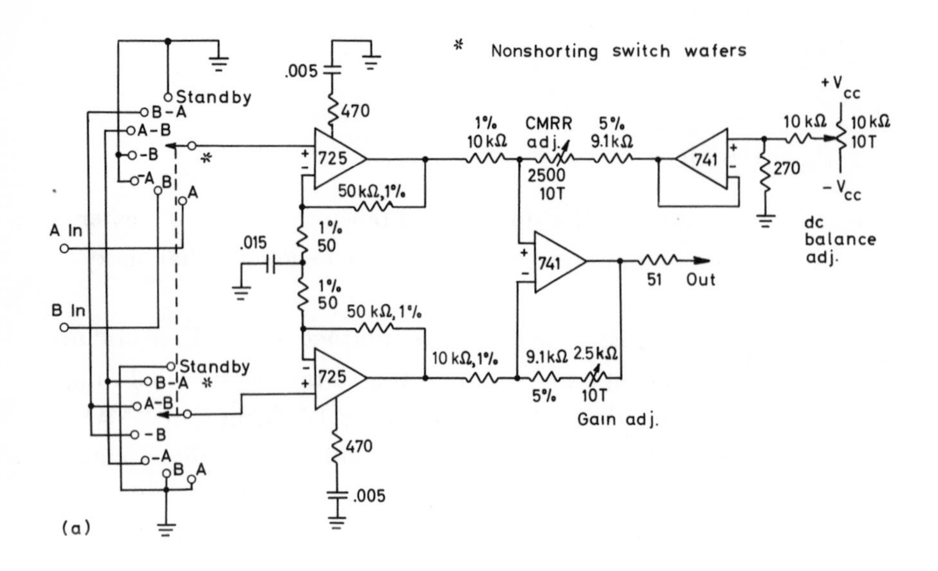

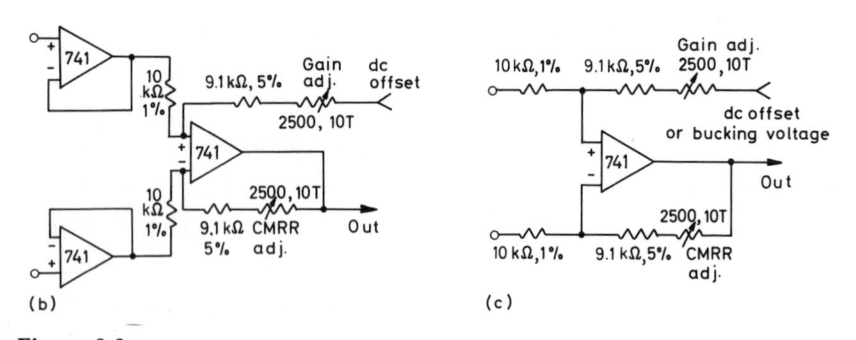

Figure 9.6

Differential input stage of general-purpose amplifier: (a) 30 MΩ input Z, × 1000 gain; (b) 100 kΩ input Z, × 1 gain; (c) 10 kΩ input Z, × 1 gain; (d and e) 725 op amp characteristics (from data sheet: μA725 *Instrumentation Operational Amplifier*, 1970, by Fairchild Semiconductor. Used with permission of Fairchild Camera and Instrument Corp.).

CONNECTION DIAGRAM
(TOP VIEW)

OFFSET NULL, TAB, 8, 1, 7, V+, INVERTING INPUT 2, 6 OUTPUT, OUTPUT FREQUENCY COMPENSATION, NON-INVERTING INPUT 3, 4, 5, V−

NOTE: Pin 4 connected to case

ABSOLUTE MAXIMUM RATINGS

Supply Voltage	±22 V
Internal Power Dissipation (Note 1)	500 mW
Differential Input Voltage (Note 2)	±22 V
Input Voltage (Note 3)	±22 V
Voltage between Offset Null and V+	±0.5 V
Storage Temperature Range	−65°C to +150°C
Operating Temperature Range	−20°C to +85°C
Lead Temperature (Soldering, 60 seconds)	300°C

NOTES:
(1) Rating applies for case temperatures to +85°C; derate linearly at 6.5 mW/°C for ambient temperatures above 75°C.
(2) Rating applies for 5 ms pulses with 10% duty cycle, derate to ±5 V for continuous operation.
(3) For supply voltages less than ±22 V, the absolute maximum input voltage is equal to the supply voltage.

ELECTRICAL CHARACTERISTICS ($V_S = \pm 15$ V, $T_A = 25°C$ unless otherwise specified)

PARAMETER	TEST CONDITIONS	MIN.	TYP.	MAX.	UNITS
Input Offset Voltage (Without external trim)	$R_S \leq 10$ kΩ		0.5	1.0	mV
Input Offset Current			2.0	20	nA
Input Bias Current			42	100	nA
Input Noise Voltage	$f_o = 10$ Hz		15		nV/$\sqrt{Hz}$
	$f_o = 100$ Hz		9.0		nV/$\sqrt{Hz}$
	$f_o = 1$ kHz		8.0		nV/$\sqrt{Hz}$
Input Noise Current	$f_o = 10$ Hz		1.0		pA/$\sqrt{Hz}$
	$f_o = 100$ Hz		0.3		pA/$\sqrt{Hz}$
	$f_o = 1$ kHz		0.15		pA/$\sqrt{Hz}$
Input Resistance			1.5		MΩ
Input Voltage Range		±13.5	±14		V
Large Signal Voltage Gain	$R_L \geq 2$ kΩ, $V_{out} = \pm 10$ V	1,000,000	3,000,000		
Common Mode Rejection Ratio	$R_S \leq 10$ kΩ	110	120		dB
Power Supply Rejection Ratio	$R_S \leq 10$ kΩ		2.0	10	μV/V
Output Voltage Swing	$R_L \geq 10$ kΩ	±12	±13.5		V
	$R_L \geq 2$ kΩ	±10	±13.5		V
Output Resistance			150		Ω
Power Consumption			80	105	mW
The following specifications apply for $-55°C \leq T_A \leq +125°C$ unless otherwise specified:					
Input Offset Voltage (Without external trim)	$R_S \leq 10$ kΩ			1.5	mV
Average Input Offset Voltage Drift (Without external trim)	$R_S = 50$ Ω		2.0	5.0	μV/°C
Average Input Offset Voltage Drift (With external trim)	$R_S = 50$ Ω		0.6		μV/°C
Input Offset Current	$T_A = +125°C$		1.2	20	nA
	$T_A = -55°C$		7.5	40	nA
Average Input Offset Current Drift			35	150	pA/°C
Input Bias Current	$T_A = +125°C$		20	100	nA
	$T_A = -55°C$		80	200	nA
Large Signal Voltage Gain	$R_L \geq 2$ kΩ, $T_A = +125°C$	1,000,000			
	$R_L \geq 2$ kΩ, $T_A = -55°C$	250,000			
Common Mode Rejection Ratio	$R_S \leq 10$ kΩ	100			dB
Power Supply Rejection Ratio	$R_S \leq 10$ kΩ			20	μV/V
Output Voltage Swing	$R_L \geq 2$ kΩ	±10			V

(d)

Figure 9.6 (continued)

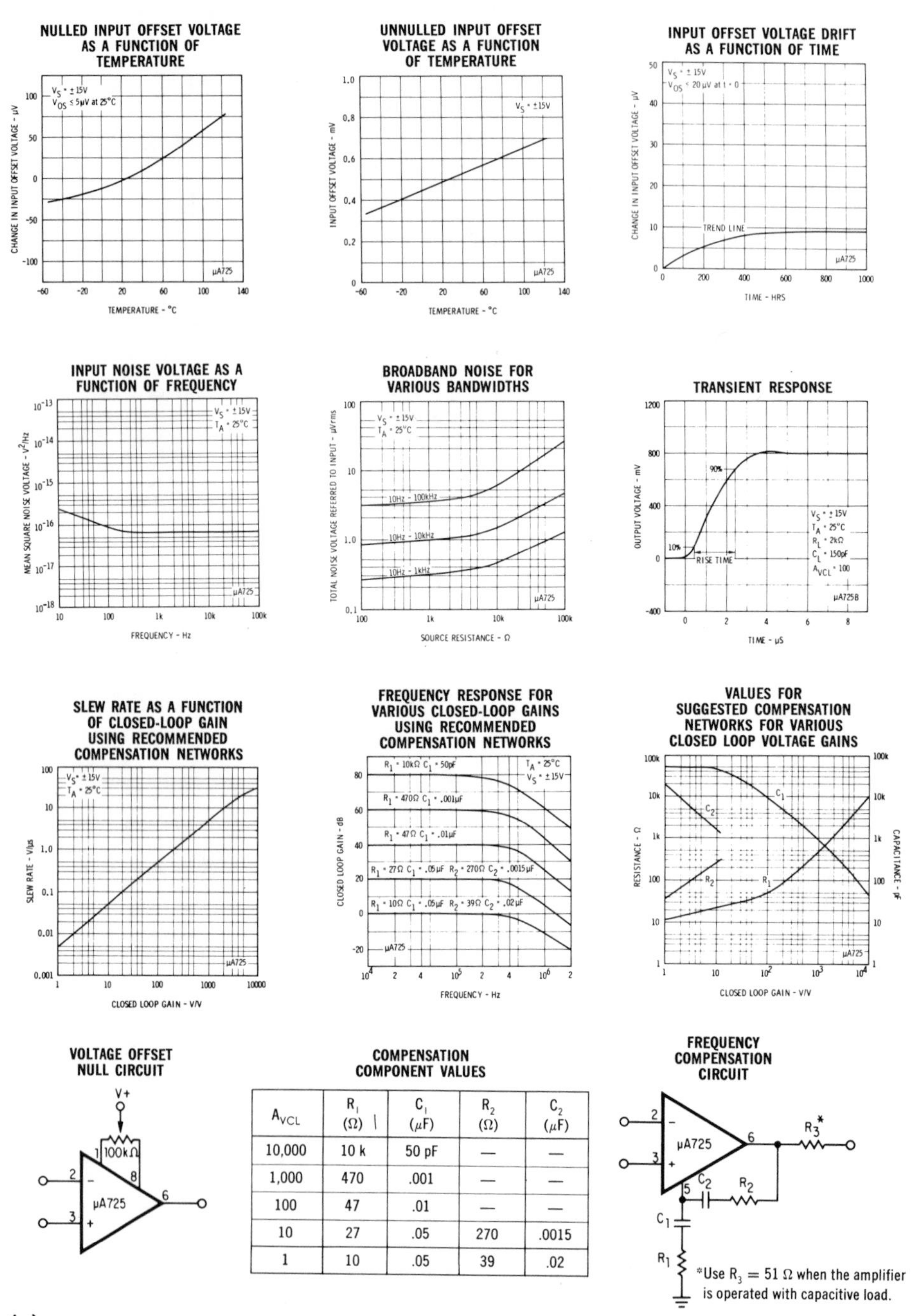

COMPENSATION COMPONENT VALUES

A_{VCL}	R_1 (Ω)	C_1 (μF)	R_2 (Ω)	C_2 (μF)
10,000	10 k	50 pF	—	—
1,000	470	.001	—	—
100	47	.01	—	—
10	27	.05	270	.0015
1	10	.05	39	.02

(e)

Figure 9.6 (continued)

We will therefore concentrate on the design of an ac amplifier with high gain, indicating various design strategies for various applications as we discuss the circuit principles.

The differential input stage (Figure 9.6) is required only if common mode rejection is not achieved earlier. The device is a variation on a commonly used configuration, and has a gain of × 1000. Unless dc is rejected prior to this stage, it should be ac coupled. Presumably, little additional gain would be needed after this stage. If unity gain is adequate, with intermediate input impedance, 741 unity-gain followers can be used to replace the 725s (Figure 9.6b). If source impedances are under 100 Ω, the adder-subtracter 741 will suffice (Figure 9.6c).

The 725 op amps of Figure 9.6a require frequency compensation. We will include the compensation networks recommended for our designs; the network must be modified for different feedback resistors. The properties of the 725 are summarized in Figure 9.6d and e (data reproduced courtesy of Fairchild Camera and Instrument Corp.).

In order to adjust the common-mode rejection, apply a 1000/sec square wave of 1 V amplitude to the two inputs, or to whatever combination of inputs and headstages will be used in the recording setup. Adjust for a minimum output signal.

To adjust the gain, apply the 1000/sec square wave to the positive input, and to one input of a differential oscilloscope. Divide the output with a resistor network to obtain unity gain. Apply the amplifier output to the other input of the differential oscilloscope. Adjust for minimum amplitude of the oscilloscope trace. Then repeat the procedures for common-mode rejection adjustment and gain adjustment until an optimum combination is achieved. Of course, the oscilloscope common-mode rejection must be adequate for this adjustment.

The gain stage module of Figure 9.7 uses the 725, although 741s are adequate for some applications, for example if a differential input stage with gain is used ahead of it. The 741 has inadequate frequency response at gains of 100 or more.

The gain of each amplifier is varied by switching input resistors rather than feedback resistors, in order to use only one compensation network for all gains and to allow dc offset adjustment to be accurate for all gains. Gain is achieved in single-ended stages rather than the differential stage in order to simplify resistor networks. The entire circuit will fit on a single card. To adjust offsets, ground the input to the module, and with the gain switch of A3 set to 1, adjust the offset for A2, switching the gain multiplier on A2 back and forth until the output voltage is unaffected by the gain multiplier. Next adjust the offset of A3 for no output voltage. Finally set the A2 gain to 100 and readjust both offsets at this higher resolution.

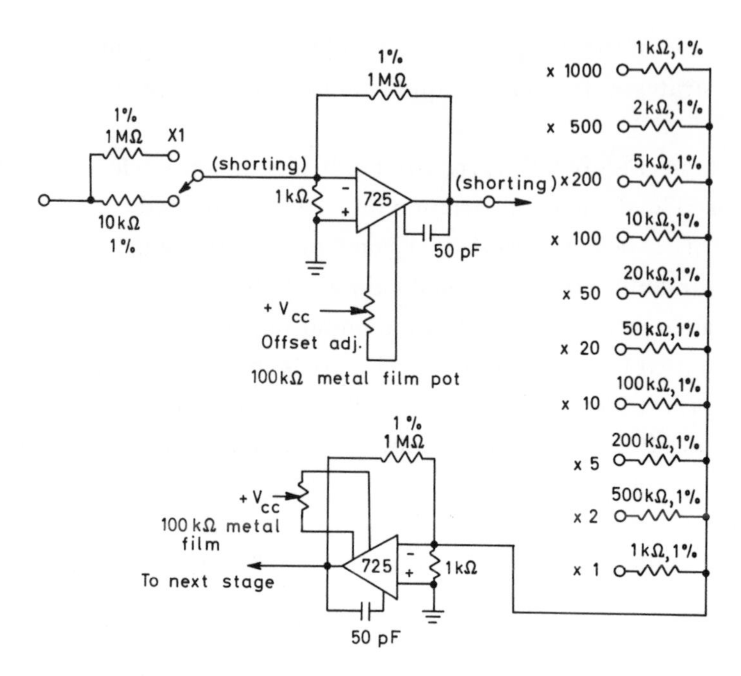

Figure 9.7
Gain stage for general-purpose amplifier.

Note that, because dc coupling is used, any dc voltage on the output of the differential input stage will be amplified. If this is large enough, the output of the gain stage will saturate, and ac portions are lost. Therefore, it is common to place the high-pass filter stage before the gain stage, or at least to ac-couple with a long time constant to the gain stage.

Location of filter stages is largely a function of the nature of unwanted frequency components after common-mode rejection. Obviously, it is desirable to achieve gain as early as possible in order to avoid addition of amplifier noise. However, if interfering signals are anticipated that are larger than the input signal, limitations are imposed on the amount of gain that can be achieved without clipping. This is particularly true of 60-cycle interference. If the desired signal is 500 μV in amplitude and an output of 1 V is needed, then there must be less than 5 mV of interference on the signal going into the gain stage or the interference will cause clipping and possible distortion of the output. If interference cannot be reduced below this level, it must be filtered out before amplification, or at least after initial preamplification and before full gain is achieved. The solution of achieving $\times$ 10 gain at the common-mode rejection stage thus has an added advantage as a compromise between maximum input voltage range and maximum noise reduction.

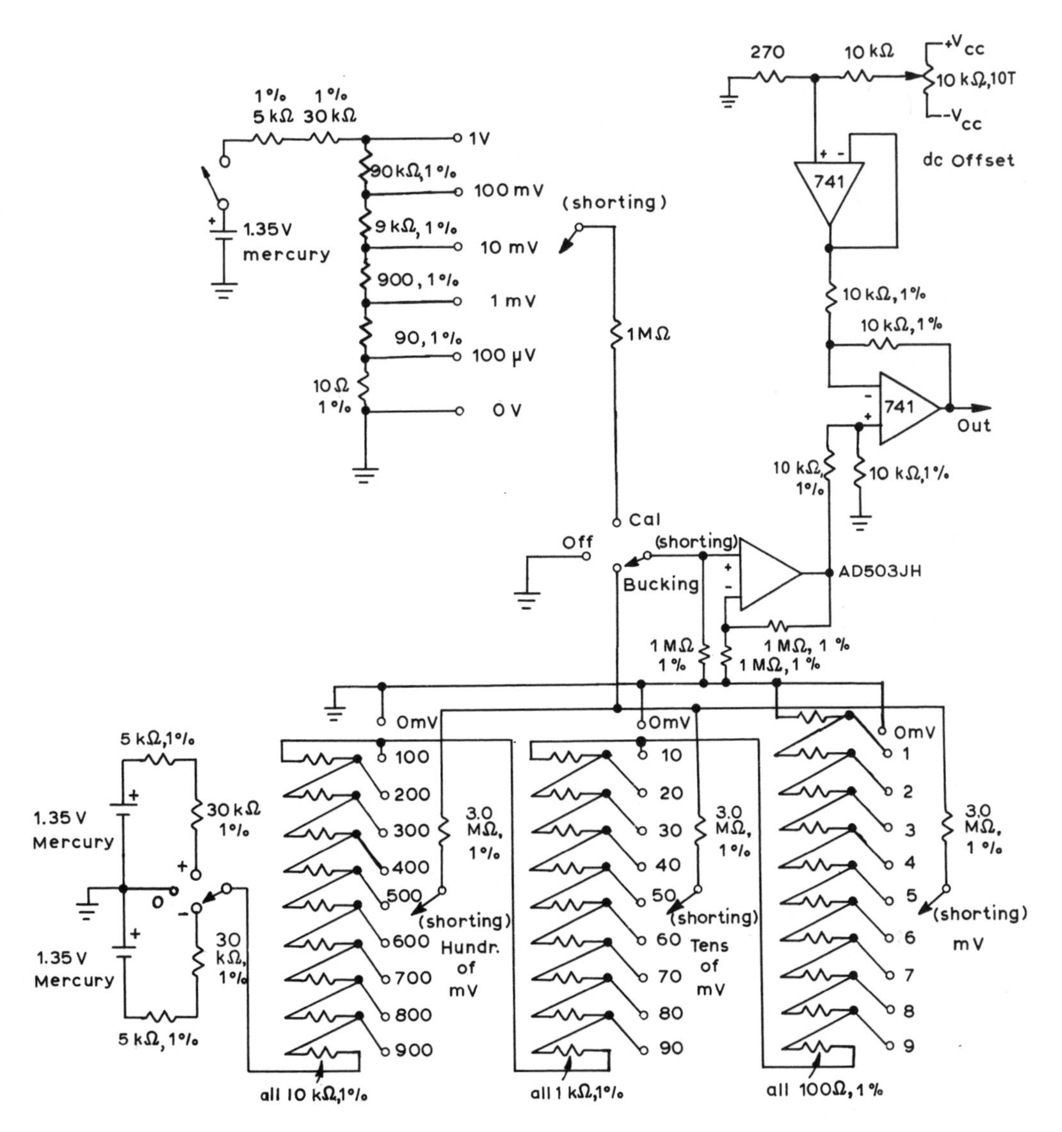

Figure 9.8
Calibration and bucking voltage module.

Figure 9.8 illustrates the configuration of the calibration and bucking voltage circuits. Offset is adjusted by using a 0 V setting on the bucking voltage with the CAL voltage off and adjusting for a 0 V output. Use good silver solder connections, because the series effects of all the solder junctions can be significant in the bucking resistor network. The batteries are 1.35 V mercury cells. A voltage reference circuit may be substituted for the batteries. The output of this module is fed to the adder-subtracter of the input stage. Correct for input gain, if any.

The filter stage module (Figure 9.9), like the others, fits on one card. Each stage has an offset of around 10 mV. If this is too great, each offset may be trimmed to zero. This is accomplished by grounding the input to each filter stage and adjusting the output offset to a tolerable value. The adjustment need be made only once, because offset drift with time is negligible.

The 60 Hz filter is a simple twin-tee notch filter that can be inserted into the signal path or bypassed. In some environments, it is useful to add a 120 Hz filter as well. Cut resistance values in half to select 120 Hz. Design equations from Chapter 5 (Figure 5.15a to c) were used. Trimming of resistors may be necessary for proper tuning.

The high-pass and low-pass Butterworth filters were constructed by using the design equations from Chapter 5, Equations 5.13 and 5.14. The high-input-impedance LM310 allows the resistors to be switched rather than the capacitors, minimizing recovery time and eliminating unpleasant switching noise, as well as reducing the physical size of the circuit considerably. The 100 pF capacitors paralleling the resistors in the high-pass amplifier prevent instability when the large resistors are switched in. Bandpass of the high-pass amplifier is still 200 kHz, even with the 100 pF capacitors in place.

The 100 pF capacitor in the low-pass section also serves to provide improved stability.

When these high impedances are used, equivalent input noise can be several hundred microvolts, peak-to-peak; therefore, they should be inserted in the signal path only after the signal is at least 10 mV, preferably 100 mV, in amplitude. If lower noise is desired, use smaller resistors and larger capacitors; this will limit the range of cutoff values possible, unless the more conventional method of switching capacitors, with consequent exasperating switching transients, is used.

The 60 Hz filter can be used for signals of 1 mV or higher, preferably at least 10 mV, because the resistors are large enough to contribute perhaps 100 μV of noise. Properties of the LM310 are illustrated in Figure 9.9d.

The output module of Figure 9.10 utilizes the versatile and inexpensive 741s to drive a push-pull output pair of transistors. Three outputs are available: a

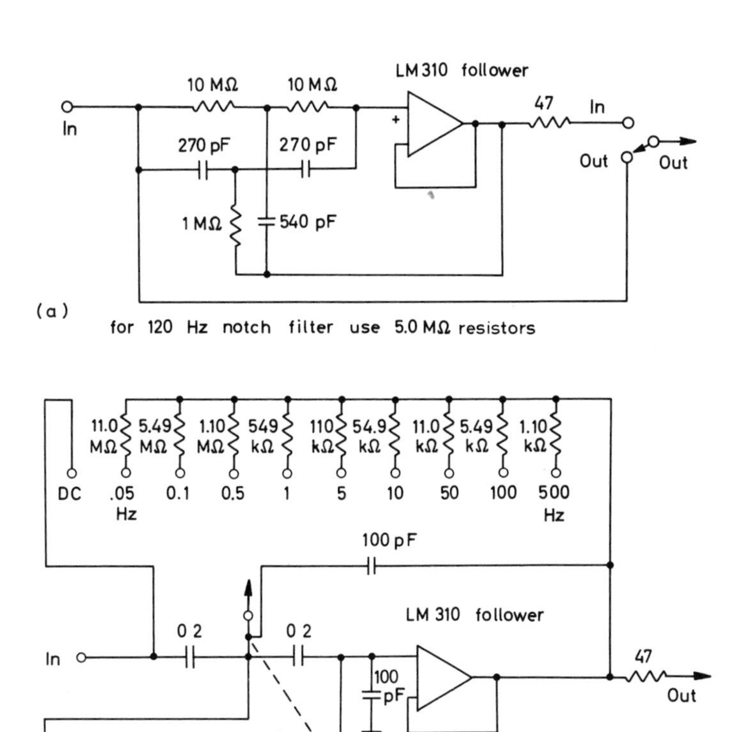

Figure 9.9
Filter module. (a) 60 Hz notch filter; (b) low-pass section; (c) high-pass section; (d) properties of LM310 follower (from *Linear Integrated Circuits*, 1971, by National Semiconductor. Used with permission of National Semiconductor).

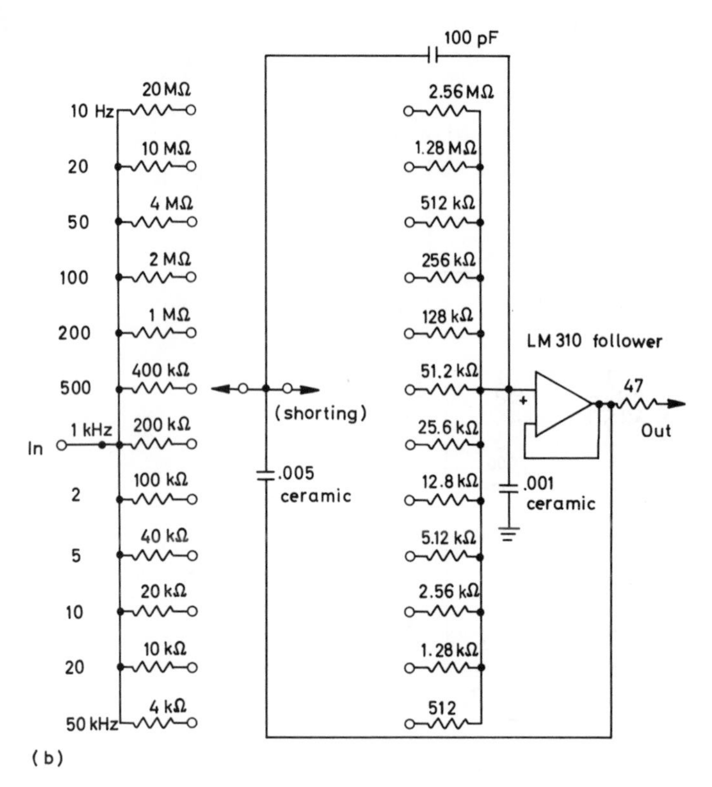

Figure 9.9 (continued)

positive and negative differential pair, either of which can be used referenced to ground, and a loudspeaker outlet for an audio monitor, with volume control. If complete independence of volume and amplifier gain is desired, use the output of the unity-gain differential input stage (Figure 9.6), if available, to drive a separate audio gain stage. Generally, if such independence is desired, a separate audio amplifier, which can be used to monitor any signal, is advisable. Adjust the offsets on the outputs to zero with the module input set to 0 V. Note that the output series resistors constitute the output impedances and provide short-circuit protection. The power transistors should be mounted on extruded aluminum heat sinks, on the back of the device chassis, with good air circulation. If the amplifier need not have such low output impedance, the emitter-follower push-pull output stages are not necessary.

The general-purpose amplifier should be built in a single chassis. Leave room for additional modules if desired. Decouple power voltages on each card. If high gain accuracy and dc stability are required, use metal film or noninductive wire-wound resistors; use precision resistors in the common-mode rejection circuits, in any case. Carefully shield the circuits with a metal chassis, and use shielded leads to the headstage amplifiers. Separate high-voltage signals from low-voltage

absolute maximum ratings

Supply Voltage	±18V
Power Dissipation	500 mW
Input Voltage	±15V
Output Short Circuit Duration	Indefinite
Operating Temperature Range	0°C to 70°C
Storage Temperature Range	−65°C to 150°C
Lead Temperature (Soldering, 10 sec)	300°C

electrical characteristics

PARAMETER	CONDITIONS	MIN	TYP	MAX	UNITS
Input Offset Voltage	$T_A = 25°C$		2.5	7.5	mV
Input Bias Current	$T_A = 25°C$		2.0	7.0	nA
Input Resistance	$T_A = 25°C$	10^{10}	10^{12}		Ω
Input Capacitance			1.5		pF
Large Signal Voltage Gain	$T_A = 25°C$, $V_S = \pm15V$ $V_{OUT} = \pm10V$, $R_L = 8k\Omega$	0.999	0.9999		V/V
Output Resistance	$T_A = 25°C$		0.75	2.5	Ω
Supply Current	$T_A = 25°C$		3.9	5.5	mA
Input Offset Voltage				10	mV
Offset Voltage Temperature Drift			10		μV/°C
Input Bias Current				10	nA
Large Signal Voltage Gain	$V_S = \pm15V$, $V_{OUT} = \pm10V$ $R_L = 10k\Omega$	0.999			V/V
Output Voltage Swing	$V_S = \pm15V$, $R_L = 10k\Omega$	±10			V
Supply Voltage Rejection Ratio	$\pm5V \le V_S \le \pm18V$	70	80		dB

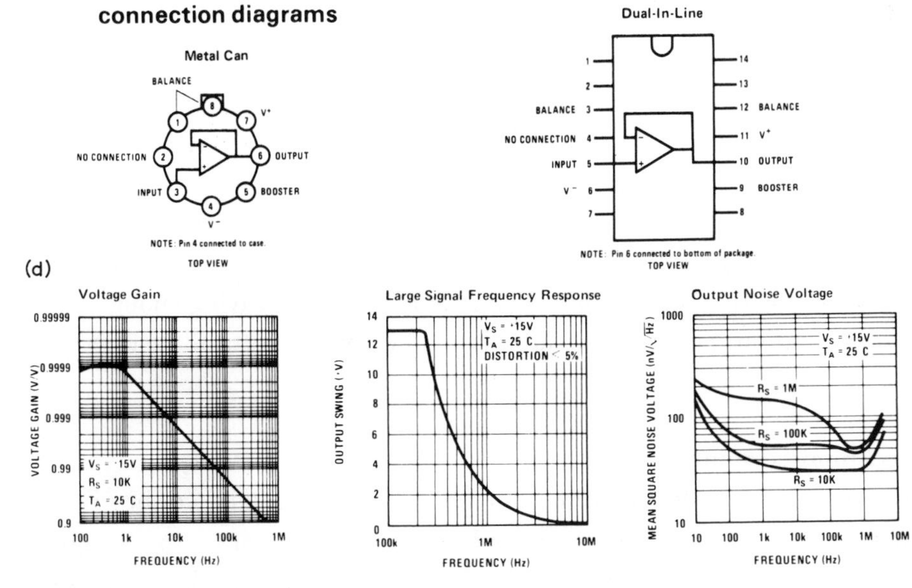

Figure 9.9 (continued)

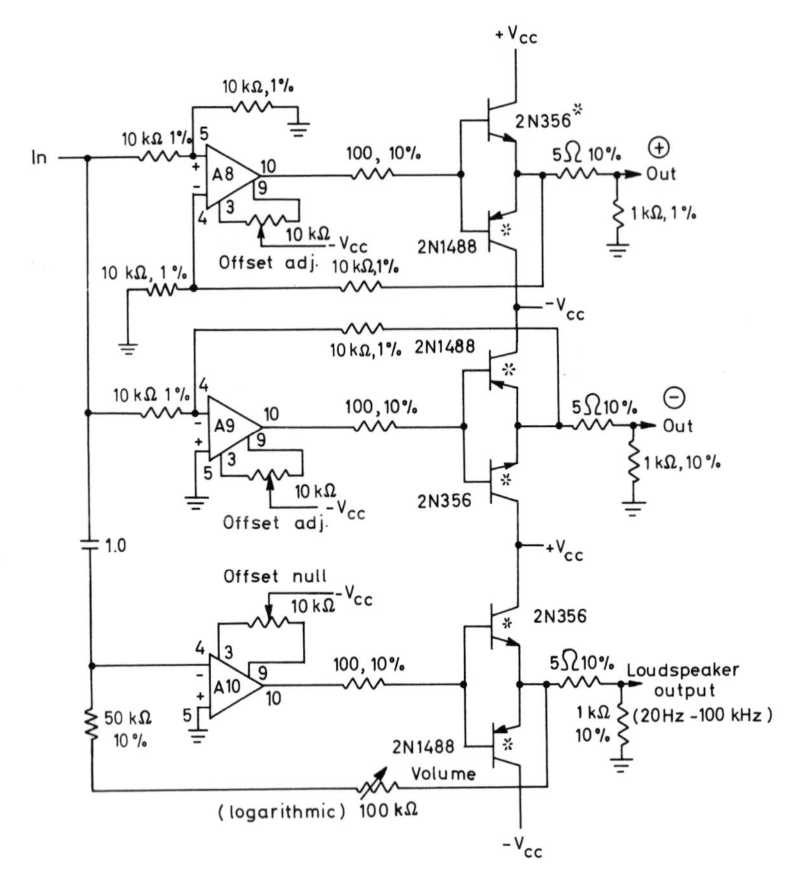

Figure 9.10
Output stage for general-purpose amplifier.

signals in order to prevent undesirable interactions, and carefully avoid ground loops. Try to establish a good ground plane on each card. Although the amplifiers have good power supply rejection, use a well-regulated supply. If the exposed power transistors on the back of the chassis could be shorted to ground inadvertently, guard them with a mesh or punched-hole metal cage, leaving enough openings for air circulation. Fins on heat sinks should be aligned vertically for best air circulation.

9.3 Spike Enhancement

When recording single units, occasions often arise where the spikes to be discriminated are barely larger than the noise level. Although filter settings can be optimized for noise suppression, much of the noise may be of neural origin, and

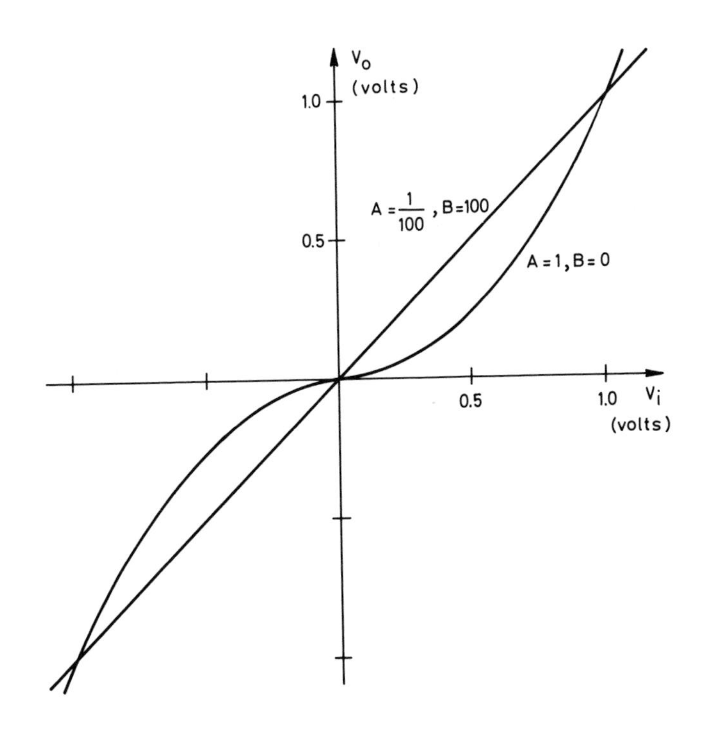

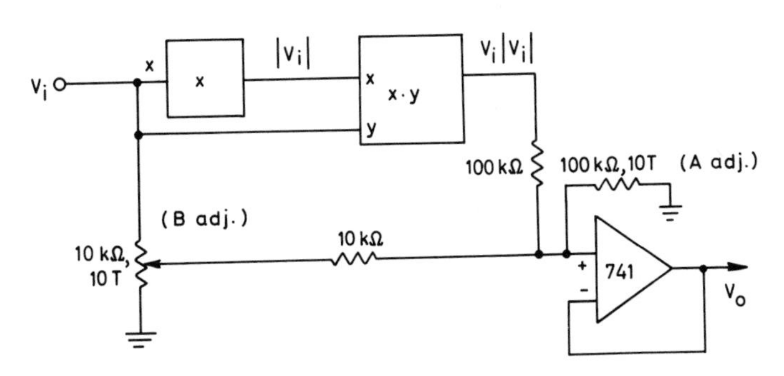

Figure 9.11
Spike enhancement. $V_o = A(BV_i + V_i|V_i|)$

hence of much the same bandwidth as the signal. In order to facilitate discrimination and in order to maximize signal-to-noise ratio when tape recording, the signal may be passed through a *spike enhancer*. Such a device should exaggerate the relative height of the spikes, and it should compress the noise if the spikes are larger than the noise in the first place. The input-output relation must therefore be continuous but nonlinear. One simple function that can be used is that graphed in Figure 9.11:

$$V_o = A(BV_i + V_i\,|V_i|).$$

A block diagram is presented in Figure 9.11. The absolute value circuit of Figures 3.13 and 3.14 and a 795 multiplier can be used. Adjust gain A for the desired dynamic range at the output, using the slope adjustment B to determine the degree of nonlinearity.

One advantage of the function chosen lies in the fact that the order of amplitudes of different single units is maintained and the original signal can be retrieved by the inverse of the operation.

9.4 Beam Intensification

Often, when photographing action potentials from the oscilloscope screen, the rapidly rising phase is not displayed as intensely on the oscilloscope as the more slowly moving portion. This is due to the fact that the beam intensity varies with the amount of energy imparted to the phosphors. The light intensity at a point is a function of the anodal acceleration of the electron beam and the amount of time during which the beam impinges on that point. Thus, if the beam sweeps across some points more rapidly than across others, the former points will emit less light than the latter. In real-time displays, there is of course no way to reproduce faithfully the wave form and simultaneously maintain a fixed writing rate. However, we can compensate for variations in speed of beam traverse by proportionally varying the acceleration of electrons. On most modern oscilloscopes, it is possible to vary the cathode voltage, at least briefly, via a capacitor-coupled input on the back of the oscilloscope, thus varying the acceleration of the electron beam. Manufacturers provide schematics for modifying the intensification circuit for external modulation, in oscilloscopes that do not have this option. The differentiator of Figure 9.12 can be used to modulate the beam intensity. The faster the rate of change of the voltage (and hence the faster the movement of the CRT beam across the phosphors), the greater the magnitude of the derivative. Since we wish to intensify for either direction of movement, an absolute-value circuit is used to drive the output. External cathode inputs to Tektronix oscilloscopes generally

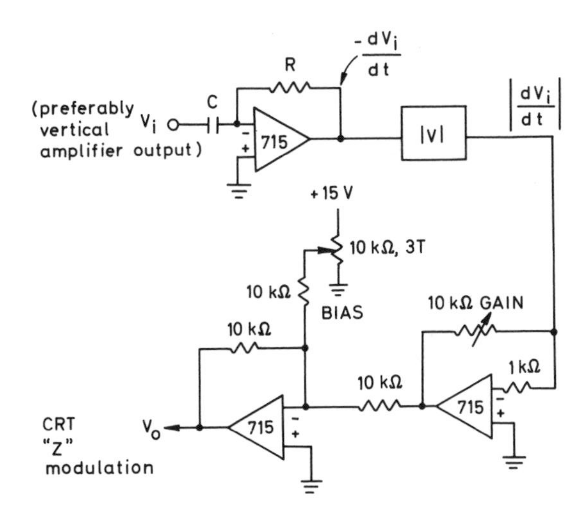

Figure 9.12
Beam intensification. $V_o = -A + B|dV_i/dt|$.

require from +3 to +30 V for intensification. Since they are capacitor-coupled, the full range of ±10 to ±15 V of standard op amps is adequate. Choose amplifiers with adequate frequency response; the 715 op amp would be adequate for most purposes. In order to allow variation of oscilloscope vertical gain, use the actual voltage on the upper vertical deflection plate or the difference between upper and lower plates. This is available as a vertical amplifier output on the back of some oscilloscopes and may be added to other oscilloscopes as a simple modification, according to instructions available from the manufacturer.

9.5 Measuring Electrode Resistance

Several techniques are available for measuring electrode resistance or impedance. It is usually not necessary to have a high degree of accuracy for such measurements, because good impedances are empirically determined, depending on the type of electrode and the recording situation. However, the technique should give results that are reproducible to, say, ±10%.

Figure 9.13 illustrates three techniques for measuring electrode impedances.

All three circuits rely on the generation of a constant-current signal that produces a voltage across the microelectrode proportional to the electrode resistance. This can be accomplished by using a constant-current stimulator such as the ones discussed in Chapter 8 or by using the simple circuits of Figure 9.13. The circuits of (a) and (b) are probably the most commonly used measurement techniques that pass small enough currents (particularly the Lettvin circuit of Figure 9.13) such that they do not excite tissues and can be used to measure *in situ*. An optional

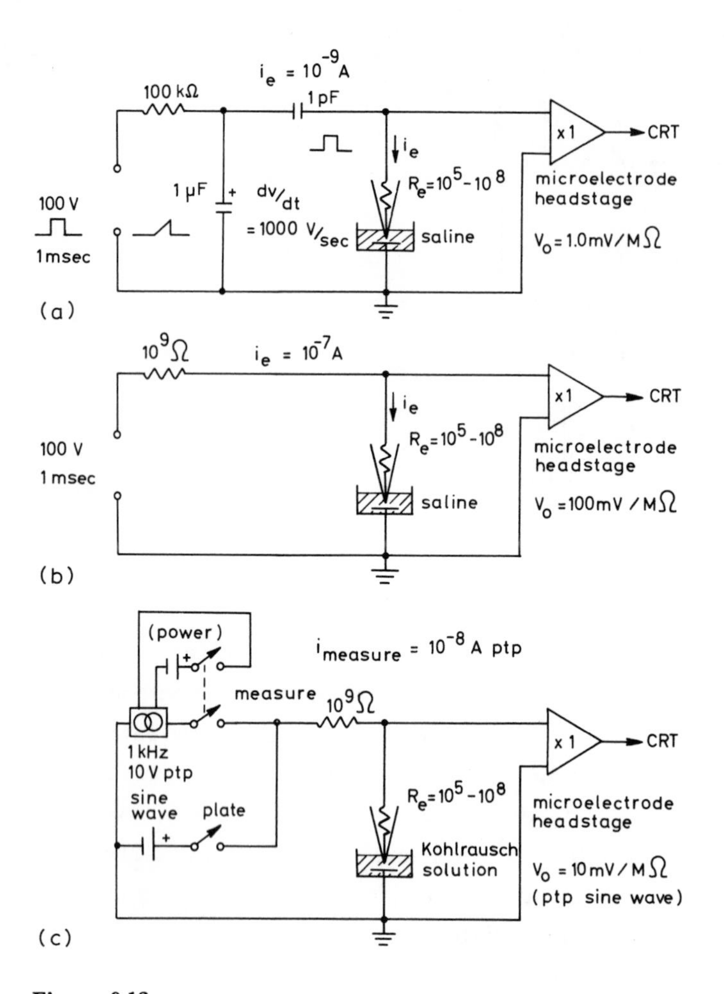

Figure 9.13
Electrode impedance measurement. (a) Lettvin technique using ac-coupled constant-current source. (b) 10^9 Ω Resistor used to simulate perfect current source. (c) Circuit for monitoring resistance while plating electrode.

capacitor (C, in b) can be added to round the edges of the test pulse and prevent activation of excitable elements.

The Lettvin network uses the 100 kΩ × 1 μF RC circuit to integrate the 100 V, 1 msec pulse into a ramp with dV/dt = 1000 V/sec (1 V/msec). This ramp is further differentiated in the R_e × 1 pF network, producing a constant current of $i_e = 10^{-9}$ A through R_e. Therefore, the voltage across the electrode is $V_e = i_eR_e = 10^{-9}R_e$ V, or 1 mV/MΩ. This circuit has an advantage over the other two, in that there is no dc path to the electrode, and hence the input resistance is not lowered; this means electrode measurement can be accomplished during recording. The circuit should be calibrated, however, because stray capacitances may alter sensitivity. Use known resistors over the range 100 kΩ–100 MΩ.

The circuit of Figure 9.13b provides approximate constant current by applying a 100 V pulse to a series 10^9 Ω resistor. The sensitivity of the device is therefore represented by V_e/R_e = 10 mV/MΩ.

In Figure 9.13c, a method is presented for plating metal microelectrodes with platinum or other metal to reduce the tip impedance, while directly monitoring the impedance. A 10 V ptp sine wave (1 kHz) is applied through 10^9 Ω for measurement purposes, with a sensitivity of 1 mV/MΩ. Any desired plating voltage can be applied independently or simultaneously to plate metal onto the tip. The decreasing impedance can be monitored on the oscilloscope (use ac coupling) with both circuits on, and when the desired impedance is attained, the plating current is turned off.

9.6 Physiological Monitoring

Most neurobiology experiments require minimal recording of physiological parameters. We will consider some of those that are most commonly used. Monitoring the state of the eye (position, pupil diameter, and accommodative state) is described in Chapter 9, where appropriate stimuli for these systems are also discussed.

When recording any physiological parameters from humans, special precautions must be taken to prevent shock hazards or other health hazards. Some of the references at the end of this chapter discuss elimination of shock hazards (for example, Morrison, 1967, Strong, 1970, and Geddes and Baker, 1968).

Probably the most commonly monitored physiological parameter is the EKG. A good differential amplifier such as the one of Section 9.2 can be used for this purpose, or cheaper variants without as many of the functions of the general-purpose amplifier can be applied for this specialized application. An inexpensive EKG amplifier is diagrammed in Figure 9.14. Be sure to shield the circuit and

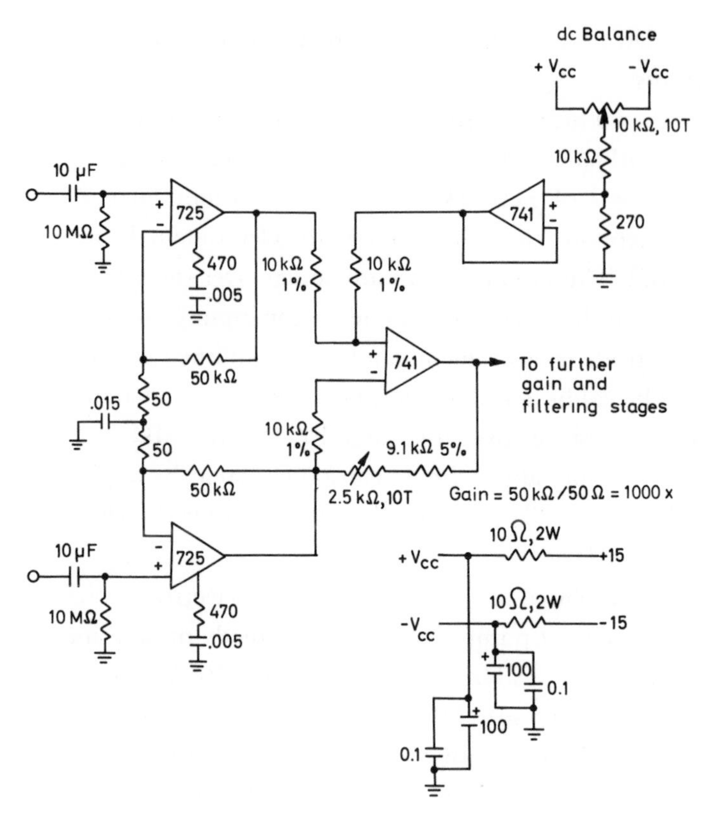

Figure 9.14
High-gain, low-noise ac amplifier for EEG recording.

input leads, decouple supply voltages, and use the appropriate frequency compensation for the 725 amplifier. A filtering stage can easily be added. EKG frequencies are mostly contained in the band from 0.5 to 100 Hz. The same device may be used for EMG recording.

EEG records can be obtained with the same amplifier as that used for EKG recording. Since EKG signals are of the order of 1 mV and EEG records are of the order of 20–500 μV, additional, adjustable gain may be required. Bandpass filtering is essential to reduce noise as much as possible. EEG frequencies fall in the frequency band from 0.5 Hz to 30 Hz; therefore, 12 dB/octave filters similar to those in Figure 9.9 should be suitable. Evoked cortical responses and ERG can be recorded with devices of the same design, using different bandpass filter settings.

Blood pressure is easily monitored with one of the many commercially available pressure transducers. Strain-gauge, piezoelectric, and even dynamic (moving coil) transducers are available. The piezoelectric types include versions small enough to cannulate major vessels directly. Circuit sophistication need not be particularly great; variants of the EKG amplifier of Figure 9.14 are generally more than adequate.

For measuring thoracic volume a flexible length of rubber tubing is generally wrapped around the thorax with a sensitive pressure transducer inserted in the contained air compartment, which is sealed at both ends. As chest circumference varies, the air is compressed to greater or lesser degree. For actual intrathoracic pressures, cannulate the pleural cavity, observing the same precautions as observed for any pneumothorax, and ensuring an air-tight seal. Strain-gauge or piezoelectric monitors are inexpensive and reliable.

Temperatures are commonly monitored by using miniature thermocouples to generate small temperature-dependent voltages, or by measuring current resulting from a fixed voltage across a temperature-dependent resistor (thermistor), or by dividing current from a known voltage across a fixed resistor and a thermistor and measuring the voltage across either the thermistor or the fixed resistor. The resulting temperature-dependent voltage or current is amplified and used to drive a meter. Thermistors of the necessary sensitivity, linearity, and temperature range are now quite inexpensive; use an op amp with sufficiently high input resistance to prevent shunting the temperature-sensitive element. Calibrate with water baths of various temperatures within the desired range, using an accurate thermometor as a reference.

9.7 Voltage Discrimination

If the wave form of a signal, such as an action potential, is irrelevant to the variable being analyzed, such as spike timing, it is convenient to convert the variable and complicated action potential voltage sequence into a series of uniform pulses. This is accomplished by voltage discrimination.

We will use TTL pulses for several purposes in this section and in the chapter on data analysis; therefore, we will first discuss a practical method of discriminating voltages with an added feature, *pulse height analysis.* A pulse height analyzer is a device that has a threshold *window*, consisting of an upper and lower (usually adjustable) voltage threshold; when a signal crosses the lower threshold, into the window area and back out, without crossing the upper boundary of the window, a pulse of fixed duration appears at the output of the pulse height analyzer. Such a device is very useful in signaling the presence or absence of discriminable spikes that are of smaller amplitude than the largest spikes in a multiunit recording. Pulse height analyzers with multiple windows can be constructed on the same principles as those employed in the design considered here.

Figure 9.15 presents a design for a pulse height analyzer. The inputs are fed to

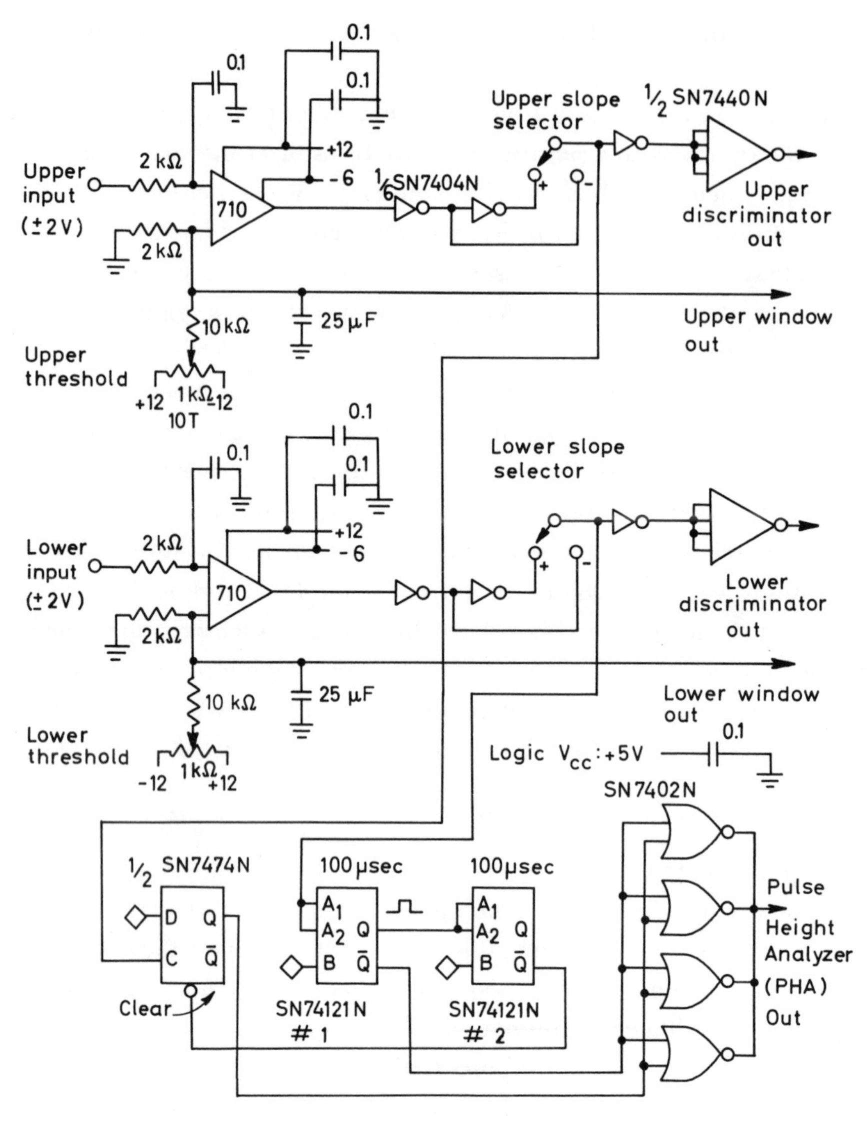

Figure 9.15
Pulse height analyzer. Select input bypass capacitor for desired frequency cutoff.

two discriminators, consisting of 710 comparators with variable filtered dc comparison voltages. The 0.01 μF capacitor shunts high-frequency noise, making such noise common mode to the comparator inputs; this prevents multiple high-frequency pulses from occurring at the discriminator output as a noisy action potential crosses threshold.

Well-regulated supply voltages must be used, with good decoupling at each 710. In the absence of such precautions, current transients due to 710 output transitions can cause feedback effects, introducing undesirable instabilities.

It is assumed that input voltages range from +2 V to −2 V; for a larger input range, divide the input voltage with a divider similar to that used for the comparison voltage. Different capacitors (C_1 and C_2) will probably be necessary if such a divider is used. If the relatively low input impedance (10 kΩ) is too low for the device driving it, use an input buffer amplifier and adjust the gain for desired voltage range. If a negative feedback inverter is used, switch the 710 inputs; that is, the input signal should go to the negative input, and the comparator voltage goes to the positive input. The 710s may be replaced by a 741 or 715 op amp in the open-loop inverting or noninverting mode with diode feedback for TTL compatibility. See Figure 4.35 for this type of comparator design. The use of an op amp alleviates the need for the separate 710 supply voltages.

The comparison voltage is simply the output of a 10-turn pot connected between +15 V and −15 V, filtered with a 25 μF capacitor to ground. The resistor divider limits the comparator voltage to ±2.5 V. This range brackets the ±2 V input range, and the 710 differential input limit of ±5 V is never exceeded.

The comparator outputs are buffered and inverted and led to slope selector switches, which provide alternate polarities of the discriminator outputs. These outputs are further buffered and made available in order to use the discriminators independently, if desired. A positive level appears at a discriminator output, if the input is more positive than the threshold (positive slope) or more negative than the threshold (negative slope), and lasts as long as the input bears the proper relation to the threshold.

Fancier designs include a multiplexer at the output; by using a chopping frequency of 50–100 kHz, an analog switch can be used to generate a "chopped dual-beam" display on an oscilloscope, using only one oscilloscope beam. This permits easy comparison of input signal and threshold level. The oscilloscope must have adequate frequency response for following the chopper frequency, of course. However, if the multiplexed output is used as input to a chopped-beam oscilloscope, provision must be made to avoid beat frequency effects in which part of one multiplexer channel or the other may vanish for part of the sweep. Unless

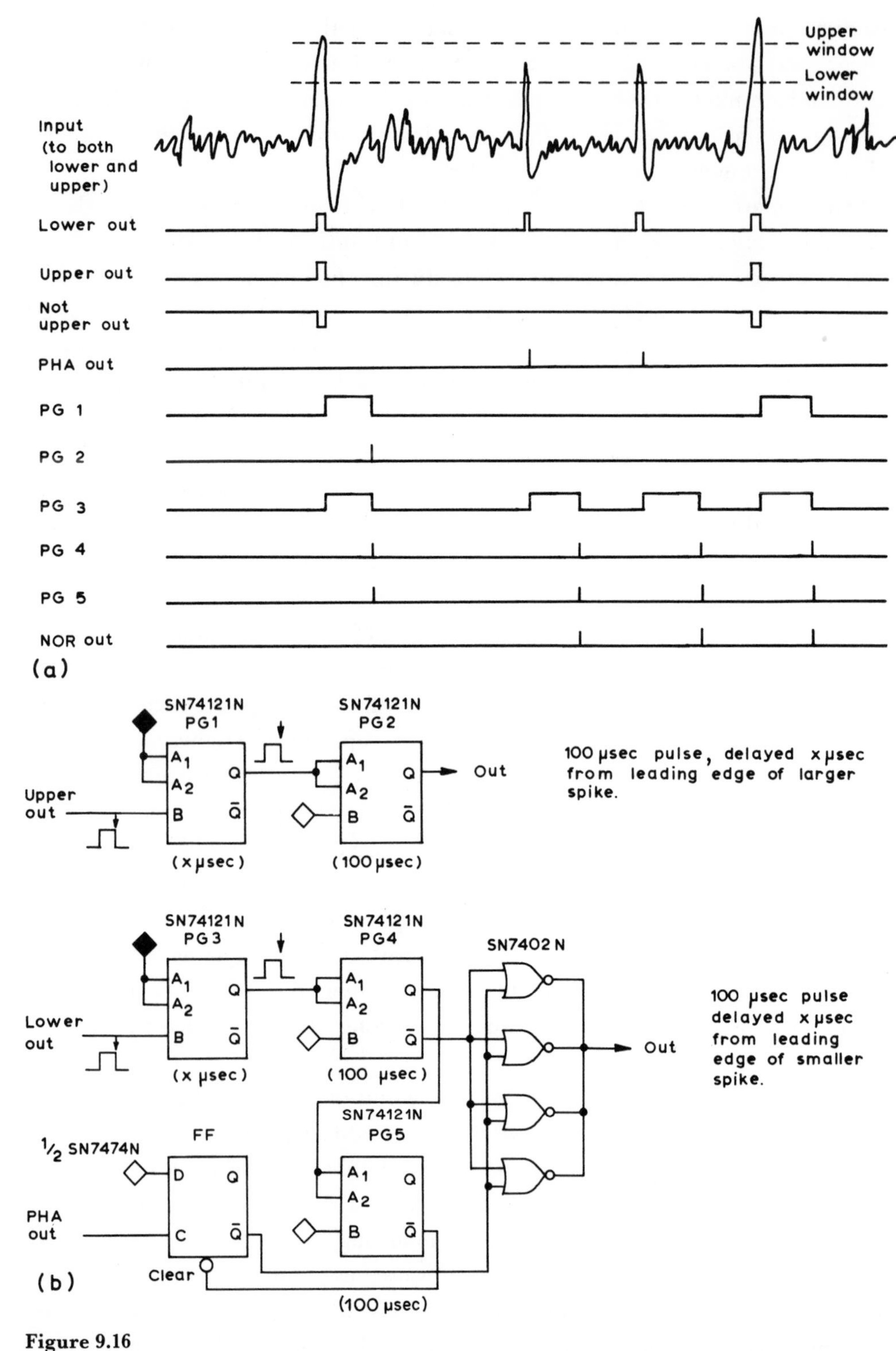

Figure 9.16
Delay equalizer for pulse height analyzer. (a) Wave forms for figure 9.15, and for P.G. 1–5 of this figure. (b) Delay circuits.

a variable multiplexing frequency is available or the oscilloscope multiplexer is oscillating at a much higher frequency, it is good practice to avoid multiplexing inputs on a chopped-beam oscilloscope channel.

The discriminators can be used as the upper and lower boundaries of a pulse height analyzer window if the inputs are connected in parallel; both slope selector switches are set for the same polarity, and the upper threshold is set for a larger voltage, of the same sign, as the lower threshold. For ease of expression we refer to the input as exceeding threshold of either boundary if the corresponding discriminator output is positive.

There is only one condition for which we want a pulse to appear at the pulse height analyzer output: when an action potential, or other transient event, crosses the lower boundary and enters the window, and recrosses the lower boundary, "defenestrating," without first crossing the upper boundary. This immediately implies that the output pulse cannot occur until the defenestration, that is, on the falling slope of the action potential. Since the event to be detected is determined at that time, the pulse duration cannot possibly correspond to the action potential "intrafenestral" duration unless some sort of "memory" is used to program a pulse width. Although this can be done, there is no real reason to do so. Therefore, we will generate a fixed duration (100 μsec) pulse upon the occurrence of both of two conditions: (1) defenestration, and (2) the absence of a positive output from the upper discriminator at any time since the previous defenestration.

The additional logic required is very simple: one D-flipflop, two pulse generators, and a NOR gate. One pulse generator (#1) fires whenever defenestration occurs and triggers another pulse generator (#2) on the trailing edge. Both monostables are set for approximately 100 μsec. The delayed pulse clears the flipflop with its NOT output during the period starting 100 μsec after defenestration and ending 200 μsec after defenestration.

The flipflop output and #1 pulse generator NOT output are NORed, which is equivalent to ANDing pulse generator #1 output and the NOT output of the flipflop. This will generate the desired output, because the flipflop ON condition represents a memory of a positive transition of the upper boundary discriminator since the last defenestration (when the flipflop was last cleared). This is achieved by setting the flipflop on the positive transition of the upper discriminator.

There is a delay of the pulse height analyzer output relative to the output of a simple discriminator. The latter triggers on the leading edge, and a pulse height analyzer triggers on the trailing edge. There are two simple solutions to the problem of eliminating this delay, illustrated in Figure 9.16. Note that both the PHA and NOT LOWER go positive on the trailing edges of the respective spikes.

Therefore, the PHA and NOT LOWER can be used. If this is acceptable it is the simplest solution. However, it often is not acceptable, especially when the durations of the two spikes are grossly different, and the more complicated method of Figure 9.16b must then be used. The solution consists of delaying an output pulse generated by an UPPER OUT and a LOWER OUT, enough for PHA to occur or not occur and to enable the delayed lower pulse if PHA occurs. Delaying the upper pulse is easy enough; the UPPER OUT positive transition triggers a pulse generator (PG1) to fire for X μsec, and another MVB (PG2) fires a fixed 100 μsec pulse on the trailing edge of the X μsec pulse. The 100 μsec pulse is thus delayed X μsec from the leading edge of UPPER OUT. The LOWER OUT is used to fire an X μsec pulse (PG3), which triggers a 100 μsec pulse (PG4). The NOT pulse of PG4 is inhibited by the NOR gate, however, if a PHA pulse has not arrived at the flipflop (FF) at any time since the previous LOWER OUT pulse. If PHA fires, the FF is set on the leading edge of PHA OUT and its Q goes low, enabling the delayed 100 μsec pulse. At the end of the 100 μsec PG4 pulse, a brief (1 μsec) pulse is triggered at PG5 to clear FF for the next sequence. Thus a 100 μsec pulse appears at the output delayed X μsec from the leading edge of the smaller spike but not if the large spike occurs, and the delay is the same as for UPPER OUT's delay. The simpler delay circuit can be used for any other leading edges whose timing relative to the leading edge of the smaller spike must be accurately monitored, such as synchronization pulses indicating onset of a stimulus, and so forth. The value of X should be selected to be longer than the lower spike plus 101 μsec and less than the minimum interval of the smaller spike minus 101 μsec. Therefore 400–500 μsec is probably a good value of X for many applications.

A word of caution: Unless the times of occurrence of the large and small spikes are constrained by their natural interactions or by interactions within a common network, their durations may overlap. If this occurs the resulting potential wave form is difficult to predict. It is safe to predict, however, that these circuits will not simultaneously signal the arrival of both action potentials. Such a possibility must be kept in mind when interpreting relative timing data for the two single units. Only sophisticated pattern recognition programs using high-speed digital computers will suffice to detect coincidence of both spikes.

9.8 Data Transmission Techniques

It is frequently necessary to transmit electrical signals over long distances. Figures 9.17, 9.18, and 9.19 illustrate simple transmission techniques for audio (intercom), video (computer oscilloscope display), and digital data, respectively.

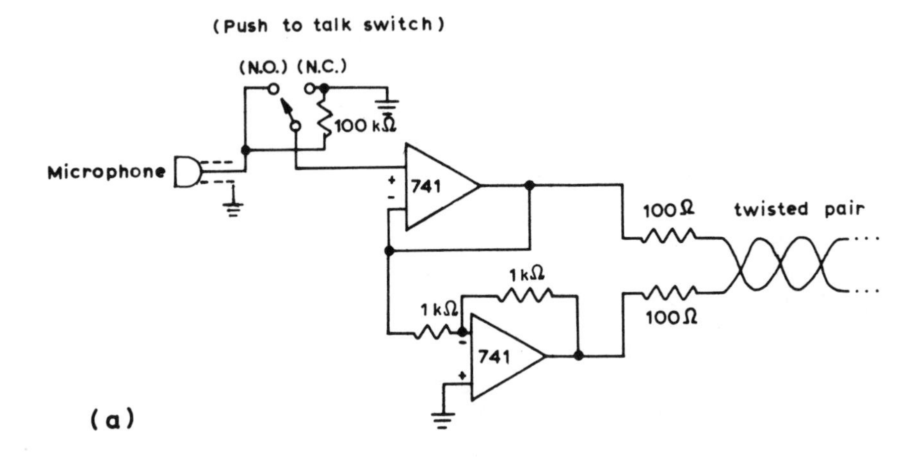

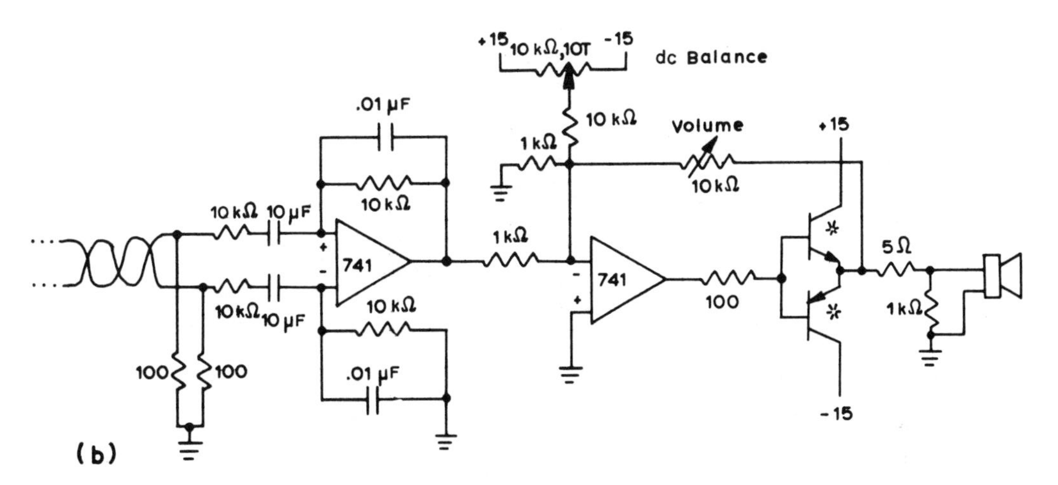

Figure 9.17
Intercom stations. (a) Transmitter; (b) Receiver. *PNP = 2N376A, NPN = 2N1488 (both on heat sinks).

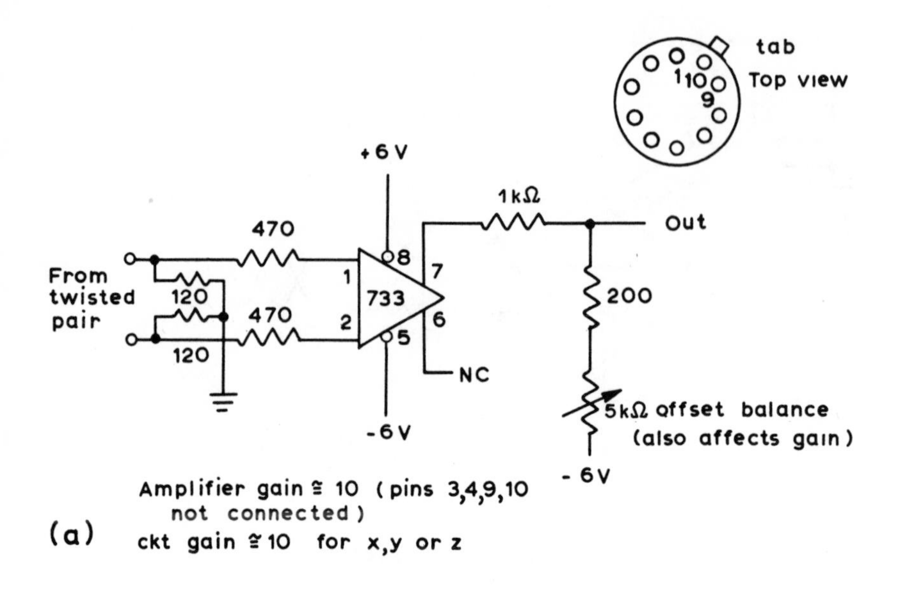

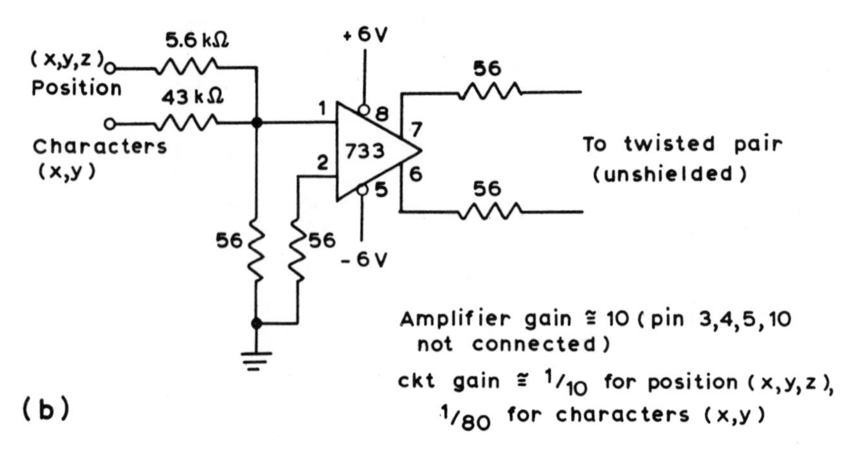

Figure 9.18
Video cable interface. (a) Receiver; (b) Transmitter.

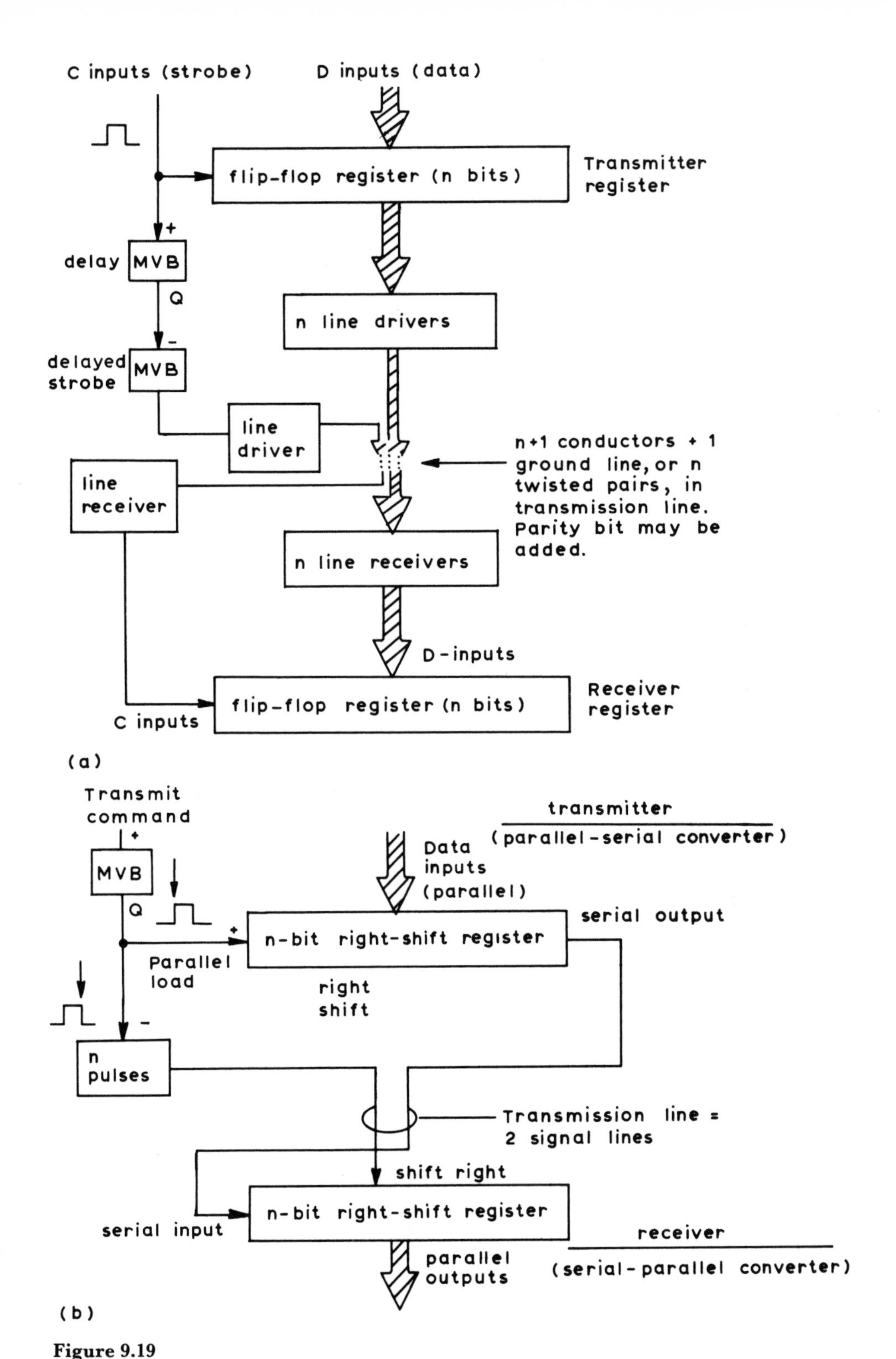

Figure 9.19
Digital cable interfaces. (a) Parallel transmission. (b) Serial transmission on two wires. (c) Serial transmission on one wire. In (c), the n pulses at the receiver are timed to strobe 2nd through $(n + 1)$th bits into the n-bit receiver. The transmission complete pulse occurs at the end of MVB inhibit and the receiver MVB is once again enabled for transmission of the next data word.

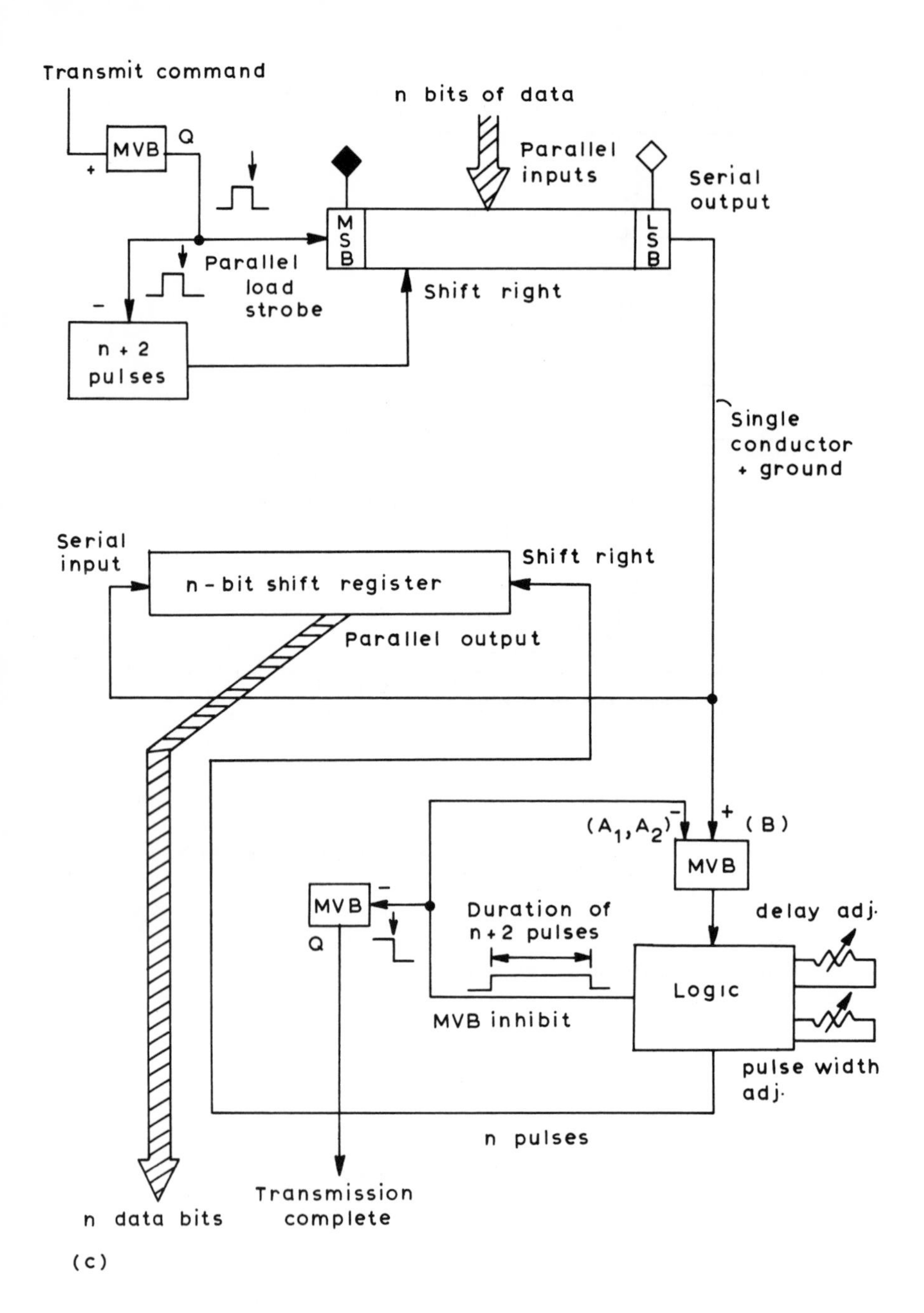

Figure 9.19 (continued)

The intercom of Figure 9.17 consists of a unity gain follower used to lower the effective impedance of a push-to-talk microphone, a resistor terminated twisted pair, and a receiver consisting of a variable-gain, high-current amplifier. For two-way transmission, use another twisted pair or use the push-to-talk switch to connect the receiver or transmitter to the twisted pair. The series resistors of each transmitter prevent damage to the follower amplifiers in the latter configuration, even when both users press the push-to-talk buttons on their microphones simultaneously. Often a single ground-referenced line is adequate for transmissions; this results in a saving of one wire if a ground is already carried through on another line.

The video transmitter of Figure 9.18 consists of a fixed-gain video amplifier with a resistor divider at the input for mixing position and character generation voltages (these are often separately produced by a computer display processor). Keep the input resistances (R_1 and R_2) high, and the source resistances (R_3 and R_4) to the 733 low in order to minimize crosstalk and noise, respectively. If this results in too small a signal for $\times 10$ operation, simply use one of the higher gains available for the 733: $\times 40$ or $\times 100$, depending on external connection of gain-adjustment pins. The receiver end differentially amplifies the signal, and the output mixer compensates for the common-mode dc offset characteristic of the 733.

Twisted pairs are generally used for such transmission lines, because they are cheaper than coaxial cable, and high-frequency losses are not as great. Differential amplification removes common-mode pickup, which constitutes virtually the entire source of noise.

Digital signals are generally transmitted as parallel (Figure 9.19a) or serial (Figures 9.19b, c) configurations. The former is faster but requires more wires. An extra wire is included for strobing the other levels (the bits to be transmitted). Parity checking is often useful, especially in noisy environments. Once again, twisted pairs should be used, although coax and single wires work for some configurations. Digital line drivers and receivers are available in IC form, such as the Texas Instruments SN75110 and SN75107, respectively.

Serial transmission is more complicated but still relatively easy to accomplish. Two wires can be used (Figure 9.19b) with one for a shift clock signal and the other for the serial data bits, or a single wire can be used (Figure 9.19c) if an extra bit is transmitted at the beginning of data (*synch*) in order to trigger strobing of data bits during successive clock cycles. In this case, the data level should be 0 before the next strobe bit. Therefore, a shift register two bits longer than the receiver is used: one bit for initiation, which goes on to initiate the timing sequence, and one bit for termination of transmission, which is always off.

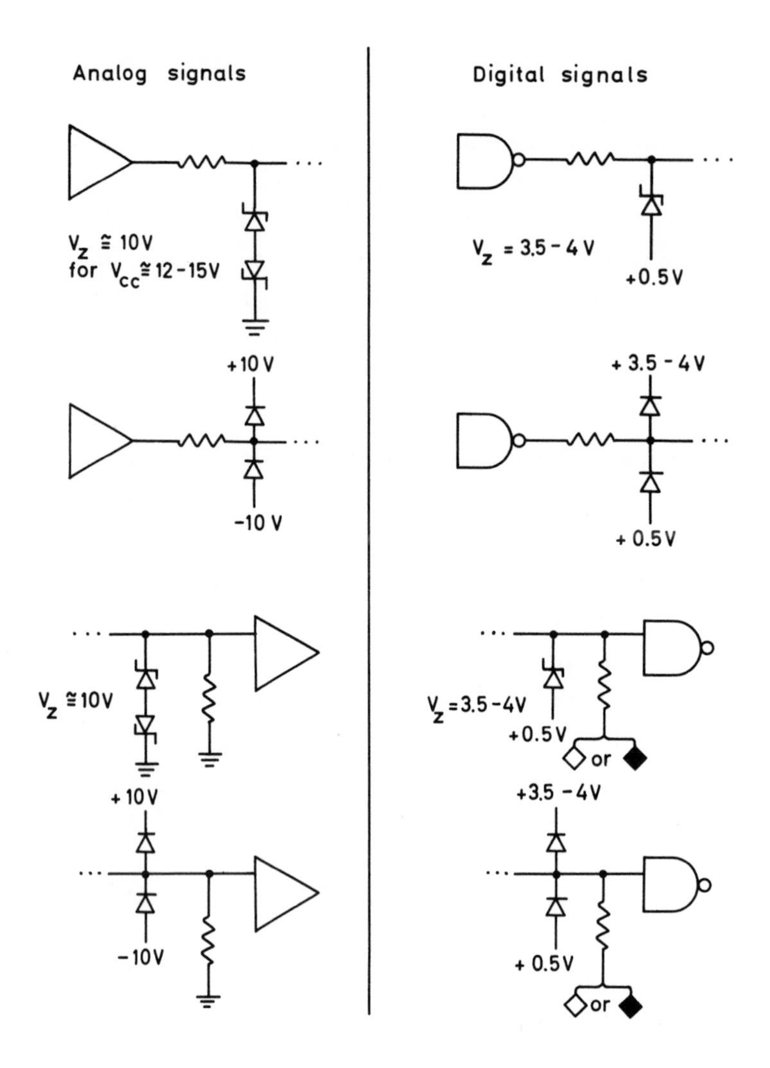

Figure 9.20
Protection of cable interfaces.

Cable transmitters and receivers sometimes require protection of their inputs and outputs from overvoltages picked up in the cable. If there is any chance of such overvoltages occurring, use diodes to protect them, as illustrated in Figure 9.20.

Selected References

Bureš, Jan, Mojmir Petráň, and Josef Zachar. 1967. (P. Hahn, translator). *Electrophysiological Methods in Biological Research.* New York: Academic Press.

Fairchild Semiconductor. 1970. Data Sheet: *μA725 Instrumentation Operational Amplifier.* Mountain View, Calif.: Fairchild Camera and Instrument Corporation.

Fein, H. 1966. Passing current through recording glass micropipette electrodes. *IEEE Trans. Bio.-Med. Engr. BME-13:* 211.

Geddes, L. A., and L. E. Baker. 1968. *Principles of Applied Biomedical Instrumentation.* New York: John Wiley & Sons.

Huntsman, L. L., and G. L. Nichols. 1971. A low-cost high-gain amplifier with exceptional noise performance. *IEEE Trans. Bio.-Med. Engr. BME-18:* 301.

Morrison, Ralph. 1967. *Grounding and Shielding Techniques in Instrumentation.* New York: John Wiley & Sons.

Nastuk, William L. 1964. *Physical Techniques in Biological Research*, Vol. V: *Electrophysiological Methods, Part A*, and Vol. VI: *Electrophysiological Methods, Part B.* New York: Academic Press.

National Semiconductor. 1971. *Linear Integrated Circuits.* Santa Clara, California: National Semiconductor Corporation.

Silverman, Robert W., and Donald J. Jenden. 1971. A novel high performance preamplifier for biological applications. *IEEE Trans. Bio.-Med. Engr. BME-18:* 430.

Strong, Peter. 1970. *Biophysical Measurements.* Beaverton, Oregon: Tektronix, Inc.

Wyland, D. C. 1971. FET cascode technique optimizes differential amplifier performance. *Electronics 44*, 2: 81.

10 DATA ANALYSIS TECHNIQUES

Paul B. Brown

There are many aspects of neural activity that cannot be deduced conveniently from an oscilloscope trace. Most of these are statistical measures, requiring some condensation of an otherwise indigestible mass of information. Although digital computers are essential for computation of most statistical measures, there are many aspects of neuronal activity that can be extracted by simple electronic circuits. We will describe these techniques as well as the design of two types of computer interface that conveniently transform the original data into a digital format, which is compatible with most data processing computers.

10.1 Voltage as a Function of Time

Although it is possible to represent any time-varying voltage as a graphic display of voltage *vs.* time, it is frequently advantageous to use electronic methods to focus on specific aspects of the signal. One method of monitoring signals is by displaying the time-varying power average with an rms meter. Fluctuations of the signal's average power over time are indicated, without regard to the actual detailed wave form. The rms meter is simply a full-wave rectifier followed by a low-pass RC filter. Variants on this device will be used as frequency meters and interval meters later in this chapter.

Whereas the simple display of voltage as a function of time is an approximation of the idealized "time domain" representation of all frequencies, it is often important to visualize the "frequency domain" representation of the signal. The fact that a finite duration is used simply defines the lower limit of the bandwidth that can be sampled, just as the properties of real electronic components limit the bandwidth during amplification and recording of a time-varying signal.

Frequency domain measurement, also called spectrum analysis, wave analysis, or harmonic analysis, is used in order to determine the relative amplitudes of frequency components of a signal. For example, during the construction of a sine wave generator for auditory stimulation, it is necessary to ensure that harmonics of the fundamental frequency are sufficiently attenuated to prevent neural or behavioral responses to the unwanted harmonics. Similarly, the output of a balanced modulator must be checked during the balancing procedure, to maximize suppression of the carrier frequency. In both of these examples, the suppression of the unwanted signal cannot be measured to the necessary degree of precision by simply inspecting the oscilloscope trace.

An electrical wave form can be analyzed into its component frequencies with a commercial harmonic analyzer, or by a computer program that processes the digitized time-varying voltage. Harmonic analyzers are relatively expensive, but they are too difficult to construct and calibrate using ICs. However, we can describe the principles of operation of harmonic analyzers and related devices. They consist of narrow-band tunable filters with precisely calibrated tuning frequency, low-distortion electronics, and amplification circuits used to drive meters or other output devices. The circuit of Figure 10.1a is a simple analyzer. The narrow-band

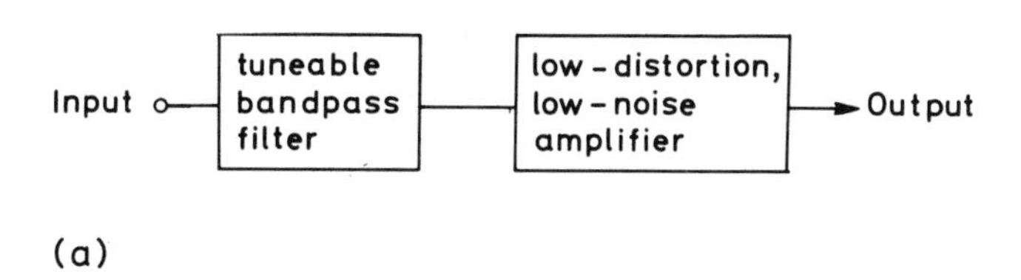

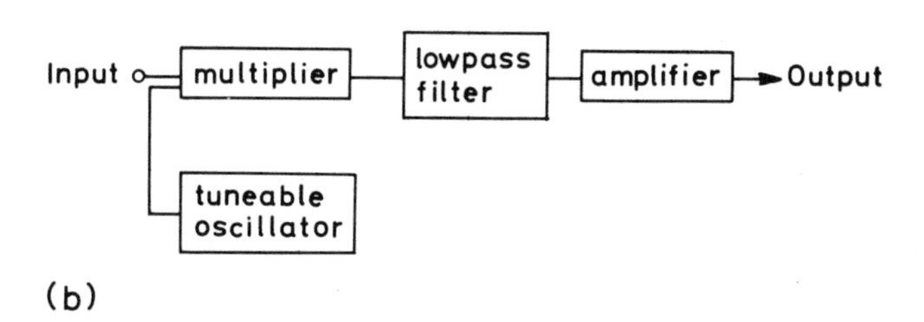

Figure 10.1
Two methods of harmonic analysis: (a) simple filter technique; (b) heterodyne technique.

filter selects the frequency component to be measured, and the amplifier corrects for attenuation at the center frequency of the notch filter. The output can be used to drive an rms meter or a penwriter. This type of analyzer has a sensitivity that, depending on the characteristics of the notch filter, has some fixed number of db/octave roll-off on both sides of the center frequency.

A much sharper frequency selectivity is accomplished by balanced modulation of the input with a precisely controlled sine wave frequency. This method is illustrated schematically in Figure 10.1b. The different frequencies are then passed through a filter; thus, if the input signal is multiplied by a 1000 Hz sine wave and the low-pass filter is set for dc-10 Hz with 6 dB/octave roll-off, the output reflects the intensity of the portion of the input spectrum from 990 to 1010 Hz with 6 dB/10 Hz roll-off on both sides of this bandwidth.

The Hewlett-Packard 3590A Wave Analyzer (Figure 10.2: reprinted by permission of Hewlett-Packard) is an example of a highly versatile device that can be used to "sweep" across a selected band of frequencies, producing a pair of output voltages, corresponding to intensity and frequency, which can be used to drive an *X-Y* oscilloscope or plotter; alternatively, a fixed frequency can be monitored. A panel meter display allows monitoring directly without any external display device. The device has selectable bandwidths of 10, 100, 1000, and 3100 Hz, as well as selectable sweep rate. Automatic scanning of frequency bands provides detailed information concerning harmonic distortion (Figure 10.2a) and intermodulation distortion (Figure 10.2b), as in the auditory stimulation examples described above. An internal BFO (beat frequency oscillator) output provides a pure sine wave of fixed amplitude at the frequency to which the analyzer is tuned, in order to excite passive or active devices and determine their bandpass characteristics (Figure 10.2c).

Although our description of the workings of the wave analyzer will not do justice to the design, it should give some indication of the methods used to obtain precise frequency-selective properties.

Figure 10.2d is a simplified block diagram of the 3590A Wave Analyzer, after a similar diagram in the operating manual. The input signal is attenuated and amplified, with compensation for subsequent frequency losses in the low-pass filter and input mixer. The low-pass filter eliminates image or spurious signals above the selected frequency range (dc-620 kHz or dc-62 kHz, selectable). The output of the filter is mixed with the local oscillator (LO) output, from the plug-in unit (we will describe the 3593A plug-in below). This can vary from 1.28 MHz to 1.90 MHz. The difference frequency corresponding to 1.28 MHz will be selectively tuned, to provide an intermediate frequency (i.f.). Thus, a 1.28 MHz LO frequency corresponds to a selected input frequency of 0 Hz and a 1.90 MHz LO frequency corresponds to a selected input frequency of 620 kHz. Since all input frequencies above 620 kHz have been removed, we know that the frequencies out of the mixer can vary only from 1.28 MHz to 2.56 MHz. The 1.28 MHz signal, proportional in amplitude to the tuned frequency component, is attenuated to control the input level to the active bandpass filters, either manually or automatically. The active bandpass filters will determine the "selectivity" of the device, that is, the bandpass tuning of the analyzer.

The i.f. signal, tuned at 1.28 MHz, is converted to two separate signals with a 180° phase difference, and each is mixed with a precisely tuned 1.28 MHz oscillator sine wave. The resulting frequency range at the inputs of the active bandpass filters is 0 Hz $\pm$ a roll-off bandwidth on both sides of 0 Hz. The filter channels each have three cascaded active filters, arranged to provide low pass from dc to 10, 100, 1000, or 3100 Hz. Within this range the spectral response of the preceding stages is essentially flat. The low-pass filters provide a flat response out to the corner frequency, with sharp roll-off above that frequency. The dc is rejected, however, in order to discard the 1.28 MHz carrier frequency from the i.f. band. There is therefore a sharp notch at the center of the pass band. Dual-channel filtering is used to filter out undesirable sidebands resulting from the double heterodyning (up and down) process, and to provide a tuning reference for the automatic frequency control (AFC) circuit, described below. After filtering, the two signals are heterodyned back up to i.f., by using their outputs as differential input to a mixer which mixes them with the 1.28 MHz oscillator. A 1.28 MHz low-pass filter is once again used to eliminate spurious high frequencies This signal is further attenuated and amplified to be detected and provide a dc signal used to drive the meter, log converter, and auto ranging circuits. The log converter provides a dc voltage proportional to the logarithm of the dc detector voltage, for logarithmic Y axis output to a plotter or for a decibel meter. The auto ranging circuit is used to automatically control the internal attenuators in one mode of operation.

The restored output is obtained by mixing the i.f. signal from the meter amplifier with the LO signal from the plug-in, to provide an output at the tuned input frequency at an amplitude which is proportional to the strength of that frequency component.

The BFO (beat frequency oscillator) output is obtained by mixing the LO with a 1.28 MHz oscillator, which is slightly offset to prevent the BFO output from falling into the 0 Hz notch of the internal filters. The BFO is thus a useful output for testing the transfer characteristics of various devices, such as filters and amplifiers. This is a consequence of the fact that the sweeping LO will always

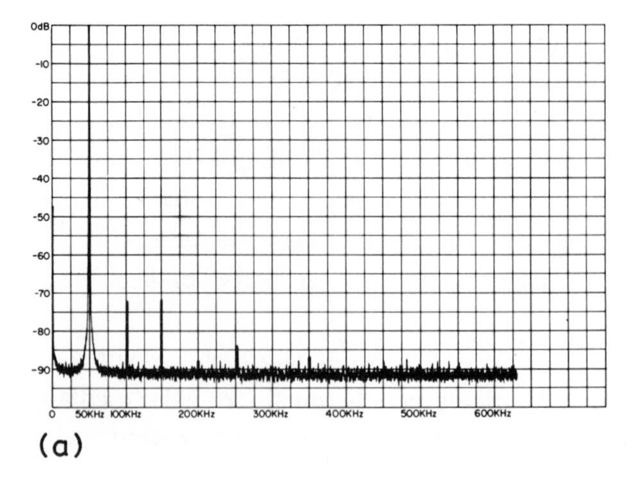

(a)

Harmonic distortion of an oscillator is easily resolved using recordings generated by the 3590A. To make this recording, the Y-axis LOG and X-axis LINEAR recorder outputs were used.

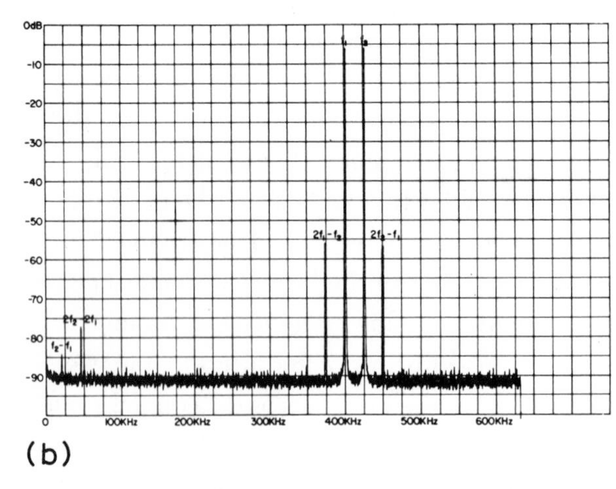

(b)

Intermodulation products can be readily measured using the recorder outputs generated by the 3590A. In the case shown two signals, 400 kHz and 425 kHz, were injected into an amplifier and then the resulting distortion products were measured. The recording shown is using the Y-axis LOG with X-axis LINEAR.

The recorder output may also be used to display filter shapes. On the left is the 3590A's 10 Hz active bandpass filter shape. On the right is a typical 5 Hz crystal filter shape. To make this recording, the Y-axis LOG and X-axis LINEAR recorder outputs were used.

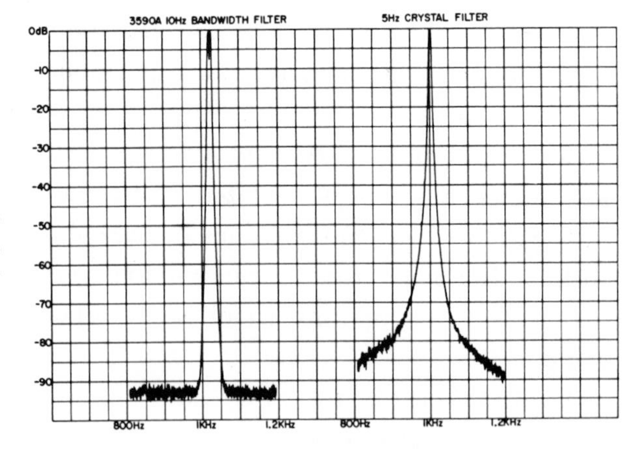

(c)

Figure 10.2
Applications of Hewlett-Packard 3590A Wave Analyzer (from *Operating Service Manual*, *Wave Analyzer 3590A*, 1970, by Hewlett-Packard. Used with permission of Hewlett-Packard). (a) analysis of harmonic distortion; (b) analysis of intermodulation distortion; (c) analysis of filter characteristics; (d) block diagram of 3590A.

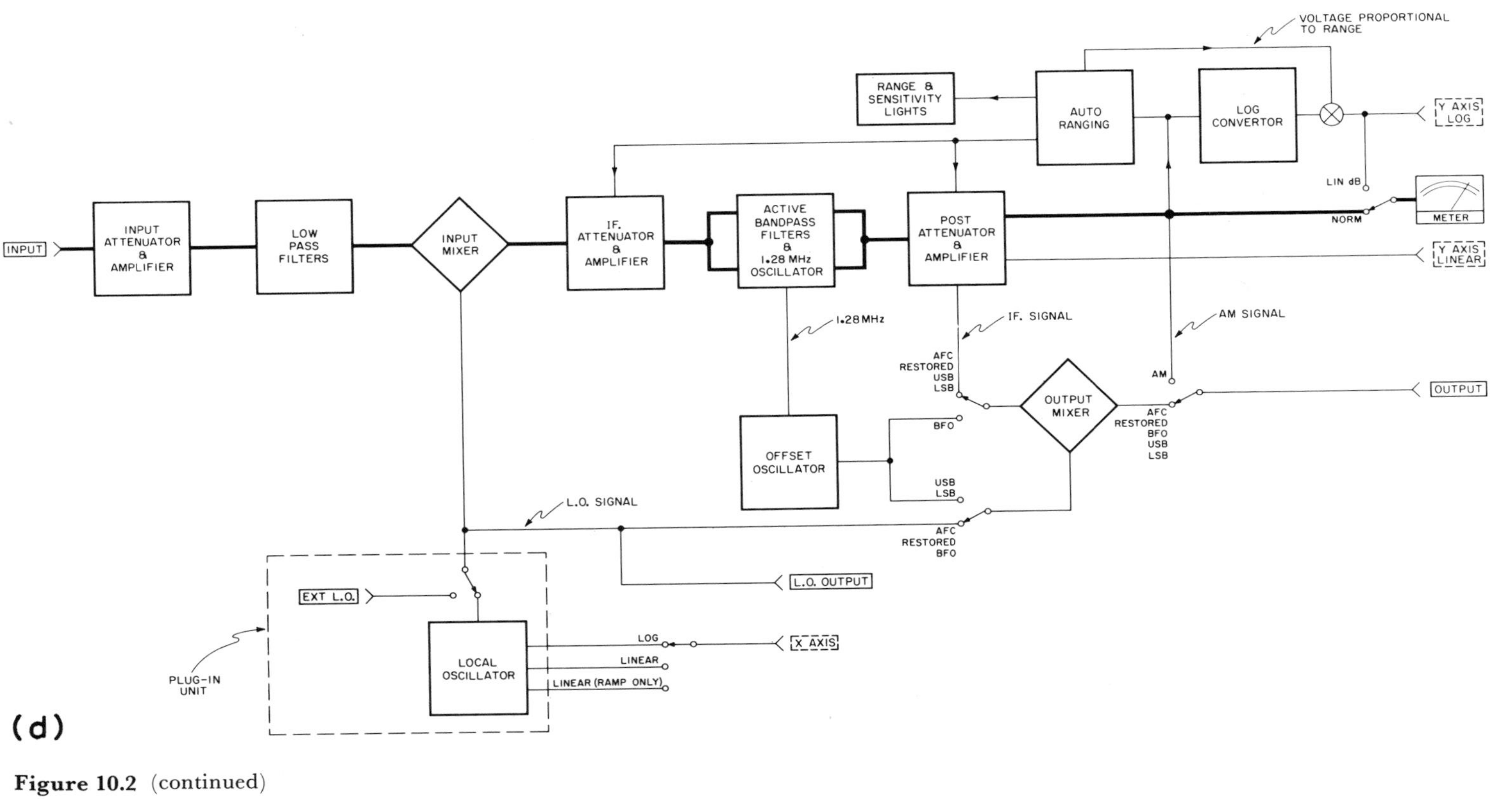

Figure 10.2 (continued)

provide a BFO that is offset by about 2 Hz, and therefore within the bandpass of the analyzer, that is, outside the 0 Hz notch of the filters.

The AFC output is a restored output whose frequency is slightly offset from the input frequency, by the same frequency difference as the difference between the 1.28 MHz and offset oscillators.

When the 10 Hz passband is used, the AFC option uses the offset oscillator to continually tune the analyzer out of the dc notch, which is approximately 2 Hz wide, into the flat region of the selected passband. Therefore, the strategy for tuning a harmonic (when using manual tuning to locate it) is to use the 100 Hz passband in order to manually locate it; then switch to 10 Hz passband and *very slowly* tune it more accurately. Once located, use the AFC to lock in on the selected harmonic for further measurement and testing. The precise frequency of the harmonic can be determined by tuning the analyzer with AFC off, until the harmonic falls in the notch, at which time the meter reading will drop to a low value. Tuning a small amount in either direction should result in a higher meter reading, indicating a local minimum.

The 3593A Sweeping Local Oscillator is simply a voltage controlled oscillator (VCO) that varies over a 620 kHz range from 1.28 MHz to 1.90 MHz or a 62 kHz range from 1280 kHz to 1900 kHz, depending on which is selected. The minimum frequency corresponds to a modulator voltage of 0 volts, and the maximum, to +15.5 V (250 mV/kHz ± 5%). Internal or external sweeping or tuning is possible and digital readout of tuned frequency is present. The *X*-axis for an *X-Y* display in conjunction with the 3095A mainframe *Y*-axis output is also accessible.

Devices of greater or lesser complexity and precision than the 3590A can be obtained. Simpler devices include analyzers that are essentially carefully calibrated tunable filters with very linear characteristics. More complicated devices include analyzers that generate three-dimensional representations of frequency and amplitude *vs.* time, used to produce "voice-print" representations of spoken words, whale songs, bat cries, and bird calls. These are particularly useful in studies of vocal communication and echo-ranging in various species.

The presence of temporal correlation between two time-varying quantities is a minimal criterion used for determining the presence of a causal relation between the two, or for detecting the existence of a third factor that causes both. Electronic methods can be used to digitize voltages, and a digital computer can then generate cross correlograms based on the digitized data.

Variations of this technique which are frequently useful in neurophysiology can be implemented electronically. For example, wave-form averaging, in which analog-to-digital (A/D) conversion is used to digitize the potential sequence following a stimulus or other time-reference event, can be used to extract time-locked events. The principle of wave-form averaging is a simple one: the time-varying sequence of voltage occurring after the event believed to be the source of a consistent voltage variation is sampled by digitizing the voltage at a high rate and storing the resulting series of digital numbers in a memory array. The synchronizing event for each digitizing sweep is an electrical pulse triggered by a stimulus or a discriminable event occurring somewhere in the nervous system. The voltage sequence that is digitized is one that is believed to contain some response to the stimulus or the discriminated neuroelectric event used to trigger the sweep. The signal to be averaged is sampled at regular intervals, starting at the synchronizing pulse or at some constant interval after it; sampling interval is generally controlled by a precision oscillator. This process is repeated, summing the ordered array with another array, in which a running total of all sweeps is accumulated. Any coherent signal (that is, one which is time-locked to the sample-synchronizing event) will tend to grow (that is, the sum will get larger) in direct proportion to the number of summed repetitions. Noise (that is, that portion of the signal which is not time-locked to the synchronizing event) will, on the average, only grow as the square root of the number of trials, as explained in Chapter 3, in the discussion of random noise. Therefore, if we assume no effects of digitizing rate, sampling aperture width, or resolution, the signal-to-noise ratio should be enhanced by the square root of the number of repetitions. Thus, although the signal-to-noise ratio should be improved tenfold with 100 trials, 10,000 trials will be required for a further tenfold increase. This "diminishing returns" effect places a practical limit on the signal enhancement which can be obtained, as do limitations due to resolution, digitizing rate, and aperture width.

Generally, averaging is used to enhance evoked potentials or other stimulus-locked events, using the stimulus to synchronize the averaging sweep, wherein the voltage is digitized at some fixed rate for a fixed length of time. Figure 10.3, reproduced by permission of The MIT Press from Rosenblith (1959), illustrates the use of this technique in averaging a visual evoked potential recorded at the cortex. Discriminated action potentials can be used to synch the sweep (Brown and Tapper, work in progress), in order to study any effects at another recording sight which are elicited by the discriminated spike. The averaged signal need not be a neuroelectric event: It can be any voltage suspected to vary as a function of the synchronizing event, such as the output of a transducer (for example, blood pressure or GSR monitor) or signal processor (such as a spike-frequency meter).

A technique described by Casby et al. (1963) for extracting activity of a restricted conduction group from a whole nerve recording, consists of multiplying the signal recorded upstream after a delay corresponding to conduction time of the desired conduction group, by the signal recorded downstream in the same nerve. Those

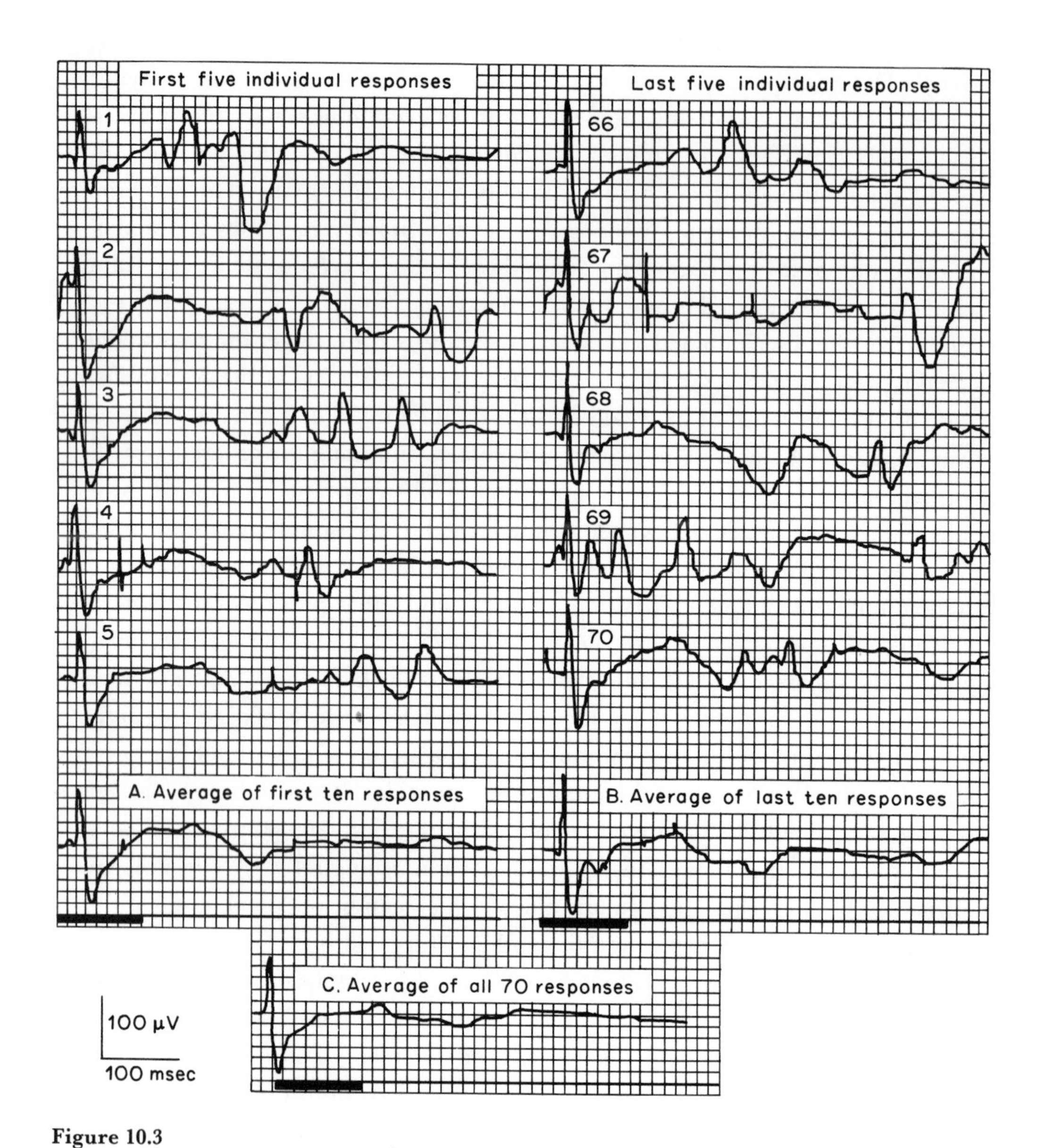

Figure 10.3
Averaging visual evoked potential from cortex. An early averaged evoked potential study. Cortical responses to periodic light flashes recorded from an anesthetized cat. Light pulses were about 100 msec long: The lower traces in A, B, and C show flash duration. Seventy repetitions, at once per five seconds. (From Figure 2.3, in *Processing Neuroelectric Data*, 1959, by Walter A. Rosenblith, ed. Used with permission of MIT Press.)

components of the signal that are traveling at the desired conduction velocity will be enhanced, whereas those that are not will be minimized. This technique is particularly effective if the cross-correlated signal is averaged.

Depending on the magnitude of the calculated delay (distance/conduction velocity), a commercial delay line (delays up to at least 10 msec are available) or a tape loop with adjustable speed or distance between recording and playback heads can be used to generate the delay. Of course, if analog-to-digital (A/D) conversion (that is, generation of a number code for voltages at the input of the converter) is available, in conjunction with a digital computer, the process is greatly simplified.

Since D/A (digital-to-analog) conversion is essential for some A/D techniques, we will describe D/A conversion first. A block diagram of a 4-bit D/A converter is presented in Figure 10.4. The circuit provides voltages proportional to the numerical value of each bit by successive division of a fixed reference V_{ref}, by a factor of 2, and addition of those which are turned on by the analog multiplexer. Resistance values are such that the successive voltages are successively higher powers of 2 multiplied by the bit 1 resistor (R_1). Thus the resistance R_i, where the i-bit voltage is taken off the top of R_i, is expressed as

$$R_i = 2^{(i-1)}R_1, \qquad i > 1. \tag{10.1}$$

The voltage at the top of each resistor is thus

$$V_i = V_{ref}/2^{n-i}, \tag{10.2}$$

where n is the total number of bits.

It is essential, in order for output error to be small relative to the least significant bit (LSB), for each resistor to be accurate to within R_1E/n, where E is the maximum permissible absolute voltage error.

The parallel resistors leading to the multiplexer (MPX) switches must be large in order to prevent shunting the divider. Generally, it is adequate to use resistors equal to $2^n(10\ R_n)$. If they are more than 100 kΩ use a FET input op amp.

The analog MPX consists of MOSFET switches driven by bit drivers. Voltages from the different resistor junctions are summed at the noninverting input of a voltage follower. The off resistances of the MOSFETS should be at least $2^n \times 10$ times as high as the parallel resistors.

The current adder of Figure 10.4b is more commonly used, because it requires fewer resistors. The device consists of four resistors gated through a 4-channel analog multiplexer. The current through R (bit 4) is

$$i_R = V_{ref}/R,$$

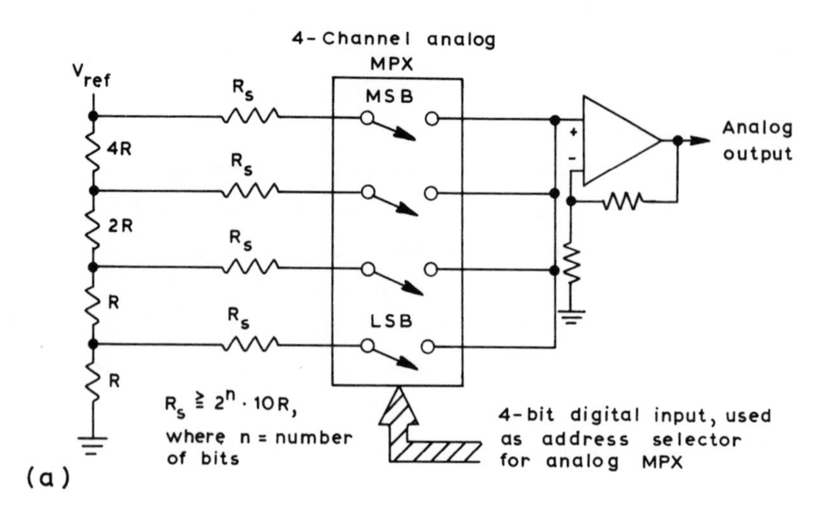

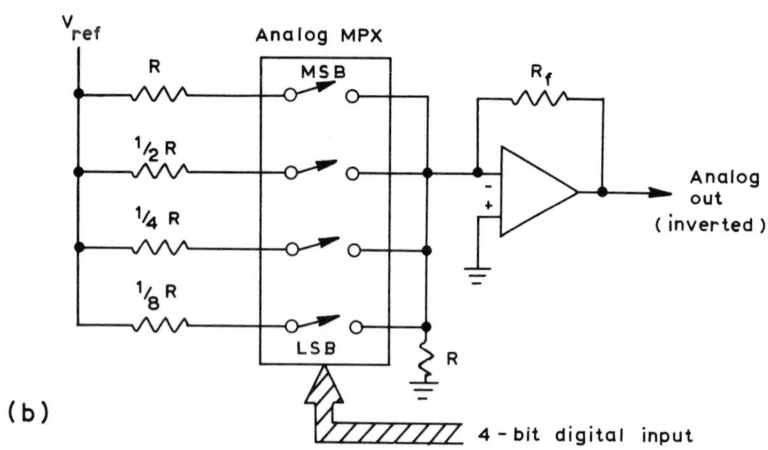

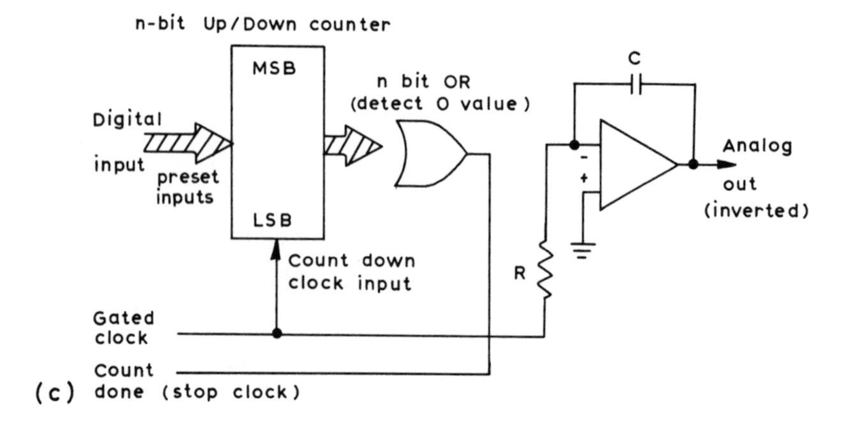

Figure 10.4
D/A conversion: (a) 4-bit D/A converter using voltage addition; (b) current addition; (c) counter technique.

because the negative input of A is a virtual ground. The current through $R/2$ is therefore twice that through R_1; the current through $R/4$ is four times that for R_1; current through $R/8$ is eight times that through R. Therefore, if R is led to the lowest-order MPX channel, $R/2$ to the next, and so forth, the currents will be proportional to the numerical values of their corresponding MPX input bits, the digital input. More generally, for an n-bit D/A converter, assume there are n resistors R_i in the ladder, labeled

$$R_i = R_1 \cdots R_n,$$

where R_n is the largest-valued resistor R_{LSB}. Now assume that

$$R_i = 2^{i-1} R_1,$$

where R_1 is the lowest-valued resistor R_{MSB}, for the most significant bit.

Therefore, since the inverting op amp input is a virtual ground,

$$i_i = a_i V_{\mathrm{ref}}/(2^{i-1} R_1),$$

where i_i is the current through R_i and a_i is the value of the ith bit of the digital input word. If $a_i = 1$, the ith MPX switch is closed. The output V_o is therefore

$$V_o = -\sum_{i=1}^{n} i_i R_f. \tag{10.3}$$

Consider the instructive example where $R_f = R_1/2$:

$$V_o = -\frac{V_{\mathrm{ref}}}{2} \sum_{i=1}^{n} a_i/2^{i-1} = -V_{\mathrm{ref}} \sum_{i=1}^{n} a_i 2^{-i}.$$

A digital input of 0 would produce a zero-volt output, because all a_i would be zero. The largest possible input number $2^n - 1$ would produce an output voltage of

$$V_{\max} = -V_{\mathrm{ref}} \sum_{i=1}^{n} 2^{-i},$$

because all a_i are ones. Converting to terms with identical denominators,

$$V_{\max} = -\frac{V_{\mathrm{ref}}}{2^n} \sum_{i=1}^{n} 2^{n-i}.$$

The sum can be expressed as

$$\sum_{i=1}^{n} 2^{n-i} = \sum_{i=1}^{n} 2^{i-1},$$

which is simply the expression for the largest n-bit number:

$$\sum_{i=1}^{n} 2^{i-1} = 2^n - 1.$$

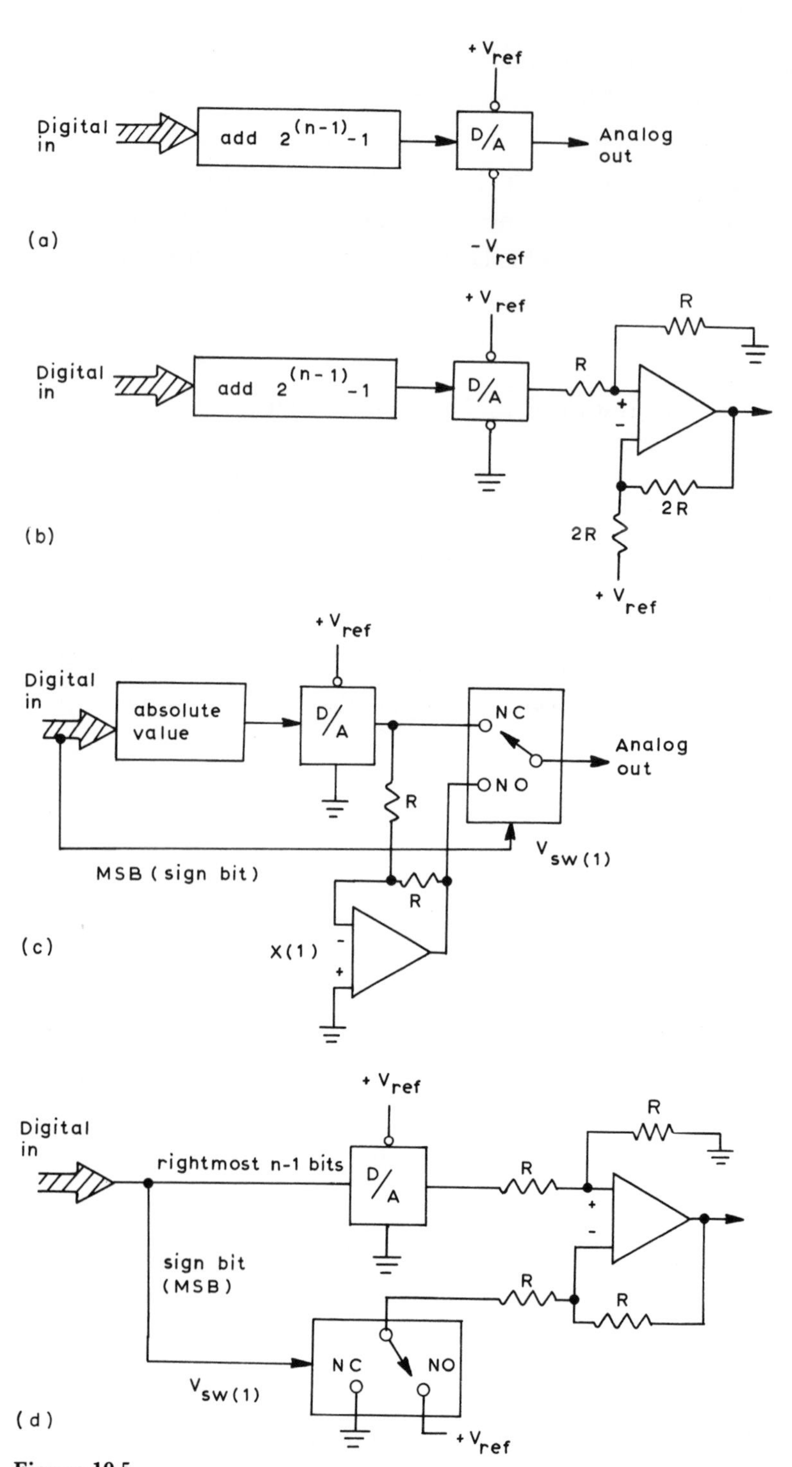

Figure 10.5

Methods for conversion of signed digital numbers into signed analog output: (a, b) transform signed numbers to unsigned numbers, then convert; (c, d) convert magnitude, use analog circuits to restore sign.

Therefore,

$$V_{max} = -V_{ref}\frac{2^{n-1}}{2^n} = V_{ref} - \frac{V_{ref}}{2^n}.$$

We know $V_{LSB} = -2^{-n}V_{ref}$; therefore,

$$V_{max} = -(V_{ref} - V_{LSB}).$$

The sum of Equation 10.3 therefore represents a voltage range of 0 to $-(V_{ref} - V_{LSB})$, the upper limit converging to $-V_{ref}$ as $n \to \infty$.

The problem of resistor selection can be avoided by using one of the many ladder networks which are commercially available. However, the prices of D/A converters in modular form are dropping rapidly, to the point where it is already more economical to buy most types of D/A converter modules than to build one's own. Many are available in DIP packages.

Alternative methods for D/A conversion are possible. For example, the up-down counter method of Figure 10.4c can be used. The counter is loaded with the digital number, and clock pulses are used to increase an analog memory (integrator) while decreasing the counter. The pulses are stopped when the count reaches zero. This device is less convenient than the ladder network in that it is slower, harder to implement, and requires an output analog memory device (see sample-and-hold amplifier, below) to hold the analog output while the next analog value is being generated. We will use the ladder network method wherever D/A conversion is required.

The D/A converters we have examined so far can convert positive numbers or negative numbers, but not both. The solutions of Figure 10.5 can be used to implement signed output. The simplest method, that of Figure 10.5a and b, is to convert the binary code used to represent the number by adding $2^{n-1} - 1$ to the original signed number. The output code is transformed as described in Table 10.1.

Table 10.1
Conversion of input voltages with variable polarity.

Original 2s complement number, represented as unsigned binary		Output after addition (modulo 2^{n-1}) of $2^{n-1} - 1$, represented as unsigned binary
positive range:	1 to $2^{n-2} - 1$	2^{n-1} to $2^n - 2$ ($2^n - 1$ illegal)
zero:	0	$2^{n-1} - 1$
negative range:	$2^{n-1} + 1$ to $2^n - 1$	0 to $2^{n-1} - 2$

This code and other "offset binary" codes similar to it are often used for D/A and A/D converters: 0 represents the most negative value, $2^{n-2} - 1 = 0$ V, and $2^n - 2$ represents the most positive value. This is particularly convenient, in that digital processors can handle the numbers as absolute (unsigned) numbers within an arbitrary voltage range that centers around 0 V. It is inconvenient in that processors that use signed numbers must convert A/D numbers in offset binary to signed equivalents and signed numbers to offset binary D/A equivalents. Generally, the code corresponding to the processor system is selected. In Figure 10.5a, the number is converted over the range $-V_{ref}$ to $+V_{ref}$. In Figure 10.5b, it is converted over the range from 0 to $-V_{ref}$, doubled, and $+V_{ref}$ is subtracted.

Another method for handling signed digital numbers is that of Figure 10.5c, where the digital number is converted to an absolute value and D/A converted to a positive voltage. This is inverted and the inverted or noninverted voltage is gated to the output by an analog switch driven by the sign bit. This technique, although it requires additional logic, is relatively fast, and it can be quite accurate.

The method of Figure 10.5d consists of converting the $n - 1$ rightmost bits as though they were a positive number and shifting by a level equal to $-V_{ref}$ if the sign bit is on. This is equivalent to the method of Figure 10.5a, except the shift is accomplished by the analog circuit rather than by the digital processor generating the digital number. The technique is rarely used because it is difficult to obtain a high degree of accuracy.

An A/D conversion is accomplished by any of a number of different techniques, depending on the degree of precision and the conversion speed desired. One of the simplest methods is that of Figure 10.6, where the input voltage modulates a voltage-to-frequency converter (FM modulator). Resolution is determined by the digitizing interval and frequency:

$$r = 1/IF \tag{10.4}$$

where r = resolution (reciprocal of number of possible values), I = counting interval, and F = output frequency modulation range. Thus, if the modulator

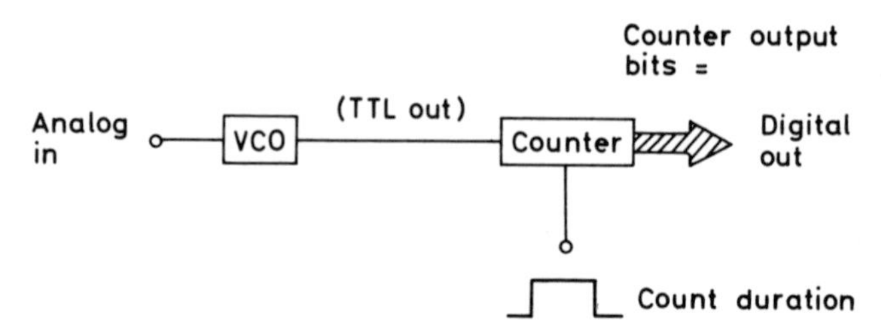

Figure 10.6
A/D conversion technique using voltage-controlled oscillator.

produces an output range of 10 MHz $\pm$ 5 MHz for an input voltage of $\pm$10 V and the counter is read and reset every 1 msec, the count must be 10,000 + 5000 or

$$r = 1/(10^{-3}\ \text{sec} \times 10^{7}\ \text{sec}^{-1}) = 10^{-4}.$$

The resolution can be expressed as a voltage V_r:

$$V_r = r(V_{max}^{+} - V_{max}^{-}).$$

Thus for the above example $V_r = 20/10^4 = 2 \times 10^{-3}$, or 2 mV. Actually, this is a means of expressing the "digitizing error," $\pm\frac{1}{2}$ the resolution, and we can express all such digital values as $\pm$ this value. For binary outputs this is $\pm\frac{1}{2}$ LSB.

Such a device would be more than adequate for a digital voltmeter (DVM). In fact for most such applications much less temporal resolution is still acceptable. There are situations, however, where faster conversion with higher precision is required. For such applications one of the techniques illustrated in Figure 10.7 is necessary. These all convert positive voltages, with 0 V = 0, $V_{max} = 2^n - 1$, where there are n bits. The serial return-to-zero (RZ) converter consists of a clock-driven counter that counts up from zero until the D/A output of a converter operating on the counter output exceeds V_i. The clock is then stopped, and the digital output is greater than V_i and less than V_i + 1 LSB. By adjusting input offset to $\frac{1}{2}$ LSB, output is accurate to $\pm\frac{1}{2}$ LSB. The number of steps (clock cycles) required is the count; hence maximum conversion time for V_{max} is $2^n - 1$ times the clock frequency. For 10 bits and a 10 MHz clock this could be as great as 0.1023 msec, providing a maximum digitizing rate of slightly less than 10 kHz (see, however, the discussion on sample-and-hold amplifiers, below, for an examination of errors due to slew rate in input signals).

The serial nonreturn-to-zero (NRZ) converter (Figure 10.7b) utilizes an up-down counter to "track" the voltage from one state to the next. If the "tracking rate" (expressed as $\Delta V/\Delta t$) is greater than the slew rate of the input voltage, the counter will always be within 1 LSB of the correct value and a CONVERT COMMAND could be used to strobe the counter output into the digital processor at any time.

This means that *sampling rate* can be as high as 10 MHz, for a single input. The *tracking rate* of this device (the most rapid change of voltage over time that it can follow) is simply

$$\left(\frac{\Delta V}{\Delta t}\right)_{max} = \frac{V_{LSB}}{1\ \text{clock period}} = \frac{V_{max}/2^n}{0.1\ \text{msec}}$$

$$= \frac{(10\ \text{V}/1024)}{10^{-7}} \cong 10^5\ \text{V/sec},$$

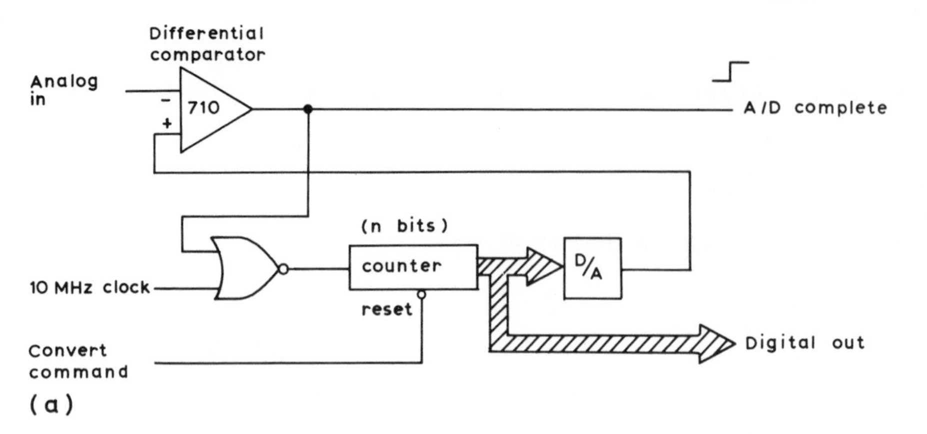

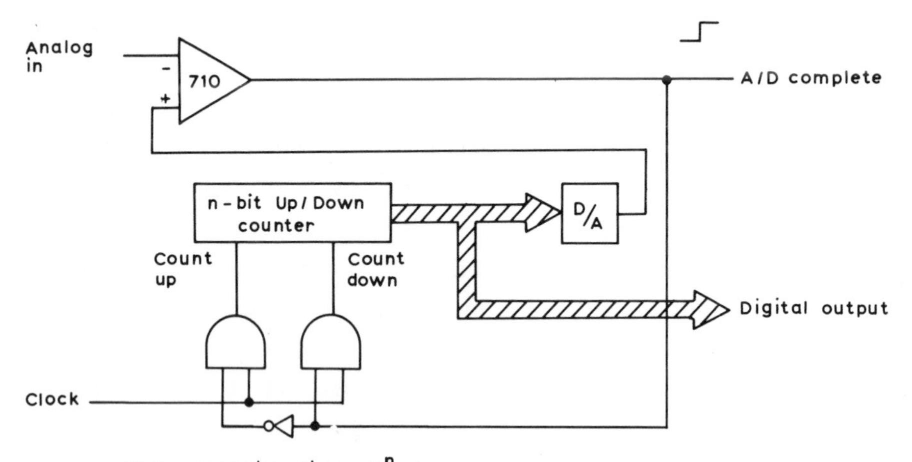

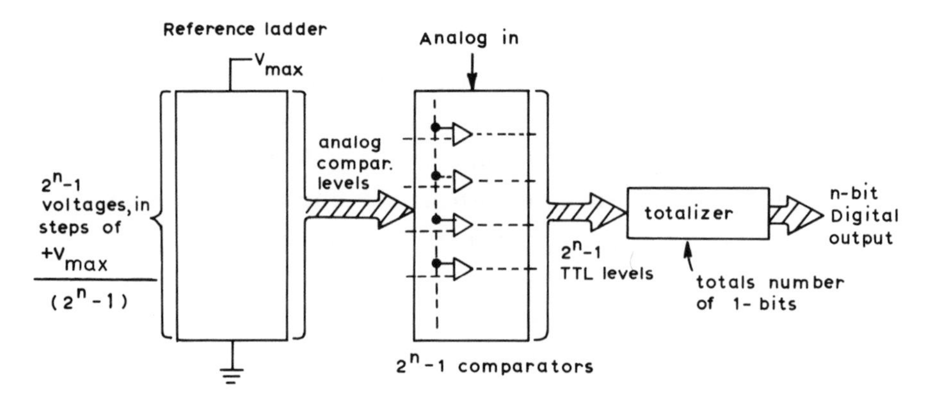

Figure 10.7
A/D conversion methods using comparators: (a) serial return-to-zero (RZ); (b) serial nonreturn-to-zero (NRZ); (c) simultaneous conversion; (d) successive approximation method.

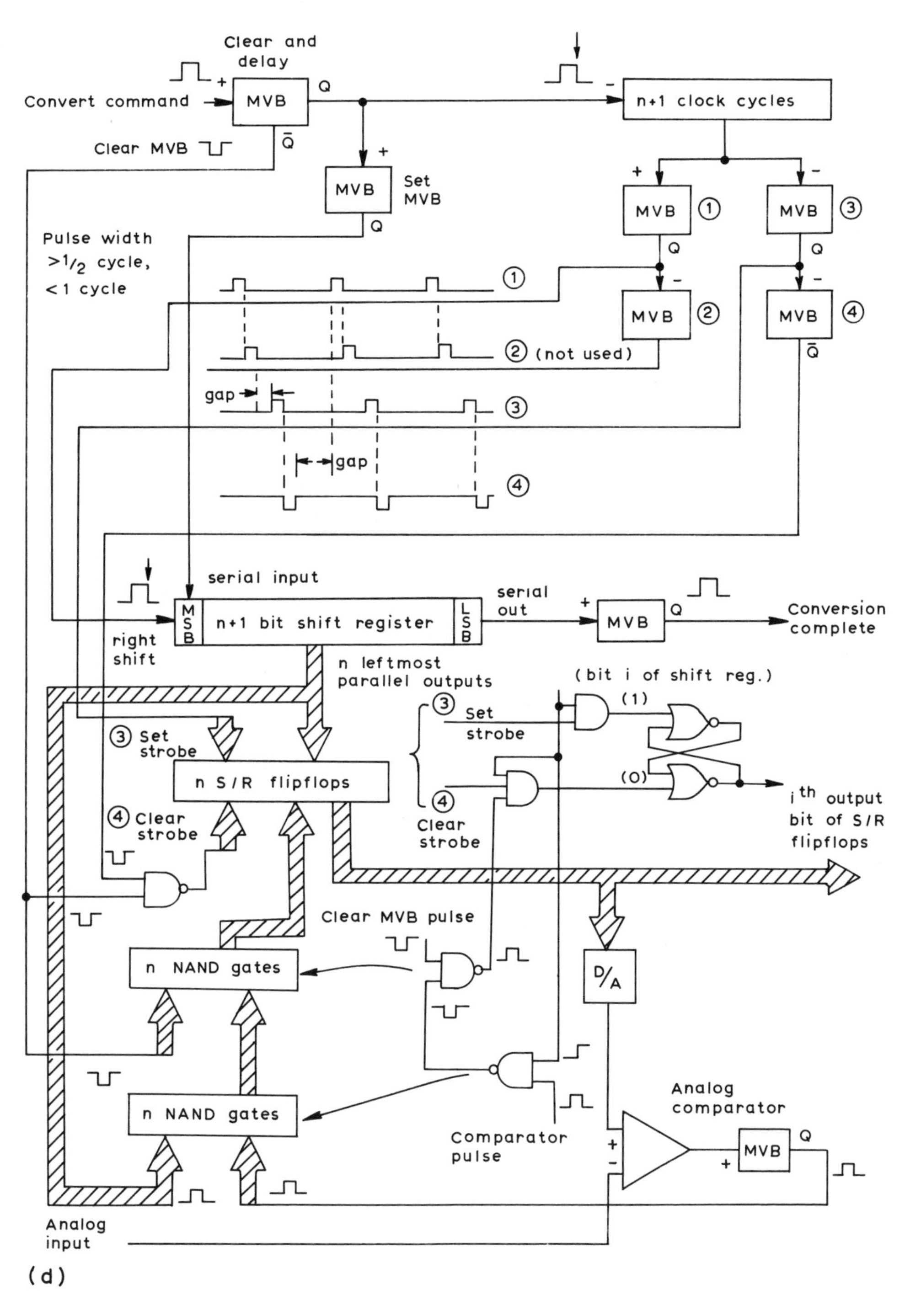

Figure 10.7 (continued)

for a V_{max} of 10 V, 10 MHz clock rate, and 10-bit accuracy. This would be adequate to track a full-scale signal up to frequencies of about 1.5 kHz, because

$$(dV/dt)_{max} = (dV_{max}(\sin \omega t)/dt)_{max} = (V_{max}\omega \cos \omega t)_{max}$$
$$= 2\pi f V_{max},$$

and therefore,

$$f_{max} = \frac{(\Delta V/\Delta t)_{max}}{2\pi V_{max}} = \frac{10^5 \text{ V/sec}}{2\pi(10 \text{ V})} \cong 1.5 \text{ kHz}.$$

Such an A/D converter is said to be *slew rate limited*, because the highest frequency it can resolve is determined by its tracking rate. Theoretically, a bandpass signal can be resolved if the sampling rate is at least double the highest frequency component in the input signal. The tracking speed can be increased by decreasing n. A twofold frequency gain is accrued for each sacrificed bit. Of course, if the device is used to digitize signals from multiple multiplexer channels it would have to count up or down from one voltage to another (presumably unrelated) voltage. In that case, digitizing time is not 0.1 μsec but can be as much as for the RZ serial A/D converter of Figure 10.7a: 0.1 msec. This will still allow digitizing at rates approaching 10 kHz (see, however, the note on effect of input signal's slew rate in the section on sample-and-hold amplifiers).

The simultaneous A/D converter of Figure 10.7c is theoretically the fastest device illustrated; it is also the least practical, because it requires $2^n - 1$ comparators, a very precise resistor divider network to provide comparison voltages, and extensive encoding gates at the output. Each comparator detects the presence or absence of $V_i > V_j$, where

$$V_j = j(V_{max}/2^n),$$

if i = input voltage and j = comparator number. The encoding gates essentially indicate how many comparators are on, producing the digital output. The conversion time is limited by the settling times of the comparators and the switching speed of the gates.

Probably the most popular A/D design is the successive approximation converter, Figure 10.7d. The device uses a simple algorithm:

1. $i = 1$. Set all n bits to 0.
2. Set bit i (numbering bits from left to right, 1 to n).
3. Is the corresponding D/A voltage generated by all n bits larger than the analog input voltage? If so, reset bit i to 0. If not, leave the bit set to 1. In either case D/A voltage is less than analog input at the end of this step.

4. Is i equal to n? If so, conversion is done. If not, increment i and go to step 2 above.

Now consider the operation of the circuit of Figure 10.7d in detail. The CONVERT COMMAND triggers a MVB, which clears the output (*RS* flipflop) bits; at the end of the clear pulse, a clock circuit is enabled, to produce $n + 1$ square-wave clock cycles. The clock cycles are broken up into four sets of successive pulses (1, 2, 3, 4) for strobing purposes. Note that there is no gap between 1 and 2 or 3 and 4, but there are gaps between 2 and 3, and 4 and 1. Pulse 1 is used to right-shift a 1 bit (SET MVB) into the MSB of a right-shift register of $n + 1$ bits. Before the next shift pulse the SET MVB goes to 0; therefore, a single 1 bit will be shifted through the register, appearing at the LSB on the last shift. When it appears in the LSB, the conversion will be complete, and a CONVERSION COMPLETE pulse is generated.

After each shift, pulse 3 is used to strobe the ith bit into the ith *RS* flipflop. The outputs of the *RS* register bits drive a D/A converter, the output of which is compared with the analog input. If the D/A output exceeds the analog input a MVB is triggered to fire long enough for coincidence with pulse 4 in order to reset the ith bit of the *RS* flipflop register. There is a time gap between the reset pulse and the next set pulse to allow settling.

The successive-approximation converter is a highly flexible and accurate device. Simple switching allows selection of n for trade-off of conversion time versus resolution.

Assembly of A/D converters from discrete components or even op amps is generally not practical. A large number of manufacturers supply a wide variety of A/D and D/A modules that are quite reliable. Some are in standard IC packages, particularly D/A converters, many of which come as DIPs. Many manufacturers provide modular systems constructed of standard modules selected according to the buyer's specifications. These are inexpensive compared to the discrete component devices or preassembled converters available from many other suppliers.

For many neurophysiological applications simple A/D conversion is not enough in itself. For example, with a successive approximation converter the rate of change of the analog input need not be very high for considerable errors in digitization to occur. This can occur even for small signals and quite low frequencies as a consequence of the fact that the signal is changing during the conversion process. In order to "freeze" the analog voltage during conversion, an analog memory or "sample-and-hold amplifier" is used to sample the analog voltage for a very short time and store it as a fixed value long enough for conversion. A sample-and-hold amplifier is diagrammed in Figure 10.8a. Most sample-and-hold devices are some-

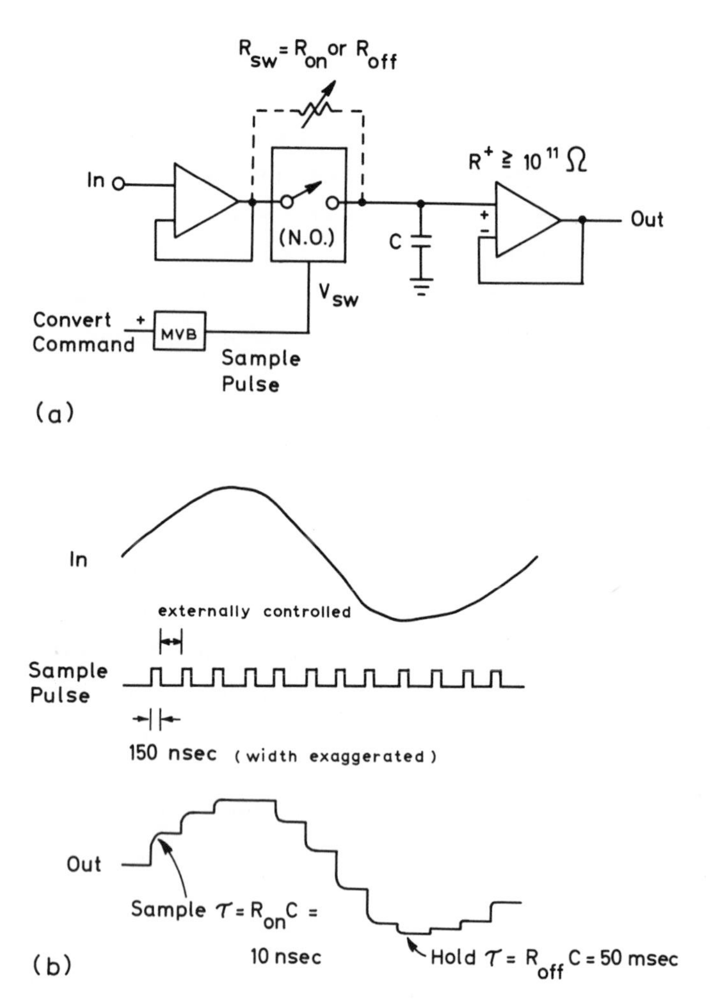

Figure 10.8
Sample-and-hold amplifier; (a) simplified schematic; (b) signal wave forms.

what more complicated than this in order to compensate for switching spikes and "droop" of the stored voltage. The most elementary device, that of Figure 10.8a, consists of an input follower amplifier used to charge a capacitor during the time it is connected to the capacitor by the analog switch, and an output follower amplifier that monitors the voltage across the capacitor. The output amplifier is assumed to have a higher input impedance than the switch "OFF" impedance for simplicity; the time constant for charging is therefore $R_{on}C$, and the time constant for leakage through the switch is $R_{off}C$. With a good switch these time constants can have a ratio of 10^7 or more. The capacitor is charged to the value of the input signal during the brief (say, 150 nsec) sample command, and the voltage is held by the capacitor. This permits the A/D converter to digitize a *fixed* voltage, eliminating incorrect values; the input signal would have to have a very high slope to introduce any significant error.

Unfortunately such a technique exaggerates the disadvantage of discontinuous sampling: the tendency to miss brief events occurring between samples. This can be at least partially alleviated by integrating the input between samples and resetting the integrator briefly after each sample. Such a device is illustrated in Figure 10.9.

The simplest version, Figure 10.9a, consists of an RC network with a long time constant (1 msec, in this example), which is unaffected by the OFF resistance of the analog switch used to discharge the capacitor. The RESET command is typically issued at the completion of a sample-and-hold (or, if no sample-and-hold is used, at the end of an A/D conversion). The capacitor essentially integrates the input voltage if the period between resets is kept short (say, one-twentieth of the time constant). This means that the output is attenuated. Since the capacitor should be buffered through an amplifier in any case, an amplifier with appropriate gain can be used as the output buffer.

If greater linearity is required, the op amp integrator of Figure 10.9b can be used; of course the op amp must be capable of handling the fast signals with low noise levels. Whatever integration method is used, the output is not, strictly speaking, the average of the input although it is proportional to the average if the integrating time is always of the same duration. If the integrating time is variable, the digital processor that controls the A/D converter must perform the appropriate scaling, or the scheme of Figure 10.9c can be used. In this configuration, the integrated voltage is divided by another voltage, which is proportional to the integration time. The divisor voltage is obtained by integrating a constant voltage over the same period as the analog voltage input integration. For this reason, both integrators are reset and enabled simultaneously. The analog divider must have adequate frequency response and low enough noise level; most cheap multiplier/dividers can handle audio frequencies; to approach 1 MHz, larger, more expensive modules must be used.

Figure 10.10a diagrams a multichannel A/D converter with sample and hold. The configuration was provided by Analog Devices, Inc. The device automatically samples the selected channel and converts the analog voltage at the appropriate input to a digital number of 8, 10, or 12 bits, depending on the specific analog to digital converter used. An INITIATE SEQUENCE COMMAND from the digital controller initiates the conversion. With the control logic used here, the multiplexer address should not be changed during the conversion sequence, and

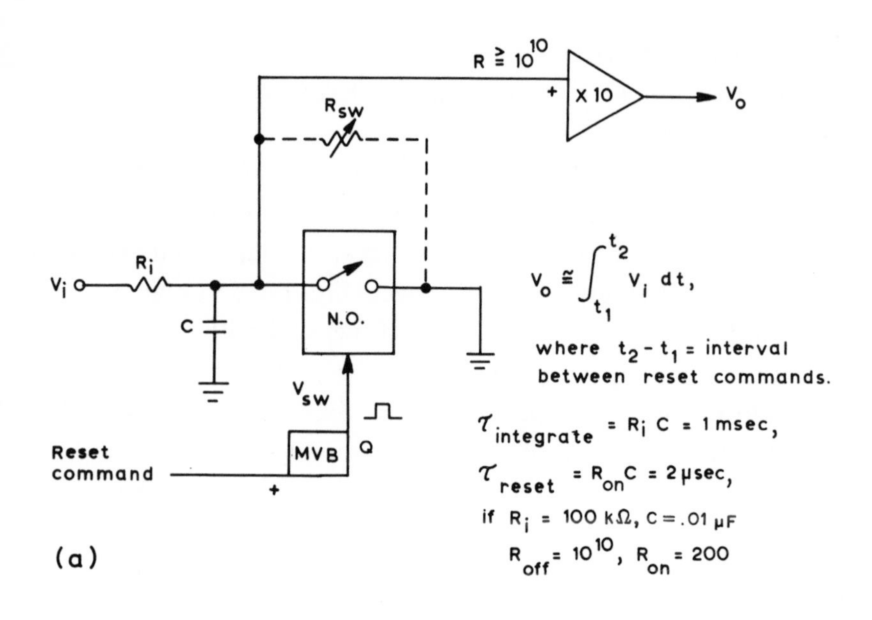

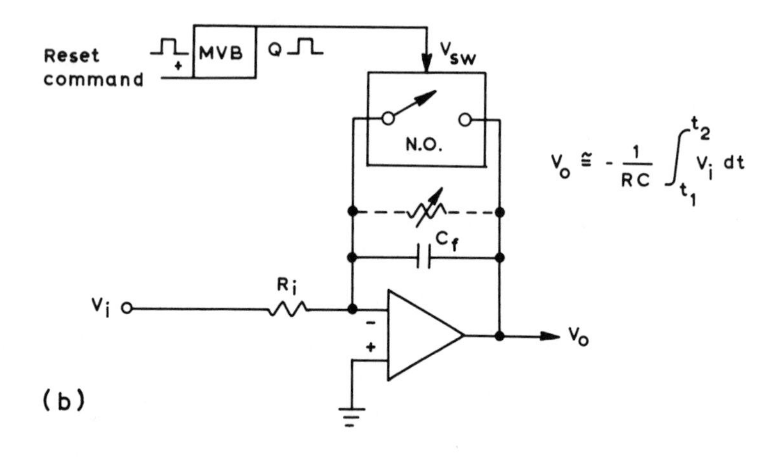

Figure 10.9
Integrating inputs for A/D conversion: (a) RC integrator; (b) op amp integrator; (c) true-average integrator.

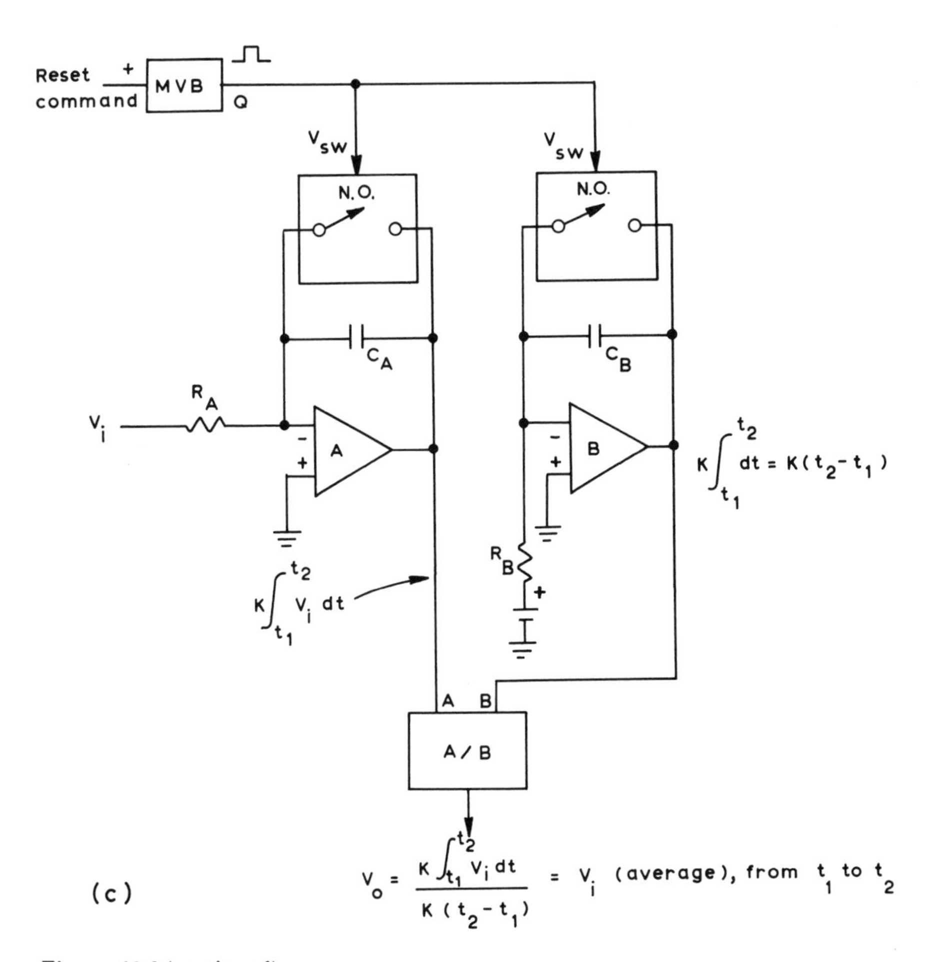

Figure 10.9 (continued)

the INITIATE CONVERSION COMMAND should not be issued earlier than 2 μsec after a multiplexer address change takes place, because the multiplexer takes 2 μsec. (worst case) to settle. The Analog Devices MPX-8A multiplexer is used for this design (Figure 10.10b and c).

The control logic (Figure 10.10g) consists of a string of nonretriggerable MVBs, which initiate the sample-and-hold and A/D conversion and which transmit a pulse back to the computer (CONVERSION DONE) when the conversion is done. The first MVB (MVB1) has a pulse width equal to, or greater than, the maximum sequence time, which is partly dependent on the conversion time (dependent on number of bits). The leading edge of this pulse triggers the SAMPLE TIME MVB (MVB2), which generates the S/H COMMAND. While this pulse is high, for 5.1 μsec, the SHA IA (Figure 10.10d and e) module is in the "sample" mode: 5.0 μsec are required for charging the internal capacitor to within 0.01%

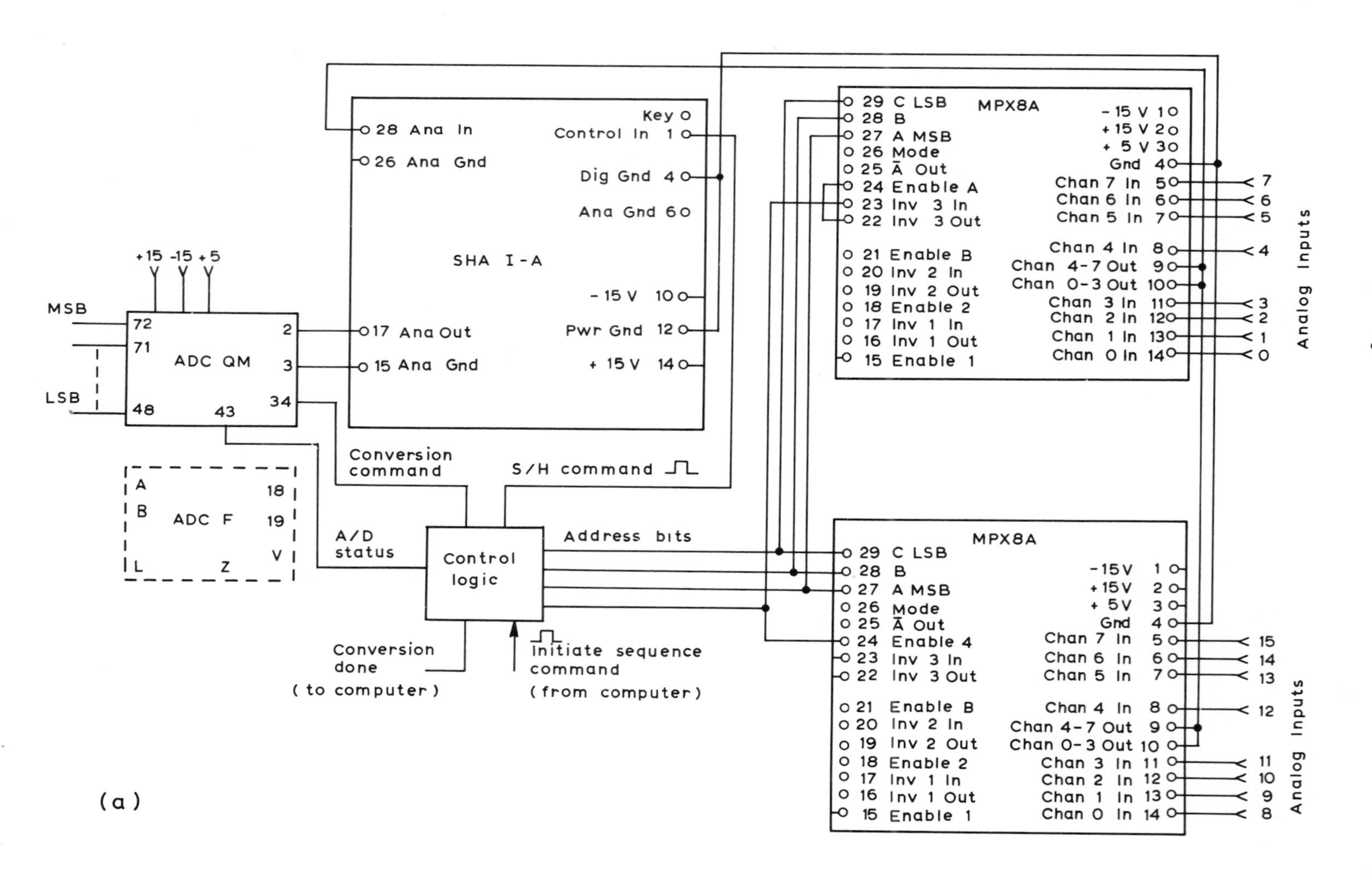

MSB
LSB
+15 -15 +5
ADC QM
72
71
48
43
2
3
34
ADC F
A
B
L
Z
18
19
V
SHA I-A
28 Ana In
26 Ana Gnd
17 Ana Out
15 Ana Gnd
Key 0
Control In 1
Dig Gnd 4
Ana Gnd 6
- 15 V 10
Pwr Gnd 12
+ 15 V 14
Conversion command
S/H command
A/D status
Control logic
Address bits
Conversion done (to computer)
Initiate sequence command (from computer)
MPX8A
29 C LSB
28 B
27 A MSB
26 Mode
25 Ā Out
24 Enable A
23 Inv 3 In
22 Inv 3 Out
21 Enable B
20 Inv 2 In
19 Inv 2 Out
18 Enable 2
17 Inv 1 In
16 Inv 1 Out
15 Enable 1
- 15 V 1
+ 15 V 2
+ 5 V 3
Gnd 4
Chan 7 In 5
Chan 6 In 6
Chan 5 In 7
Chan 4 In 8
Chan 4-7 Out 9
Chan 0-3 Out 10
Chan 3 In 11
Chan 2 In 12
Chan 1 In 13
Chan 0 In 14
7
6
5
4
3
2
1
0
Analog Inputs
MPX8A
29 C LSB
28 B
27 A MSB
26 Mode
25 Ā Out
24 Enable 4
23 Inv 3 In
22 Inv 3 Out
21 Enable B
20 Inv 2 In
19 Inv 2 Out
18 Enable 2
17 Inv 1 In
16 Inv 1 Out
15 Enable 1
-15V 1
+15V 2
+ 5V 3
Gnd 4
Chan 7 In 5
Chan 6 In 6
Chan 5 In 7
Chan 4 In 8
Chan 4-7 Out 9
Chan 0-3 Out 10
Chan 3 In 11
Chan 2 In 12
Chan 1 In 13
Chan 0 In 14
15
14
13
12
11
10
9
8
Analog Inputs

(a)

Figure 10.10
16-channel A/D converter with sample-and-hold: (a) block diagram (courtesy of Analog Devices, Inc.). (b and c) Analog Devices MPX8A Analog multiplexer (from *Model MPX-8A Multiplexer*, 1970, (d and e) Analog Devices SHA-IA sample and hold amplifier (from *SHA-IA Sample and Hold Module, 1971*, by Analog Devices, Inc. Used with permission of Analog Devices, Inc.). (f) Analog Devices ADC QM A/D converter (from *Model ADC-QM Analog-to-Digital Converters*, 1970, by Analog Devices, Inc. Used with permission of Analog Devices, Inc.). (g) suggested control logic.

	Pulse Durations (μsec)				
Number of bits	MVB1	MVB2	MVB3	MVB4	A/D conversion time
8	23.8	5.1	0.4	0.2	18
10	27.8	5.1	0.4	0.2	22
12	30.8	5.1	0.4	0.2	25

MODEL	MPX-8A
CHANNELS	8 Single-ended, or 4 Differential (programmable by user)
VOLTAGE RANGE	
Normal Operating	−10V to +10V
Overvoltage Protection	−15V to +15V
CROSSTALK	$\lessapprox$ −80dB
TRANSFER ACCURACY	Determined by following Amplifier. Values to $<$0.01% readily attainable
INPUT IMPEDANCE	Determined by following Amplifier. Values to 10^{10} ohms readily attainable
COMMON MODE REJECTION	Determined by following Amplifier. Values to 120dB available
ANALOG SWITCHES	MOSFET Transistors
SWITCH CHARACTERISTICS (EACH CHANNEL)	
ON Resistance	1000 ohms
OFF Resistance	1000 megohms, min
Input Capacitance	10pF
Leakage Capacitance (OFF Channels)	$<$3pF
ON Input Leakage Current	
@ +25°C	10nA, max
@ +70°C	100nA, max
Settling Time to 0.01%	
−10V to +10V	$<$400ns
+10V to −10V	$<2\mu s$
THROUGHPUT RATE	Rates to 500kHz. Practical high limit is determined by accessory equipment, as well as nature of signals
FAULT PROTECTION	1. Binary address selection makes it impossible to select more than one channel at a time 2. MOSFET switches return to "OFF" state whenever power is lost or removed
ADDRESS CONTROL	
Code	Binary
Logic	TTL/DTL Compatible
"1"	E $>$ +2.4V @ +40μA, or Open Circuit
"0"	E $<$ +0.8V @ −1.6mA
Channel Address	3-bit Binary Code turns on one of 8 Switches
Mode Control	Jumper at module terminals determines whether module operates as 8-channel single-ended, or 4-channel differential switch
Address Extender (4 input AND gate)	All Inputs at Logic "1" enables module addressing. Provides for system expansion to 64 channels, either single-ended or differential
Logic Inverters (3, uncommitted)	Provide all logic elements required for full expansion of system
Module Disable	A logic "0" at any input of extender gate opens all switches in module
POWER	+15V ±1V @ 6.2mA −15V −1V + 0 @ 4mA +5V ±10% @ 102mA
TEMPERATURE	
Operating	0°C to +70°C
Storage	−65°C to +150°C
SIZE	2″ × 2″ × 0.4″ Module

PIN DESIGNATION

TOP VIEW
ACTUAL LABEL

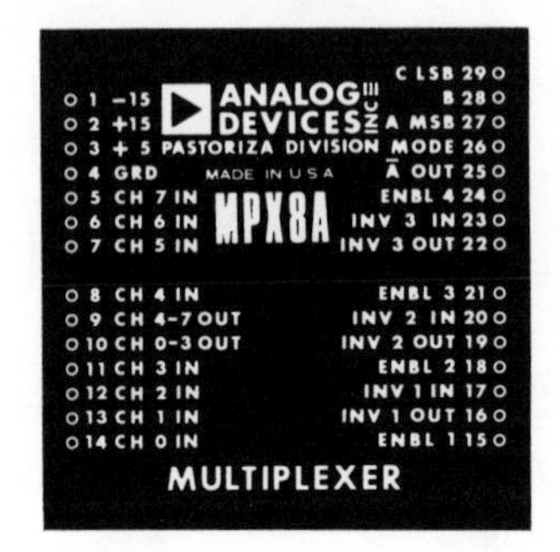

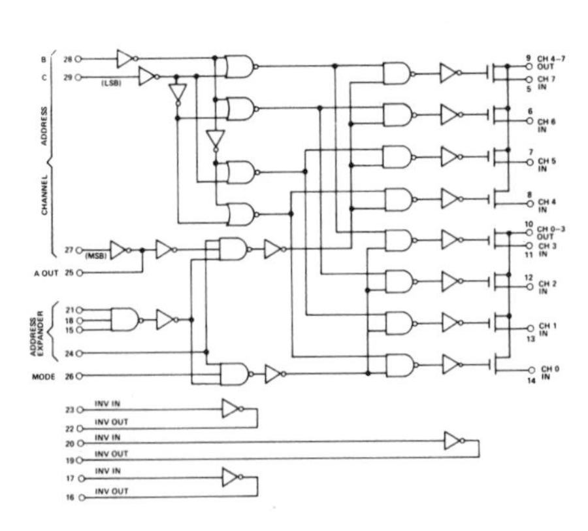

LOGIC FLOW DIAGRAM – MPX-8A

(b)

Figure 10.10 (continued)

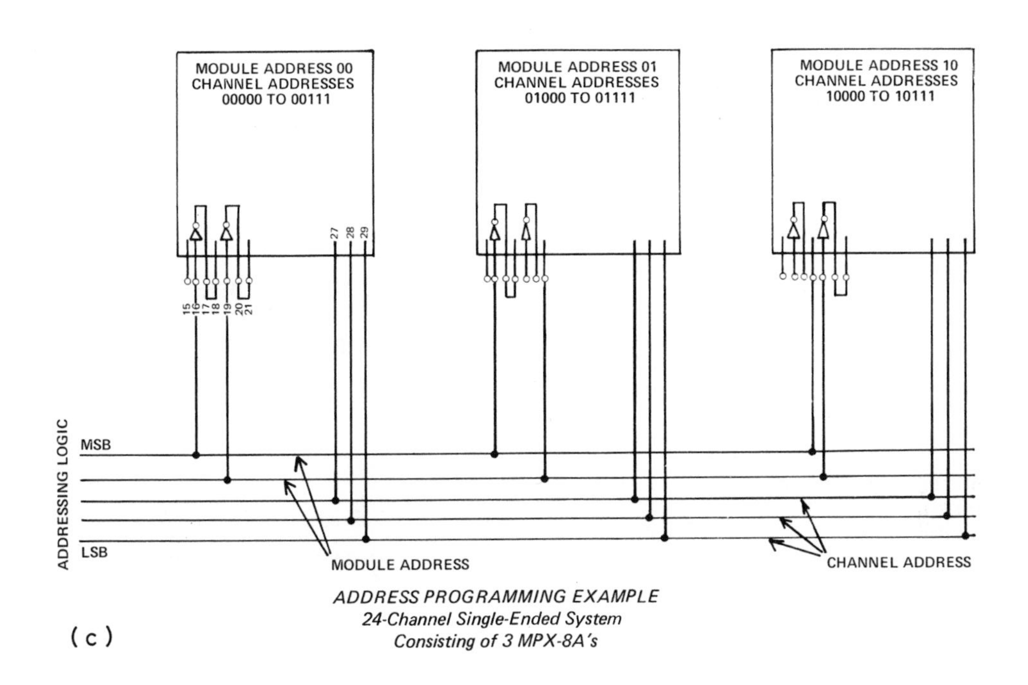

ADDRESS PROGRAMMING EXAMPLE
24-Channel Single-Ended System
Consisting of 3 MPX-8A's

(c)

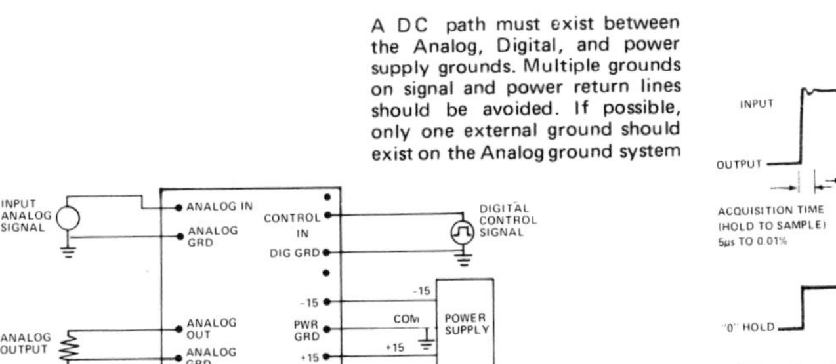

Fig. 1 SHA IA Connections and Grounding

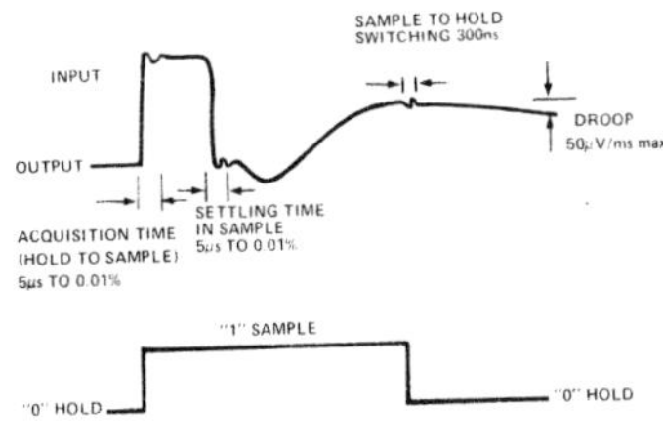

Fig. 2 Illustration of Dynamic Specifications (not to scale)

(d)

Figure 10.10 (continued)

SHA IA

SPECIFICATIONS (typical @ +25°C and nominal supply voltages, unless otherwise noted)

ACCURACY	
Gain	+1
Gain Error	+0.0,-0.05% max
Total Throughput Non Linearity (Includes Gain and Sample to Hold Offset Non Linearities)	2mV max over ±10V input range 1mV max over 0 to +10V or 0 to -10V input range
FREQUENCY RESPONSE IN SAMPLE MODE	
Small Signal-3dB	500kHz min
Slew Rate	4V/μs
Settling Time to 0.01% for 20 Volt Input Step	5μs max
SAMPLE TO HOLD SWITCHING	
Aperture Delay Time	40ns max
Jitter (Cycle to Cycle Variance in Delay)	5ns peak
Switching Transient Settling Time (to ±1mV)	300ns
HOLDING CHARACTERISTICS	
Droop Rate	50μV/ms max
Droop Rate vs. Temp.	X2/10°C
Feedthrough (10kHz, 20V p-p input)	0.005% max
HOLD TO SAMPLE SWITCHING	
Acquisition Time to 0.01% of Full Scale	5μs max
INPUT CHARACTERISTICS	
Input Resistance	10^{12} ohms
Input Capacitance	5pF max
Input Bias Current	10nA max, 1nA typ
Initial Input Offset	1mV max
Offset vs. Supply	100μV/%
Offset vs. Temp.	25μV/°C max
Input Voltage, Max. Safe	±15V
Input Voltage, Normal Operation	±10V
OUTPUT CHARACTERISTICS	
Output Voltage, Current	±10V min at ±20mA min
Maximum Load Capacitance at Output	500pF
DIGITAL CONTROL	
Logic Levels (DTL/TTL Comp.)	
("1") Sample	+2V to +5.5V at 40nA
("0") Hold	-0.5V to +0.8V at 20μA
POWER REQUIREMENTS	±15VDC at +10mA,-15mA (±3% tolerance on voltage)
TEMPERATURE RANGE	
Rated Accuracy	0°C to +70°C
Storage	-55°C to +85°C

OUTLINE DIMENSIONS AND PIN CONNECTIONS

(In Inches)

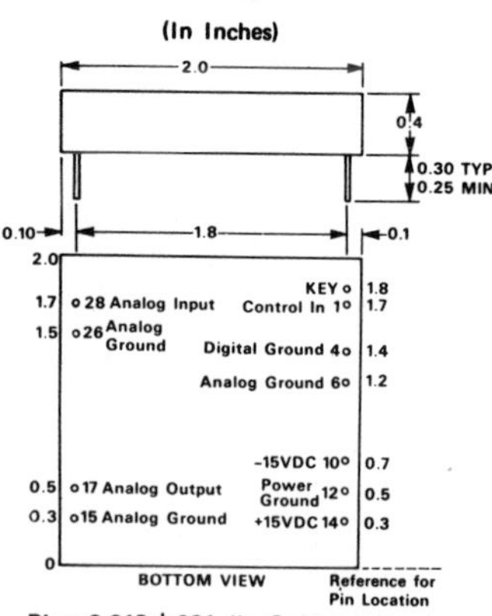

Pins: 0.019 ±.001 dia, Gold plated rodar, per MIL-G-45204 Class 1, type 2

Markings appear on top surface of module, and are shown here on bottom view for reference only.

(e)

Figure 10.10 (continued)

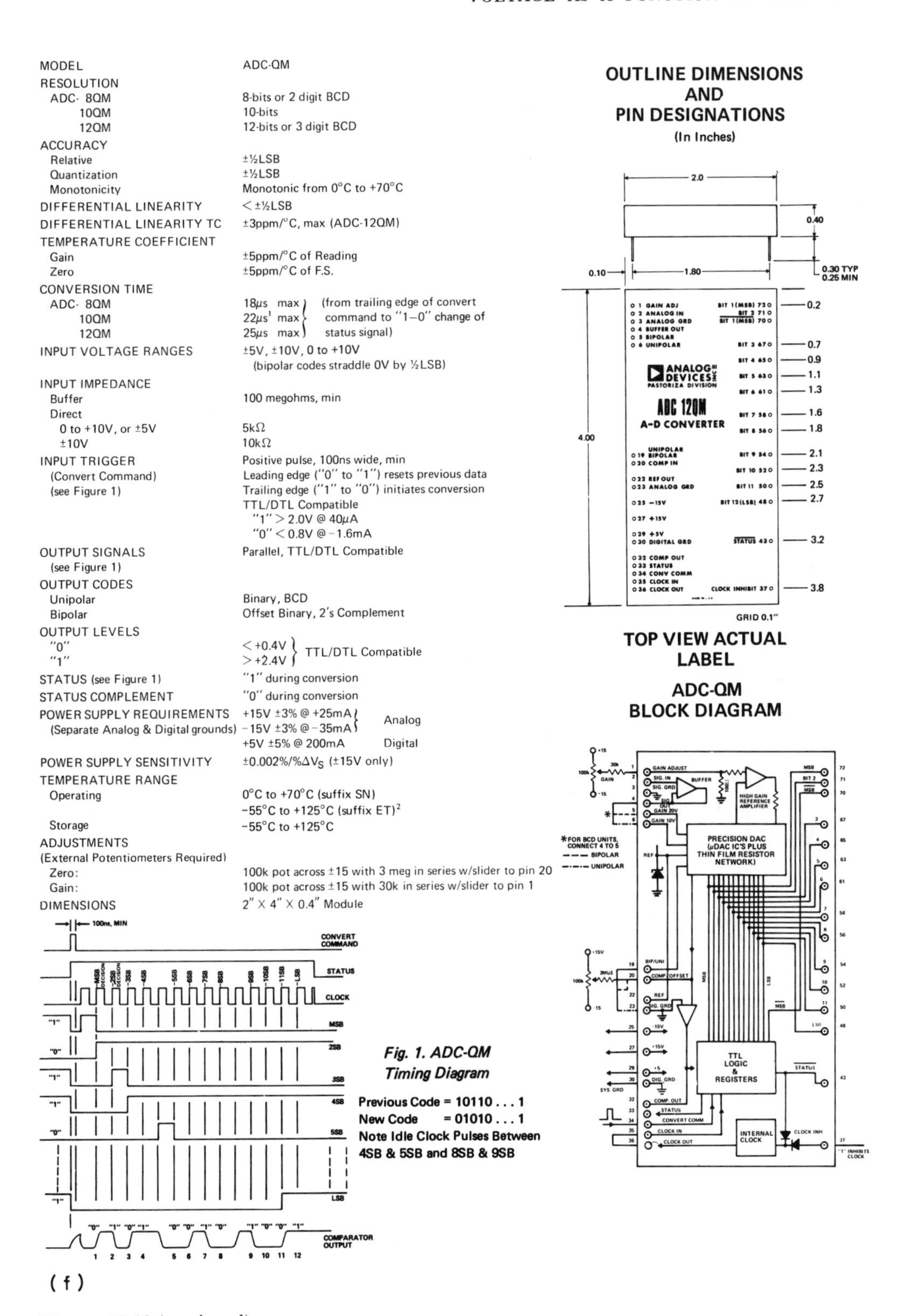

MODEL	ADC-QM
RESOLUTION	
ADC- 8QM	8-bits or 2 digit BCD
10QM	10-bits
12QM	12-bits or 3 digit BCD
ACCURACY	
Relative	±½LSB
Quantization	±½LSB
Monotonicity	Monotonic from 0°C to +70°C
DIFFERENTIAL LINEARITY	< ±½LSB
DIFFERENTIAL LINEARITY TC	±3ppm/°C, max (ADC-12QM)
TEMPERATURE COEFFICIENT	
Gain	±5ppm/°C of Reading
Zero	±5ppm/°C of F.S.
CONVERSION TIME	(from trailing edge of convert command to "1—0" change of status signal)
ADC- 8QM	18μs max
10QM	22μs[1] max
12QM	25μs max
INPUT VOLTAGE RANGES	±5V, ±10V, 0 to +10V (bipolar codes straddle 0V by ½LSB)
INPUT IMPEDANCE	
Buffer	100 megohms, min
Direct	
0 to +10V, or ±5V	5kΩ
±10V	10kΩ
INPUT TRIGGER (Convert Command) (see Figure 1)	Positive pulse, 100ns wide, min Leading edge ("0" to "1") resets previous data Trailing edge ("1" to "0") initiates conversion TTL/DTL Compatible "1" > 2.0V @ 40μA "0" < 0.8V @ −1.6mA
OUTPUT SIGNALS (see Figure 1)	Parallel, TTL/DTL Compatible
OUTPUT CODES	
Unipolar	Binary, BCD
Bipolar	Offset Binary, 2's Complement
OUTPUT LEVELS	TTL/DTL Compatible
"0"	< +0.4V
"1"	> +2.4V
STATUS (see Figure 1)	"1" during conversion
STATUS COMPLEMENT	"0" during conversion
POWER SUPPLY REQUIREMENTS (Separate Analog & Digital grounds)	+15V ±3% @ +25mA, −15V ±3% @ −35mA: Analog +5V ±5% @ 200mA: Digital
POWER SUPPLY SENSITIVITY	±0.002%/%ΔV_S (±15V only)
TEMPERATURE RANGE	
Operating	0°C to +70°C (suffix SN) −55°C to +125°C (suffix ET)[2]
Storage	−55°C to +125°C
ADJUSTMENTS (External Potentiometers Required)	
Zero:	100k pot across ±15 with 3 meg in series w/slider to pin 20
Gain:	100k pot across ±15 with 30k in series w/slider to pin 1
DIMENSIONS	2" X 4" X 0.4" Module

(f)

Figure 10.10 (continued)

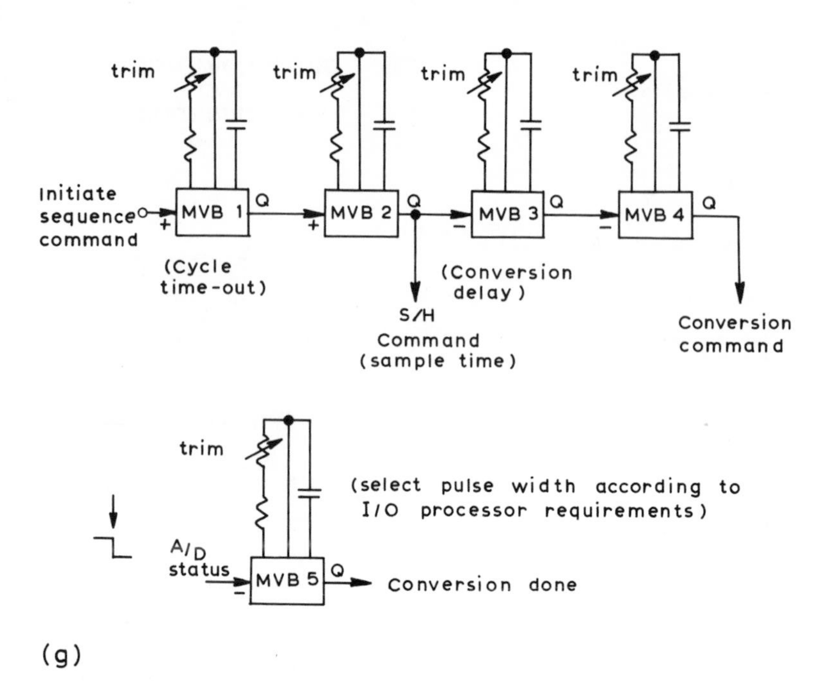

Figure 10.10 (continued)

of the input voltage (worst case). The MVB3 triggers on the trailing edge of the S/H COMMAND, delaying the CONVERSION COMMAND pulse by 400 nsec, allowing time for the SHA IA to switch to the "hold" mode. The CONVERSION COMMAND (MVB4) pulse occurs on the trailing edge of the MVB3 pulse, initiating conversion, and turning on the A/D STATUS output from the ADC-QM A/D converter (Figure 10.10f). When this output goes off again, the conversion is complete, and a CONVERSION DONE pulse of any desired length is generated by MVB5.

Total conversion time, then, is about 33 μsec, from the time that MPX address change occurs to the completion of a 12-bit A/D conversion. For most purposes, this is adequate, and the system is an inexpensive, easily constructed, easily modified one that offers a welcome alternative to the slower, more expensive A/D converters offered as peripherals by most computer manufacturers. The same design principles can be used with more expensive, faster converters such as the ADC-F module, indicated in broken lines in the block diagram of Figure 10.10a. This module, although more expensive, allows much faster conversion, because a 10-bit conversion takes only 1.0 μsec. Faster multiplexers and S/H modules are also available.

10.2 Interval as a Function of Time

In neurophysiological studies, the variation of signal voltage with respect to time is often of incidental importance, if the relative timing of action potentials is being examined. In this case, a discriminator or pulse height analyzer is used to transform the data into a series of uniform pulses, and these pulses are examined with respect to their timing. Many processing techniques for condensing interval data in a meaningful way are available, and some of the more useful ones are discussed here.

One simple analysis consists of counting spikes. A general purpose TTL counter is a useful device in any case. It can range in complexity from a simple manual-reset continuous counter through sophisticated devices with gated inputs, automatic reset, preset count, and different modes of display. Counting techniques and preset counting have already been reviewed; therefore, let us go directly to a flexible general-purpose design, illustrated in Figure 10.11.

The device consists of n decade counters in serial-count configuration (D-output of each decade counter provides A-input of next more significant digit), whose BCD outputs drive an n-digit display consisting of Hewlett Packard 5082-7300 7-segment TTL compatible decoder-driver-displays. These devices are probably the simplest, most versatile numeric display elements presently available; their characteristics are illustrated in Figure 10.12 (data courtesy of Hewlett-Packard).

Let us consider first the different features we would like to incorporate in the general-purpose counter, in order to simplify the task of modular design.

1. Three counting modes:
   a. Interval timing
      (1) START–STOP intervals
      (2) START–EVENT intervals
      (3) EVENT–STOP intervals
      (4) GATE duration
   b. Frequency measurement
   c. Event counting
2. Preset count capability, with preset count of
   a. Elapsed time
   b. Number of external events
3. Versatile display, with
   a. Display of either elapsed time (timer) or events (counter)
   b. Different display entry modes, such as
      (1) Manual entry
      (2) Continuous display

(3) Strobed entry at end of each count cycle, retention of count in display until next strobe

c. Back-panel BCD output, slaved to display and display strobing logic.

4. Different reset modes:
   a. Manual
   b. External TTL
   c. Internal
5. Different count enable modes
   a. Start and stop pulses (TTL) input
   b. Manual
   c. Gate TTL level input
6. Modular construction, ease of expansion and modification

Actually, a device of this complexity is rarely required, and operation of the counter is made complicated by the presence of so many options. The options chosen for this example are those most commonly employed, and the exercise in design should be adequate to prepare anyone to specify his own, simpler, variation. This particular design is presented only as an exercise and is not recommended for actual laboratory use, due to the complexity of operation.

The three counting modes are easily achieved. Interval measurement is accomplished by counting a clock during the interval to be timed. Interval resolution is determined by selection of one of a set of decade-variable clock rates, from 1 Hz to 1 MHz, with the SAMPLING FREQUENCY/INTERVAL RESOLUTION SELECTOR (Figure 10.11d). The 10 MHz clock is divided by these decade dividers from one TIMER ZERO-RESET pulse to the next: the TIMER ZERO-RESET pulse is generated once per measured interval. The divided clock frequency, DIVIDED CLOCK H, is gated by COUNT ENABLE H, discussed below, and further gated (Figure 10.11h) in the INTERVAL mode to provide COUNT INPUT H, the input to the counter. When not in the PC (preset count) mode, the interval timing continues as long as the count is enabled. In the PC mode, the PC DONE signal resets the time. Generation of PC DONE is discussed below. The INTERVAL DURATION H level is generated in a different fashion for each of the different interval modes (Figure 10.11i); a START/STOP high level is generated by a flipflop set by a START TTL input and reset by a STOP TTL input. The START/EVENT mode and the EVENT/STOP mode are based on the generation of analogous *R-S* flipflop outputs. The EVENT/EVENT mode is maintained as the $\bar{Q}$ output of a 50 nsec MVB triggered by the high TTL pulses at the EVENTS input. Finally, the GATE DURATION level is simply the COUNT GATE H level derived directly from the GATE input (Figure 10.11c). GATED

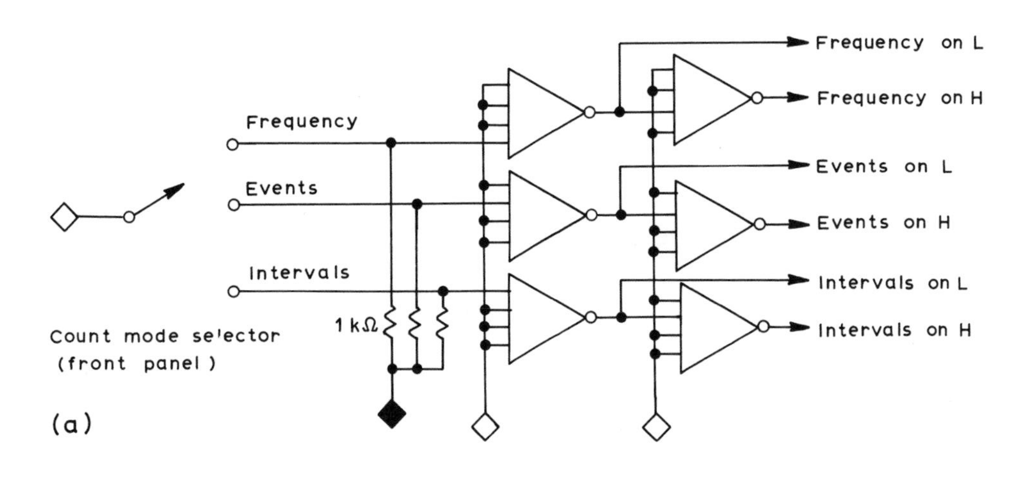

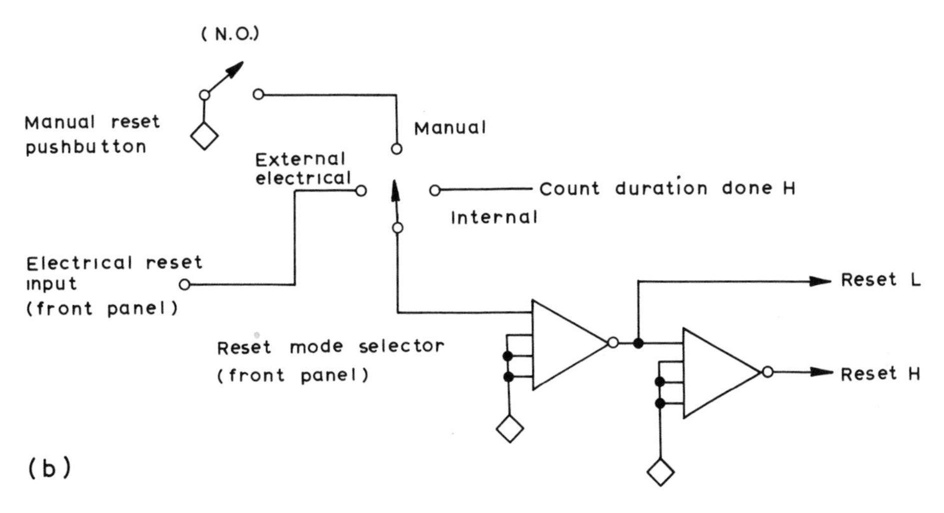

Figure 10.11
General-purpose counter: (a) count mode selection; (b) reset mode selection; (c) count enable mode selection; (d) timer section; (e) counter and display section; (f) display enable section; (g) display entry mode selection; (h) count-input gating; (i) interval selection; (j) display contents selection; (k) count duration done, timer zero-reset; (l) display BCD input bit gating; (m) preset count mode selection.

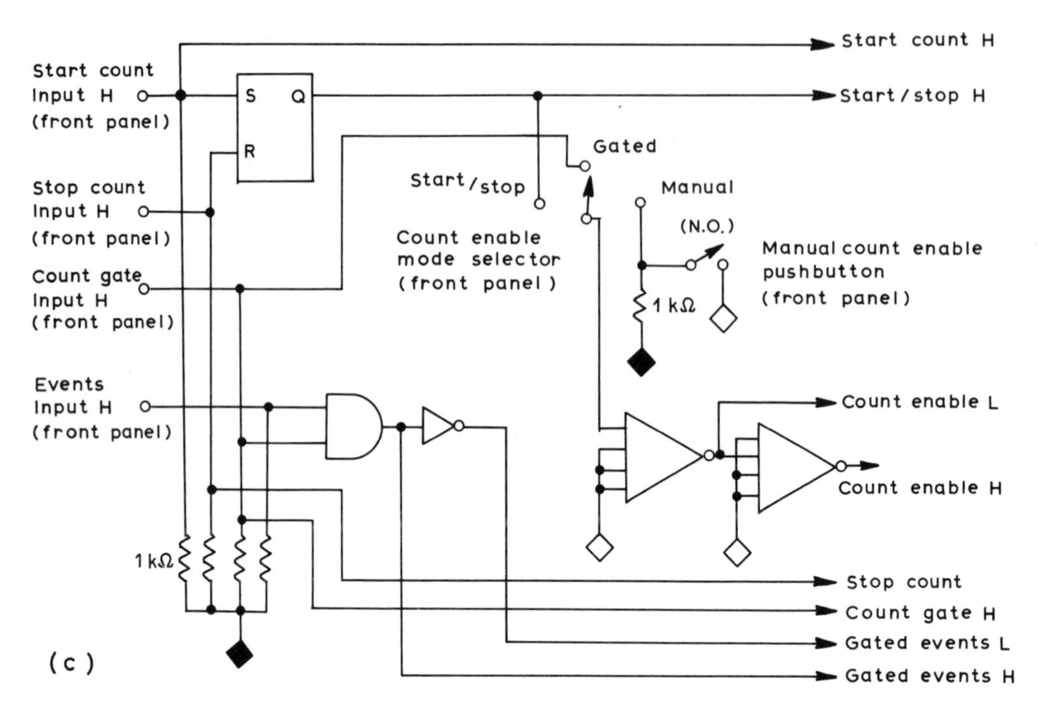

Figure 10.11 (continued)

INTERVAL DURATION H is derived from COUNT ENABLE H ∧ INTERVAL DURATION H, in order to measure intervals only during the COUNT ENABLE period, described below. The GATED INTERVAL DURATION H is then ANDed with INTERVALS ON H (Figure 10.11k) and this signal is used to generate COUNT DURATION DONE H, which is used to reset and strobe counter values.

INTERVALS ON H, FREQUENCY ON H, and EVENTS ON H are mutually exclusive high levels generated by the COUNT MODE SELECTOR switch (Figure 10.11a). These levels are used by the internal logic to determine mode of operation. Thus, the COUNT DURATION DONE H is determined only by GATED INTERVAL DURATION H, as long as the INTERVAL mode is selected and no preset count is used (Figure 10.11k). The switch also determines location of the decimal point on the display (10.11f) and which of the three mode indicator lights is illuminated. Note that choice of indicator light and location of decimal point are also determined by whether the display is of elapsed time, or of the counter contents, depending on selection of COUNTER or TIMER by the DISPLAY CONTENTS switch (Figure 10.11j).

Frequency measurements of EVENT inputs are accomplished by counting the number of EVENTs during some decade multiple of 1 μsec. The display (if

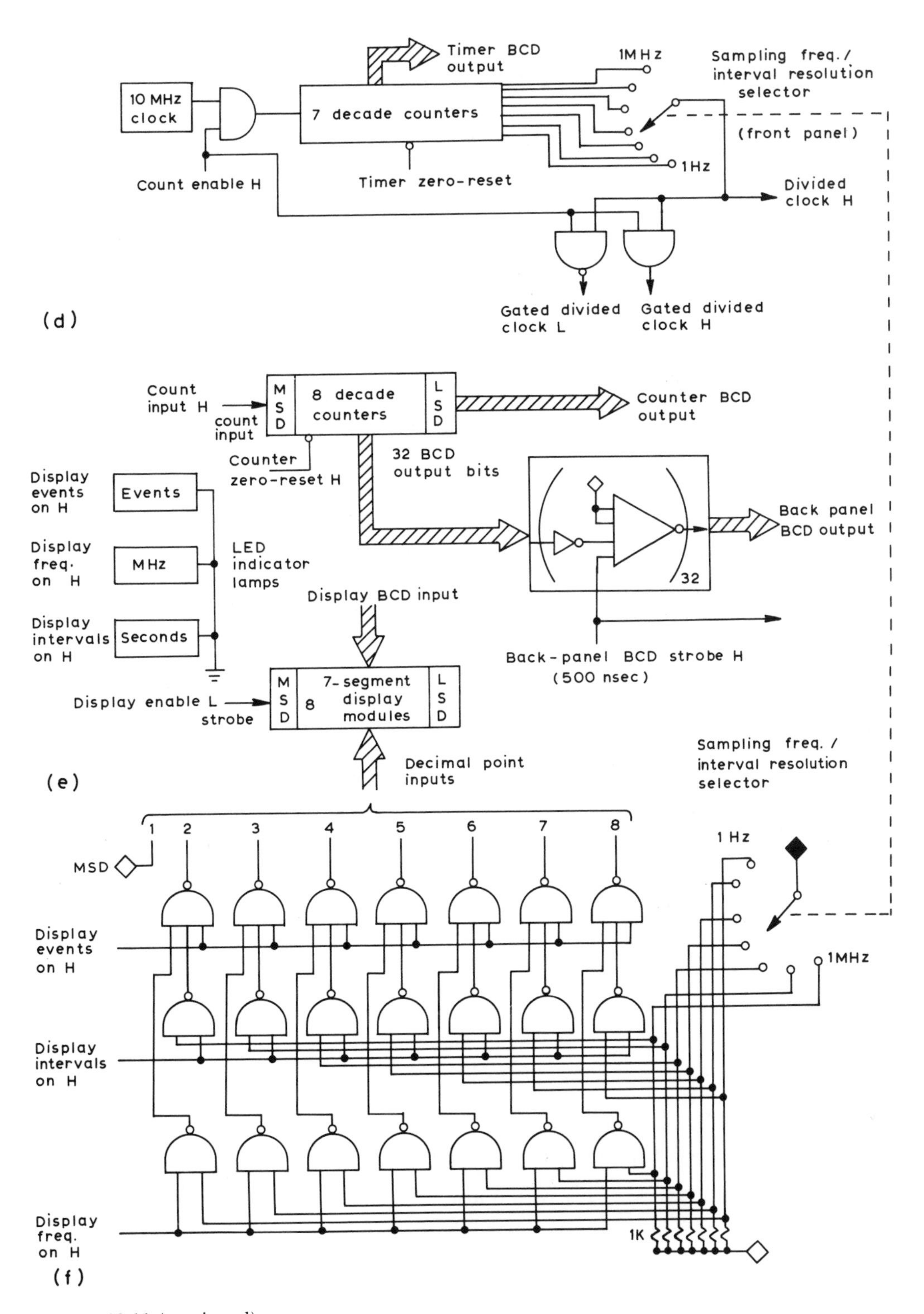

Figure 10.11 (continued)

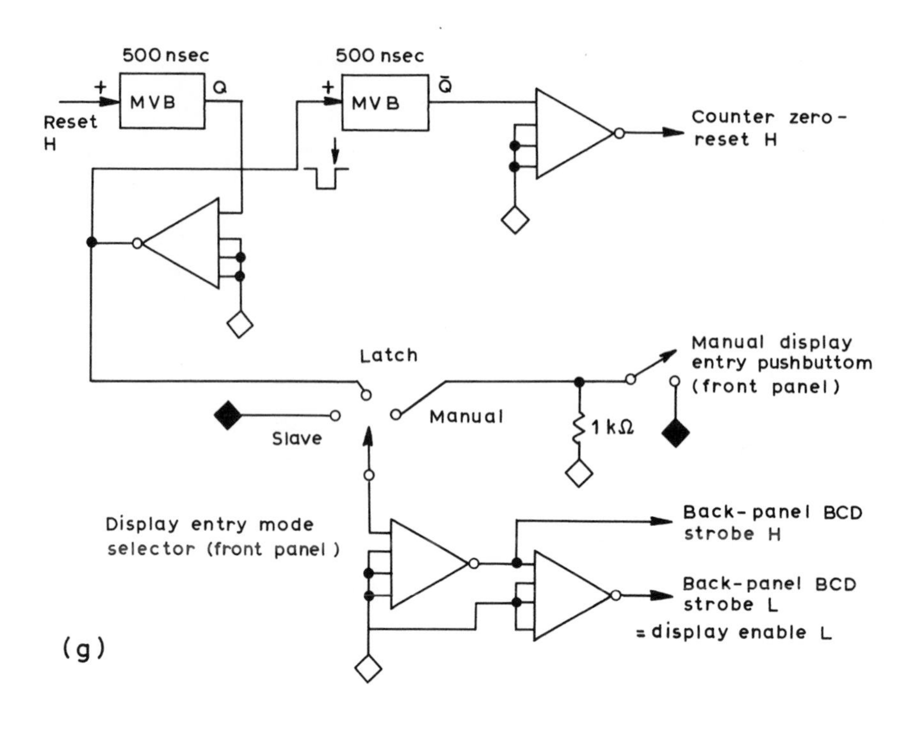

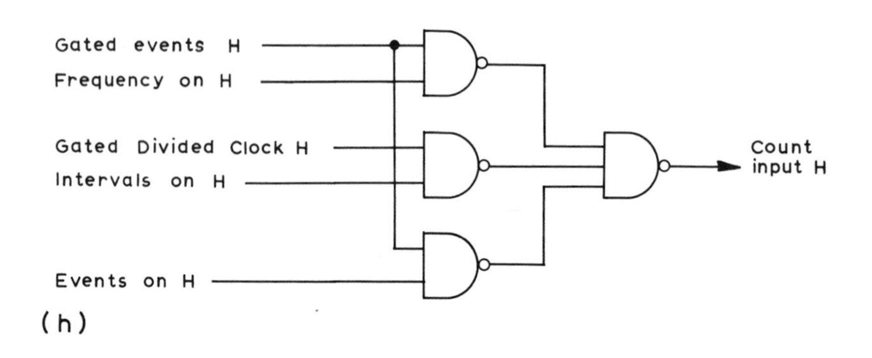

Figure 10.11 (continued)

COUNTER is displayed) is in number of MHz, with decimal point location determined by the SAMPLING FREQUENCY/INTERVAL RESOLUTION switch (Figures 10.11d, f). This switch also determines the units used for interval measurements; INTERVAL RESOLUTION is decade variable from 1 μsec to 1 sec, with automatic adjustment of decimal point. In the FREQUENCY mode, the number of GATED EVENTS (Figure 10.11c) during each cycle of GATED DIVIDED CLOCK is counted (Figure 10.11k) and displayed at the end of the cycle. This is determined by COUNT DURATION DONE H. Note interaction

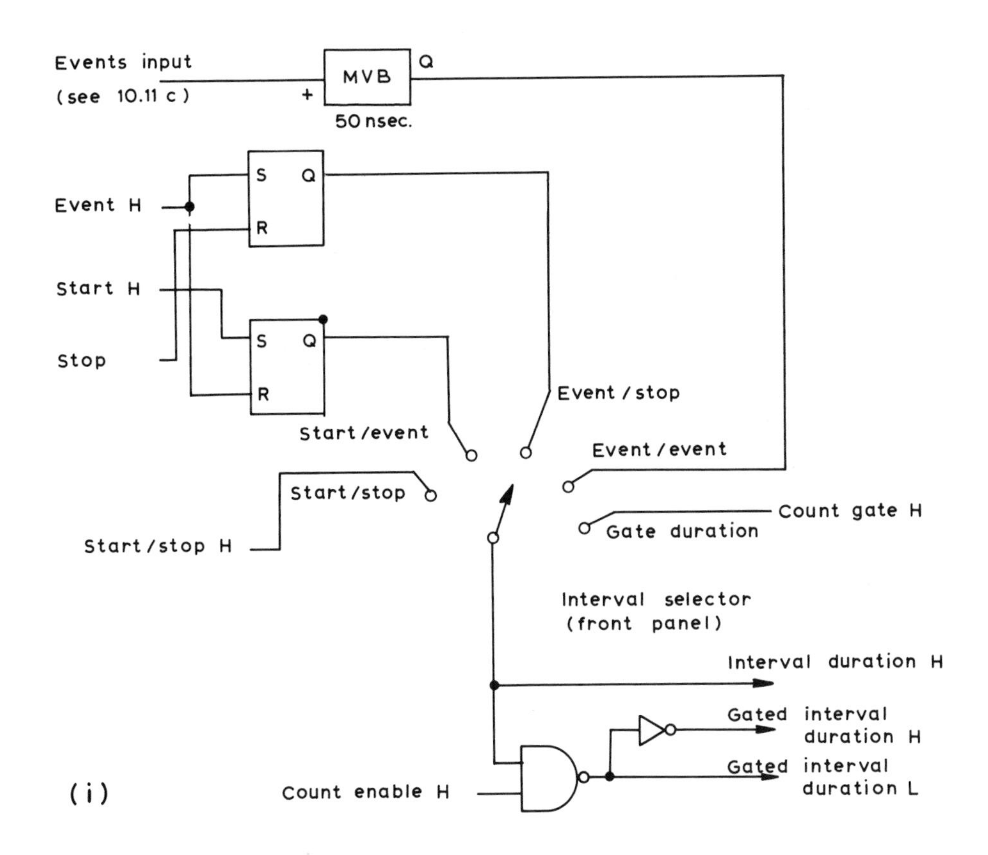

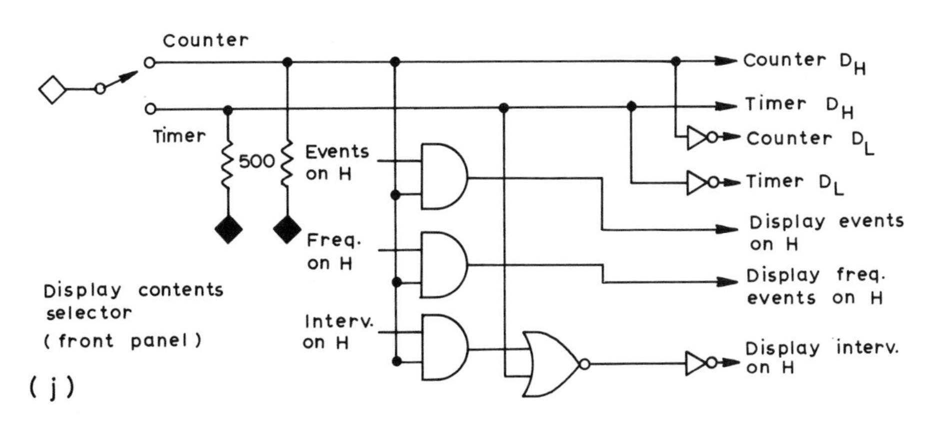

Figure 10.11 (continued)

of COUNT ENABLE H and DIVIDED CLOCK; if a fractional DIVIDED CLOCK INTERVAL is terminated by the COUNT ENABLE H going low, the last frequency count will be in error. If a running frequency sample over a longer period than the required period is used, this last measurement can simply be thrown out.

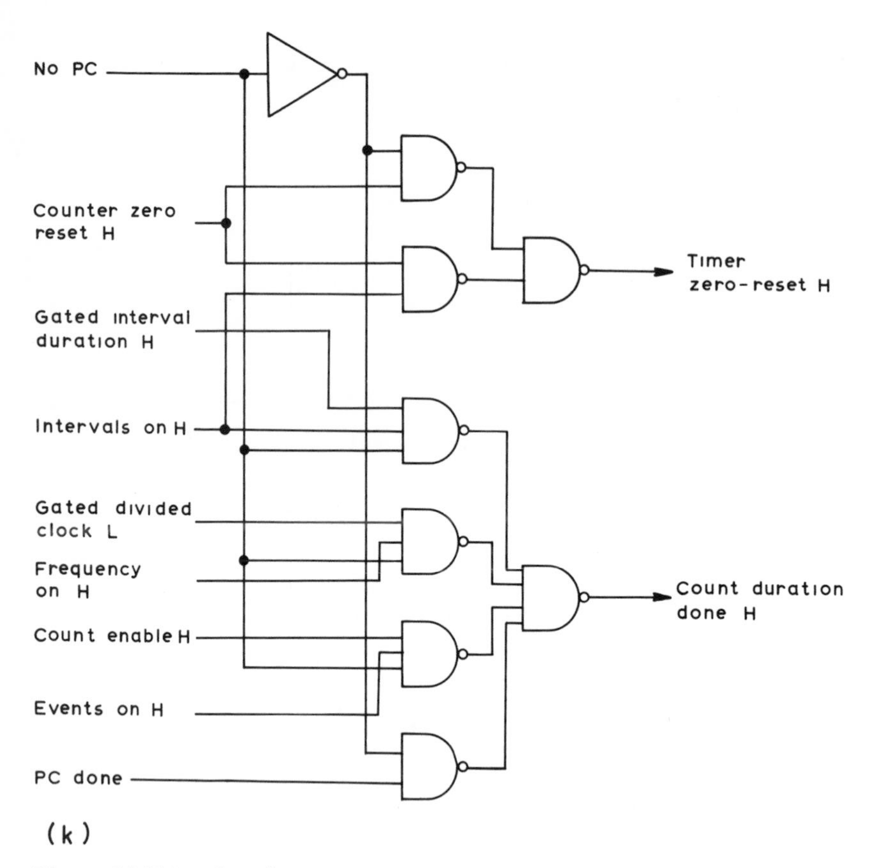

Figure 10.11 (continued)

In the EVENTS counting mode, the GATED EVENTS are counted as long as COUNT ENABLE H is on. At the end of each COUNT ENABLE H gate, the counting period is terminated, via COUNT DURATION DONE H (Figure 10.11k).

In any counting mode, the COUNT DURATION DONE H positive transition can serve to strobe the COUNT and reset the counter and timer, depending on the RESET MODE (Figure 10.11b) and DISPLAY ENTRY MODE (Figure 10.11g). The former selector switch also allows MANUAL or EXTERNAL ELECTRICAL reset. Whenever a RESET H positive transition occurs, a 500 nsec MVB pulse is triggered, which is used to strobe (LATCH) the count into the display, before a second 500 nsec pulse is triggered to reset the counter. This delayed pulse is also used to reset the timer in the INTERVAL mode, or when the PRESET COUNT option is enabled.

The count can be strobed manually, or it can be slaved to the counter or timer (whichever input is being displayed), depending on the position of the DISPLAY

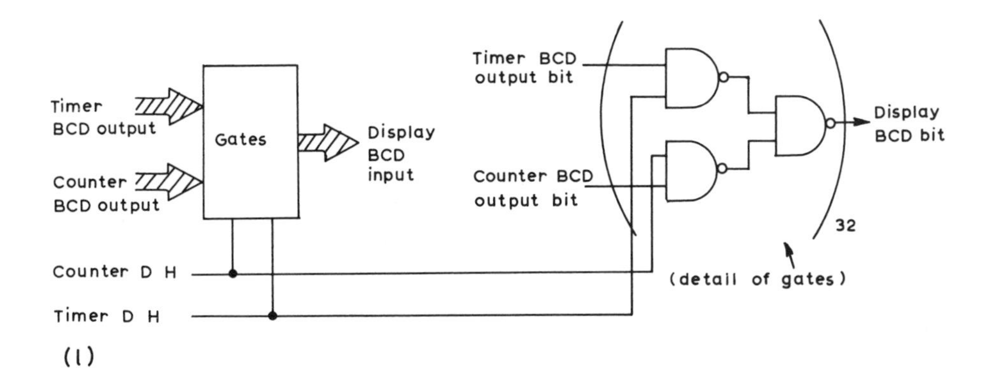

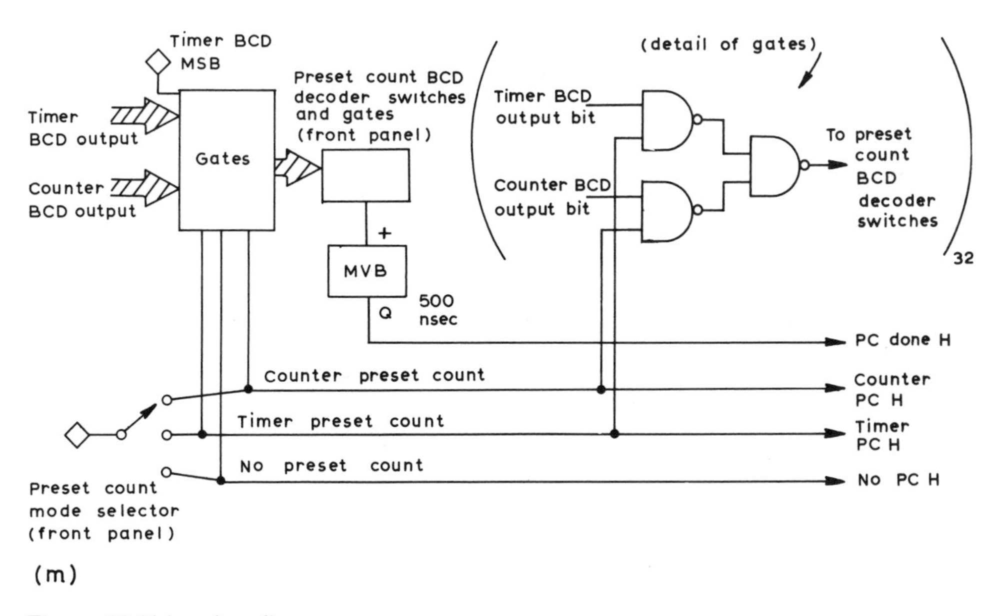

Figure 10.11 (continued)

ENTRY mode switch. The BACK-PANEL STROBE, used for parallel BCD output strobing, is the same signal as that used to strobe the count into the display, DISPLAY ENABLE L. These modes do not affect the RESET circuitry.

In the PRESET COUNT mode, counting is terminated by PC DONE, when either a preset timer or counter value is attained. Choices of either of these options (Figure 10.11m) forces COUNT DURATION DONE H and TIMER ZERO-RESET H on when PC DONE occurs.

Note that it is possible to select combinations of options that are contradictory, in which case incorrect results will be obtained. If a device of this complexity is really required, error-detection logic should be incorporated to energize alarm

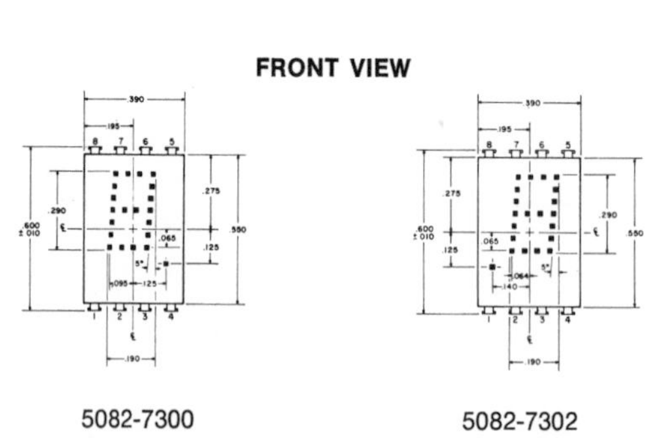

FUNCTION	PIN	
	5082-7300	5082-7302
	Right hand decimal point	Left hand decimal point
Input 1 (A)	8	8
Input 2 (B)	1	1
Input 4 (C)	2	2
Input 8 (D)	3	3
V_{CC}	7	7
V_E (Latch)	5	5
Decimal point	4	4
Ground	6	6

Display contrast can be improved by placing a long wave pass band filter between the display devices and the viewer. Plexiglas #2423 material is suitable for this application.

Use TTL supply voltage, TTL digital input. Loading: 1 unit load for each input.

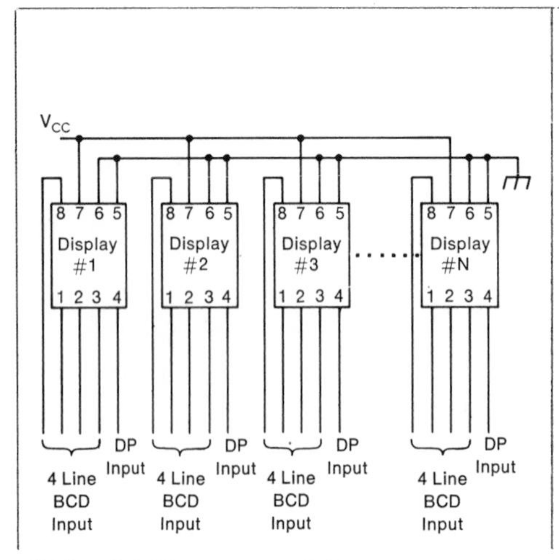

Bit Parallel, Character Parallel Input Data.

To address each display with character information in parallel, all memory enable input lines should be connected to ground. In this mode the device will display as a real time function the BCD and decimal point inputs.

The decimal point status information is processed by a latch in the same manner as the BCD inputs. The decimal point convention is negative logic — decimal point voltage low corresponds to the decimal point illuminated. The decimal point latch and the BCD latches are controlled by the same enable line. The enable line ("latch") causes the display to follow inputs when it is low. When the enable level goes high, the current display is "latched" and held until the next time the enable input goes low, regardless of changes at the data inputs.

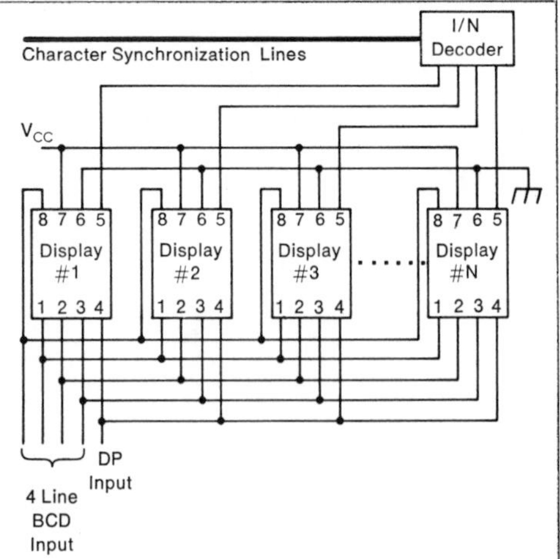

Bit Parallel, Character Serial Input Data.

The on-board latches can be used to store data presented in a character serial format, as shown in Figure 9. Selective activation of the display enable lines steers the data into the appropriate latches. Each display input is equivalent to 1 U.L., so that a standard 54/74 TTL output will provide enough drive for 10 display modules in parallel. A 1/N active low decoder can be used to generate the enable line signals.

Figure 10.12

5082-7300/7302 numeric decoder-driver-display integrated circuits (from 5082-7300/7302 Numeric Display data sheet, 1972, by Hewlett-Packard. Used with permission of Hewlett-Packard).

lights when such combinations are selected. With proper selections of options, the device is a powerful tool, capable of constructing PST histograms (if output is appropriately recorded), interval data, latency measurements, response magnitudes, and many other functions. Modification is easily accomplished because of the modular organization.

There are other analyses of interval data that are possible with a minimum of hardware. For example, a running average of pulse frequency (using uniform TTL pulses triggered on spikes) can be obtained by using a low-pass filter to give a smoothed curve of frequency versus time (Figure 10.13). It can be used to drive a meter, to deflect an oscilloscope or penwriter, or even as input to an A/D converter.

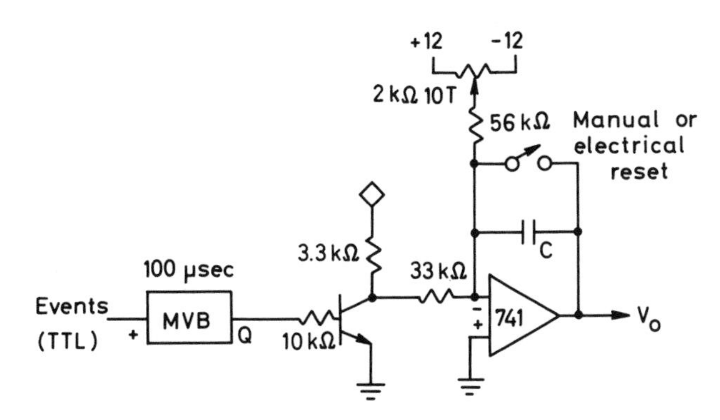

Figure 10.13
Spike frequency-to-voltage converter.

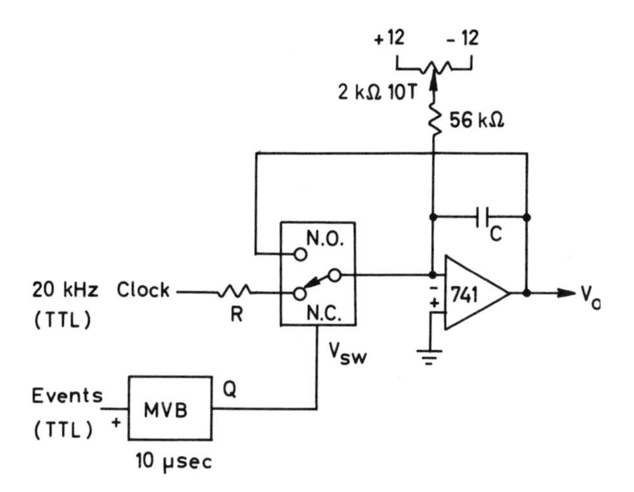

Figure 10.14
Spike interval-to-voltage converter.

A similar approach can be used to convert interspike intervals into corresponding voltages (Figure 10.14). A clock frequency is integrated, resetting on each spike. The peaks of the integrator ramps represent the interval lengths. If desired, these peaks can be successively strobed into a sample-and-hold amplifier or A/D converter, or they can be low-pass filtered to provide a smoothed curve of interspike interval versus time.

Figure 10.15a illustrates a setup for generating a dot-pattern display. The leftmost column of dots represents the synchronization pulses used to start successive sweeps (generated by synch pulses initiating the stimulus). Subsequent dots in each row represent times of occurrence of action potentials (or other discriminable events). Each row of dots represents a new stimulus, or if synchs are available for each phase of a periodic stimulus, each row may represent a successive cycle of the stimulus.

Spikes and synchs are discriminated and led to the inputs of a NOR gate. The "off" pulse from the NOR is inverted and amplified, to generate +30 V pulses for the unblanking (*Z* axis), which is applied to the external cathode circuit via the back-panel input on a Tektronix oscilloscope. Adjust the intensity for no visible beam with unblanking off, and for a well-focused dot with unblanking on. The synch pulse discriminator also triggers two sawtooth generators, either those of Chapter 6, Tektronix wave-form generators, or even an oscilloscope horizontal sweep (if EXTERNAL HORIZONTAL OUTPUT is available). Sawtooth 1 generates the scope sweep and should be adjusted for the desired sweep duration (the external trigger and internal sweep of the scope may be used). Adjust the EXTERNAL HORIZONTAL INPUT gain for the desired sweep length on the CRT face, if an externally generated sawtooth is used. Sawtooth 2 is used to generate a slow downward deflection. Although the rows of dots will be slightly tilted, this will not be objectionable if the sweep duration is brief compared to the total duration of sawtooth 2, especially if the sweep duration is brief compared to intersweep interval. If the tilt is a source of annoyance, the sawtooth generator of Figure 10.15b should be used.

The vertical deflection can be obtained by an alternative method: A binary counter can be used to count trials, and the counter output can be used to drive a D/A converter. Since D/A converters of up to 8 bits are relatively inexpensive, this is an economical technique; also, the rows are perfectly horizontal, and problems of drift associated with integrators can be avoided. This technique is illustrated in Figure 10.15c.

To view the entire pattern, use a storage oscilloscope or photograph the display, holding the camera shutter on "bulb," during the generation of the entire dot pattern.

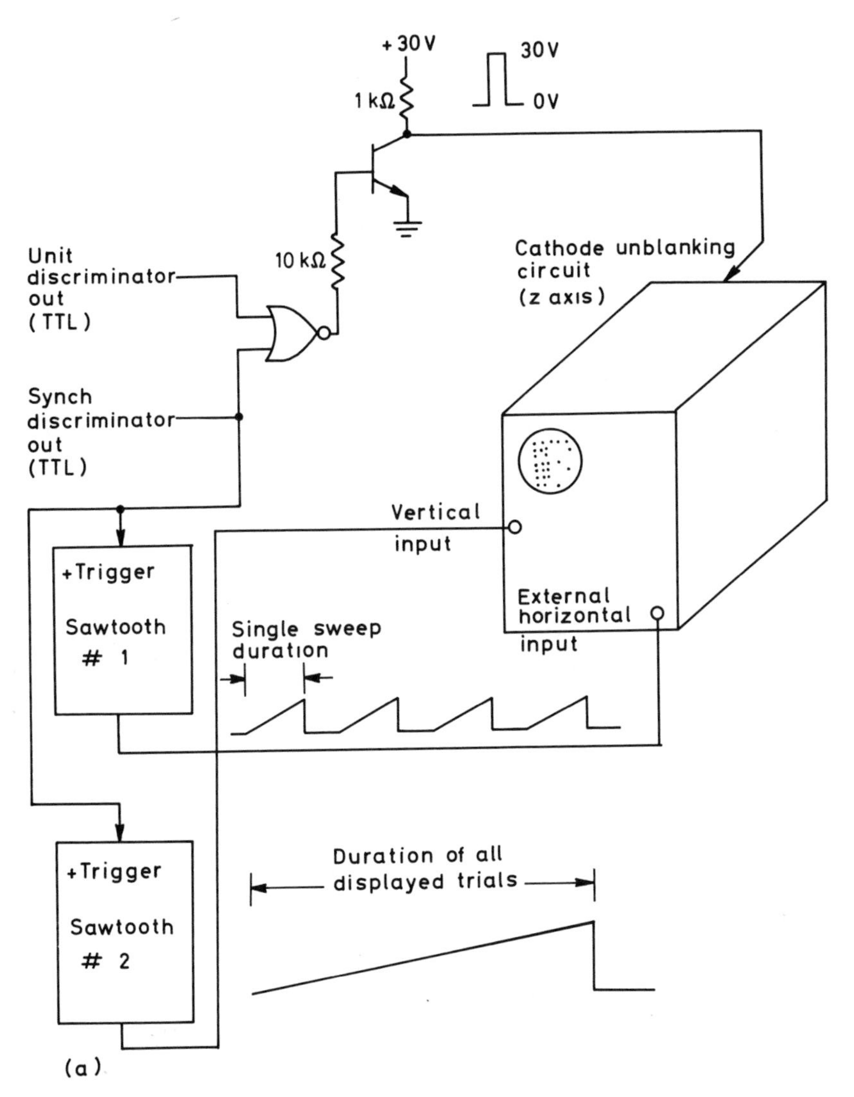

Figure 10.15
Dot pattern display: (a) block diagram, integrator method; (b) modification of sawtooth generator #2 and internal waveforms; (c) use of binary counters and D/A converter for generation of vertical deflection voltage.

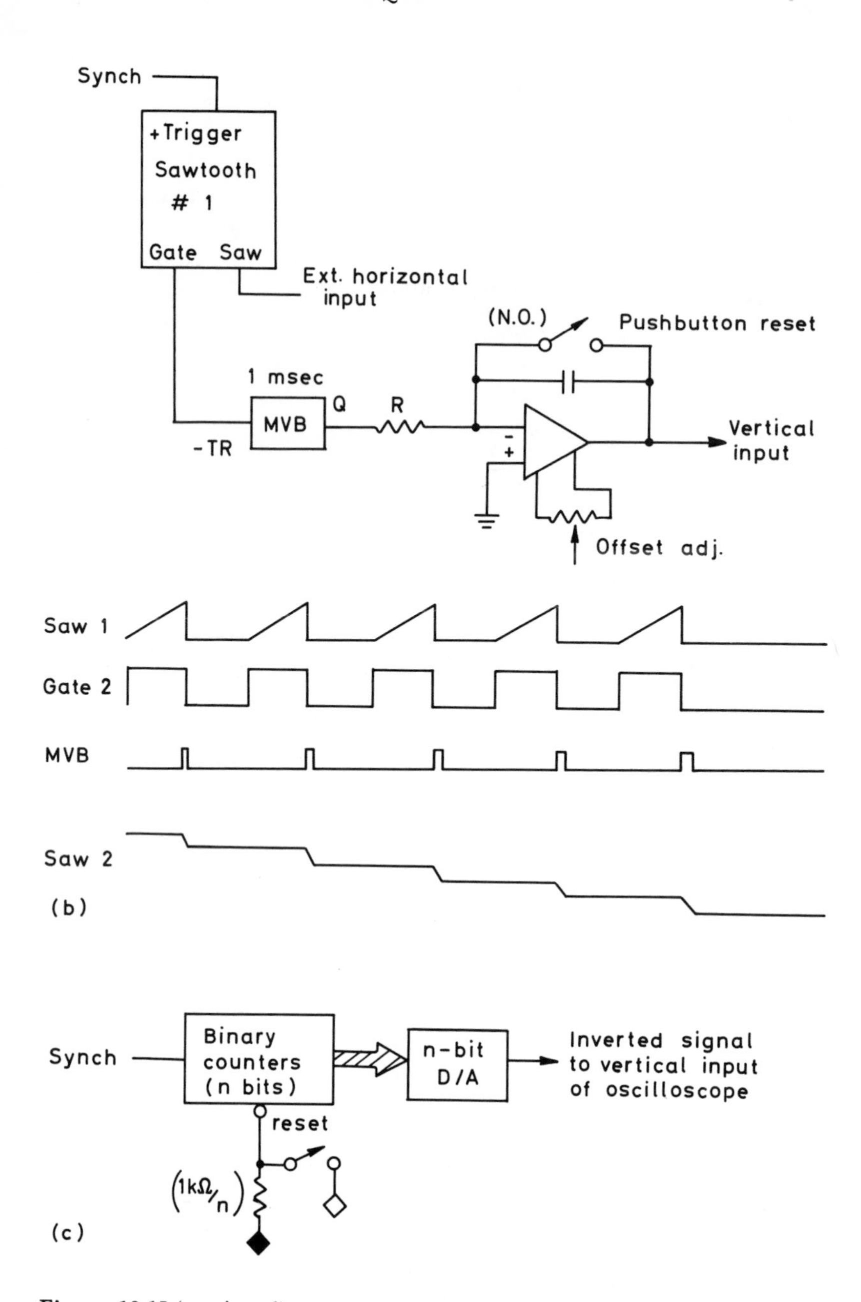

Figure 10.15 (continued)

A trial-by-trial PST histogram is obtained with the circuit of Figure 10.16. The sweep begins with the synch, and points are displayed as frequency (vertical) versus time (horizontal). For a graph of average frequency versus time, use the output of the frequency meter described earlier in this chapter for the vertical deflection, with beam unblanked during the entire sweep. Single-trial PSTs and even multitrace recordings of these are not nearly as useful as a real accumulated PST. The reason for this is entirely analogous to the advantage of voltage averaging over a photograph of superimposed oscilloscope traces. The wave form of the response, recorded as spikes/sec/bin, consists of ongoing random firings (except where there is no spontaneous activity), and a variable (in most cases) response to some input to the cell under study. The PST wave form can be averaged (although it is usually just summed) over several trials, enhancing the signal/noise ratio by the square root of the number of trials. Just as in voltage averaging, a response that is entirely buried in noise may become visible, and the "true response wave form" may emerge from a noise-distorted trace. The technique has the same diminishing return effect with increased number of trials as does the voltage wave–form averaging method. Accumulated PSTs require some form of memory, however.

To generate an interval scattergram, use the arrangement of Figure 10.17. A memory is required for interval histogram generation. If average interval versus time is desired, use the output of the interval meter previously described for the vertical deflection, with the beam unblanked during the entire sweep.

A joint interval distribution scattergram is obtained with the circuit of Figure 10.18a. The X-axis is the ith interval length, and the Y-axis is the $(i + 1)$th interval length. Two digital integrators consisting of counters and D/A converters alternate in timing the ongoing interspike interval, and each one is used first to deflect the Y-axis and then to deflect the X-axis on the subsequent spike. The initialization flipflop suppresses display of the first interval. The technique is useful for spotting serial correlations among intervals. Wave forms are illustrated in Figure 10.18b.

Obviously, similar methods can be used for measurement of latencies, phase distribution relative to the stimulus, and other useful indices of neuronal spike timing. With the addition of an appropriate memory and the use of digital rather than analog representations, detailed histograms can be constructed. Although it is generally wiser to use a small general-purpose computer, if one is available, histogram modules consisting of digital input logic, digital memory, and display output may become available in the very near future; such modules could serve as powerful tools in the laboratory, for investigating any of a number of timing properties, depending on the user's input hardware. It should be noted that online PSTs are extremely useful during experiments, to indicate the presence or absence

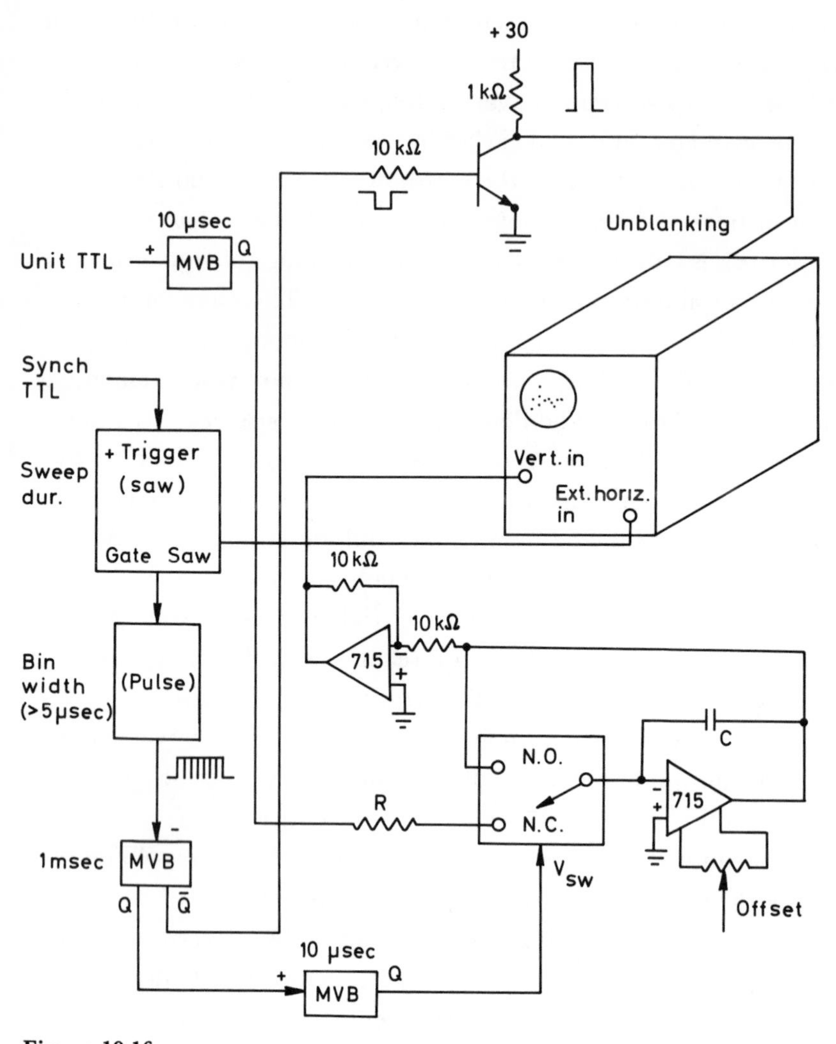

Figure 10.16
Trial-by-trial PST histogram. Internal oscilloscope horizontal sweep may be used instead of external horizontal input: in that case, trigger on SYNCH TTL.

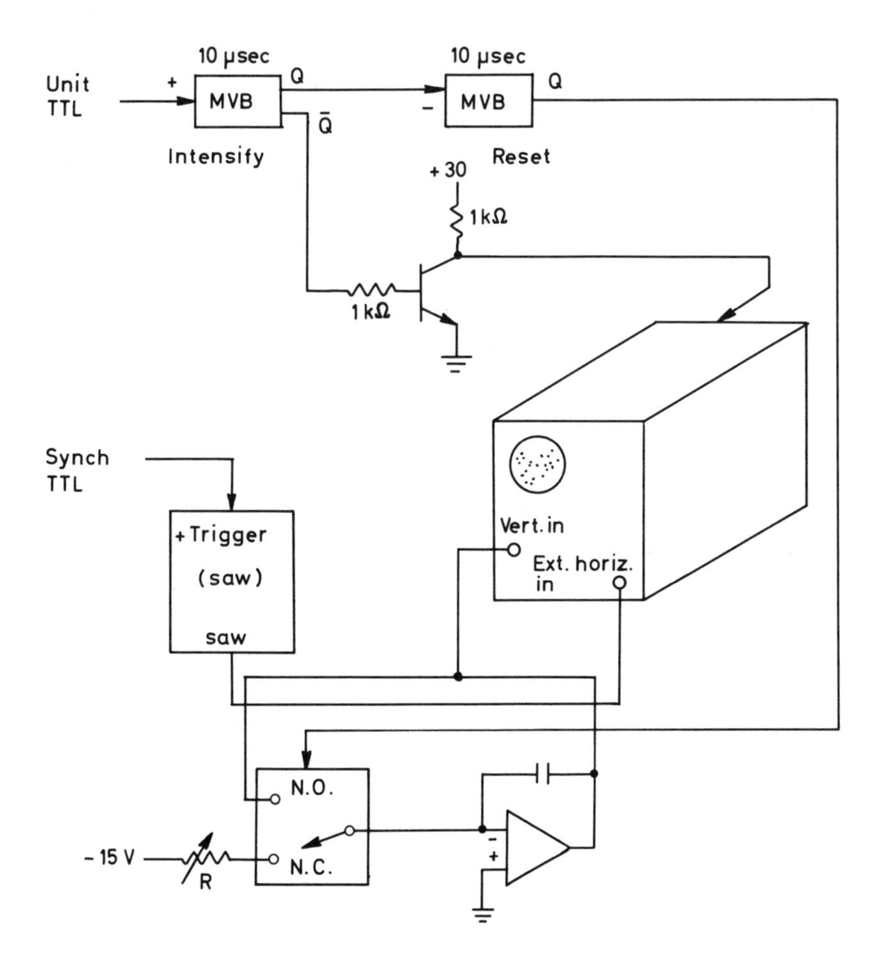

Figure 10.17
Interval versus time dot display.

of a response or to determine the response wave form. The cost of most commercially available histogram generators is less than the corresponding computer user charges for, say, 200 to 500 hours of online use, and any laboratory that needs such online feedback and must pay user charges for online data processing would benefit from the use of such a machine, with one drawback: No commercially available histogram machines provide a convenient bulk-storage output, such as a digital magnetic tape or cassette recording. Although a PST is a useful representation of data, most research would benefit from other computer analyses as well. In order to obtain these, data must be recorded on analog tape and digitized offline for computer analysis, an uneconomical use of personnel time, or interval data must be digitized online, an uneconomical use of computer time. In either case it is necessary to convert intervals to numbers. We will therefore discuss the process of digitization of interval data for computer analysis.

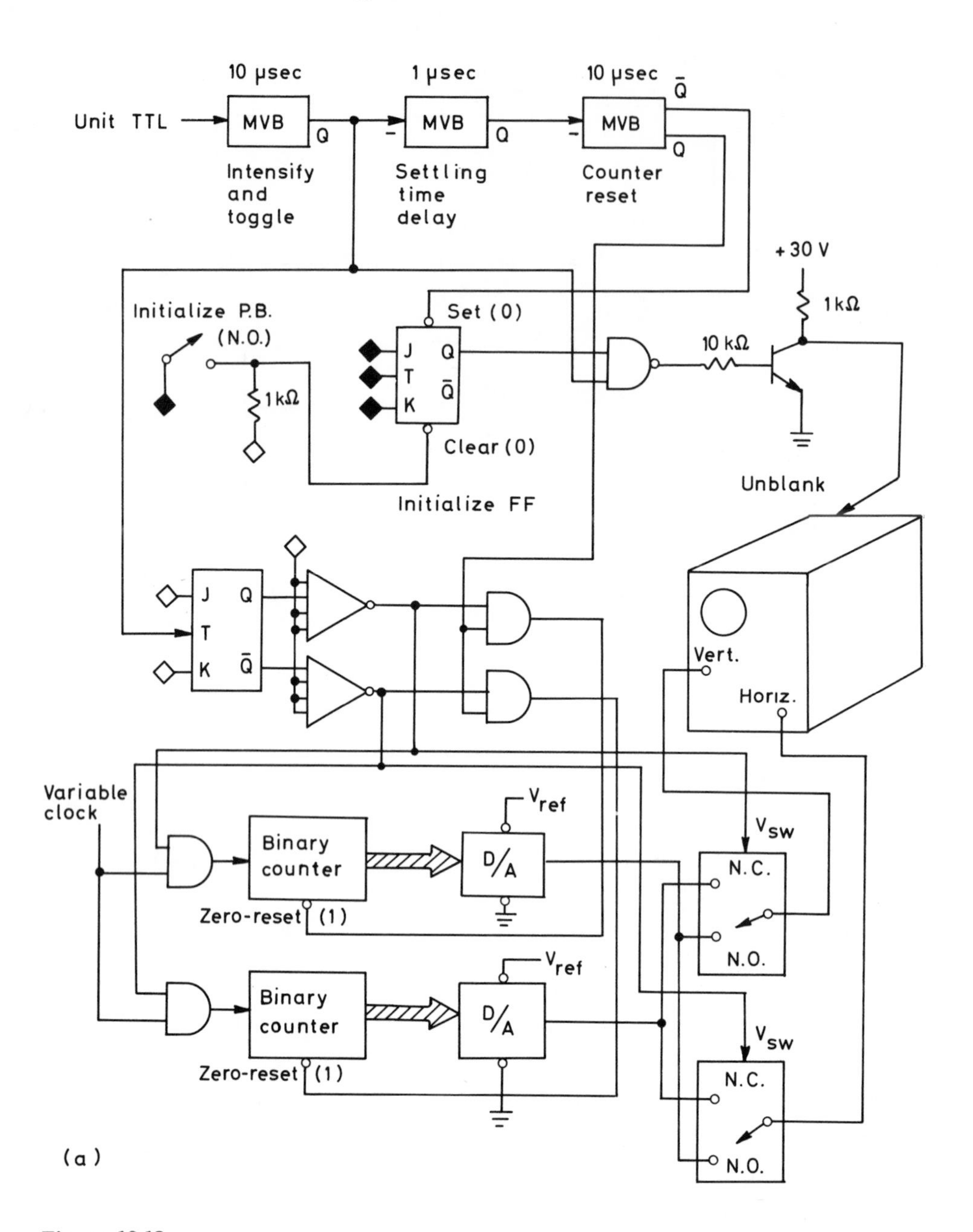

Figure 10.18
Joint interval scattergram: (a) block diagram; (b) timing diagram (delay to RESET exaggerated).

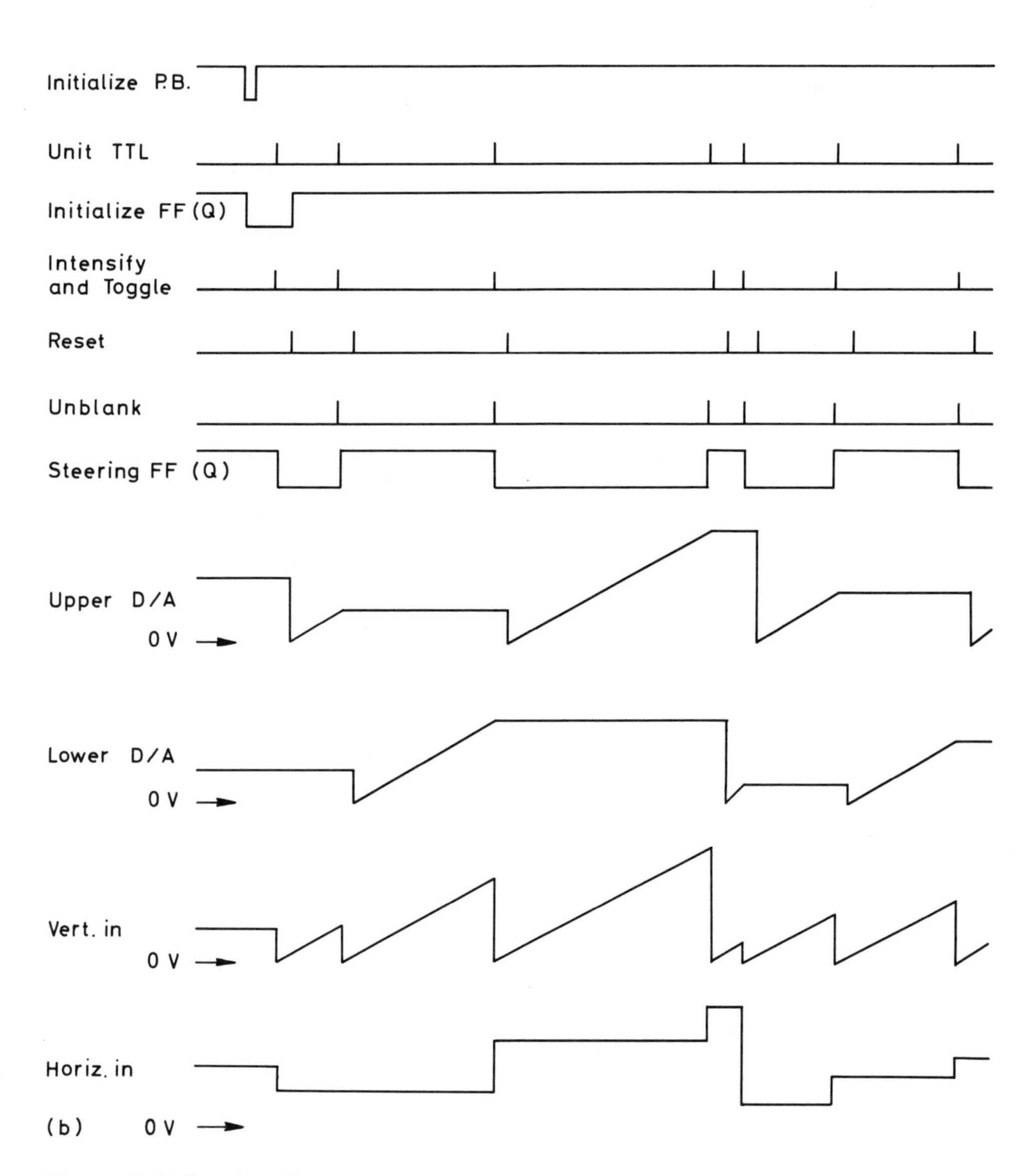

Figure 10.18 (continued)

Several approaches have been used in the past few years for computer analysis of the precise timing of biological events such as the occurrence of action potentials recorded from single nerve cells. In general, these methods have been variants on two types of approach: (1) a special-purpose computer is used, which has been designed for the specific purpose of analyzing intervals between external input signals, or (2) a general-purpose computer is used, and timing is accomplished by programmed timing loops or by some external hardware.

The latter approach is especially practical, in view of the fact that a small general-purpose computer need not be much more expensive than the special-purpose devices and is much more versatile. At somewhat higher cost, magnetic tape bulk storage can be added, providing the opportunity for reanalysis using digitized data rather than real-time data, which would have to be discriminated and digitized each time an analysis is performed. Thus, a five-minute sample can be analyzed using magnetic tape data in a period of time ranging from a few seconds to a minute, and setup time is reduced to that required to load the program and data tape, eliminating time-consuming adjustment of discriminators and location of the data on an analog tape. Most, if not all, data-acquisition computers cannot easily provide sufficient time resolution and buffering of intervals through the use of program loops or program-controlled clocks. To date, few researchers in the biological sciences could design and construct their own time-digitizer (pulse interval timer, PIT), and a low-cost, high-resolution timer has not been commercially available.

Such a PIT should have at least the following characteristics: (1) ability to detect multiple input events, with buffered digital output for computer processing and unique flags for each type of event; (2) high resolution, balanced against the need to conserve core space; (3) interrupt-generating or data-break capability; and (4) low cost and easy assembly.

The PIT described here has a timing resolution of 10 μsec per bit with independently buffered output for two external events. Four event flags are provided, with one interrupt signal (or data channel strobe) for all four.

The design is based on principles similar to those incorporated in a device designed by J. M. Goldberg and constructed by Digital Equipment Corporation (DEC). The PIT described here was constructed for use in the laboratory of D. N. Tapper at Cornell University, as an input interface for the DEC PDP-15.

The PIT provided an interrupt level (which can also be used for strobing data via a data channel) and flags to indicate the occurrence of any of four events, three of which come from sources external to the timer: (1) a positive voltage transition indicating the occurrence of an event (called *SYNCH* or *S*) such as the onset of a stimulus; (2) a similar external event called *UNIT* (or *U*) such as the onset of a behavioral or neural response; and (3) an event (called *END* or *E*) that could be used to indicate termination of the stimulus or the sampling sequence. The *U* and *S* flags are accompanied by a digital number in the output buffer, which is available to the computer for parallel access through some digital input. If no parallel access exists for the computer input, appropriate shift registers and other logic can easily be incorporated for serial transmission of bits to the computer. The third external event, the *END* signal, does not generate an interval at the output. *UNIT* and *SYNCH* reset the timer, so that the interval time is that interval since the last occurrence of a *SYNCH*, a *UNIT*, or a fourth, internally generated flag, *OVERFLOW* (*O*). The *OVERFLOW* flag is raised whenever the timer counter reaches its maximum value without occurrence of *U* or *S*, and cycles to zero. Without such a flag, all intervals would be modulo the maximum timer value, an unworkable situation.

The actual timer consists of a 15-bit binary counter driven by a clock. The number of bits is easily changed for other word lengths. The *U*, *S*, and *E* flags may be incorporated as bits in the data word. The *O* need not be coded, because it is the only event that produces an interval equal to the maximum timer interval. However, the interval must be stored; hence an *O* flag is included to notify the computer of the need to transfer a data word.

Any combination of *U*, *S*, *E*, or *O* will produce a corresponding combination of flags at the output, if they occur within the same clock cycle (10 μsec). At the end of the clock cycle, the interrupt level is turned on. Later events are prevented from generating flags until the pending flags are cleared by the computer. Queuing of flags up to a queue length of four is possible in this design.

Clock frequency, word length, number of flags, queue length, number of buffered outputs, and the computer-controlled enabling of flags are all easily modified.

A separate section, called PS (for PIT SYNCH), generates an interrupt flag for detection of *SYNCH:* The logic is designed to detect (a) the first *SYNCH* after clearing the level under computer control or (b) the first *SYNCH* after occurrence of an *END*. This allows synchronization of other processes, such as averaging sweeps.

The computer must generate pulses for controlling the PIT and PS, as follows:

PITCLR Clear all flags and registers, stop PIT. No effect on PS.
PITGO Start the PIT. No effect on PS.
PSGO Enables PS, clear PS. No effect on PIT.

PSSTOP Clear and disable PS. No effect on PIT.
PWRCLR Clear and disable PIT and PS when computer is turned on.
TRANSMISSION COMPLETE H Shifts queue one level forward, clearing output level and bringing in pending level.

The cable inputs from the laboratory discriminators or logic devices are buffered by SN74121N MVBs (Figure 10.19); the zeners protect against transients that could damage the interface logic, if the device is coupled to a cable. The resulting 1 μsec pulses (*S IN H*, *U IN H*, and *E IN H*) are used as inputs to both PIT and PS.

In Figure 10.19, PS consists of two RS flipflops, two gates, and an MVB. One RS flipflop serves as an "enable"; it is set by *PSGO L* and reset by *PSSTOP L*

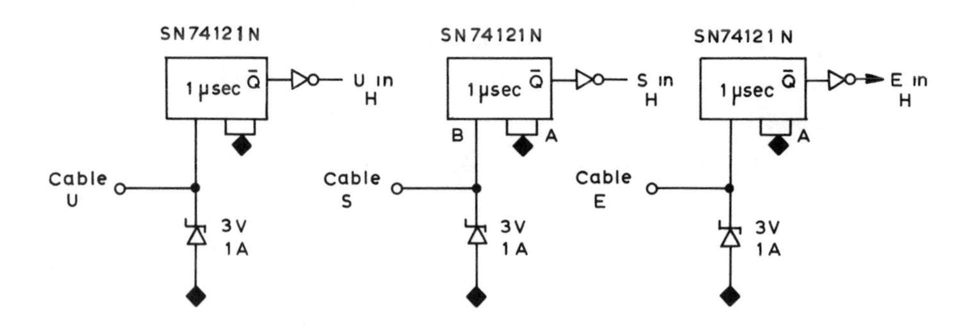

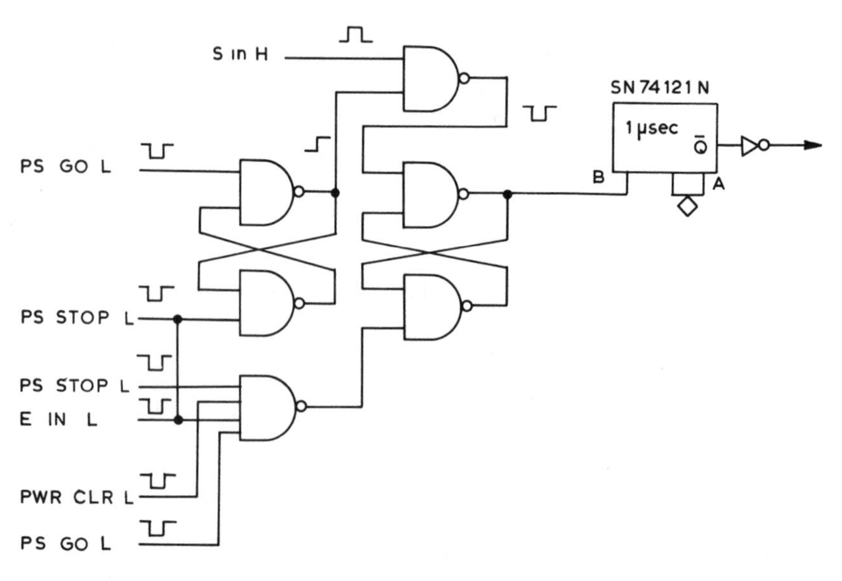

Figure 10.19
PIT cable inputs, PS.

and conditions a gate that passes *S IN H* only if the enable FF is set. The resulting low pulse sets the second RS FF, triggering a 1 μsec pulse, *PS H*, which is transmitted to the computer. If a level is preferred the MVB may be omitted. The second FF is reset by either *PSSTOP L, E IN L, PSGO L*, or *PWRCLR L*. The last of these occurs when general IO reset conditions obtain at the computer: these generally occur when the power is turned on, during power failures, and at turnoff. Some computers also have provisions for manual generation of the same pulse when the operator depresses an appropriate console switch, or for program initiation through a software command.

The PIT consists of several sections, but the functioning of the device is simple in concept. A clock is used to generate timing pulses; these divide real time into 10 μsec "bins," each of which is subdivided into several different phases, for control of timing of the many events that take place within single timing bins, in the internal logic of the PIT. These 10 μsec bins are the units of time which are counted by the timer. Whenever an *S* or *U* occurs, the timer value is strobed into an *S* or *U* buffer register, and the timer is reset. The pending output number is a function of which event or combination of events (*U*, *S*, *E*, or *O*) is pending for computer transmission, and the magnitude of the interval terminated by that event or combination of events.

Under most circumstances, the computer will respond to the request to transmit data after a variable length of time, either by effecting a transfer under program control or by automatic transfer via a data break or similar facility. Therefore, it is necessary to buffer event flags and their corresponding interval values. Furthermore, if the input events are independent, pairs of events may occur with any timing relationship, and a "queue" must be established in order to hold them and to push them forward for transfer to the computer in the order of their occurrence, under computer control. It is assumed that the computer can always process an event, *X*, (such as *U*) before the next occurrence of *X*, even though it cannot always process *X* before another type of input, *Y* (such as *S*), occurs. Therefore, a 4 × 4 matrix is needed for the queue in order to handle all possible timing relations among *U*, *S*, *E*, and *O* allowed within these constraints. If an input event occurs during a given timer bin (10 μsec), it is pushed forward in the queue to a level just behind the most recently filled queue level, if there is any pending event for transmission. If there is no event already pending, the flag is pushed all the way through to the output level. Events occurring during the same 10 μsec bin are advanced through the queue in such a fashion as to ensure that they are always on the same level at any time.

There is another occasion upon which queue advancing occurs: At the end of a

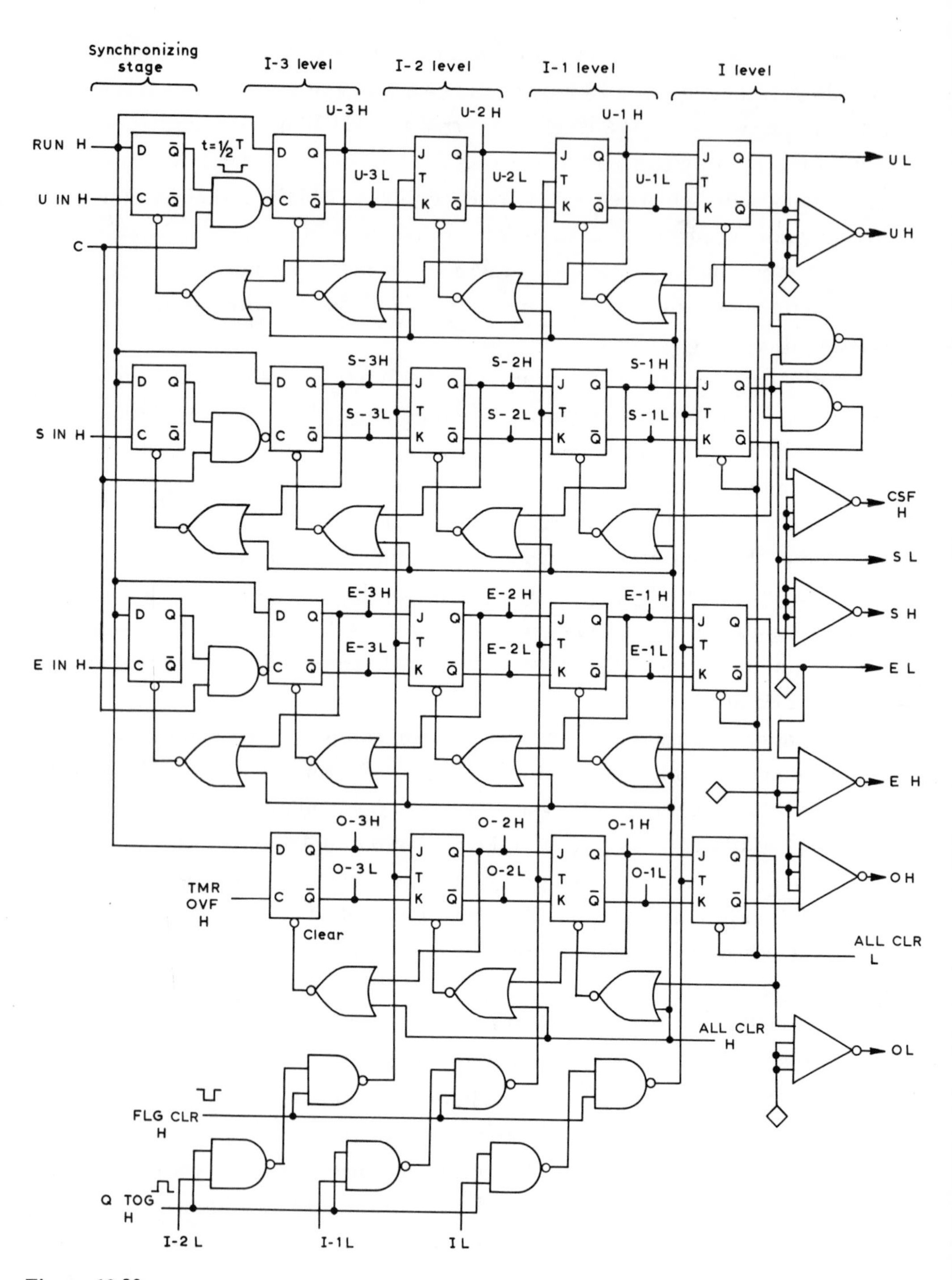

Figure 10.20
PIT queue, flag generation.

data transfer, the computer generates *TRANSMISSION COMPLETE H*, causing the entire queue to advance exactly one step, shifting the previous output flags out the end and entering the flags from the next level back, if there are any. The different queue levels are referred to as the *I*, *I-1*, *I-2*, and *I-3* levels (Figure 10.20); there is an earlier level for *U*, *S*, and *E*, for purposes of synchronizing their entry into the queue with the timer clock cycle. The *OVERFLOW* (*TMR OVF H*) is already synchronized with the clock cycle, and hence this level is not required for *O* flag queueing.

The queue consists of four specially designed right-shift registers, relying on two-phase shifting. A shift occurs on every *FLG CLR L* pulse (which occurs at the end of a data transmission), or on every *Q TOG H* (which occurs five times every clock cycle, timed so it never coincides with *FLG CLR L*). The two-phased shifting on *Q TOG H* is inhibited beyond the last unoccupied level, by "level busy" inhibit levels, called *I-2 L*, *I-1 L*, and *I L*. These are low if their corresponding queue levels are occupied. Generation of these levels is explained in detail below. They are required to "hold off" queue flags until the next level is cleared by a data transmission. At that time, *FLG CLR L* shifts all levels forward one place; *FLG CLR L* is not inhibited by the "level busy" low levels.

Each *I*-level flipflop is used as an output "flag" to the computer. Thus, if *U*, *S*, and *E* arrive during the same timer cycle, they are shifted forward together, and eventually *U H*, *S H*, and *E H* go on, to be transmitted on the next transfer to the computer.

Each flipflop is cleared under one of two conditions: (a) transfer of its contents to the next queue level (direct clearing by feedback from the next level) or (b) an *ALL CLR H*, a pulse generated by one of several conditions described below. The output flipflops are an exception to this rule: They are cleared by advancing the previous level's contents—because of the feedback clearing of the previous level—this means that any output level flipflop is cleared on level advancing if it was set in the first place. It may either remain off or be set, depending on the *I-1* level flag in that channel, if it was initially off. The output level is also cleared by *ALL CLR L*, which is simply the inverse of *ALL CLR H*, and will be described later. If *RUN H* is off (when the PIT has been stopped), no entries to the queue are possible, because *RUN H* provides the *D* inputs for the synchronizing level and the *I-3* level. Also, any condition that turns off *RUN H* also generates an *ALL CLR H* and *L*, which will clear every flipflop in the queue.

The operation of the queue will be discussed again after the operation of the timer clock and the timer are described. The clock (Figure 10.21) consists of a 2 MHz crystal oscillator whose output, *M*, is divided by an SN7490N decade divider

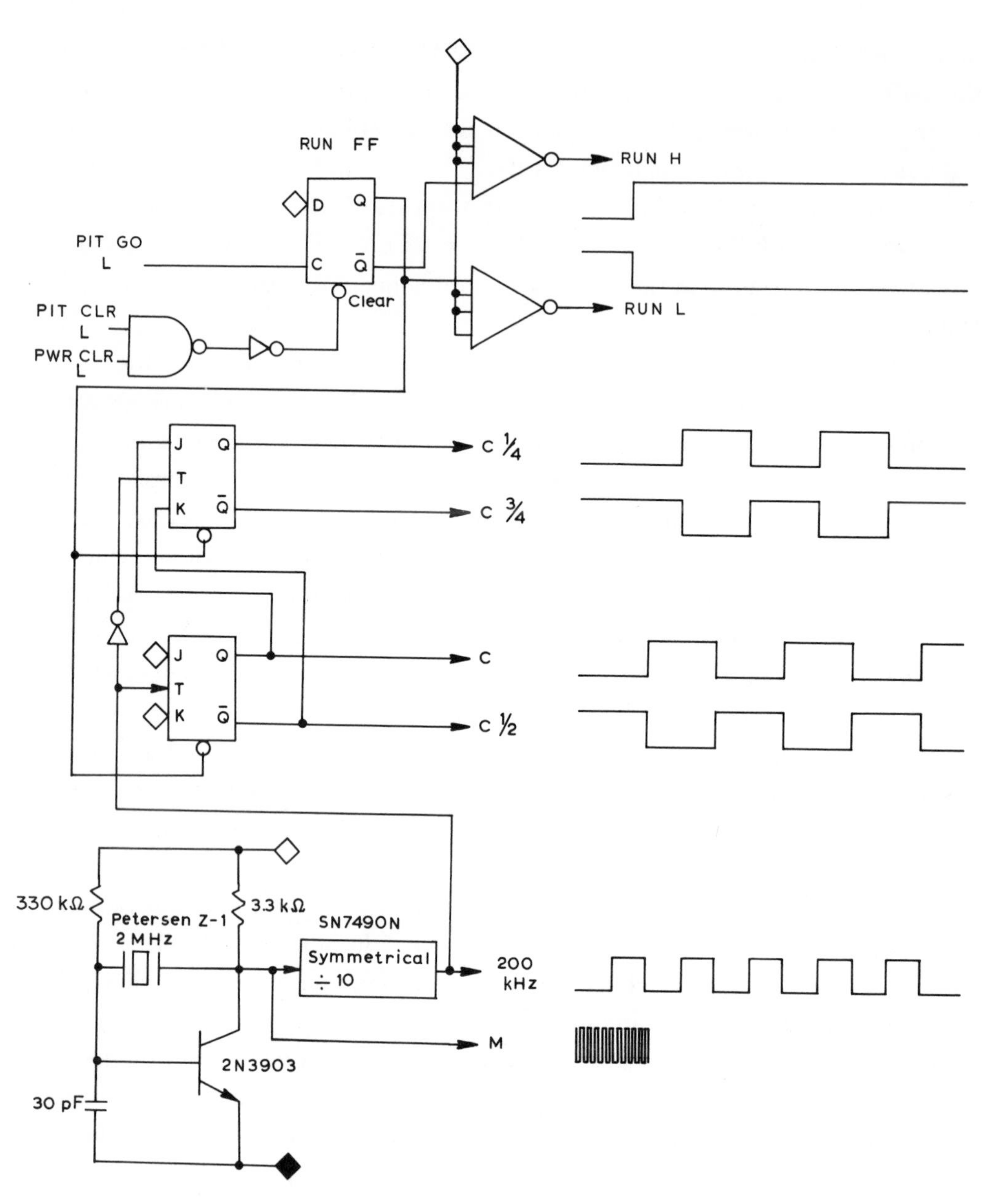

Figure 10.21
PIT clock frequency generator.

to produce a 200 kHz signal. This is coupled to a pair of flipflops configured to generate four separate 100 kHz signals separated from each other by quarter-cycle phase delays. These are labelled C, $C\frac{1}{4}$, $C\frac{1}{2}$, and $C\frac{3}{4}$. We will call the clock period T, the length of time it takes C to complete one cycle: 10 μsec. Positive transitions of C, $C\frac{1}{4}$, $C\frac{1}{2}$, and $C\frac{3}{4}$ will be said to occur at $t = 0\ (= T)$, $\frac{1}{4}T$, $\frac{1}{2}T$, and $\frac{3}{4}T$, respectively. These different signals will be used to control the relative timing of multiple events occurring within single C cycles.

We use *PITGO* to set the RUN FF, which generates *RUN H* (1) when it is on. When the FF is off, the clock-generating FFs are disabled, and the synchronizing level and I-3 queue level are disabled. The RUN FF is turned off by *PITCLR L* or *PWRCLR L*.

The timer section of the PIT (Figure 10.22) consists of four 4-bit binary counters and associated logic. The C is input to the counter generating the four least significant bits, and the D-output of that timer drives the next counter, continuing in series to the MSB, the fifteenth bit (the sixteenth bit is not used). We will use these fifteen bits as the timer value; count transitions occur at $\frac{1}{2}T$. Timer overflow is detected when the timer value goes to 77777_8, by ANDing all fifteen bits, using two 8-input NAND gates and a two-input NOR gate, to trigger a 100 nsec *TMR OVF H*.

The timer is allowed to count whenever C is running, and is reset by *PITCLR L* ∨ *PWRCLR* L ∨ (*USS* H ∧ *C*) ∨ *TMR OVF L*. The *USS H* occurs whenever a timer value is strobed into the U or S buffer, and ANDing it with C causes clearing on $t = 0$. Thus, whenever an interval is strobed into a buffer, the count goes to 00001 on the next clock cycle negative transition. Otherwise, an event occurring in the next cycle would be timed at an interval of 00000, which would be incorrect. Similarly, the *TMR OVF L* pulse causes the timer to be cleared immediately on a 77777_8 timer value, in order to allow the timer to go to 00001 on the next cycle.

The *ALL CLR H* and *L* are generated by either *PITCLR* or *PWRCLR*. Thus the timer is reset to zero, the clock is stopped (Figure 10.21), *RUN* goes off (Figure 10.21), and all queue FFs are cleared (Figure 10.20), as well as all the "level busy" flags (Figure 10.22). These flags are used to inhibit queue level entry into any already occupied levels, and *I H* is also used to request transfer of output to the computer. These flags are turned on by *LEV ADV L*, after each queue shift is completed, to inhibit shifting of new flags into those queue levels already occupied. Hence, the D-inputs of the FFs are derived from the NANDed low levels of the four FFs at that level, for example, the *I-1* FF is set on *LEV ADV L* if *U-1*, *S-1*, *E-1*, or *O-1* is on. Clearing of each flag except the *I*-level flag occurs on the

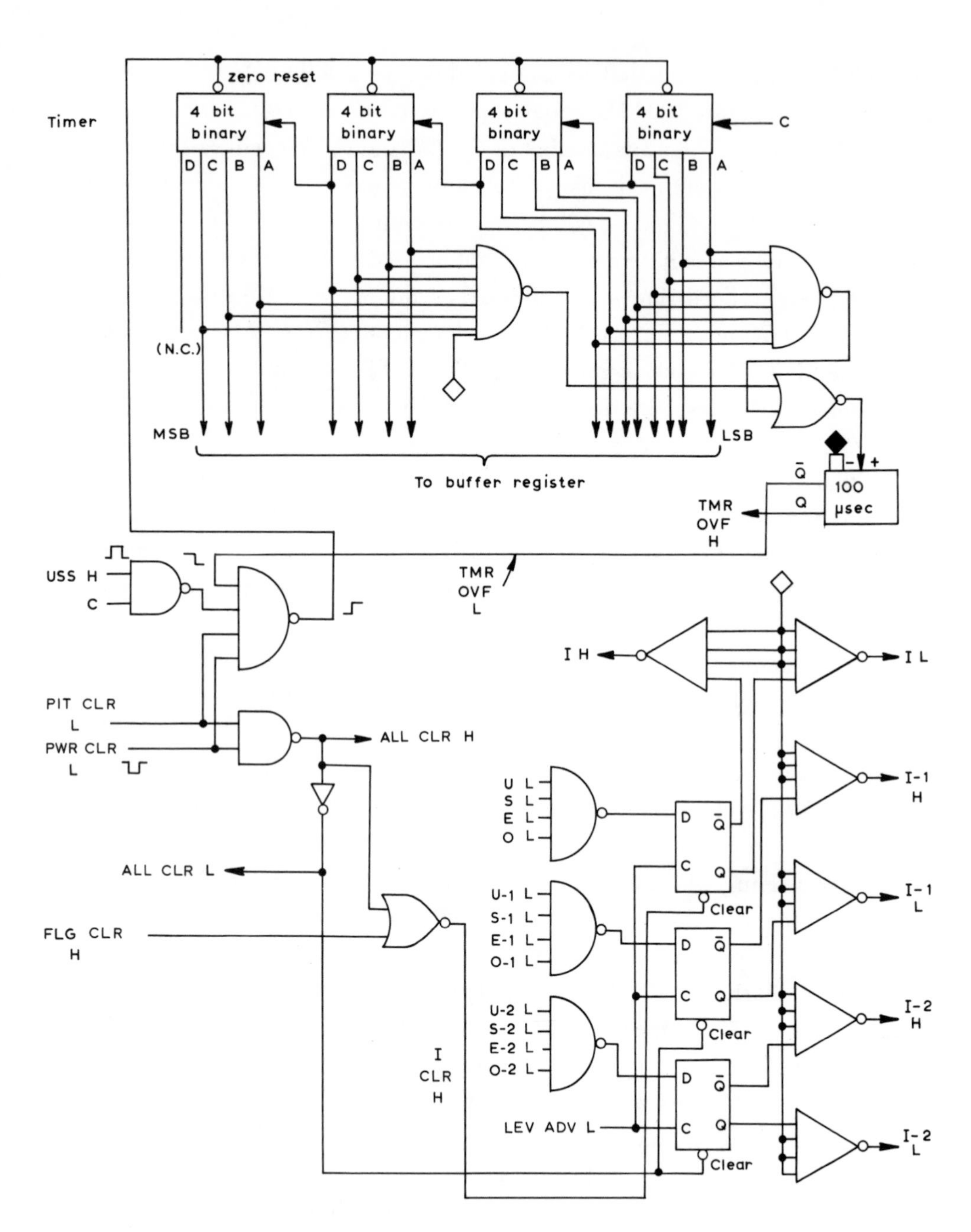

Figure 10.22
PIT timer, queue level flag generation, TMR OVF, ALL CLR.

first *LEV ADV L* after that level becomes unoccupied, since the preceding level cannot have had that channel on (because of feedback clearing in the queue), or on *ALL CLR L*. The *I*-level FF is cleared directly not only by *ALL CLR*, but also by *FLG CLR*. This is accomplished by using *ALL CLR H* $\overline{\vee}$ *FLG CLR H* to produce *I CLR L*, which is applied directly to the clear input. Thus, if the *I-1* level is occupied at the time of *FLG CLR*, *I H* goes off during *FLG CLR*, and back on at the end of *LEV ADV L*; this is necessary in order to achieve a new positive transition, signalling a new output for transmission to the computer. Otherwise, the output would not go off, and it would not signal readiness for the next transmission.

The *LEV ADV L* must occur after shifting is completed and prior to any subsequent shift. It is therefore generated on the trailing edge of *FLG CLR L* and *Q TOG H*, and a low pulse is used so settling can occur before the positive transition to the C-inputs of the *D* FFs of Figure 10.22. This process is illustrated in Figure 10.23, as is the generation of *Q TOG H* and *FLG CLR L*.

The *Q TOG H* is generated five times per clock cycle, as a 100 nsec pulse that fires on every positive transition of $M \overline{\wedge} C\frac{1}{2}$ (MC), that is, during the $C\frac{1}{2}$ *H* clock half-cycle ($t = \frac{1}{2}T$ to T), every 500 nsec. After each *Q TOG H* pulse, a *LEV ADV L* pulse occurs. Thus, any inputs which have set the synchronizing level and *I-3* level FFs before $t = \frac{1}{2}T$, will advance in parallel through their respective queue channels, to the right-most unoccupied level. On the last *Q TOG H* pulse and *LEV ADV L* pulse, the rightmost previously unoccupied level inhibit signal is on.

The synchronization of inputs to the queue occurs as follows: *U IN H*, *S IN H*, or *E IN H* will set the corresponding synchronizing level FF as long as the corresponding *I-3* level FF is off. At the next *C* negative transition, that flipflop level is NANDed with *C* to produce a positive transition to the *C* input of the corresponding *I-3* level FF setting it. The synchronizing level is reset by direct feedback via the NOR gate; since the *C*-input to the *I-3* level FF stays on once the synchronizing level FF goes off, there is no danger of losing the advancing bit during the 1-phase shift. In subsequent queue levels, 2-stage shifting is used. Thus *I-3* level FFs are set at $t = \frac{1}{2}T$ (Figure 10.20), before *Q TOG H* (which oscillates from $t = \frac{1}{2}T + 100$ nsec to $t = T$) and after $t = \frac{1}{4}T$, which is when the *FLG CLR L* shift pulse occurs, if it occurs. Since *TMR OVF* occurs at a *C* negative transition, it is always synchronized with the queue entry gating. Hence *TMR OVF H* is used to set the *O-3* FF directly.

The *FLG CLR L* occurs for 100 nsec, starting at $t = \frac{1}{4}T$. This is accomplished by synchronizing the *TRANSMISSION COMPLETE* pulse with a flipflop and a gate, in a fashion similar to the method used for synchronization of levels at the

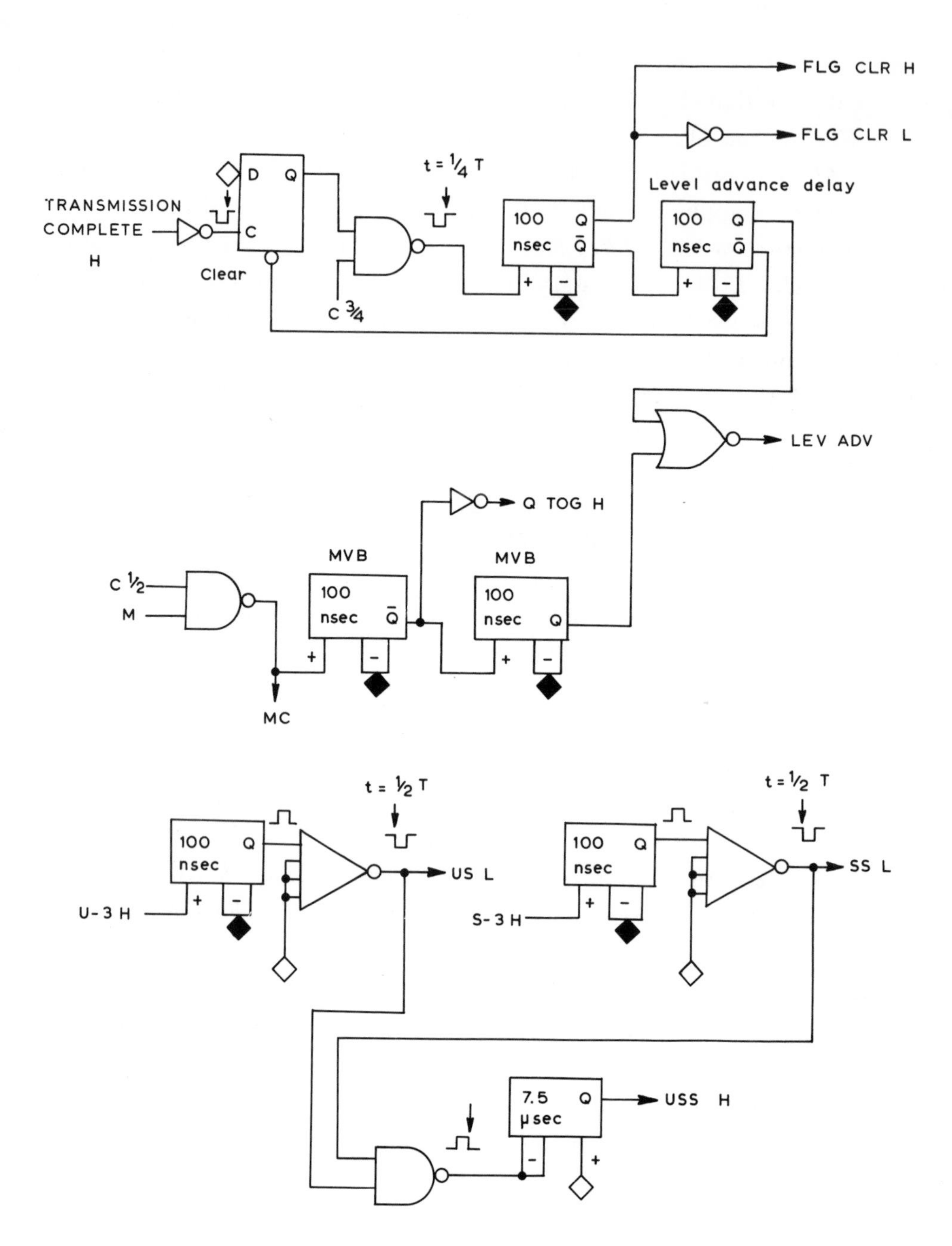

Figure 10.23
PIT FLG CLR, LEV ADV, Q TOG, unit and synch strobes.

queue. The *FLG CLR L* pulse is followed by the *LEV ADV L* pulse, which advances the "level occupied" flags.

The timer value must be strobed into the *U* output buffer or *S* output buffer (described below) during the half clock cycle after the *I-3* level is entered on the *U* or *S* channel because resetting occurs at $t = T$. Therefore (Figure 10.23) the *U-3 H* or *S-3* level positive transition triggers a 100 nsec pulse at about $t = \frac{1}{2}T$, and a low pulse positive transition (*US L* or *SS L*) is used to strobe the timer bits into the *U* or *S* buffer register, respectively, about 100 nsec after the *C* negative transition. Also, a 7.5 μsec MVB is triggered on the trailing edge of *US L* or *SS L*. This pulse, *USS H*, lasts from $t = \frac{1}{2}T$ to $t \cong T\frac{1}{4}$. This is NANDed with *C* (Figure 10.22) to clear the timer from the next $t = 0$ to $t \cong \frac{1}{4}T$, in time for the next *C* negative transition at $t = \frac{1}{2}T$ to increment the timer to 00001. This all occurs independently of subsequent shifting through the queue. The MVB used to generate *USS H* is ready for retriggering by the next *US L* or *SS L*.

The output buffer logic (Figure 10.24) consists of 15 *D*-flipflops for the *U* buffer, 15 *D*-FFs for the *S* buffer, and 45 gates for selecting the buffer (if any), which is gated to the output, for transmission of the appropriate interval value to the computer.

The 15 timer output bits are used as inputs to the *D*-inputs of the *U* and *S* 15-bit buffers. *US L* and *SS L* positive transitions, around 100 nsec after the timer increment, jam the timer bits into the corresponding buffer. Once the *U* or *S* flag comes on at the *I* level, the *U H* or *CSF H* flag will gate the corresponding *U* or *S* buffer bits through to the output. The *CSF* flag (Figure 10.20) is generated if *S H* and *U L* are both 1; that is, if both *U* and *S* are on, the *U*-buffer output is gated through to the *PIT OUTPUT* bits and not the *S* buffer.

Note that if *O H* is on, regardless of *S* or *U*, *O L* forces the three-input gates at the *PIT OUTPUT* on, regardless of *U* or *S* buffer values. This ensures that the output is 77777_8 when *O* is in the *I* level, regardless of the values in *U* or *S*. Indeed, *U* or *S* could generate 00000 in the corresponding buffer output when simultaneous with *TMR OVF*, because *TMR OVF* resets the timer potentially early enough for *US L* or *SS L* to strobe 00000 into the *U* or *S* buffer register. Also, since *E* generates no interval of its own accord, 00000 appears at the *PIT OUTPUT* if *E* occurs alone, which is convenient in the use of software elapsed-time counters used to measure cumulative intervals of various types, because the 15-bit timer value may always be added to the previous total interval and produce the correct total elapsed time. If *E* arrives simultaneously at the *I*-level with some other flag, the output interval is unaffected by *E*. Note also that the *PIT OUTPUT* value is held to 00000 when there is no pending output flag at the *I* level in the queue.

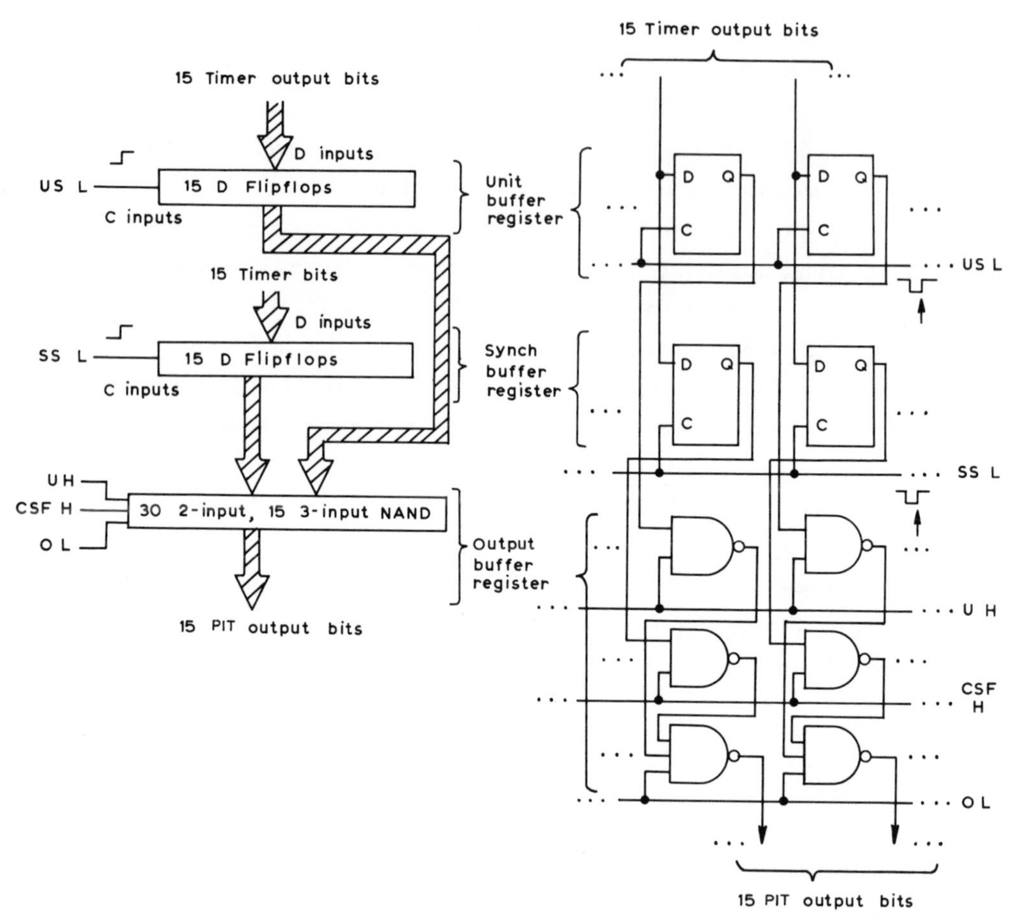

Figure 10.24
PIT output buffer resistor.

With no external input to the *PIT*, and with *RUN H* on, *O H* occurs every 32,767 clock cycles rather than every $2^{15} = 32{,}768$ cycles, because the timer goes from 32,767 to 1 instead of from 32,767 to 0. Zero is thus an illegal interval, as it must be for proper timing. The PIT, with no external input, will therefore generate *I H* with an *O H* flag, and transmits 77777 once every 327.67 msec. Thus, software cumulative-time variables may be updated by adding in the 15-bit number, regardless of the event leading to it. This is an economical choice of maximum interval value, because core filling is slow at this rate, and data are efficiently stored, mostly as nonoverflow values, since neural discharge rarely drops below one spike per 327 msec in mammalian neurons that have significant spontaneous activity or that are discharging in response to synaptic or sensory input. Although the 10 μsec resolution may seem excessively fine, some auditory neurons have been demonstrated to preserve certain aspects of stimulus timing with a precision of 50 to 100 μsec. Even in systems with less precisely timed discharges, the 10 μsec resolution is useful in the elimination of annoying "digitization artifacts" that can arise in the generation of histograms using timers with less resolution. If a larger unit of interval resolution is desired, adjust the 2 MHz clock rate and all MVB pulse duration values by multiplying by a factor equal to the new interval/10 μsec.

Although many details of programming are functions of the particular computer installation and the user's applications, some guidelines must be followed:

1. The program and the I/O controller must be able to handle worst-case sequences to the extent that flags which are held up in the *I-3* position advance to the next queue position before another input occurs. If occasional pile-ups are anticipated, an error-detecting flag might be useful. Further, the SYNCH or UNIT buffer value must be processed before the next input transition to the SYNCH or UNIT queue, respectively, or a new value will be strobed into the corresponding buffer, and the value for the first interval will be lost; the computer will then conclude that both intervals were of the same length, because it will read the same number both times.

2. The present enable circuits do not allow individual control of queue channel enable levels; obviously the user must distinguish between data to be sampled and inputs which occur between sample periods.

3. Only 15 bits were used out of 18 available in the particular computer used (DEC PDP-15) for coding interval values. Bit 0 (the sign bit) was used for coding *U*; the *S* (1) was coded as bit 1 (1); and the *E* (1) was coded as bit 2 (1). Since, in this system, 000000 is an illegal code, 000000 is used by the program to code end-of-data, allowing variable-length strings of bulk storage records to be used.

Selected References

Analog Devices, Inc. 1970a. *Model ADC-QM Analog-to-Digital Converters*. Cambridge, Mass.: Analog Devices, Inc.

——— 1970a. *Model MPX-8A Multiplexer*. Cambridge, Mass.: Analog Devices, Inc.

——— 1970b. *SHA-IA Sample and Hold Module*. Cambridge, Mass.: Analog Devices, Inc.

Blackman, R. B., and J. W. Tukey. 1958. *The Measurement of Power Spectra from the Point of View of Communications Engineering*. New York: Dover Publications.

Casby, J. U., R. Siminoff, and T. R. Houseknecht. 1963. An analogue cross-correlator to study naturally induced activity in intact nerve trunks. *J. Neurophysiol. 26:* 432–446.

Goldman, Stanford. 1968. *Frequency Analysis, Modulation and Noise*. New York: Dover Publications.

Gordon, Bernard M. 1970. Digital sampling and recovery of analog signals. *EEE 18*, 5: 65–75.

Hewlett-Packard Co. 1968. *Operating and Service Manual. Sweeping Local Oscillator 3593A/3594A*. Loveland, Colo.: Hewlett-Packard Co.

——— 1970a. *Operating and Service Manual. Model 3590A Wave Analyzer*. Loveland, Colo.: Hewlett-Packard Co.

——— 1970b. *Theory and Applications of Wave Analyzers*. Loveland, Colo.: Hewlett-Packard Co.

Hoeschle, David F., Jr. 1968. *Analog-to-Digital/Digital-to-Analog Conversion Techniques*. New York: Wiley-Interscience.

Hybrid Systems Corp. 1970. *Digital-to-Analog Converter Handbook*. Burlington, Mass.: Hybrid Systems Corp.

Langenthal, Ira M. 1970. Correlation and probability analysis. *Saicor Signals, TB14*. Hauppauge, New York: Signal Analysis Industries Corp.

Moore, George P., Jose P. Segundo, Donald H. Perkel, and Herbert Levitan. 1970. Statistical signs of synaptic interactions in neurons. *Biophys. J. 10:* 876.

Perkel, Donald H., George L. Gerstein, and George P. Moore. 1967. Neuronal spike trains and stochastic point processes. I. The single spike train. *Biophys. J. 7:* 391.

——— 1967. Neuronal spike trains and stochastic point processes. II. Simultaneous spike trains. *Biophys. J. 7:* 419.

Rosenblith, Walter A. 1959. *Processing Neuroelectric Data*. Cambridge, Mass.: MIT Press.

Saicor. 1971. *Modular Approach to Measurement of Cross Spectral Density and Other Statistical Parameters*. Hauppauge, N.Y.: Signal Analysis Industries Corp.

Smith, Bruce K. 1970. Digital-to-analog converters and their performance specifications. *EEE 18*, 11: 54–59.

11 POWER SUPPLIES

Bruce W. Maxfield

This chapter is devoted to a discussion of methods that are used for converting the 60 Hz line voltage to direct current.

11.1 Rectification

Rectification is the conversion of an ac voltage into a dc voltage (or current). One means of achieving rectification is shown in Figure 11.1; the two diodes are arranged to permit the flow of current in only one direction through the load resistor connected between the output terminal and ground. Since both the positive and negative going portions of the ac input voltage are directed by these diodes to flow through the load, the circuit is called a *full-wave rectifier*. The input and output wave forms are shown in Figure 11.2. Actually, the peak output voltage is slightly smaller than the peak input voltage, because there is always one diode in series with the load. With the diodes connected as shown, the output

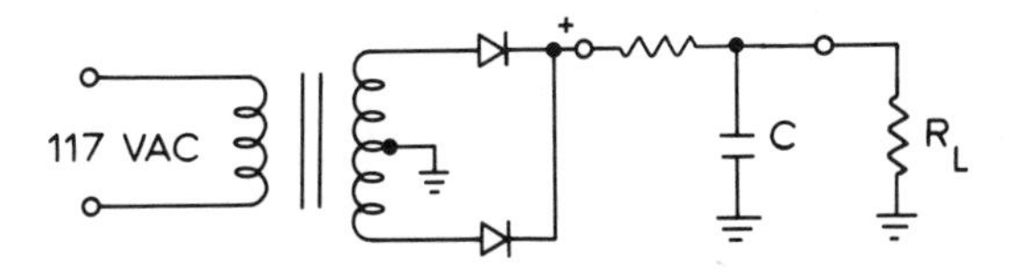

Figure 11.1
A full-wave rectifier.

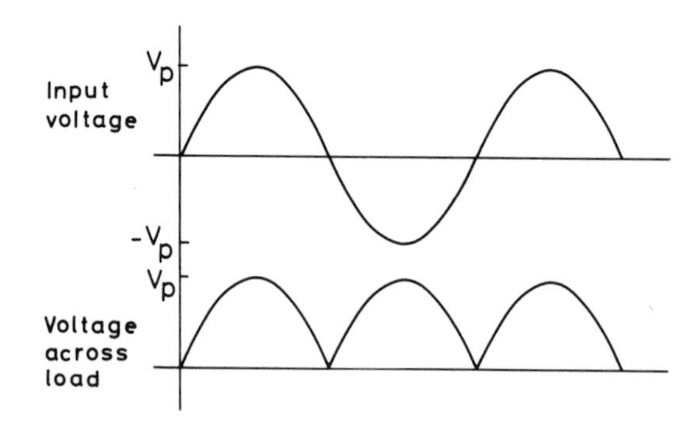

Figure 11.2
Input and output voltages from the full-wave rectifier shown in Figure 11.1.

is positive with respect to ground. Reversing the diode polarity reverses the output polarity. The peak output voltage appears across each diode when it is reverse biased. Therefore, these diodes must have a peak inverse voltage (PIV) rating at least as great as the peak voltage. Because of internal heating, all diodes have a limited current capacity. It is usually necessary to heat sink power diodes. Since the diode forward resistance is small, the current delivered by a rectifier is determined almost completely by the load resistance.

A bipolar power supply, that is, one having both a positive and negative output voltage with respect to ground, can be obtained using two of the full-wave rectifiers shown in Figure 11.1 with each set of two diodes connected to provide the correct polarity. Of course, each set of diodes can be driven from the same center-tapped transformer. Such a circuit, often called a *full-wave bridge rectifier*, is discussed later (see Figure 11.5). Bridge rectifiers are available as single units.

11.2 Filtering and Regulation

For a full-wave rectifier to be a useful source of voltage and current, the output must be filtered (smoothed). The residual ac voltage left in the dc output is called *ripple*. It is also usually desirable to have a voltage or current source whose output is reasonably independent of the load; that is, some form of regulation is necessary. Regulation is usually specified in terms of drift (very low frequency changes in the output) at constant load and output changes when either the input or load are changed suddenly (line and load regulation, respectively).

11.2.1 A Simple RC Filter

If the load will remain constant and if a few percent ripple and the normal few percent drift in output voltage due to heating and aging effects can be tolerated, then active transistor regulation may not be necessary. The relatively large output impedance of an RC filter can be tolerated simply because the load is constant.

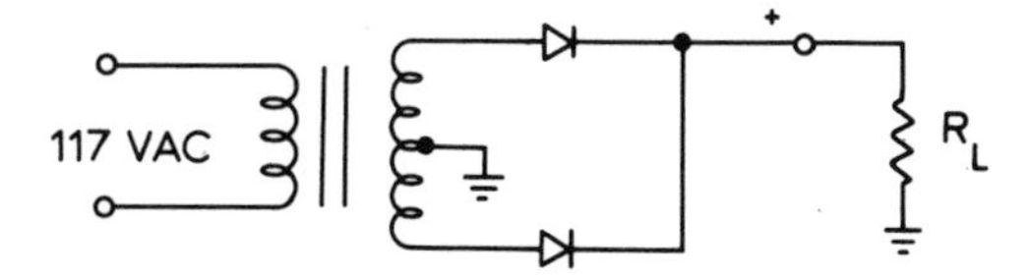

Figure 11.3
A full-wave rectifier with output smoothed by a low-pass RC filter.

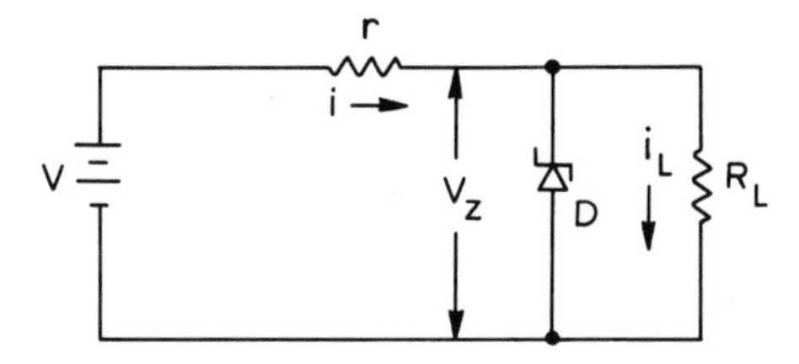

Figure 11.4
A Zener diode used as a voltage regulator.

Under these conditions, a simple RC low-pass network on the output of a full-wave rectifier is adequate and the circuit shown in Figure 11.3 may be an acceptable power source. The output resistance of this circuit is approximately equal to R. The load resistance should be at least a few times R if the filtering action is to be determined primarily by RC. Power supplies using a simple RC filter have poor load regulation and ripple characteristics and are therefore of very little use in powering most electronic equipment.

11.2.2 A Zener Diode Voltage Regulator

A simple Zener diode voltage regulator circuit is given in Figure 11.4. The battery V represents any source of dc voltage (not necessarily steady), and r represents its output resistance. In particular, V and r could be replaced by the rectifier and filter network in Figure 11.3. The voltage across the load is determined by the breakdown voltage of the Zener diode (it should be clear that $V > V_Z$ is a necessary condition for regulation). Because V_Z has a small current dependence, the output impedance is quite low; typical values range from about 100 Ω in 1-W Zener diodes to about 1 Ω in 50-W units. Note that the Zener diode must be able to handle the maximum load current.

A transistor can be used to improve the regulation of a Zener diode by further lowering the output impedance. A Zener having a power rating sufficient to handle the base current instead of the total load current can be used. This permits the use of Zener diodes having a much lower temperature coefficient. Figure 11.5 shows a bipolar power supply that can be used for the power requirements of many op amps and other ICs when the best possible circuit performance is not

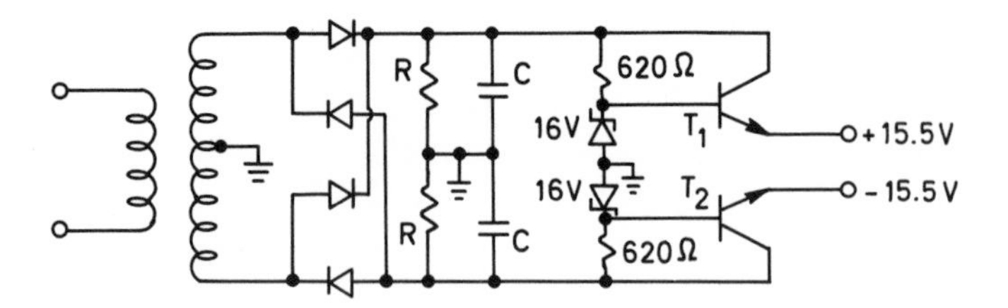

Figure 11.5
A Zener regulated bipolar power supply. The transformer output can range from 18-0-18 to about 28-0-28 (all rms values). Voltages shown are for 18 V input.

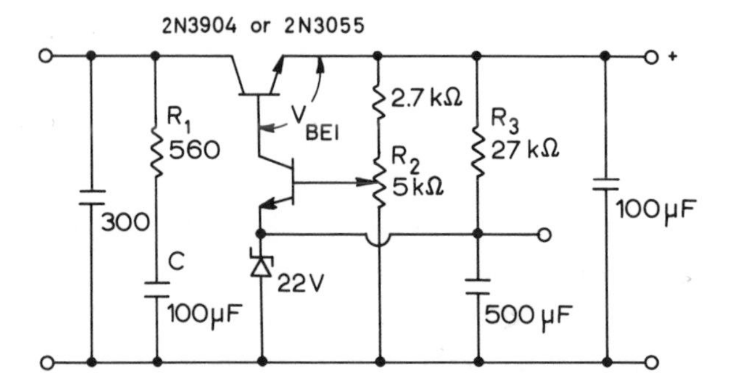

Figure 11.6
A series type transistorized voltage regulator using negative feedback to lower the output impedance. Voltages are measured values under open circuit output conditions and 36 V dc input.

required. The output current must not exceed the maximum collector currents, of either T_1 or T_2.

11.2.3 Transistorized Voltage Regulator

When smaller ripple or better load regulation than is available using either of the two previous methods is required, electronic methods incorporating much more negative feedback must be used. A fairly simple yet practical voltage regulator using two transistors and a reference Zener diode is shown in Figure 11.6. This circuit will give about 1% load regulation for load currents up to 200 mA. Larger currents can be obtained by using a higher wattage transistor in place of T_1. The output impedance is about 1 Ω. There is nothing critical about the transistor types used in this circuit. T_1 should have a collector breakdown voltage at least 20 percent larger than the maximum dc output voltage. Maximum load current requirements determine the maximum collector current through T_1. Transistors of large β are available with collector currents up to about 100 mA. Larger load currents will require a transistor of β smaller than the 2N3904 and will therefore result in slightly poorer regulation.

The Zener diode fixes the emitter potential of T_2. The setting of potentiometer R_2 determines the base voltage on T_2 and hence controls V_{BE2}. The base current for T_1 is supplied primarily through R_1. If T_1 has a collector current of 200 mA and $\beta = 100$, only about 2 mA flows through R_1. Since this produces about a 1-V drop, the base and collector are at about the same potential. The collector current, I_{C1}, is controlled by V_{BE1} which, in turn, is controlled by V_{BE2}. If the output voltage decreases, then V_{BE2} decreases, causing $V_{C2} = V_{B1}$ to increase. An increased forward bias on T_1 decreases the voltage drop across T_1 and increases the current through T_1. Thus the error signal fed to the base of T_2 tends to compensate for the initial decrease in output voltage. This negative feedback applies equally well to ripple (and other "noise"), output changes due to varying load conditions and changes in the input voltage (due to line voltage changes). Negative feedback increases the effective capacitance in the filter section if the loop gain is large at the ripple frequency. Capacitor C_2 decreases the loop gain as the frequency increases, and C_3 prevents ripple from producing a compensating change in V_{BE2}.

The control potentiometer R_2 permits some adjustment to be made in the output voltage since it determines the voltage drop across T_1. Regulation is limited by the temperature stability of the Zener diode, the temperature coefficient of V_{BE1} and the finite loop gain. Common carbon composition resistors are sufficiently stable that they should not limit the performance of this regulator. The R_3 fixes the current through the Zener diode at some value near the recommended Zener current I_Z. Neglecting the small emitter current in T_2, we obtain $I_Z = (V_o - V_Z)/R_3$. A large output current can destroy T_1 so the circuit should not be operated with the output shorted.

11.2.4 Voltage Regulators Using Operational Amplifiers

When line and load regulation better than about 1% or very small ripple (less than about 1 mV) is required, it is necessary to use a negative feedback amplifier having a large loop gain. The circuit in Figure 11.7 is one means of obtaining a stable bipolar power supply. Component values and voltages are given for outputs of ± 15 V. Circuit operation is similar to that discussed previously in Figure 11.6. The positive output voltage V_o^+ is determined by

$$V_o^+ = V_Z(R_1 + R_3)/R_1, \tag{11.1}$$

and the negative output voltage V_o^- by

$$V_o^- = -V_o^+(R_2/R_4). \tag{11.2}$$

The positive output requires npn transistors and the negative output pnp transistors.

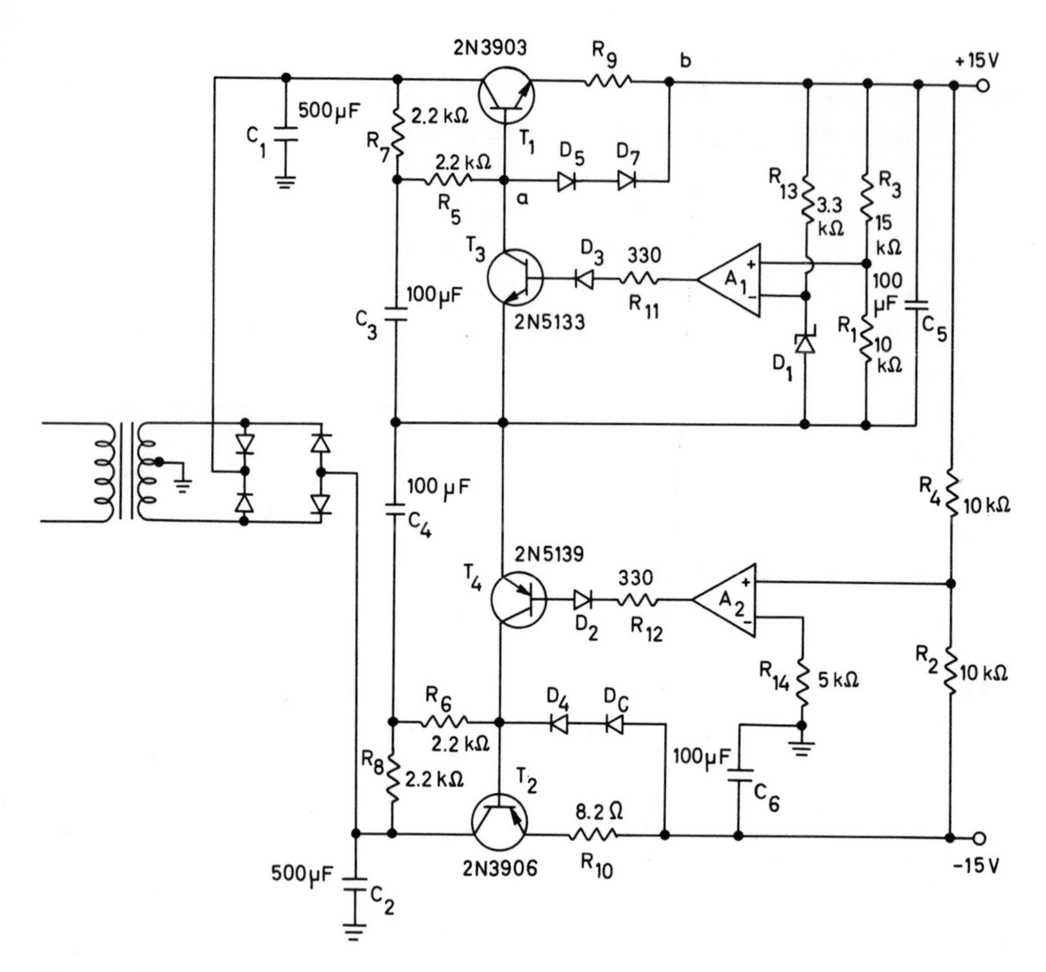

Figure 11.7
A bipolar, constant voltage supply. Component values and voltages (with respect to ground) are shown for an output of ±15 V and an output current of 75 mA.

Diodes D_2 and D_3 protect transistors T_2 and T_4, respectively, from a large base-emitter reverse bias, and they reduce drastically the loop gain if an output surge causes the feedback to become positive momentarily. Capacitors C_5, C_6 reduce the loop gain at high frequency and therefore help to ensure that the feedback is always negative. The R_5 and C_3 roll off the current gain of T_3 above $\omega_{CL} = 1/R_5C_3$, and R_6 and C_4 serve to stabilize the loop gain of T_4. Resistors $R_7 + R_5$ and $R_8 + R_6$ supply the base current requirements of T_1 and T_3, respectively.

Silicon diodes D_5, D_7, and resistor R_9 serve to limit the positive output current. Because of the two series diodes between the base and the output side of the emitter resistor R_9, the maximum dc potential difference between points *a* and *b* is the forward drop across these two diodes or about 1.2 V. There is a drop of about 0.6 V across the base-emitter junction of T_1 so the maximum drop across R_9 is about 0.6 V; this limits the output current to about

$$I_{\text{max}} = \frac{0.6 \text{ V}}{R_9} \tag{11.3}$$

or about 75 mA for the component values shown. The output current cannot exceed this value; if it tries to, the diodes short out some of the base current so as to maintain about an 0.6 V drop across R_9. Short-circuit protection such as provided by D_5, D_7, and R_9 is extremely easy to add to any regulator using a series output transistor (such as T_1). Both the output transistor and external circuitry are thereby protected from excessive currents. Diodes D_5 and D_7 can be quite low power, because they must carry, at most, the collector current of T_3. Similar arguments apply to diodes D_4, D_6, resistor R_{10}, and transistor T_2.

The output current of this supply can be increased by reducing R_9 and using higher-power transistors for T_1 and T_2. Since the output voltage is also used to power the op amps, it must be kept within a specified range. For the 741 op amp, this is between ± 12 and ± 22 V.

11.2.5 Modular Power Supplies

A number of modular power supplies featuring op amp (IC) regulation are available. These normally require a specified ac input voltage (from a center-tapped transformer if it is a bipolar supply). A set of voltage, current, line, load, drift and ripple characteristics are specified for each unit. Modular power supplies are often epoxy encapsulated and so are nearly impossible to repair. They are, however, very convenient and compact.

GLOSSARY

A
Ampere.

Absolute maximum ratings
Ratings for operating parameters of a circuit that must never be exceeded to avoid damage to the circuit.

Absolute-value circuit
A circuit that produces an output signal proportional to the absolute voltage of the input signal. An ideal full-wave rectifier is an absolute-value circuit.

ac
Alternating current.

ac Voltmeter
A voltmeter designed to measure rms ac voltage.

Accommodation Q
The reciprocal of the distance for which the eye is focused, q.

Active components
Elements such as transistors and vaccuum tubes, which have a conductance that may be varied by means of an externally applied control signal, and which therefore can be used as amplifiers.

Active filters
Filters that are constructed with active elements.

A/D conversion
Analog-to-digital conversion.

Adder-subtracter, analog
Circuit whose output voltage is proportional to the sum of inverted and noninverted input voltages.

Adder-subtracter, digital
Circuit whose digital output is the sum or difference of two or more digital input numbers.

Address, multiplexer
Digital specification of multiplexer channel (input). Every input has a unique address, although some addresses may not represent any existing input. *See also* Multiplexer.

Admittance Y in ohm^{-1}
Inverse of impedance Z.

AFC
Automatic frequency control.

AGC
Automatic gain control.

AM
Amplitude modulation.

American Wire Gauge
Standardized nomenclature for describing wire diameters.

Ammeter
Meter for measuring current.

Ampere
Unit of current, defined as 1 coulomb/sec.

Amplifier
Any device that, within practical limitations, can be specified as multiplying the input voltage, current, or power by a fixed or controllable factor. An ideal amplifier has no other effect.

Amplitude modulation AM
Control of a circuit's gain by means of a control voltage (modulator signal), in order to vary the envelope of a higher frequency signal, the carrier. Analog multiplication.

Analog
Continuously variable, capable of a stable level at any of an infinite number of values over a finite range. Term applied to signals and circuits that process them. *See also* Digital.

Analog computer
A computer whose working elements are analog circuits. *See also* Computer, Digital Computer, Hybrid Computer.

Analog multiplexing
Switching of analog signals under digital control to produce an output which is equal to the selected input channel. *See also* Multiplexer.

Analog-to-digital (A/D) conversion
Representation of an analog quantity, usually voltage, as a digital number, usually in the form of a binary signal.

AND
A dyadic logical operation. A AND B is true if and only if A is true and B is true.

AND gate
Digital device whose output is a logical 1 if and only if all of its inputs are logical 1.

AND/NAND fluidic gate
Digital fluidic device with two outputs, one of which is logical 1 if and only if all the inputs are logical 1; the other output is the inverse: It is 0 if and only if all the inputs are 1.

Angular frequency ω
In rad/sec $= 2\pi f$.

Anode
The terminal of a device that is the most positive; *i.e.*, the positive-voltage terminal of a battery, the end of a diode that is relatively positive during forward-bias operation.

Antilog circuit
A circuit whose output is proportional to the antilogarithm of the input.

Astable multivibrator
A binary device whose output alternates periodically between 1 and 0.

Audio
Pertaining to sound. Audio frequencies are the audible frequencies. An audio signal is either derived from a sound or is intended to produce a sound, and audio circuits are specifically intended for processing audio signals.

Autocorrelation function
A function describing the degree of periodicity of a signal. Defined as

$$C(\tau) = \lim_{T\to\infty} \frac{1}{T} \int_{-T/2}^{T/2} X(t) \cdot X(t + \tau)\, dt.$$

Automatic gain control AGC
Feedback control of a circuit's gain, to maintain a fixed output voltage or signal power.

Available output noise power N, in watts
$N = N_g G = ktBG$, or the anticipated output noise power of a circuit. *See also* Available input noise power, Available power gain, Effective bandwidth.

Available power gain G, in watts
$G = S/S_g$, or the ratio of available output power to available signal power, for the middle of a network's pass band.

Available signal power s, in watts
Maximum power that can be delivered by a signal generator.

AWG
American Wire Gauge.

B
Susceptance.

Balanced modulation
Suppressed carrier modulation. A balanced modulator produces the product of two ac signal voltages, the carrier and the modulator. Usually the carrier has a fixed frequency and amplitude, and the modulator is time-varying, with an upper cutoff frequency that is substantially lower than the carrier frequency.

Bandpass filter
Filter that has a fixed gain, usually unity, for all frequencies within a specified band and that attenuates frequencies above and below the bandpass limits.

Bandpass noise
Noise that is equivalent to white noise put through a bandpass filter. The spectrum is flat over the passband and monotonically decreases at frequencies above and below the bandpass limits.

Base
The control region of a bipolar transistor.

BCD
Binary Coded Decimal.

Beat frequency oscillator BFO
An oscillator whose output frequency is the difference between two input frequencies.

Bernoulli series
Series of 1s and 0s which are randomly related to each other. A series of coin tosses is a Bernoulli series.

BFO
Beat frequency oscillator.

Bias circuit
A circuit used to control or offset the baseline (dc component) of a signal.

Bias current
For a differential amplifier, the common-mode offset current required to bring the output to zero volts.

Bias voltage
For a transistor, the dc offset applied to the input signal to set the operating point. For a differential amplifier, the common-mode offset voltage required to bring the output to zero volts.

Bimorph
A two-layered piezoelectric device, usually constructed so the axes of the two layers point in opposite directions, in order to produce bending of the device upon application of a voltage, or voltage generation upon bending.

Binary arithmetic
Arithmetic using numbers in the binary number system, which has a modulus (radix, base) of 2.

Binary coded decimal BCD
A method of representing decimal digits as 4-bit binary numbers.

Binary logic
Two-valued logic.

Bipolar integrated circuit
An integrated circuit using bipolar (*pn*) junctions for all active devices.

Bipolar junction transistor
A transistor using two *pn* junctions: a *pnp* or *npn* transistor. The bias across the base-emitter junction controls the flow of current from emitter to collector.

Bistable multivibrator
A device that has two stable output states and that will switch from one to the other in response to an appropriate input signal.

Bit
A binary digit.

Blur
Decreased sharpness of an image; for example, the smoothing of an originally sharp dark-light boundary by moving the plane of a projection out of the focal plane of the projecting optics.

Boltzmann's constant k
The proportionality between pressure and temperature of an ideal gas: $k = \frac{P}{nT}$, where P is pressure, T is temperature, and n is number of particles per unit volume. Useful in statistical mechanics and thermodynamics.

Breadboard
A device used to interconnect and disconnect quickly electronic components to test circuit designs or construct temporary working circuits.

Bridge circuit
A circuit composed of at least four elements in a loop, with an input applied across two alternate nodes and output taken from two other nodes.

Bridge rectifier
A full-wave rectifier, constructed from diodes in a bridge circuit. An ideal bridge rectifier is an absolute-value circuit.

C
Capacitance, in farads (electronic).

C
Capacitance, in square inches (fluidic).

Calibration
(a) Setting of circuit adjustments in order to cause circuit performance to meet specifications. (b) Comparison of measured circuit parameters against a standard, in order to tabulate or graph a conversion chart or *calibration curve*, or to mark dials on controls.

Capacitance C in farads
In electronics, the ability of a device to store a charge under an applied voltage. Defined by the equation $C = q/V$. An ideal capacitor has infinite resistance and zero inductance. 1 F = 1 coulomb/volt.

Capacitor
A device used to introduce capacitance, with a minimum of inductance and conductance. Practical limits are 1 pF to 10^4 μF.

Capacitor coupling
Interposing a capacitor in a signal path, to pass ac and block dc.

Carbon resistor
Resistor made from a carbon composition. These are the cheapest variety, ranging from a few ohms to 10^8 Ω, with common tolerances of 1, 5, 10, and 20%.

Carrier
(a) The physical entity which moves under the influence of an applied emf, and hence the vehicle for current. (b) The frequency, usually fixed, whose amplitude is modulated by a signal, the modulator, in amplitude modulation. *See also* Amplitude modulation.

Cathode
The negative end of a device; for example, the negative terminal of a battery, or the end of a diode that is relatively negative when the diode is forward biased.

Channel, multiplexer
One of the inputs to a multiplexer. *See also* Multiplexer.

Characteristic polynomial
A polynomial used to describe the generating (feedback) function for a shift-register pseudorandom noise generator.

Chip
The substrate carrying a semiconductor device, or sometimes, the device itself, not including the mounting leads or package.

Clipper circuit
A circuit whose output is proportional to the input within specified limits, and which is equal to the output limit voltage whenever the input voltage exceeds the output limit divided by the circuit gain. Clipping may be of either polarity, or both.

Closed-loop gain m' (dimensionless)
The gain of a circuit using an operational amplifier with feedback. *See also* Open-loop gain.

Closed-loop gain error (dimensionless)
The deviation of the closed-loop gain from theoretical closed-loop gain for an ideal operational amplifier, expressed as percent of theoretical closed-loop gain.

CML current-mode logic
A form of digital logic that relies on the switching of current paths, using circuitry which is not driven to saturation or cutoff.

Coanda effect
See Wall-attachment effect.

Cold solder joint
A solder joint which has crystallized due to improper cooling, a cold soldering iron, or movement during cooling. Cold solder joints are unreliable, both electrically and mechanically.

Collector
In a forward-biased bipolar transistor, the terminal that is the sink for the charge carriers migrating across the base region. *See also* Base, Emitter.

Collector characteristics
A set of curves describing collector current as a function of collector-emitter voltage, given various base currents.

Color coding
(a) Method of coding the properties of a component, especially the resistance and tolerance of a resistor. (b) Method of coding functions of wires used to interconnect components or modules.

Common base configuration
One-transistor circuit configuration of a four-terminal device in which the base of the transistor is one terminal for both output and input.

Common collector configuration
One-transistor circuit configuration of a four-terminal device in which the collector of the transistor is one terminal for both output and input.

Common drain configuration
One-transistor FET circuit configuration of a four-terminal device in which the drain of the field effect transistor is one terminal for both output and input.

Common emitter configuration
One-transistor circuit configuration of a four-terminal device in which the emitter of the transistor is one terminal for both output and input.

Common gate configuration
One transistor FET circuit configuration of a four-terminal device in which the gate of the field effect transistor is one terminal for both output and input.

Common mode rejection
Cancellation of a signal that is common to two terminals, by differential amplification.

Common-mode rejection ratio CMRR (dimensionless)
A measure of common-mode rejection, expressed as the ratio of output signal of a differential amplifier, to expected amplitude of that signal if amplified single ended. Usually expressed in dB. Usually expressed for large voltages: the common-mode signal required in order to produce a maximum output voltage, divided by the single-ended voltage required to produce the same output.

Common mode voltage
That portion of a differential signal that is common to both terminals.

Common source configuration
A one-transistor FET configuration of a four-terminal device, in which the source of the field effect transistor is one terminal for both output and input.

Comparator
A device whose output signals the sign of the difference between two inputs. Usually, an analog comparator's output is logical 1 if the positive input is more positive than the negative input, and a digital comparator's output is logical 1 if the signal input bits correspond to a larger binary number than the reference input bits.

Complex numbers
Composite numbers of the form $a + bi$, where a and b are real numbers and i is the square root of -1; bi is an *imaginary number*.

Computer
A device that can perform a sequence of operations, specified by a *program*, on a set of *input data* and/or data stored in *memory*, to produce a set of output data, and/or new data stored in memory. The data and the program are variable. *See also*, Analog computer, Digital computer, Hybrid computer.

Condenser
Capacitor.

Conductance G
Inverse of resistance, in mhos ℧, defined as $G = 1/R = I/E$. 1 amp/volt $=$ 1 ohm^{-1} $=$ 1 mho.

Conductor
A device used to approximate an ideal conductor, which has zero resistance, zero capacitance, and zero inductance. Typically made of materials with resistivities of around 10^{-8} Ωm.

Conservation of charge
The inability of chemical or physical processes to alter the total net positive or negative charge in a closed system. This means that current past a point results from the accumulation of the same amount of charge at the sink as is supplied by the source, according to the equation

$$\int_{t_1}^{t_2} i\,dt = -\int_{t_1}^{t_2} \frac{dq_{\text{source}}}{dt} = \int_{t_1}^{t_2} \frac{dq_{\text{sink}}}{dt}.$$

Constant-current source
A source of specifiable current, either fixed or controllable, that within its operating limits will deliver the specified current into any load.

Constant-temperature reservoir
Any object whose temperature is invariant, regardless of heat flow into or out of it, within specified operating limits.

Control port
The hole in a fluidics device through which the input is coupled.

Controlled rectifier
See Silicon controlled rectifier.

Corner frequency f_0
Frequency at which $V_0/V_i = -3$ dB, on the skirt of a device's transfer function.

Correlation
In statistics, the degree of deviation from a random relation between one variable and another: A correlation of -1 indicates a perfect linear relation with negative slope, a correlation of 0 indicates a totally random relation, and a correlation of $+1$ indicates a perfectly linear relation with a positive slope.

Coulomb
Unit of charge.

Counter
Any device which will keep a record of the number of input events.

Cross-correlation
A measure of temporal correlation between two signals. Defined as

$$C_{XY}(\tau) = \lim_{T\to\infty} \frac{1}{T}\int_{-T/2}^{T/2} X(t)\cdot Y(t+\tau)\,dt.$$

Crossover distortion
Distortion produced by a push-pull amplifier or a crossover network.

Crystal oscillator
Oscillator whose output frequency is primarily determined by a quartz crystal used as a capacitor in a resonant circuit.

CTR
Current transfer ratio.

Current I in amperes
Rate of flow of charge past a point, or rate of change of total charge dq/dt, in coulombs/sec.

Current boost amplifier
An amplifier used as an impedance transformer, to lower the source impedance of a signal and hence increase the current capability of the signal source. Voltage gain is usually unity.

Current divider
A parallel resistor network used to controllably divide input current into a set of output currents, in a known proportion.

Current feedback
Feedback of current from output to input. The current feedback is proportional to output voltage, as in negative feedback to a virtual ground.

Current loop
A current path within a circuit that can be traced from a node, through components and nodes,

back to the starting node. A current loop can pass through any number of nodes and components as long as it does not cross itself, and it may be composed of smaller current loops.

Current transfer ratio CTR
Ratio of output current to input current.

Cutoff
Reduction of a bipolar transistor's collector current to a minimum by appropriate base bias.

dB
Decibel

dc
Direct current.

DCTL Diode-Capacitor-Transistor Logic
A type of digital logic.

de Morgan's theorem.
$-(A \wedge B) = \bar{A} \vee \bar{B}$; and $-(A \vee B) = \bar{A} \wedge \bar{B}$.

Dead-zone amplifier
An amplifier whose output voltage is proportional to input voltage, minus a constant, for outputs greater than the constant times circuit gain, and whose output voltage is zero for inputs less than the constant times circuit gain.

Debugging
A term borrowed from computer-programming jargon, meaning the detection and elimination of design or construction errors, or *bugs*.

Decade counter
A counter used to count events in the decimal system, usually with BCD elements.

Decibel dB
Logarithmic unit of gain and attenuation (dimensionless). Twenty decibels (power) is a ratio of 10:1 between input and output, 0 dB is unity gain. Attenuation is represented as negative dB, amplification as positive dB.

Decoupling
Increasing impedance between two signal paths to the point where there is negligible interaction, either for the entire signal(s), or for specified frequency components.

Delay line
A network used to produce a delay between input and output signals, with negligible effect on other characteristics of the signal.

Depletion mode
Operation of a field effect transistor with a bias that diminishes the available carriers relative to the unbiased state.

Differential amplifier
An amplifier whose output closely approximates the gain times the difference between the non-inverting (positive) and inverting (negative) inputs, within its bandpass range: $V_o = (V^+ - V^-)m$. The output may be differential or single ended.

Differential comparator
A comparator which measures the difference between two inputs, and whose output is logical 1 if the difference is positive, and logical 0 if the difference is negative.

Differential signal
A signal in the form of a voltage difference across two conductors, neither of which is necessarily held at ground potential.

Differentiation, analog
Production of an output signal that is proportional to the derivative of the input signal.

Differentiator-integrator, analog
A circuit that acts as a differentiator of low-frequency signals and an integrator of high-frequency signals.

Digital
Capable of only a finite number of stable values. *See also* Analog.

Digital computer
A computer whose working elements are digital circuits.

Digital fluidics
Fluidic devices used for digital processing.

Digital multiplexing
Selection of digital signals through electronic control. *See also* Multiplexer, Analog multiplexing.

Digital-to-analog (D/A) conversion
Representation of a digital number by a proportional voltage or current.

Diode
A device which has a higher conductance for current flowing in one direction (forward current) than for current flowing in the opposite direction (reverse current).

Diode equation
Equation describing relation of forward current to forward bias, in a diode. See Equation 2.4, in text, for details.

DIP
Dual-Inline Package.

Direct current dc
The average current (or voltage) of a signal; that component having zero frequency.

Discrete
Pertaining to *individual* circuit components, such as single transistors, resistors, and diodes, as opposed to *integrated*. *See also* Integrated circuit.

Discriminator
A device used to detect signals which exceed a specified threshold. Usually a logical 1 is produced for the full time during which threshold is exceeded. Threshold may be a positive or negative difference between input and comparison voltage, and comparison voltage may be constant or controllable. A discriminator is an analog comparator. Sometimes used to refer to a pulse height analyzer. *See also* Comparator, Pulse height analyzer.

Distortion
Unwanted signal components, caused by pickup of another signal (crosstalk, intermodulation distortion) or nonlinear distortion of the input signal (harmonic distortion).

Documentation
Thorough description of the circuit theory, construction (including schematics and pictorial diagrams of circuit layout), specifications, and operation of a device.

Dot pattern
Representation of events (usually spikes) on a horizontal axis representing time, by dots placed at points corresponding to their times of occurrence. Repeated observations (usually successive stimulus presentations) may be represented as successive rows of dots lined up one under another.

Drain
The carrier-sink electrode of a field effect transistor.

Drift
Change of baseline voltage over time, either spontaneously or as a function of temperature.

DTL Diode-Transistor Logic
A type of integrated circuit digital logic.

Dual-Inline Package DIP
An integrated circuit package in which the leads emerge from two sides, bend downward, and are spaced at 0.100 in. intervals along each side; the rows are 0.300 in. apart. Most common configuration is 14 or 16 pins.

Duty cycle
That fraction of interpulse interval that must not be exceeded by the pulse duration. Specified for a monostable MVB. Attempt to exceed the duty cycle may result in decreased pulse width, inaccurate timing, or erratic performance.

DVM
Digital voltmeter.

Dyadic relation
Relation between two elements. AND, NAND, OR, NOR, and EOR are dyadic relations.

Earth
Primary ground, the potential of the earth. Often called "ground."

Edge-mount card connectors
Connector sockets or male connectors consisting of rows of spring-loaded contacts (in sockets) or finger-shaped pins or conductive strips on PC boards, used to mechanically mount and electrically connect to PC boards.

EEG
Electroencephalogram.

Effective bandwidth

$$B = \frac{1}{G}\int G_f \, df,$$

where G is the available power gain, and G_f is the gain at frequency f. *See also* Available power gain.

EKG
Electrocardiogram.

Electrical isolation
Lack of any coupling of one signal or circuit with another; sometimes used to refer to lack of all coupling except one path, as in *stimulus isolation*, where attachment of the stimulator to an animal restores coupling to the recording system.

Electrocardiogram EKG
Recording of the electrical activity of the heart.

Electroencephalogram EEG
Recording of the electrical activity of the brain.

Electrolytic capacitor
A capacitor in which one electrode consists of a set of interconnected metal surfaces with a thin insulation, and the other electrode consists of an electrolyte filling the interstices, to provide a high capacitance in a small volume. Typical range: 0.1 to several thousand microfarads.

Electromagnetic interference EMI
Interference in the form of an unwanted signal picked up by inductive or capacitive pickup.

Electromotive force emf
Force applied to a charge by an electric field.

EMI
Electromagnetic interference.

Emitter
The carrier-source of a transistor.

Emitter-coupled pair
Two transistors connected with coupled emitters. The circuit can be used as a differential amplifier.

Emitter follower
A transistor connected in the common-collector configuration; used as an impedance transformer to lower output impedance with a gain which is nearly unity.

Energy storage rating
The total amount of energy which can be delivered by a battery.

Enhancement mode
Operating a field effect transistor with a bias that increases the number of charge carriers in the channel.

EOR
Exclusive OR, ⊕.

Equivalence, logical
A dyadic logical operation. A is equivalent to B if and only if A is true and B is true, or A is false and B is false.

Equivalent input ripple voltage
Amount of differential input ripple voltage which would produce observed output ripple if an operational amplifier were operated open-loop, given 1 V of supply ripple.

Even parity
See Parity bit.

Exclusive OR, EOR, ⊕
A dyadic logical operation. A EOR B is true if and only if A is true and B is false, or B is true and A is false.

Extender card
A PC board or perf-board with a male card connector at one end and a female card connector at the other with corresponding pins on the two connectors tied together. Used to space a PC card away from its connector for easy servicing.

Extrinsic semiconductor
A semiconductor with selected impurities added, in order to introduce extra holes or electrons for conduction. The process, called *doping*, produces an n type semiconductor if higher-valence *donor* impurities are added, or a p type semiconductor if lower-valence *acceptor* impurities are added.

f
Frequency, in sec^{-1} or Hz (Hertz).

F
Farad.

f-
Femto-.

f_0
Corner frequency.

Fan out
Number of unit loads which can be driven by the output of a digital device.

Farad F
Unit of capacitance, defined as the ratio of charge, in coulombs, stored in a capacitor, to the voltage across the capacitor, in volts: $C = q/V$.

Faraday cage
A grounded conductive shell, often double-walled, placed around a piece of apparatus to prevent interference.

Feedback
Coupling between the output of a circuit and an earlier stage.

Feedthrough
Coupling between a signal source and the input of a receiver.

Femto-; f-
Prefix meaning 10^{-15}.

FET
Field effect transistor.

Fiber optics
Optical transmission system consisting of one or more "light pipes," which are stiff or flexible glass or plastic rods that propagate light with small loss, using internal reflection to keep the light inside the pipe. Bundles of fine glass or plastic fibers can be used to transmit images.

Field effect transistor FET
One of two types of transistors, the insulated gate FET or the junction FET. *See also* Insulated gate, Unipolar junction transistor.

Filter
In electronics, a linear device specifically selected to provide a desired transfer function. *See also* Bandpass filter, High-pass filter, Low-pass filter.

Flat-pack
An IC package with leads coming straight out from the sides, which is smaller than a DIP but more difficult to use.

Flicker noise
Low-frequency noise; the power of a frequency component is proportional to $1/f$.

Flipflop
A bistable multivibrator; in digital logic, used to preserve at its output a record of an event or events at its input.

Floating electrical stimulation
Stimulation with a signal that is not coupled to ground or any other electrical circuit, except for unavoidable coupling through the animal.

Floating reference or indifferent
The circuit common, or signal return path, also called the reference or indifferent, is not coupled to ground or common of some other apparatus, or earth.

Fluidics
The use of gas pressures and flows through circuits, called *fluidic circuits*, for the purpose of signal generation, transmission, or modification. Often used for control functions in environments where electronic control is undesirable.

Flux, solder
Material used to promote intimate contact between solder and metal, to allow formation of an alloy junction. Acid flux should never be used for electronic circuitry. *See also* Rosin flux, Stainless steel flux.

FM
Frequency modulation.

Forward bias
Bias of a rectifying junction to produce current in the direction of least resistance. *See also* Diode.

Four-quadrant multiplier
Analog multiplier capable of signed multiplication.

Frequency analysis
Determination of the amount of power contained in each of the frequency components of a signal, or in small frequency bands.

Frequency compensation
Addition of passive filters, usually in feedback loops specifically designed for the purpose, in order to provide a flat frequency response and stable operation of a device, usually an operational amplifier.

Frequency modulation FM
Control of a signal's frequency by means of an applied voltage, the *control* or *modulator* signal, which has frequency components all of which are less than the unmodulated *center* frequency.

Frequency response
A specification of the transfer function of a linear device, often simply specification of the −3 dB points at both ends of the pass band.

Frequency-to-voltage conversion
Production of an output voltage which is proportional to an input frequency.

Fundamental frequency
Lowest frequency component of a repeating signal, which is equal to the reciprocal of the period of repetition, regardless of wave form.

Fuse
A conductor that has a low resistance until its current limit is exceeded, at which point the heat generated by the current causes it to melt. Used to prevent harmful surges of current through electrical devices.

G
Conductance.

g-
Giga-.

Gain a (dimensionless)
The ratio between output and input. *See also* Closed-loop gain, Open-loop gain.

Gain bandwidth product, in Hz
Product of the unity-gain bandwidth times the bandpass gain.

Gain error
Deviation of observed gain from theoretical gain, usually expressed as percent of theoretical gain.

Gain margin
Ratio of open-loop gain to theoretical closed-loop gain. The closed-loop gain error is approximately equal to the reciprocal of the gain margin.

Gate
A digital device whose output is the resultant of a logical relation among its inputs. *See also* AND gate, AND/NAND gate, Inhibited OR gate, NAND gate, NOR gate, OR gate, OR/NOR gate.

Giga-, g-
Prefix meaning 10^9.

Ground
Common, reference. Return path for a single-ended signal, often understood to be earth, which is the potential of the earth.

Ground loop
A conductor loop attached to ground at one point. Currents induced in this loop will produce a voltage drop across the loop impedance to ground.

Ground plane
A plane established by the presence of ground conductors, all running within that plane. A useful means of minimizing interaction of signals within a circuit.

H
Henry, unit of inductance.

Harmonic analysis
See Frequency analysis.

Harmonic distortion
Nonlinear distortion, resulting in the production of harmonics (overtones) of the input frequency components.

Harmonic frequencies
Frequencies which are integral multiples of a *fundamental* frequency. *See also* Fundamental.

Harmonic oscillator
A stable sine-wave oscillator.

Heat capacity
The rate of change of heat as a function of the rate of change of temperature. Defined as $C = dq/dT$, where C = heat capacity and q = heat. Note similarity to capacitance.

Heat pump
A device used to transfer heat from one object to another object that has a higher temperature. Energy must be expended in the process.

Heat reservoir
(a) A heat source. (b) A constant-temperature reservoir.

Heat sink
A device used to dissipate heat.

Heat source
A device used to generate heat.

Henry H
Unit of inductance. Defined by the equation: 1 henry = 1 V/amp/sec.

High-pass filter
Filter that has a fixed gain, usually unity, for all frequencies above a specified frequency and that attenuates all frequencies below that frequency.

Hybrid circuit
(a) A circuit using both vacuum-tube and solid-state active components. (b) A circuit using both analog and digital components. (c) A circuit composed of more than one integrated circuit, or an integrated circuit and some other components, packaged as a single device, often in a standard integrated circuit package. For example, most FET-input operational amplifiers are hybrids composed of a bipolar operational amplifier and a FET pair on separate chips. This is the case with most circuits composed of both MOS and bipolar components.

Hybrid computer
A computer made up of both analog and digital computing elements.

Hysteresis
A dual-valued portion of a function, wherein the path across the region in one direction along the *x*-axis is different than the path in the other direction.

Hz
Hertz

I
current in amperes.

i
instantaneous current, in amperes.

i_C
Current into a capacitor.

i_f
Feedback current.

i_i
Input current.

i_L
Current through a load or an inductor.

i_o
Output current.

i_R
Current through a resistor.

i^+
Current into or out of positive input or output.

i^-
Current into or out of negative input or output.

IC
Integrated circuit.

Ideal available input noise N_g, in watts
The ideal available output noise power divided by circuit gain.

Ideal operational amplifier
An amplifier whose only effect is to multiply an input voltage by an infinite gain.

Iff
Abbreviation for "if and only if."

IGFET
Insulated gate field effect transistor.

Imaginary numbers
Any number that is a product of a real number and i, the square root of -1. Sometimes j is used to represent $\sqrt{-1}$ rather than i, to avoid confusion with i, instantaneous current.

Imaginary part of impedance
Reactance. Nonresistive impedance, either inductive reactance or capacitive reactance.

Impedance
Any quantity Z that is independent of applied current or voltage and is a proportionality between current and voltage: $i = \xi/Z$.

Impedance matching
Adjusting the output impedance of a signal source and the input impedance of a signal receiver to equal values, for maximum power transfer.

Independent current loop
A current loop that cannot be subdivided into smaller, constituent current loops.

Inductance L, in Henries
In electronics, the proportionality between voltage developed across a device and the rate of change of current through the device.

$$1 \text{ Henry} = \frac{1 \text{ volt}}{1 \text{ amp/sec}}$$

Inductor
A device used to introduce a specified inductance. An ideal inductor has zero resistance and zero capacitance.

Input characteristics
Properties of the input terminals of a device, such as input impedance, resistance, capacitance, bias current, and voltage. Also, electrical contributions to output voltage, such as offset current and voltage, voltage range, supply voltage rejection ratio.

Instantaneous current i, in amperes
The current flowing at an instant in time.

Instrumentation
Devices used for transduction, measurement, storage and retrieval, modification, or generation of signals.

Insulated gate field effect transistor
A field effect transistor consisting of a channel of p or n substance whose effective channel width is controlled by the potential on an insulated control electrode, the *gate*. *See also*, Field effect transistor.

Integrated circuit
A collection of components, often comprising a functional circuit or circuits, fabricated on a single semiconductor substrate. *See also* Discrete, Hybrid circuit, Large-scale integration, Medium-scale integration, Small-scale integration.

Interference
Unwanted signals picked up from the environment by electrostatic or electromagnetic coupling.

I/O
Input-output.

Irreducible polynomial
A polynomial which cannot be factored.

j
$\sqrt{-1}$.

JFET
Junction field effect transistor.

Johnson noise
See White noise.

Joint interval plot
A scattergram in which the x-coordinate of the ith point is the ith interval (between the ith and $(i + 1)$th events) and the y-coordinate is the $(i + 1)$th interval (between the $(i + 1)$th and $(i + 2)$th. events).

Junction rule
See Kirchhoff's rules.

Junction transistor
A transistor whose function depends on junctions between p and n semiconductors. *See also* Bipolar junction transistor, Unipolar junction transistor.

Kilo-, k-
Prefix meaning 10^3.

Kirchhoff's rules
Two rules, stating: (1) The algebraic sum of all currents into a junction at any instant must be zero; (2) The algebraic sum of all voltage sources in any closed loop must equal the algebraic sum of the voltage drops across all the circuit elements in the same closed loop. Rule (1) is called the *conservation of charge*, or junction, rule, and rule (2) is called the *single valuedness*, or loop, rule.

L
Inductance, in henries H (electronics).

L
Inductance, in $sec^2/in.^2$ (fluidics).

Ladder network
Network of resistors used in a D/A converter.

Lag
Later phase of one signal parameter (such as current or voltage) relative to another.

Land
A printed circuit board terminal consisting of a conductive soldering surface with a hole drilled through it and the substrate, for lead insertion and electrical connection to the rest of the circuit through attached printed circuit conduction paths.

Large scale integration LSI
Integrated circuits with large numbers of elements on the same chips, such as one-chip calculators or one-chip 1024 bit semiconductor memories.

Large-signal voltage gain
The ratio of maximum output voltage to the input signal required to produce that output voltage.

Latching
An effect caused by hysteresis, whereby the input must go more positive (or negative) to cause the output level to swing from one extreme to the other, than is required to switch it in the other direction.

Layout
(a) Arrangement of components on a circuit board, or of devices in a chassis or cabinet. (b) The physical design phase of device construction.

LED
Light-emitting diode.

Level shifting
Shifting of the baseline of a signal.

Lickometer
A device used to signal licking.

Light-emitting diode
A diode that emits light during forward conduction.

Linear device
A device whose output can be related to the input by a linear differential equation.

Log circuit
A circuit whose output is proportional to the logarithm of the input.

Log-of-ratio circuit
A circuit whose output is proportional to the logarithm of the ratio of two inputs.

Longitudinal parity check character LPCC
The last character of a transmitted, recorded, or read-back string of characters, composed of bits whose values are set such that the sum of the ith bits of all the transmitted characters, including the LPCC, is 0 (even parity) or 1 (odd parity), for any i less than or equal to the number of bits per word.

Loop rule
See Kirchhoff's rules.

Low-pass filter
A filter that has a fixed gain, usually unity, for all frequencies below a specified limit, and that attenuates frequencies above that limit.

LPCC
Longitudinal parity check character.

LSI
Large-scale integration.

M
Mega-, or meg-.

m
Open-loop gain.

m'
Closed-loop gain.

m-
Milli-.

Magnitude of a complex number
The square root of the sum of the squares of the real and imaginary parts of a complex number. The square root of the product of a complex number and its conjugate.

Maximum output swing
The peak output voltage swing, referred to zero, that can be obtained without clipping.

Medium scale integration MSI
Integrated circuits having a moderate number of components on a single IC chip, such as decade counters and binary-BCD converters.

Meg-, mega-, M-
Prefix meaning 10^6.

Metal film resistor
A resistor consisting of a thin metal film deposited on a substrate and hermetically sealed. These can have better temperature coefficients and less stray capacitance and inductance than carbon composition resistors.

Metastable state
A state that is theoretically stable in the absence of any perturbations but that requires an infinitesimal or very small perturbation to cause a transition to another state.

Mho, ohm^{-1}
Unit of conductance.

Micro-, μ-
Prefix meaning 10^{-6}.

Microelectrode
An electrode composed of a stiff, narrow insulated conductor tapering to a point. At the point an exposed area of conductor permits recording from small volumes of tissue. A pipette may have a tip size from 0.1 to 10 μ diameter, and a metal microelectrode may have an exposed tip length of 1 to 100 μ, with a tip diameter of 1 to 10 μ.

Milli-, m-
Prefix meaning 10^{-3}.

Modular design
Design of electronic (or fluidic) hardware for ease of assembly and disassembly, with substructures integrated according to function.

Modulator
A device used for AM or FM modulation. *See also* Amplitude modulation, Frequency modulation, Balanced modulation.

Module
A subassembly of a modular system. A module may be composed of smaller modules. *See also* Modular design.

Monadic relation
A logical relation with only one argument.

Monostable multivibrator
A device that has one stable state and that can be forced to depart to a quasi-stable state temporarily upon input of an appropriate "trigger" signal. A pulse generator.

MOS Metal-Oxide Semiconductor
A semiconductor made using insulated gate field effect transistors. Insulated gate field effect transistors and MOS ICs are MOS devices. *See also* Insulated gate field effect transistor.

MOS IC
An IC using MOS technology. *See also* Insulated gate field effect transistor.

MOSFET
See Insulated-gate field-effect transistor.

MSI
Medium-scale integration.

Multimeter
A meter which can be used as an ohmmeter, a voltmeter, and an ammeter.

Multiplexer
A device used to select an analog signal (analog multiplexer) or a digital signal (digital multiplexer) from one of several input channels, by specifying a unique address (usually a bit pattern) corresponding to that channel.

Multiplexer address (channel)
See Address.

Multiplier
An analog or digital circuit whose output is proportional to the product of its inputs.

Multivibrator MVB
A device which has two stable or metastable states. *See also* Astable multivibrator, Bistable multivibrator, and Monostable multivibrator.

n-
Nano-.

n-channel FET
A field effect transistor whose channel carriers are electrons.

n substance
A semiconductor substance whose majority carrier is negative, that is, electrons.

NAND
A dyadic logical relation. *A* NAND *B* is false if and only if both *A* and *B* are true.

NAND gate
A binary device whose output is logical 0 if and only if all of its inputs are logical 1.

NAND/NOR gate, fluidic
A binary fluidic device with one output that is logical 0 if and only if all inputs are logical 1 (NAND) and with another output that is logical 1 if and only if all inputs are logical 0 (NOR).

Negative feedback
Coupling from the output of a circuit to a point in the circuit where the feed-back signal tends to decrease the magnitude of the output relative to the open-loop value. *See also* Positive feedback.

Negative logic
Digital logic in which 1 is represented by a voltage that is more negative (less positive) than 0. There is a negative logic representation for any pair of voltages chosen. *See also* Positive logic.

Node
A junction between circuit elements that obeys Kirchhoff's junction rule. *See also* Kirchhoff's rules.

Noise
Unwanted signal. Frequently used to refer to random electrical fluctuations. *See also* White noise, Pink noise.

Noise figure F
A measure of the ratio of observed output noise to ideal output noise.

Noise immunity
Insensitivity to noise, either that which is embedded in the signal or noise in the environment.

Nonlinear circuits
Circuits that cannot be completely described by a linear differential equation.

Nonreturn-to-zero A/D conversion
A form of A/D conversion where the converter tracks the incoming signal without starting at zero at the beginning of each A/D conversion.

NOR
A dyadic logical relation. A NOR B is true if and only if A and B are both false.

NOR gate
A binary logic device whose output is logical 1 if and only if all of its inputs are logical 0.

Notch filter
A filter with uniform gain, usually unity, over its entire passband, except for a very narrow, deep "notch" in its transfer function. Used to selectively attenuate a specific frequency or narrow frequency band.

npn transistor
A bipolar junction transistor with a base region composed of *p*-type semiconductor, and emitter and collector regions composed of *n*-type semiconductor. *See also* Bipolar junction transistor.

NRZ
Nonreturn-to-zero type of A/D conversion.

Octal numbers
Numbers in an arithmetic with a modulus (base) of 8. Commonly used to represent three-bit binary numbers as single octal numbers.

Odd parity
See Parity bit.

Offset binary
A means of representing signed binary numbers as unsigned binary numbers, by adding a positive number equal to the negative limit, and thus forcing all numbers to be positive.

Offset current and voltage
Input current and voltage applied differentially to produce a zero output voltage.

Ohm Ω unit of resistance
Defined as the resistance across which a 1 V potential drop will develop when 1 A of current flows through it.

Ohmmeter
A meter used to measure resistance.

Ohm's law
$\xi = i/R$.

One shot
Astable multivibrator, pulse generator. *See also* Astable multivibrator.

Ones complement arithmetic
Binary representation of negative numbers as bit-by-bit complements of corresponding positive numbers.

Open circuit
A broken conduction path.

Open-loop gain m (dimensionless)
Gain of an operational amplifier in the absence of feedback.

Operational amplifier (op amp)
A device used to approximate as closely as possible the properties of an ideal operational amplifier, whose only effect is to multiply input voltage by an infinite gain. Used with feedback to perform specified operations on input signals.

Optical coupler
A device consisting of a voltage- or current-to-light transducer in its input circuit, an optical coupling to the output circuit, and a light-to-voltage or -current output transducer.

Optical isolator
An optical coupler, used to transmit a signal between two circuits that are floating with respect to each other.

Optical reversal, principle of
A law stating that a light ray that is reflected or refracted will retrace its original path if its direction is reversed.

Opto-isolator
An optical isolator.

OR
A dyadic logical relation. A OR B is false if and only if A and B are both false.

OR gate
A binary device whose output is logical 0 if and only if all its inputs are logical 0.

OR, inhibited, fluidic gate
A binary fluidic device whose output is logical 0 if its inputs are all logical 0, or if its inhibit input is 0, regardless of the state of the other inputs.

Oscillation
Periodic fluctuation.

Oscillator
A device that produces an oscillation at its output.

Oscilloscope
A device used to deflect a glowing spot on a screen, usually with an X-axis deflection amplifier and a Y-axis deflection amplifier, such that X-deflection and Y-deflection are some function of input voltages and/or time.

Output amplifier
Amplifier at the output of a device.

Output characteristics
Characteristics of the output stage of a device, such as output impedance and maximum output current.

Output compensation
Frequency compensation through a feedback network coupled between the output and some other point in a circuit.

Output port
The opening in a fluidic device through which the output signal is coupled.

Overflow
Generation of a binary number which exceeds the capacity of a register.

Overload
A load that draws more current than a circuit can deliver without producing distortion, reduction in output amplitude, or damage to the circuit.

Overshoot
(a) Swing of an output signal past the peak expected on the basis of input signal and gain of the amplifier. (b) That portion of an action potential which is of polarity opposite to the resting potential.

Overvoltage protection
Protection of the input of a device from voltages exceeding the absolute maximum input voltage.

P
Power, in watts.

P
Pressure, in pounds per square inch (psi).

p-, pico-
Prefix meaning 10^{-12}.

p-channel FET
A field effect transistor whose channel's majority carriers are holes.

p substance
Any semiconductor material whose majority carrier is positive; that is, the majority carrier consists of holes.

Panel layout
The physical arrangement of controls, displays, and connectors on a panel.

Parallel connection
Connection of components so they are connected across the same voltage.

Parallel impedance addition rule
The sum of all the conductances for parallel connected elements is equal to the lumped parallel equivalent conductance for the entire parallel-connected circuit. For parallel-connected elements:

$$\frac{1}{Z_{\text{peq}}} = \frac{1}{\sum_{i=1}^{n} Z_i}$$

Parallel processing
Processing items of information simultaneously via multiple processors rather than sequentially, via a single processor. Examples include multiplication of two multibit binary numbers, simultaneous averaging of multiple signals using multiple averagers, transmission of a multibit register's contents via multiple wires.

Parity bit
An extra bit in a binary number, adjusted so that when all the bits are summed modulo 2, the sum will always be 0 (even parity), or alternatively, so it will always be 1 (odd parity). Used to check for incorrect bits.

Passive circuits
Circuits built entirely from passive components.

Passive components
Components whose electrical properties are, within limits, independent of voltage and, hence, cannot be used as amplifiers. *See also* Active components.

Peak inverse voltage PIV, in volts
The maximum reverse bias voltage that can be applied to a *pn* junction without damaging it.

Peltier effect
The flow of heat across a bimetallic junction that occurs when a current flows through that junction.

Percent modulation
The percent fluctuation of the envelope of a carrier, in an amplitude modulated signal.

Perforated board, perfboard
A flat insulating material with holes in it, used to breadboard circuits or for permanent circuit construction.

Period of a signal
Recurrence time; the length of time a periodic signal fluctuates before it begins to recapitulate itself.

Phase angle ϕ
(a) The fraction of a period, in radians, between two points on its wave form. (b) The delay between corresponding points on two wave forms.

Photodiode
A diode whose leakage current can be varied by exposing the *pn* junction region to light.

Photon coupler
See Optical coupler.

Phototransistor
A transistor whose transconductance can be varied by exposing the base region to light.

pico-, p-
Prefix meaning 10^{-12}.

Pinch-off
Depletion of a junction field effect transistor channel to the point where further depletion is impossible.

Pink noise
Noise whose predominant frequencies are low frequencies.

PIT
Pulse interval timer.

PIV
Peak inverse voltage.

pn junction
A junction of a *p* semiconductor and an *n* semiconductor.

pnp transistor
A bipolar transistor whose base region is composed of *n* substance and whose collector and emitter regions are composed of *p* substance.

Poisson interval distribution
An exponentially declining distribution of intervals, with the mode in the first bin. Such a distribution results when successive intervals are independent of each other.

Port
An opening in a fluidic device used to couple signals and power supply pressures.

Positive feedback
Feedback from a circuit's output to another point in the circuit, such that the fed-back signal tends to increase the output's deviation from zero in comparison with the corresponding output in the absence of the positive feedback.

Positive logic
Binary logic representation in which 1 is represented by a voltage which is more positive (less negative) than 0. There is a positive logic representation for any pair of voltages.

Poststimulus time histogram PST
A histogram in which the *X*-axis represents time after the beginning of a stimulus, and the *Y*-axis represents number of spikes. May be accumulated for multiple presentations of an identical stimulus, in which case it is sometimes called an *average response* histogram.

Potential
Voltage.

Potentiometer
A resistor with a middle element, or *wiper*, that can make contact along the body of the resistive substance at any point from one terminal contact to the other. *See also* Voltage divider.

Potentiometric feedback
Voltage feedback, in which the feedback voltage is derived from a voltage divider connected between output and ground.

Power P, in watts
Energy per unit time. One watt is defined as the power dissipated by one ampere of current through a 1 ohm resistor.

$$P = IV = I^2R = V^2/R.$$

Power spectrum
The distribution of power in the various frequency components of a signal.

Power supply
An ac-dc converter used to provide supply voltages for a circuit.

Power transistor
A transistor designed to dissipate large amounts of power, usually more than 1 W.

Preset counter
A counter that counts to a preselected value, and then produces an output signal indicating that the preselected count has been reached.

Principle of optical reversal
See Optical reversal, principle of.

Printed circuit
A pattern of conductors etched from a metal sheet glued to an insulating substrate. Used to interconnect components whose leads are inserted through holes in the substrate and copper, trimmed, and soldered to the copper.

Proposition
A statement of fact, in which a thing, *subject*, is said to have some property, *predicate*.

Pseudorandom noise
A signal which has all of the important statistical properties of random noise, except it is periodic.

PST histogram
Poststimulus time histogram.

Pulse
A momentary deflection of a signal away from baseline, followed by a return to baseline. The pulse out of a monostable multivibrator has a fixed or controllable duration, very rapid rise and fall relative to duration, and relatively flat peak that is constant or adjustable in amplitude.

Pulse height analyzer
(a) A device with an upper and lower threshold, which produces an output pulse only when an input pulse exceeds the lower threshold but not the upper. (b) A device made up of several of the variety described in (a), using contiguous threshold pairs, or *windows*.

Pulse interval timer PIT
A device used to measure intervals between pulses.

Q
Inverse focal length, accommodation, in diopters.

Q
Quality factor.

q
Charge, in coulombs.

q
Focal length, in meters, of the lens of the eye.

q
Quantity of air, in pounds.

q
Quantity of heat, in calories.

Quality factor Q (dimensionless)
A measure of the sharpness of tuning of a resonant circuit.

R
Resistance, in ohms (electrical).

R
Resistance, in sec/in.^{2} (fluidic).

Reactance
The complex part of impedance, namely the impedance of the inductive or capacitive component. The magnitude of the reactance not only determines the magnitude of the net impedance (*See* Magnitude of complex number) but also the phase lag or lead.

Real part of impedance
The resistive component of impedance.

Rectification
Passing current in one direction but not in the opposite direction, usually for ac/dc conversion.

Rectifier
A diode used for rectification.

Recursion formula
Formula describing the feedback function of a shift-register pseudo-random noise generator.

Register
A collection of binary devices, such as gates or flipflops, used to represent a multi-bit binary number.

Regulator
A circuit used to maintain a fixed power supply voltage in the presence of supply ripple, fluctuating line voltage, or load variations.

Ripple
Amount of interference consisting of harmonics of ac line-voltage frequency, expressed as amplitude (rms or peak-to-peak) or percent of signal or power supply voltage.

Relation, logical
An operation that defines the truth value of a logical variable on the basis of the values of one, two, or more other logical variables. Also called a *copula*, or logical *operator*. The variables that are operated on are called *arguments*.

Relay
A switch controlled by an applied signal.

Resistance R, in ohms
Proportionality between the steady-state voltage across an object and the steady-state current through it. $R = E/I$.

Resistivity
A physical property of materials, expressed in ohm-cm. For a cylinder of material, with electrical contacts covering the two ends, the resistance between the contacts is equal to the length of the cylinder divided by the area, times the resistivity.

Resistor
A device used to insert a specified resistance in a circuit. An ideal resistor has zero capacitance and zero inductance.

Resonance
Frequency selectivity.

Restrictor
A fluidics resistor.

Retriggerable monostable
A monostable multivibrator with zero duty cycle. Some such devices can be retriggered during a pulse, in which case the pulse width is increased so the pulse ends one pulse duration after the last trigger.

Return pressure
Highest pressure at a binary fluidics output that is considered to be logical 0. All logical 0 outputs should have lower pressures, and all inputs should have higher thresholds.

Reverse bias
Application of a voltage across a rectifier or a rectifying junction in the direction of highest resistance.

RFI
Radio frequency interference.

Ripple
ac Fluctuations, usually power line frequency and its harmonics, on a signal which is supposed to have only a dc component, such as power supply voltage.

Rise time
Time required for a voltage step to go from 10% to 90% of its full trajectory.

rms
Root-mean-square.

Root-mean-square rms
The square root of the mean of a set of squared values, usually used to specify the quadratic mean of an ac voltage or current.

Rosin flux
Solder flux using a rosin base. Recommended for soldering electronics components. Special fluxes may be required for some metals, such as stainless steel.

R-S flipflop
A bistable multivibrator configured such that a trigger signal at one input will cause a transition to logical 1 and a trigger signal at another input will cause a transition to logical 0.

RTL
Resistor-transistor logic.

RZ
Return-to-zero A/D conversion system.

Sample-and-hold circuit
A circuit used to measure approximately the instantaneous value of a signal voltage.

Saturation
Biasing the base of a bipolar transistor to raise the transconductance to its maximum value.

Schematic diagram
Picture of a circuit in which devices and components are represented symbolically, with interconnecting wires shown as lines between the component symbols. In this book nodes are indicated as points of intersection between two or more lines, with a dot at the intersection; line crossings that do not indicate nodes are indicated as points of intersection in which the dots are omitted.

Schmitt trigger
A positive-feedback voltage discriminator.

Semiconductor
Any material with a conductance intermediate between those of conductors and insulators.

Serial A/D conversion
Use of a counter coupled to a D/A converter, to match trial values against an unknown analog input. When the D/A and unknown voltages match, the counter is stopped, and the digital value is the A/D converted value of the input voltage.

Serial processing
Processing of information in a sequence, rather than simultaneously. Examples include transmission of a multibit binary number in the form of sequential 0 and 1 signals on a single wire.

Series connection
Connection of two elements across a voltage end-to-end such that the current through each one is

the same as the total current, and the voltage drops across them sum to equal the voltage drop across the whole circuit.

Series impedance addition rule
The series equivalent impedance is equal to the sum of impedances of all the series-connected elements:

$$Z_{seq} = \sum_{i=1}^{n} Z_i,$$

for n series-connected elements.

Settling time
Time required for the output to reach a condition where it will remain within a specified percent of the steady-state value, after a sudden shift to a new state at the input.

Shield
A conductive shell around a conductor that is either grounded (ground shield) or connected to a low-impedance source of a signal identical to the potential on the conductor (guard shield), to minimize interference on the shielded conductor.

Shift register
A binary register whose bits can be shifted one place to the right and/or left, any number of times. Some shift registers have provision for strobing in a binary number and/or for reading all output bits simultaneously.

Shock hazard
Danger of electric shock from an electrically powered piece of equipment.

Short circuit
Shunt across the path between two nodes, making them equivalent to one node.

Short-circuit protection
Protection of the output of a device against overload, including short circuit.

Signal
A fluctuation of some physical variable, usually measurable at least in theory and usually containing information.

Signal to noise ratio S/N
Ratio of signal power to noise power or ratio of signal voltage to noise voltage.

Signal tracing
Using an oscilloscope probe or other signal testing device to examine the successive transformations of a signal through the successive stages of a circuit, usually in order to find a faulty component.

Silhouette, fluidic
A punched or cast flat wafer with channels for air flow and input, output, supply and vent ports, for use as a fluidic active device.

Silicon controlled rectifier SCR
A four-layer, three-*pn* junction element, used to turn diode action on and off by means of an external voltage or current.

Simultaneous A/D conversion
Use of $2^n - 1$ comparators to test each possible level which can be represented by an n-bit number, for n-bit A/D conversion. The method is impractical for large numbers of bits.

Single-ended amplifier
Amplifier with single-ended input and output, used to process a signal that is ground referenced.

Single-ended signal
A ground-referenced signal.

Single valuedness rule
See Kirchhoff's rules.

Sink
In electronics, the negative end of a voltage source. A source of electrons and a point into which positive current flows.

Skirt
The rising or falling edge of the transfer function of a device.

Slew rate
Rate of change of voltage.

Small scale integration SSI
Integrated circuits with small numbers of elements, such as quad NAND gates, hex inverters, and so forth.

Soldering lug
A terminal to which leads are soldered, to provide a mechanical support and electrical contact for a circuit node.

Source
In electronics, the positive end of a voltage source. A point from which positive current flows, into which electrons flow.

Source follower
A field effect transistor in the common-drain configuration, usually used to lower the output impedance of a circuit. The source follower has a gain that is nearly unity.

Spaghetti
Insulating tubing used to insulate bare leads and wires.

Spectrum analysis
Frequency analysis.

Spike enhancement
Exaggeration of the height of an action potential in order to enhance separation of the peak from baseline noise.

SSI
Small-scale integration.

Stainless steel flux
Solder flux used for bonding solder to stainless steel. Rosin flux will not suffice for stainless steel and some other metals, such as aluminum.

Strain gauge
A transducer that converts strain of a wire or a surface into a proportional electrical signal.

Stray capacitance and inductance
Unwanted capacitance or inductance. May be responsible for undesired frequency selectivity (filter) effects as well as pickup of interference.

Substrate
Inert surface upon which an integrated circuit or a printed circuit is constructed.

Subtracter
(a) Analog device whose output is proportional to the difference of two input signals. (b) Digital device that subtracts one binary number from another.

Successive approximation A/D conversion
The A/D conversion method wherein, starting with the most significant bit, each bit is turned on to determine if the resulting D/A converted number is larger than the input. If so, the bit is turned off. The process is repeated for all bits and the final result is the A/D converted input.

Superposition principle
Law stating that any signal can be considered to be the sum of a set of sine waves and/or cosine waves of specified frequencies, amplitudes, and phases; signals may also be decomposed into unit inpulses or unit step functions.

Supply port
Hole on a fluidics device for coupling supply pressure.

Supply voltage rejection ratio SVRR
The ratio of the change of input offset voltage to the change of supply voltage producing it.

Susceptance B, in mhos
The inverse of reactance, the imaginary component of admittance.

Switch
(a) A mechanical device used to make or break a connection between electrical contacts. (b) An electronic analog, which switches signals without any moving parts.

Switch pressure
Pressure above which a fluidic digital signal is considered logical 1. Threshold at an input must be less than switch pressure and a logical 1 output must exceed switch pressure.

Symmetrical divide-by-ten configuration
Hookup configuration of a decade counter consisting of a divide-by-two counter and a divide-by-five counter, such that it is off for five counts and on for the next five, producing a square wave output if a periodic digital signal ten times the output frequency is used as input.

Tangential noise
Noise amplitude measured by noting the baseline separation at which two noise signals begin to merge on an oscilloscope screen.

Tantalum capacitor
Electrolytic capacitor in which the metal is a tantalum alloy.

Tapping
Making threads in a hole.

Tee network (feedback)
A T-shaped resistor feedback network used to simulate a high-impedance feedback path using low impedances.

Termination, cable
Series resistor connection to the center conductor of a coaxial cable to maximize power transfer and minimize reflections.

Test point
An easily accessible circuit node whose voltage can be measured during troubleshooting in order to test performance of a portion of a circuit.

Thermal noise
Random electrical signal caused by thermal agitation of charge carriers.

Thermistor
A resistor selected for a large, reproducible temperature coefficient.

Thermode
A heat source or sink of controllable or specifiable temperature, used to heat or cool tissue.

Threading
Making threads on a rod or tube.

Threshold
Signal level at which a device ceases treating an input signal as logical 0 and begins treating it as logical 1.

Thyristor
A silicon controlled rectifier.

Time constant τ
Time required for a linear circuit to charge to $[1 - (1/e)]\,\Delta V$, when subjected to a step that will produce a total output shift of ΔV.

Tinning
Flowing melted solder on surfaces.

Toggle switch
A type of switch that is operated by flipping a lever.

Toggling
Alternating between one state and another on each occurrence of an input trigger.

Tolerance
Allowable or guaranteed maximum deviation from a specified value for a device or component property, usually expressed as percent of the nominal value.

Totem-pole output
Push-pull output of a TTL device, used to maintain low output impedance for both 0 and 1 logic levels.

Tracking rate, A/D converter
Maximum rate at which an A/D converter can follow the changes in an input signal.

Transfer function
The spectral response of a device. The output function (spectrum) is the forcing function (input spectrum) times the transfer function.

Transfer of momentum
Principle used in fluidics, whereby an air jet can be deflected by a control jet impinging on it from the side.

Transient response
Response of a system to a transient input.

Transistor
An active device made from semiconductors. *See also* Bipolar junction transistor, Unipolar junction transistor, Field effect transistor.

Transistor voltmeter TVM
A voltmeter constructed with transistors.

Transmission line
Any conductor used to transmit signals over a distance.

Triac
A device similar to a silicon controlled rectifier, except current can pass in either direction.

Trigger
Initiation of circuit action (for example, scope sweep, stimulus generation) upon occurrence of some event, such as an electrical trigger pulse. Also used for synchronization of one instrument with another.

Trimmer
Adjustable capacitor, inductor, or resistor, used to provide a fine adjustment (trim) for a component value in a circuit.

Troubleshooting
Procedures for diagnosing device failure and detecting operating faults.

Truth table
Table in which all the resultant truth values are specified for all combinations of truth values of the arguments, in order to define or examine the nature of a logical relation.

TTL
Transistor-transistor logic.

TVM
Transistor voltmeter.

Twos-complement arithmetic
Binary arithmetic in which negative numbers are represented as the ones complement plus 1. The twos complement of a number can also be obtained by inverting all the bits to the left of the right-most 1, and leaving the rightmost 1 and all bits to the right of it unchanged.

Unipolar junction transistor
A junction field effect transistor. The current through a *channel* of *p* or *n* substance is controlled by varying the effective channel width via a gate, which is a region of the opposite kind attached to the channel by a *pn* junction.

Unit load
The load equivalent to one NAND gate input.

Unity gain follower
A unity gain circuit. In this book, usually an op amp with input to the positive input and a direct connection between output and the negative input. Gain is very close to unity, and input impedance is equal to the input impedance of the op amp.

Unity gain frequency cutoff
Frequency at which the high-frequency skirt of the transfer function crosses unity.

Universal PC board
A printed circuit board printed and drilled to accept standard pin configurations of ICs. Connections are made with wire jumpers.

Up/down counter
A counter that increments or decrements its count under external control.

V
Volts, units of voltage (a unit of measure).

V
Voltage, in volts (a variable).

V_C
Voltage across a capacitor C.

V_i
Input voltage.

V_o
Output voltage.

V_L
Voltage across a load L, or across an inductor L.

V_R
Voltage across a resistor R.

V^+
Voltage at positive input or output.

V^-
Voltage at negative input or output.

Vacuum tube
See Valve.

Vacuum tube voltmeter VTVM
A voltmeter constructed with vacuum tubes.

Valve
Electron tube. An active device used in early electronic circuits. Obsolete for most electrophysiological applications except cathode ray tubes.

Valve, fluidic interface
A fluidic valve, operated by a control signal from a fluidics logic device. Used to control air flow at higher pressures and flows, or for other gases.

Vent
Fluidics port open to ambient pressure. Room pressure is reference, or ground, for most fluidics.

Video
High-frequency signal used to transmit information for television images.

Virtual ground
A node held close to ground voltage by feedback, such as the negative input of an op amp during negative current feedback.

Volt V
Unit of electromotive force.

Voltage discrimination
See Discriminator.

Voltage divider
At least two resistors in series connection, resulting in at least one node voltage intermediate between the voltages at opposite ends of the divider. A potentiometer is a variable voltage divider.

Voltage feedback
Feedback whose effect is determined by the voltage fed back rather than the current. Potentiometric feedback is an example of voltage feedback.

Voltmeter
A device for measuring the potential difference between two points.

Volt-ohmmeter VOM
A meter that can be used as a voltmeter or an ohmmeter.

VOM
Volt-ohmmeter.

VTVM
Vacuum tube voltmeter

W
Gas flow in pound/sec.

W
watts, unit of power.

Wall-attachment effect
Tendency of a gas jet to flow along a wall, requiring the application of force to deflect it away from the wall.

Wave form generation
Generation of specifiable or controllable signals, usually of relatively simple form.

White noise
Random noise with a flat spectrum, excluding dc.

Wien bridge oscillator
A sine wave oscillator using a resonant bridge circuit.

Window discriminator
A two-threshold device. *See also* Pulse height analyzer.

Wire-wound resistor
A resistor made by using a long piece of thin wire whose length and resistivity are accurately known resulting in a close tolerance and low temperature coefficient. Modern methods produce low inductances and capacitances, although not generally as low as for carbon composition or metal glaze resistors.

Wire wrapping
The process of interconnecting components, usually printed circuit connectors, by tightly wrapping the stripped ends of insulated wires around metal posts attached to the components.

Worst-case calculation
Calculation of a circuit parameter, setting all relevant variables to the worst extreme in order to determine the worst value of the calculated parameter.

X
Reactance.

Y
Admittance.

Z
Impedance.

Zener diode
A diode designed to reversibly break down when subjected to a reverse bias greater than a specified *zener voltage.*

Zener voltage
Breakdown voltage of a Zener diode.

α
Collector current.

β
Transistor current gain.

γ
Hole current in base of *pnp* transistor.

ϵ
Nonrecombined holes in base current of *pnp* transistor.

μ
Short for μm, micron, 10^{-6} meter.

μ-
Micro-.

ξ
Voltage, instantaneous.

τ
Time constant.

ϕ
Phase angle.

Ω
Ohm.

ω
Angular frequency, in radians.

$\wedge$
AND.

$\vee$
OR.

$\overline{\wedge}$
NAND.

$\overline{\vee}$
NOR.

$\neg$, $\bar{\ }$, $\sim$, $\dot{\ }$
Logical inversion INV.

$\oplus$, EOR.
Exclusive OR.

INDEX

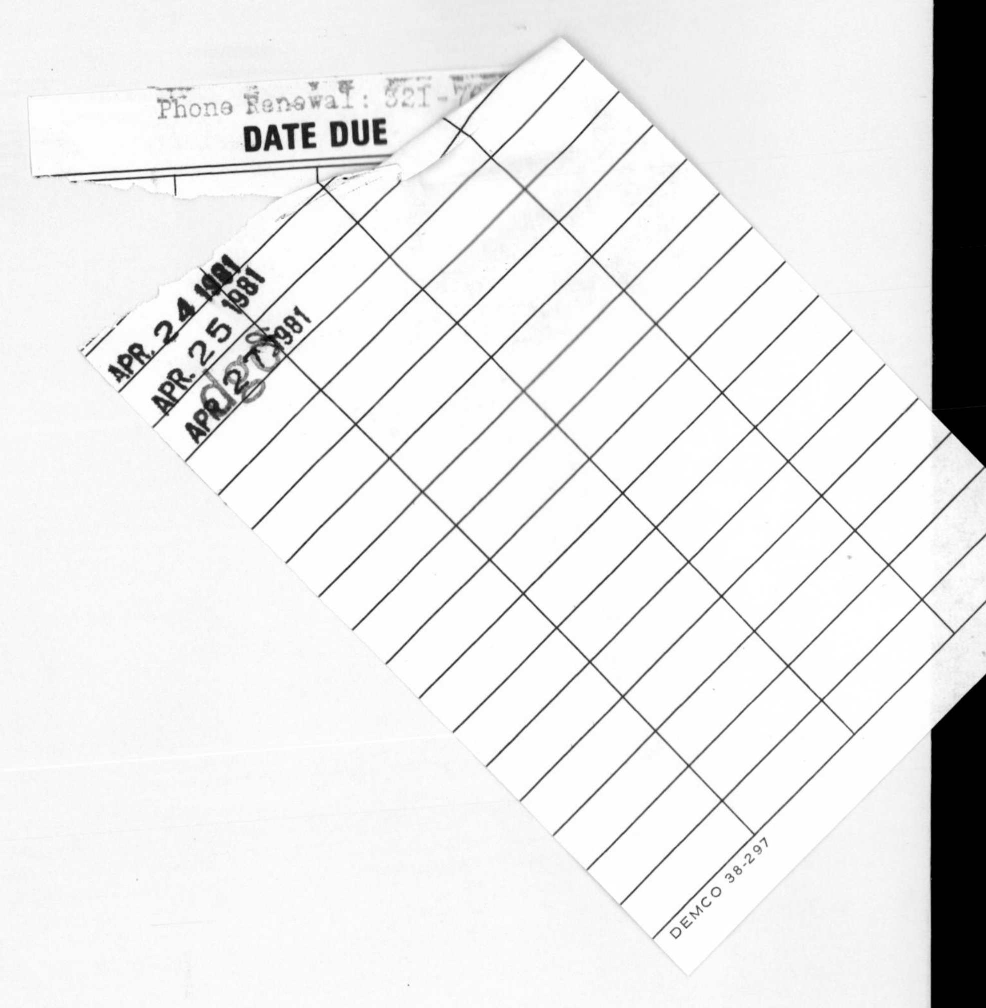
Phone Renewal: 321-
DATE DUE
APR. 24 1981
APR. 25 1981
APR. 27 1981
DEMCO 38-297